RADIOLOGY OF
Spinal cord injury

RADIOLOGY OF

Spinal cord injury

Edited by

LEONID CALENOFF, M.D.

Professor of Radiology, Northwestern University Medical School;
Chief, Outpatient Diagnostic Radiology, Northwestern Memorial Hospital;
Chief, Diagnostic Radiology, The Rehabilitation Institute of Chicago,
Chicago, Illinois

with 883 illustrations

The C. V. Mosby Company

ST. LOUIS • TORONTO • LONDON   1981

MOSBY

1906 **75** 1981
YEARS

A TRADITION OF PUBLISHING EXCELLENCE

Editor: Samuel E. Harshberger
Manuscript editor: Mary Wright
Designer: Gail M. Hudson
Production: Jeanne Bush

The C. V. Mosby Company
11830 Westline Industrial Drive, St. Louis, Missouri 63141

Library of Congress Cataloging in Publication Data

Main entry under title:

Radiology of spinal cord injury.

    Bibliography: p.
    Includes index.
    1. Spinal cord—Wounds and injuries. 2. Spinal
cord—Radiography. I. Calenoff, Leonid, 1923-
[DNLM: 1. Spinal cord injuries—Rehabilitation.
2. Spinal cord injuries—Radiography. WL 400 C149r]
RD594.3.R32   617′.48207572   80-27532
ISBN 0-8016-1114-8

C/CB/B 9 8 7 6 5 4 3 2 1   02/C/281

Contributors

HENRY B. BETTS, M.D.

Magnuson Professor and Chairman, Department of Rehabilitation Medicine, Northwestern University Medical School; Executive Vice President and Medical Director, The Rehabilitation Institute of Chicago, Chicago, Illinois

LEONID CALENOFF, M.D.

Professor of Radiology, Northwestern University Medical School; Chief, Outpatient Diagnostic Radiology, Northwestern Memorial Hospital; Chief, Diagnostic Radiology, The Rehabilitation Institute of Chicago, Chicago, Illinois

JUAN J. CAYAFFA, M.D.

Assistant Professor of Neurology, Northwestern University Medical School, Chicago, Illinois

LEONARD J. CERULLO, M.D.

Assistant Professor of Surgery (Neurosurgery), Northwestern University Medical School, Chicago, Illinois

RICHARD M. GORE, M.D.

Chief Resident, Diagnostic Radiology, Northwestern University Medical School, Chicago, Illinois

MASOUD HEMMATI, M.D.

Neuroradiologist, Department of Radiology, Michael Reese Hospital and Medical Center, Chicago, Illinois

RONALD W. HENDRIX, M.D.

Assistant Professor of Radiology, Northwestern University Medical School; Chief, Skeletal Radiology, Northwestern Memorial Hospital; Visiting Staff, The Rehabilitation Institute of Chicago, Chicago, Illinois

PAUL E. KAPLAN, M.D.

Associate Professor of Physical Medicine and Rehabilitation, Northwestern University Medical School; Attending Staff Physician, The Rehabilitation Institute of Chicago, Chicago, Illinois

LAXMAN S. KEWALRAMANI, M.D., M.S. Orth.

Associate Professor of Rheumatology and Rehabilitation, Louisiana State University School of Medicine; Director, Rehabilitation Research, Louisiana Rehabilitation Institute, New Orleans, Louisiana

PAUL R. MEYER, Jr., M.D.

Associate Professor of Orthopedic Surgery and Biological Materials, Northwestern University Medical/Dental School; Director, Acute Spinal Cord Injury; Co-Director, Midwest Regional Spinal Cord Injury Care System, McGaw Medical Center of Northwestern University, Chicago, Illinois

MICHAEL A. MIKHAEL, M.D.

Associate Professor of Radiology, Northwestern University Medical School, Chicago, Illinois; Chief, Neuroradiology, Evanston Hospital, Evanston, Illinois

RICHARD A. MINTZER, M.D.

Associate Professor of Radiology, Northwestern University Medical School; Chief, Chest and Gastrointestinal Radiology, Northwestern Memorial Hospital, Chicago, Illinois

JOHN B. NANNINGA, M.D.

Associate Professor of Urology, Northwestern University Medical School; Consulting Staff, The Rehabilitation Institute of Chicago, Chicago, Illinois

HARVEY L. NEIMAN, M.D.

Associate Professor of Radiology, Northwestern University Medical School; Chief, Angiography and Sectional Imaging, Northwestern Memorial Hospital; Visiting Staff, The Rehabilitation Institute of Chicago, Chicago, Illinois

LEE F. ROGERS, M.D.

Professor and Chairman, Department of Radiology, Northwestern University Medical School, Chicago, Illinois

JOEL S. ROSEN, M.D.

Associate Medical Director, Department of Rehabilitation Medicine, Northridge Hospital Foundation, Northridge, California; Medical Director, Southern California Spinal Cord Injury Care System; Associate Clinical Professor, Department of Rehabilitative Medicine, University of Southern California; Associate Clinical Professor, Department of Medicine, University of California, Los Angeles, Los Angeles, California; Formerly Co-Director, Midwest Regional Spinal Cord Injury Care System, McGaw Medical Center of Northwestern University, Chicago, Illinois

STEWART SPIES, M.D.

Assistant Professor of Radiology, Northwestern University Medical School; Director of Nuclear Medicine, Northwestern Memorial Hospital, Chicago, Illinois

Foreword

The care of spinal cord injured patients calls on the most humanitarian instincts of those persons involved in their care; encouragement and hope must be offered in the face of despair and optimism instilled in the face of adversity. The patients' suffering is great and their need for understanding and compassion even greater. Their requirements for medical and surgical care are considerable, without which the quality and duration of their existence are severely compromised and their chance for survival severely diminished.

The recent establishment of centers for the care of acute spinal cord injury wedded with the considerable advances in rehabilitation medicine has greatly improved the patients' prospects for a reasonably normal existence. This improvement in care has required a coupling of compassion with scientific medicine: a multidisciplinary approach that crosses many specialties, including rehabilitation medicine, intensive care, neurosurgery, orthopedics, urology, and radiology.

Diagnostic radiology plays a central role in the initial diagnosis and subsequent management of the spinal cord injured patient. Decisions regarding care are often made on the basis of some form of radiologic evaluation. This requires all facets of the diagnostic radiologic armamentarium: film radiography, computed tomography, ultrasonography, and nuclear imaging. Furthermore, the requirements cut across the various subspecialties of neuroradiology, uroradiology, and skeletal, gastrointestinal, and pulmonary radiology. In no small measure the care afforded these patients is dependent on the availability, proper utilization, and expertise in the performance and interpretation of these various radiologic procedures. There are peculiar requirements in the judicious and proper handling of these patients. The proper interpretation of the various radiologic procedures requires a significant background in the pathophysiology and pathomechanics of spinal cord injury and an in-depth understanding of the medical, surgical, and rehabilitation procedures required for the patients' care. This book brings together all facets of the problem of spinal cord injury to ensure the reader a thorough understanding of the radiologic evaluation of the spinal cord injured patient.

The radiologic services at the Rehabilitation Institute of Chicago are provided by the staff of the Department of Radiology of Northwestern University Medical School. Dr. Leonid Calenoff has served as Chief of Radiology at the Rehabilitation Institute since 1975. It became immediately obvious to Dr. Calenoff, on assuming this responsibility, that there was no appreciable radiologic literature concerning the many problems encountered in the radiologic evaluation of these patients. No text was available on this subject. I encouraged Dr. Calenoff to undertake the editorship of such a book. He did so with his accustomed enthusiasm and thoroughness. You have before you the fruits of his considerable labors. He has brought together in one volume the basic fund of knowledge required for the judicious and proper use of radiologic techniques in the evaluation and management of the spinal cord injured patient. The text details the basic pathomechanics and pathophysiology of spinal cord injury, explains the clinical problems encountered, and describes the medical and surgical treatment and role of radiologic evaluation in this entire process from acute injury through rehabilitation and long-term management of the many difficult and varied disorders that confront these unfortunate individuals.

With this book Dr. Calenoff has filled a great void not only in the radiologic literature but in the literature of surgery and rehabilitation medicine as well. He is to be commended for his efforts and congratulated for this exceptionally well-done, timely, and informative work.

Lee F. Rogers, M.D.

Introduction

The treatment of spinal cord injury and society's involvement with its consequences are relatively recent events. Gradually, however, there has developed a national momentum to give greater consideration to all disabled persons by both the lay and the medical communities. Prior to this movement for the most part persons with spinal cord injuries were discarded and were considered invalids, and even the medical community rejected them as being frustrating and boring, in favor of acute illness.

Several factors contributed to a national interest in the disabled. First, people began to live longer, thus developing more chronic illness and subsequent physical impairment. Second, with speed and industrialization, accidents (the third leading cause of death) became frequent. In addition, treatment of acute and traumatic events became more sophisticated, leading to more lives saved after accidents, but frequently these were the lives of people who consequently had physical impairment. Third, the nation came to realize the devastating economic fact of simply offering custodial care. It is far more reasonable financially to treat and rehabilitate in order to make people self-sufficient than to pay the bills in nursing homes. Finally, philosophically the United States developed a strong feeling for disadvantaged groups in general, especially minorities. The disabled, although *not* a minority group (most people will be disabled at some time in their lives), have suffered the same problems, prejudices, and anguishes as the minorities. They were therefore considered in that category as the nation took up these problems.

Persons with spinal cord injuries have been unique among the disabled in that they arrived on the American scene already as heroes. For this reason and because they tend to be young, they have had symbolically and practically a tremendous impact on society and the medical community in soliciting interest and care for *all* physically handicapped people.

The first large number of spinal cord injuries occurred "heroically" as the result of what was considered a just and noble war (World War II). People left paralyzed (or injured in other ways) were immediately welcomed home with all possible fanfare and every consideration medically and otherwise. There were such heroes in World War I (and other wars) as well, but until the discovery of antibiotics (concomitant with World War II) they died very quickly of infection. In World War I, for instance, 98% died before they returned to the United States.

The single most significant development in the treatment of spinal cord injury has been the utilization of the multidisciplinary approach. *Radiology of Spinal Cord Injury* exemplifies this development, which is characterized by the alliance between radiology, surgery, orthopedics, pulmonary medicine, physical medicine, internal medicine, urology, pediatrics, and nuclear medicine. Any team treating spinal cord injury also includes rehabilitation nursing, physical therapy, occupational therapy, chaplaincy, psychology, vocational counseling, social work, dietetics, therapeutic recreation, bioengineering, orthotics, and pharmacy. There are no more important aspects of treatment of spinal cord injury than this multidisciplinary approach and the necessity of attention to its organization. Because the paralyses are rarely totally curable, the treatment involves bringing the patient to use maximal physical strength and then teaching physical and psychologic adaptation to what residual weaknesses remain. Thus there are not only these issues of muscles, nerves, bones, *and* the psyche but also those involving religion, family, friends, community, work, and play—the total environment. Success can be achieved only by bringing the necessary professionals with skill and dedication together in a coordinated manner. These people must have not only a sense of dedication and special mission as pioneers but also the ability to communicate well—and they must have an individual able to coordinate their activities.

Radiology has had a particularly significant role in improving the care of patients with spinal cord injuries. Obviously the ability to visualize well the genitourinary and respiratory systems has saved innumerable lives and improved morbidity. Dramatic possibilities in improving care have resulted from the constantly upgraded techniques for visualizing the spine in spinal cord injury. Because of this it is possible to make an early determination relative to the severity of the injury and to appraise the pathology in light of what treatment to use. It has become possible to follow the effectiveness of surgery or conservative treatment relative to vertebral alignment and possible spinal cord compression. The utilization of computed tomography and other advanced techniques could be one of the most significant keys to the future in determining what treatment is given, establishing a prognosis, and finding complications.

The interest, dedication, and involvement of radiologists willing to devote particular attention to spinal cord injury has had a major impact at the Rehabilitation Institute of Chicago, Northwestern University Medical School, and Northwestern Memorial Hospital, which make up the Midwest Regional Spinal Cord Injury Care System. The continuing interest of radiologists in these patients and the development of more highly sophisticated techniques represent major contributions to the quality of care available to the spinal cord injured patient population. As their lives improve, they may take major leadership roles. Thus by improving care, broadening opportunities, and helping to bring those with spinal cord injuries into the mainstream, we will be bringing hope and help to millions of other disabled individuals.

Henry B. Betts, M.D.

Preface

Once considered an affliction of dismal hope for productive life, spinal cord injury has entirely different prospects today. This new outlook in spinal cord injury followed the interest of the public in general and the medical profession in particular. Public interest groups have helped establish plans for comprehensive emergency treatment, acute and rehabilitative care, as well as regional spinal cord injury care systems and numerous excellent rehabilitation centers. The interest of the medical profession in the care of spinal cord injured patients stems from the steadily increasing numbers of young spinal cord injured patients in need of medical attention, which in itself was followed by the emergence of new, sophisticated methods of treatment.

According to the National Spinal Cord Injury Foundation over 400,000 spinal cord injured individuals are living today in the United States. In addition, another 7500 new persons are added to this number every year. Modern way of life, with high speed motor vehicles, competitive sports, gunshot incidents, and other trauma to the spinal cord seems to affect an ever-younger population. Those who were lucky to survive are faced with the many years of life intimately revolving around medical care specialists such as neurologists, neurosurgeons, orthopedic surgeons, urologists, and particularly specialists in physical medicine and rehabilitation.

In this realm of multidisciplinary care of spinal cord injured patients, radiology and radiologists become involved from the moment the patient is brought to the emergency room and has his first radiograph taken. This involvement continues through the acute phase, and acute care following injury and through the continuous years of rehabilitation. Radiology with all its modalities, including neuroradiology, angiography, computed tomography, polytomography, nuclear medicine, and ultrasonography, is continuously used in the evaluation of spinal cord injured patients in relationship to the multitude of complications these patients are subjected to during their acute care and rehabilitation.

The physical organization of the Midwest Regional Spinal Cord Injury Care System with its related institutions, namely, Northwestern Memorial Hospital, The Rehabilitation Institute of Chicago, and Northwestern University Medical School, and the fact that all radiology in these institutions is performed by the same group of radiologists created an ideal opportunity to combine the total experience in a book about radiology of spinal cord injury.

This book on radiology of spinal cord injury is divided into two major parts: the acute phase and rehabilitation. In the acute phase of spinal cord injury, radiologic procedures and manifestations evolve around emergency and acute care of the spinal cord injured: evaluation of fractures and dislocations of the spine, the neuroradiologic procedures and assessment of spinal cord injury, and surgical closed reduction and open stabilization of spinal cord injury. Pulmonary, gastrointestinal, and vascular complications have a wide spectrum of radiographic manifestations important for proper care. In the rehabilitation phase a particular emphasis is placed on the neurogenic bladder, the radiologic assessment of the urinary system, and the skeletal soft tissue and joint changes in the spinal cord injury patient. Chapters on the anatomy and radiology of the spinal cord and spine are introductory to the clinical material and its proper understanding. The chapter on spinal cord injury in children is based on material from medical centers where pediatric spinal cord injuries are treated more frequently.

It is our hope that this book will shed more light on the radiologic aspects of spinal cord injury and will help not only radiologists but also physiatrists and numerous other specialists involved in spinal cord injury care to understand some of the medical problems concerning spinal cord injured patients. These problems certainly are made "visible" through the large armamentarium of modern diagnostic radiology.

• • •

Radiology of Spinal Cord Injury would not have been possible without the expertise of all contributors to whom I express my sincere appreciation. I am especially indebted to Lee F. Rogers, M.D., Professor and Chairman of Radiology, and Henry B. Betts, M.D., Magnuson Professor and Chairman of Rehabilitation Medicine at Northwestern University Medical School for their special interest, contributions, and encouragement. My special gratitude goes to Susan Sloan for her invaluable assistance. I wish also to thank Brigitte Weaver, Marianne Kaplan, and Dorothy Woodward for helping individual contributors, and Kathy Sisson and Scott Schlesser from Kascot Medi-Media for their excellent drawings and photography.

Leonid Calenoff, M.D.

Contents

PART IV

**MISCELLANEOUS ASPECTS OF SPINAL CORD
INJURY**

PART I

Anatomy and radiology
of the spinal cord

CHAPTER 1

Anatomy and vascular supply of the spinal cord

JUAN J. CAYAFFA, M.D.

A basic knowledge of the anatomy and vascular supply of the spinal cord is a prerequisite and a practical necessity for understanding spinal cord injury and for proper clinical care. This knowledge is based on the gross anatomy of the spinal cord and its relationship to the radiologically visible bony landmarks, the internal structures of the cord, the meninges, and finally the very important vascular supply.

GROSS ANATOMY OF THE SPINAL CORD*

The spinal cord (medulla spinalis [L], moelle épinière [F], Ruckenmark [G]) is the almost cylindric segment of the central nervous system. It lies within the vertebral canal surrounded by meninges and attached to the bony walls by ligaments (Fig. 1-1).

Extension. Up to the third month of fetal life the spinal cord occupies the entire length of the vertebral canal. Because of unequal growth rates of the cord and the vertebral column, the caudal tip of the cord gradually lies higher and higher. At 6 months of fetal life the caudal end lies at the lower border of the body of L3, and at birth it extends only to the lower border of L2. The cord is relatively longer in a young child than in a full-grown individual. In the adult man the caudal end of the cord is at the level of the lower border of the body of L1 or at the level of the L1-2 intervertebral disc (Fig. 1-2). In women the lower end is slightly lower, reaching the middle part or lower border of L2. Variations are to be found from T12 to L3.

Shape. The spinal cord appears as a long cylinder, somewhat flattened dorsoventrally, with two fusiform enlargements, the cervical and the lumbar, related to the innervation of the limbs. The more narrow part below the lumbar enlargement is the conus medullaris. The filum terminale is a nonnervous filament that extends from the end of the conus medullaris to the fundus of the dural sac at the level of the second sacral vertebra (Fig. 1-2).

Weight. The spinal cord weighs about 30 g, which represents 2% of the total weight of the central nervous system.

Length and regional subdivision of the spinal cord. The total length of the cord is about 45 cm in men and from 41 to 43 cm in women, while the length of the vertebral column is about 70 cm. The cord occupies approximately the upper two thirds of the spinal canal.

The spinal cord has been classically divided into five regions, whose longitudinal dimensions are as follows: upper part, 2 cm; cervical enlargement, 10 to 12 cm; thoracic part, 18 to 22 cm; lumbar enlargement, 7 to 9 cm; conus medullaris, 2 cm; and the filum terminale, 20 to 25 cm.

Spinal nerves, spinal roots, and segmental subdivision of the cord. Thirty-one pairs of spinal nerves orig-

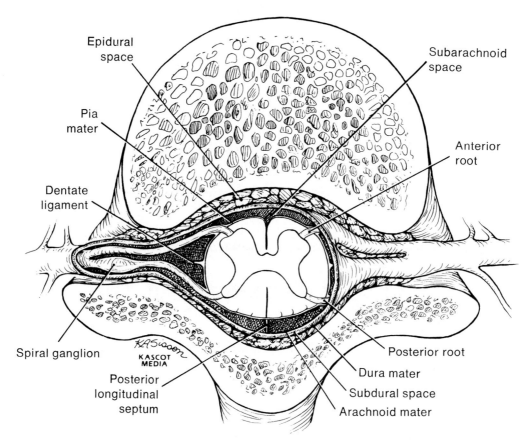

Fig. 1-1. Diagram of transverse section of cord and vertebra.

inate from the cord (Fig. 1-2). They are formed by the union of the ventral and dorsal spinal roots: eight cervical, twelve thoracic, five lumbar, and five sacral pairs and one coccygeal pair of spinal nerves. Each pair of spinal nerves corresponds to a spinal cord segment. The length of the segments varies: cervical segments, about 13 mm; midthoracic segments, 26 mm; lumbar segments, 15 mm; and sacral segments, 5 mm. Because the spinal cord is shorter than the vertebral column, the more caudal nerve roots and nerves, that is, the lumbar and sacral ones, take a progressively more oblique direction before reaching the corresponding foramen of exit, forming the cauda equina around the filum terminale (Fig. 1-3).

Enlargements. The cervical enlargement extends from C3 to T2 and the lumbar enlargement from L1 to S3.

Origin of the plexuses. The cervical plexus originates from segments C1 to C4, the brachial plexus from C5 to T1, the intercostal nerves from the thoracic segments, the lumbar plexus from L1 to L4, the sacral plexus from L4 to S2, and the pudendal plexus from S3 to S5 (Fig. 1-2).

Circumference and diameter. The regional differences in circumference and transverse and dorsoventral diameters in adults are shown in Table 1-1.

The values in Table 1-1 correspond to the maximum diameter within a particular region.[64] The greatest circumference for the cervical enlargement is found at the level of the sixth vertebra and for the lumbar enlargement at the level of the lower part of the twelfth thoracic vertebra.

The ratio of the spinal cord width to the spinal canal diameter is 3:5. The distance between the cord and the

Table 1-1. Regional differences in spinal cord circumference and diameters

Dimensions	Cervical enlargement (mm)	Lumbar enlargement (mm)	Intermediate portion (mm)
Transverse diameter	13	12	10
Dorsoventral diameter	9	9	8
Circumference	38	33	27

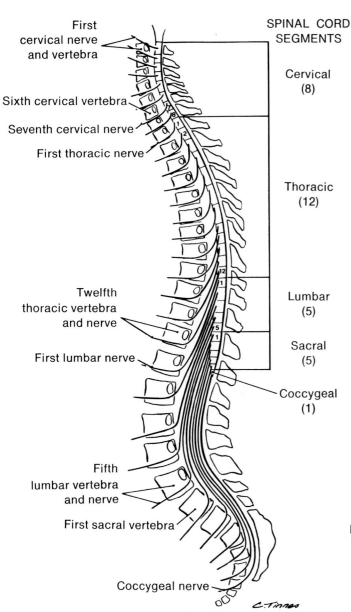

First cervical nerve and vertebra

Sixth cervical vertebra

Seventh cervical nerve

First thoracic nerve

Twelfth thoracic vertebra and nerve

First lumbar nerve

Fifth lumbar vertebra and nerve

First sacral vertebra

Coccygeal nerve

C.Tinnes

SPINAL CORD SEGMENTS

Cervical (8)

Thoracic (12)

Lumbar (5)

Sacral (5)

Coccygeal (1)

Fig. 1-2. Diagram of position and segments of spinal cord with reference to bodies and spinal processes of vertebrae.

Fig. 1-3. Posterior view of cord and nerve roots.

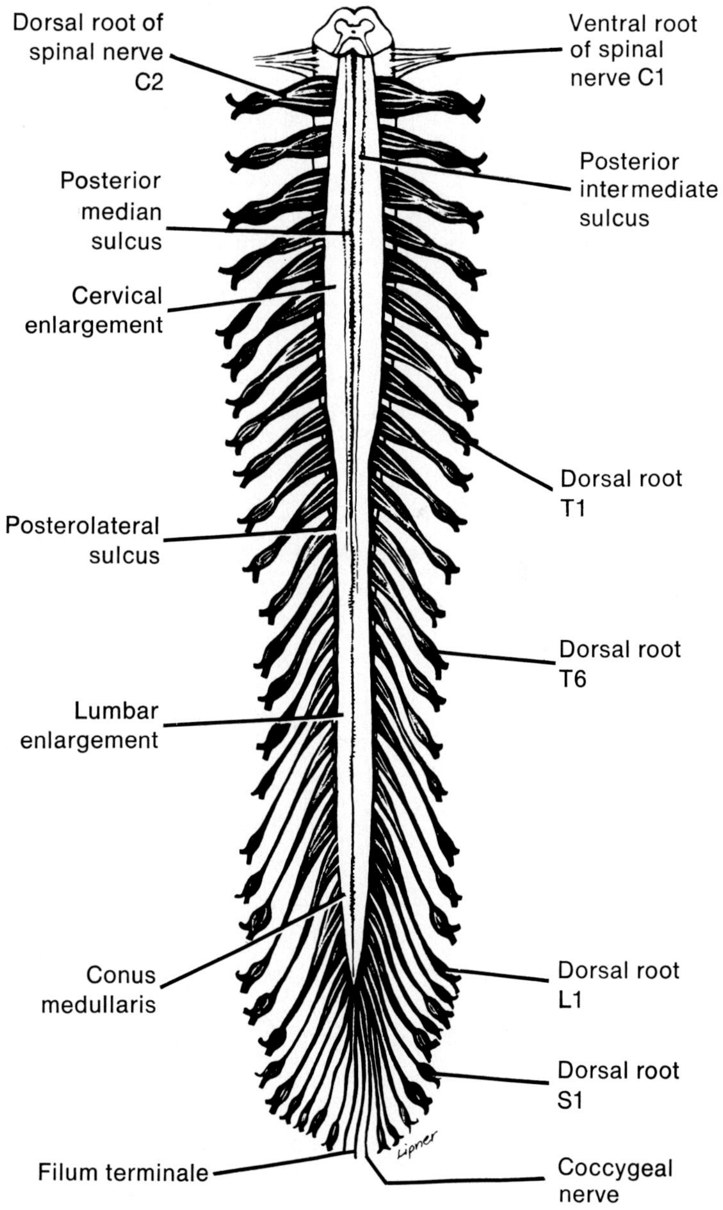

Dorsal root of spinal nerve C2

Posterior median sulcus

Cervical enlargement

Posterolateral sulcus

Lumbar enlargement

Conus medullaris

Filum terminale

Ventral root of spinal nerve C1

Posterior intermediate sulcus

Dorsal root T1

Dorsal root T6

Dorsal root L1

Dorsal root S1

Coccygeal nerve

Lipner

bony canal (perimedullary space) varies from a maximum of 8 mm at the level of the cervical region to a minimum of 3 mm in the thoracic region.[64]

Relationship between the spinal cord segments and the vertebral column. The upper cervical segments extend from the foramen magnum to the third cervical vertebra, the cervical enlargement from the third cervical to the second thoracic vertebra, and the lumbar enlargement from the ninth to the twelfth thoracic vertebra.

Relationship between the spinal cord segments and the vertebral spinous processes. The rule usually applied in determining the probable level of spinal cord damage in cord segment C2-T10 in cases of spinal column injury is to add 2 to the number of vertebral spinous process affected.

The spinous process of T10 corresponds to the T12 segment of the cord, the spinous processes of T11 and T12 correspond to the lumbar segments, and the spinous process of L1 corresponds to the sacral and coccygeal segments. This is not very accurate, but it is useful for practical purposes.

Direction. The spinal cord follows the inflexions of the vertebral column, presenting a cervical curve, convex ventrally, and a thoracic curve, concave ventrally.

External surface of the spinal cord. Fissures and sulci are seen in most of the length of the spinal cord.

The *anterior median fissure* extends through the whole length of the ventral surface of the cord and has an average depth of 3 mm (Figs. 1-3 and 1-4).

The *posterior median sulcus* is very shallow, and from it a posterior septum of neuroglia penetrates 4 to 6 mm into the substance of the cord, reaching almost to the gray commissure (Fig. 1-3).

The posterolateral sulcus is seen on each side, and along it the dorsal spinal roots enter the cord. At the level of the cervical and upper thoracic segments, the *posterointermediate sulcus* marks the position of a septum that divides each half of the posterior funiculus into two large tracts of fibers: the fasciculus gracilis medially and the fasiculus cuneatus laterally.

The *anterolateral sulcus* is shallow and corresponds to the exit of the ventral spinal roots.

Spinal roots. The *ventral spinal roots* (Fig. 1-1) consist of efferent somatic motor fibers and, at certain levels, visceral fibers (sympathetic from T1 to L2-3, parasympathetic from S2 to S4). The *dorsal spinal roots* (Fig. 1-4) present the *dorsal root ganglia*, one on each root, proximal to the junction of the root with the corresponding ventral root in the intervertebral foramen. Each dorsal root divides into six to eight rootlets which enter the cord along the posterolateral sulcus. Each ganglion nerve cell has a single short process that divides into a medial process entering the cord and a lateral process that passes peripherally to some of the sensory end-organs. The central process is morphologically an axon, and the peripheral extension is derived from a dendrite. The dorsal roots are formed by somatic and visceral afferent sensory fibers. The possible existence of autonomic parasympathetic efferent fibers has not received wide support.

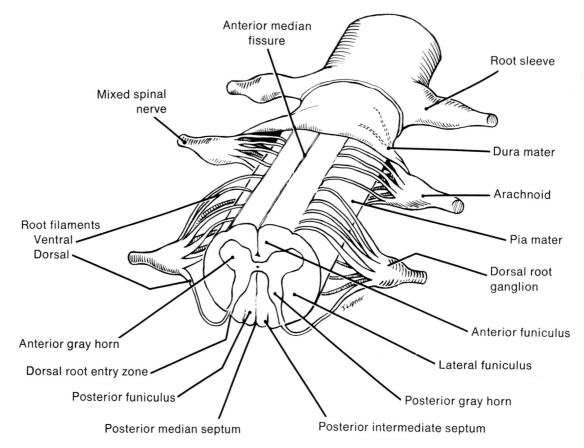

Fig. 1-4. Nerve roots and meninges.

INTERNAL STRUCTURE OF THE SPINAL CORD*
Gray and white matter

A transverse section of the spinal cord shows the central gray matter in a butterfly or letter H form surrounded by the white matter. The *gray matter* consists of symmetric masses connected by the gray commissure. A central canal traverses the commissure. On each side the central gray presents an *anterior* and a *posterior horn* and, in some segments, a *lateral* horn. The surrounding *white matter* is divided on each side into a ventral (or anterior), a lateral, and a posterior (or dorsal) funiculus or column.

In an unstained preparation the pinkish gray color of the gray matter is caused by the pigment of the nerve cell bodies, or perykarya, the lack of myelin of most of the fibers that cross the gray substance, and the abundance of capillary vessels. The color of the white matter is caused by the myelin sheath of its nerve fibers.

The gray matter includes the perikaryon of the spinal neurons, their dendrites and their axons or, in the case of the larger cells, the beginning of their axons, collateral fibers and terminal boutons from fibers that enter the gray matter, the interneuronal network or neuropil, and glial cells and vessels.

The white matter includes myelinated and nonmyelinated nerve fibers that vary in diameter from 1 to 10 μm and glial cells and vessels. The appearance and proportion of white and gray matter at different spinal cord levels are given in Fig. 1-5.

Neurons of the spinal gray matter

Motor neurons of the anterior horns. Anterior horn motor neurons[14,26] are of two types: alpha and gamma. *Alpha motor neurons* have a large perikaryon, or cell body (50 to 100 μm in diameter). These cells correspond to the Golgi type I or Deiters' neurons. They are called alpha motor neurons because their axons belong to the alpha type A of fibers in the classification of Erlanger and Gasser.[16] These axons are large fibers of 10 to 16 μm diameter covered by a thick myelin sheath. Their nerve conduction velocity is 70 to 120 m/sec. *Gamma motor neurons* have a smaller cell body (less than 30 μm in diameter). Their axons belong to the gamma type A of fibers, they are 4 to 8 μm in diameter, and their nerve conduction velocity is 15 to 40 m/sec.

Sensory neurons of the posterior horn and the dorsal nucleus of Clarke. The sensory neurons of the posterior horn and the dorsal nucleus of Clarke possess cell bodies of differing sizes and shapes.

Interneurons. Interneurons, or interstitial neurons,[3] are 30 times as numerous as motor neurons; their cell

*References 2, 5, 7-10, 13, 15, 18, 19, 24, 43, 49, 64, 68.

bodies are located within the base of the anterior horn, the intermediate zone, and the base and neck of the posterior horn. These cells are Golgi type II neurons. Their axons end on other neurons whose cell bodies are located at the same spinal cord level, ipsilaterally or contralaterally, or on neurons located in a lower or upper segmental level.[15,49]

Autonomic neurons. *Autonomic neurons* are located in the lateral part of the intermediate zone. In humans they are sympathetic neurons from T1 to L2-3, and they are parasympathetic neurons from S2-4.

Aberrant neurons of the cord. In addition to the central gray matter, there are scattered groups of cells that have migrated into the white matter.

Horns, nuclei, and lamination of the central gray matter

Horns. The dorsal horn presents a head, a neck, and a base. The ventral horn has a head and a base. The lateral horn is the lateral part of the intermediate zone from T 1 to L2 or L3.

Nuclei. Nuclei, or cell groups, found in the *dorsal horn* are the nucleus posteromarginalis, the substantia gelatinosa (of Rolando), and the proper sensory nucleus, or nucleus propius cornu dorsali (of Waldeyer).

From C1 to about C4, the gelatinous substance includes the inferior part of the nucleus of the spinal tract of the trigeminal nerve. The spinal tract of the trigeminal nerve is located within the zone of Lissauer.

The *intermediate zone* is made up of the nucleus intermediomedialis of Cajal, seen at all levels of the cord. The nucleus intermediolateralis, or lateral horn, and the nucleus dorsalis (of Clarke) are added in the thoracic and upper lumbar segments.

In the *ventral horn* there are three main divisions or nuclear groups: the *medial*, the *lateral*, and the *central* divisions. The latter is only present in the upper cervical and lumbosacral segments (see below). At the level of the cervical and lumbar enlargements the anterior horn exhibits its maximal complexity, presenting, within the *medial nuclear group*, or *division*, the posteromedial and anteromedial nuclei, and, within the *lateral division*, the anterior, anterolateral, posterolateral, and retroposterolateral nuclei.

The relationship between the nuclei of the ventral horn and the muscle territories of the limbs is shown in Figs. 1-6 and 1-7. The more medially located motor neurons are related to the proximal muscles, and the more lateral ones are related to the distal muscles of the limbs.

The *central division* at the upper cervical level includes the *phrenic nucleus*, which is best developed from C4 to C6, although it extends above and below these levels, and the *accessory nucleus*, which extends

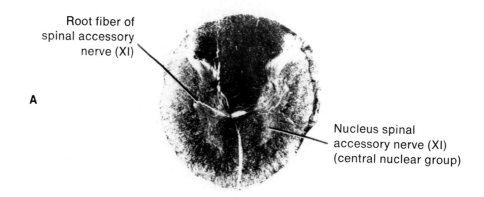

A

Root fiber of spinal accessory nerve (XI)

Nucleus spinal accessory nerve (XI) (central nuclear group)

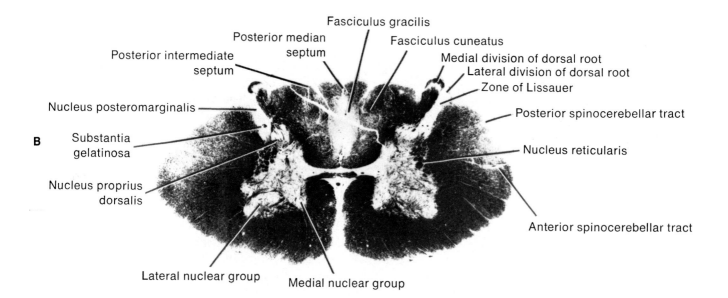

B

Posterior intermediate septum

Posterior median septum

Fasciculus gracilis

Fasciculus cuneatus

Medial division of dorsal root

Lateral division of dorsal root

Zone of Lissauer

Posterior spinocerebellar tract

Nucleus posteromarginalis

Substantia gelatinosa

Nucleus proprius dorsalis

Nucleus reticularis

Lateral nuclear group

Medial nuclear group

Anterior spinocerebellar tract

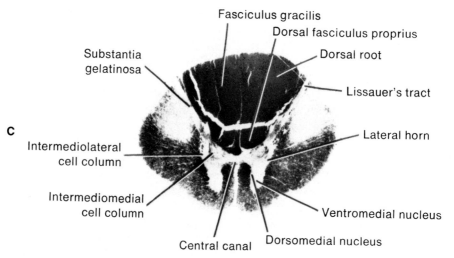

C

Fasciculus gracilis

Dorsal fasciculus proprius

Dorsal root

Lissauer's tract

Substantia gelatinosa

Lateral horn

Intermediolateral cell column

Intermediomedial cell column

Central canal

Dorsomedial nucleus

Ventromedial nucleus

Fig. 1-5. Transverse sections of human spinal cord (Weigert's stain). **A,** Upper cervical cord (C1). **B,** Cervical enlargement (C8). **C,** Thoracic level (T10).

from C1 to C5 or C6. Its caudal portion supplies the trapezius muscle, and the rostral part supplies the sternocleidomastoid muscle. The root fibers arising from this nucleus turn dorsalward and then lateralward to emerge on the lateral border of the anterior horn and form the external ramus or spinal portion of the accessory (XI) cranial nerve (Fig. 1-5, *A*).

Between the tip of the dorsal horn and the surface of the cord is the *dorsolateral fasciculus,* or *Lissauer's zone (tract).* It is formed by exogenous, or radicular, fibers and by endogenous, or spinospinal or intrinsic, fibers.

Between the lateral horn and the lateral aspect of the dorsal horn there is a prolongation of the spinal gray that intermingles with fibers of the lateral column, forming the reticular substance, or *reticular formation.* It appears at the upper thoracic and cervical levels.

Lamination of the gray matter. Based on cytoarchitectonic characteristics, the spinal gray has been divided into ten layers, or laminae (after Rexed)[54,55,65]:

Lamina I—corresponds to the posteromarginal nucleus

Lamina II——corresponds to the substantia gelatinosa

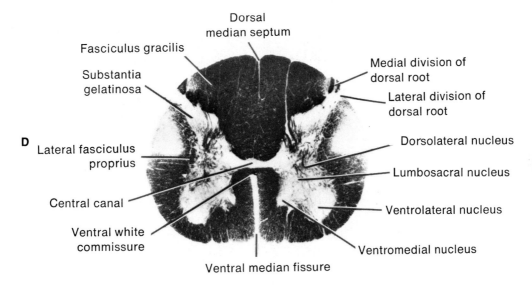

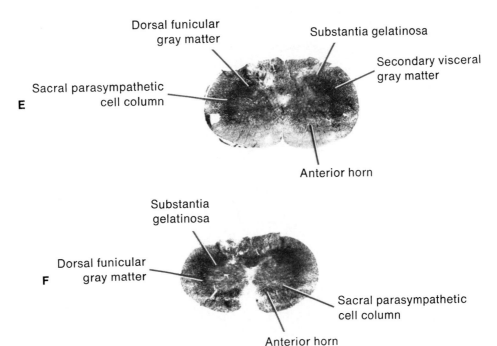

Fig. 1-5, cont'd. D, Lumbar segment (L2). **E,** Sacral segment (S2). **F,** Sacral segment (S4).

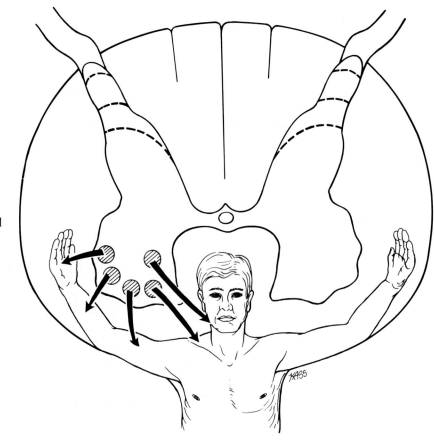

Fig. 1-6. Motor nuclei at level of cervical enlargement (see text).

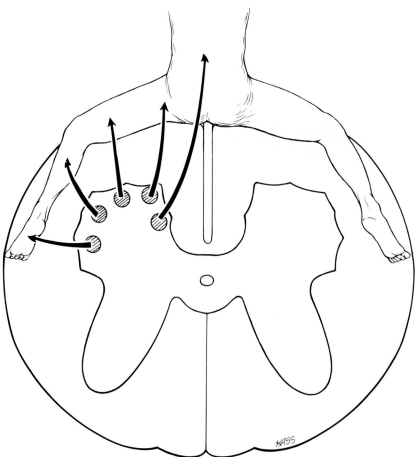

Fig. 1-7. Motor nuclei at level of lumbar enlargement (see text).

Laminae III and IV—correspond to the proper sensory nucleus

Lamina V—corresponds to the neck of the posterior horn

Lamina VI—corresponds to the base of the posterior horn

Lamina VII—corresponds to the intermediate zone

Lamina VIII—corresponds to the dorsomedial part of the anterior horn

Lamina IX—includes most of the anterior horn with the medial and lateral nuclear groups already mentioned

Lamina X—corresponds to the gray commissure

White matter

The white matter is divided into three columns of funiculi. The *anterior funiculus* is limited medially by the anterior spinal sulcus and laterally by the medial border of the ventral horn and the ventral root fibers. The *lateral funiculus* is limited medially by the lateral border of the ventral and dorsal horns and the ventral and dorsal root fibers; the lateral limit is the lateral surface of the cord. Each *posterior funiculus* is limited lat-

erally by the medial border of the dorsal horn and the dorsal root fibers, medially by the medial septum, and dorsally by the surface of the cord.

The white matter includes the following:

Descending motor (pyramidal and extrapyramidal) and autonomic fibers

Ascending sensory fibers

Interspinal fibers

Dorsal roots and the incoming sensory fibers

About 824,000 fibers enter the spinal cord through the 31 pairs of dorsal roots,[30] representing the axons of the dorsal root ganglion neurons. The other process of these neurons is connected to the peripheral receptors of the skin, subcutaneous tissue, fasciae, joint ligaments and capsules, periosteum, muscles, tendons, vessels, and viscera.

The dorsal root fibers are divided into two groups[53] (Fig. 1-8). The *lateral division* is composed mainly of thin, slightly myelinated and nonmyelinated fibers that enter the zone of Lissauer, where they divide into an ascending and a descending branch, giving rise to numerous collateral fibers. These fibers bring nerve im-

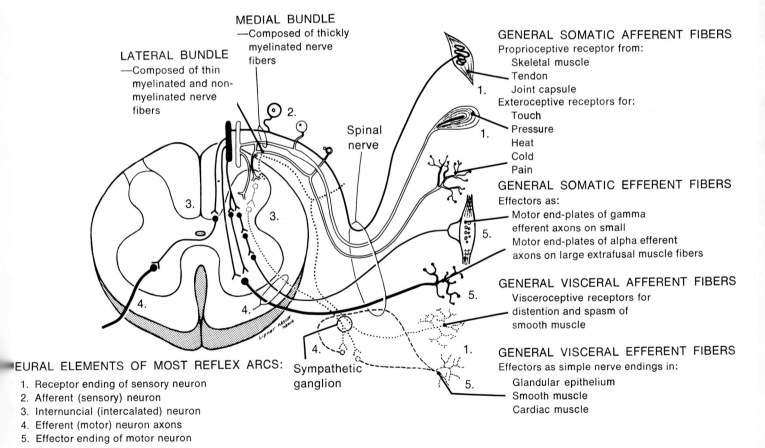

Fig. 1-8. Arrangement of dorsal root fibers.

pulses related to pain, temperature, and touch into the cord from exteroceptors, as well from visceral receptors. The incoming fibers and their collateral fibers are going to end on one of the following:

1. Sensory neurons of the dorsal horn
2. Neurons of the dorsal nucleus of Clarke
3. Interneurons of the dorsal horn, intermediate zone, or anterior horn
4. Autonomic neurons

The *medial division* is formed by large, more richly myelinated nerve fibers that pass over the tip of the dorsal horn and enter the posterolateral region of the dorsal column, where they divide into an ascending and a descending branch, both of which give rise to numerous collateral fibers. These fibers are going to end on some of the following cells:

1. Sensory neurons of the dorsal horn and the lower brain stem
2. Neurons of the dorsal nucleus of Clarke
3. Interneurons of the dorsal horn, intermediate zone, or anterior horn
4. Directly on motor neurons of the anterior horn

The incoming fibers and their collateral fibers are going to participate in three main mechanisms: sensory-perception mechanisms, cerebellar mechanisms, and reflex mechanisms of the spinal cord.

Fibers related to sensory-perception mechanisms

Fibers related to sensory-perception mechanisms make up the posterior column tracts, that is, the fasciculus gracilis and the fasciculus cuneatus (Fig. 1-9), and the lateral and ventral spinothalamic tracts.

Posterior column tracts. The posterior column tracts are formed by ascending branches of fibers that enter the cord through the medial division of the posterior roots: *fasciculus gracilis* by the ascending branches of fibers that enter the cord at the sacral, lumbar, and lower dorsal levels (up to T6) and *fasciculus cuneatus* by ascending branches of fibers that enter above T6, up to C1 (Déjerine). These ascending fibers end on second sensory neurons of nuclei gracilis and cuneatus, located in the lower medulla. The axons of these neurons cross the midline (sensory decussation), ascend as the medial lemniscus of Reil, and end in the ventroposterolateral nucleus of the thalamus (third sensory neurons), whose axons end on the fourth layer of the somatosensory cortex (area 3-1-2) in the postcentral gyrus of the parietal lobe. In this manner the nerve impulses transported by the axons become "conscious." Consciousness in neuroanatomy is equal to cerebral cortical activity.

Fasciculi gracilis and cuneatus are related to the transmission of deep sensation (deep pressure, deep

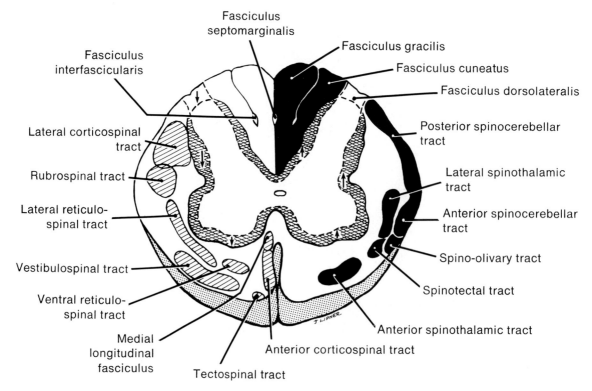

Fig. 1-9. Diagram of ascending *(solid black)*, descending *(diagonal lines)*, and interspinal *(cross-hatched)* tracts.

pain, vibration, and position sense), as well as to fine aspects of pain (localization, two-point discrimination, graphesthesia, stereognosis).

The position of the fibers within the fasciculi or lamination varies. The fibers through the inferior, sacral levels of the cord are located in the most dorsomedial portion of the posterior column, while the fibers that enter at progressively higher levels are located more and more laterally and ventrally.[64]

Lateral spinothalamic tracts. The lateral spinothalamic tracts (Fig. 1-10) are formed as follows. Terminal branches and collateral fibers from the lateral group of the posterior root fibers end on sensory neurons of the substantia gelatinosa, whose short axons end on neurons of layers VI, VII, and VIII.[50,62] The axons of the latter cells cross the midline through the anterior white commissure, arrive at the lateral funiculus, and ascend as the lateral spinothalamic tract, bringing up impulses related to pain and temperature sensation. This tract ends in the ventroposterolateral nucleus of the thalamus.

Anterior spinothalamic tract. Fibers related to touch end on the neurons of the proper sensory nucleus, whose axons end on neurons of layers VI, VII, and VIII.

The axons from these layers cross the midline through the anterior white commissure, arrive at the lateral funiculus, and ascend as the anterior spinothalamic tract (Fig. 1-9) to end in the ventroposterolateral nucleus of the thalamus. The lamination or fiber distri-

bution within the lateral and ventral spinothalamic tracts is shown in Fig. 1-11.

The so-called "extralemniscal pathways for pain"[23,51] are located as follows: one within the lateral funiculus, medial to the lateral spinothalamic tract and close to the reticulospinal tract, and the other within the lateral part of the zone of Lissauer.[12] They end in the brain stem reticular formation. Through a polysynaptic intrareticular pathway, the impulses arrive at the intralaminary nuclei of the thalamus and the posterior hypothalamus.[22,40]

Gate control theory of pain. The gate control theory of pain[42] postulates that the function of the closed polysynaptic mechanisms of the gelatinous substance control the primary afferent terminal fibers and their synaptic contact. This pool of neurons of the substantia gelatinosa receives collateral fibers of the large fibers of the posterior column, whose nervous impulses have an inhibitory effect and act as a control mechanism for the transmission of pain. Collateral fibers also arrive at the neurons of layers VI, VII, and VIII, and it is in these neurons that the lateral spinothalamic tract originates.

Visceral pain and afferent visceral or autonomic fibers. Nociceptive afferent fibers from the lower urinary and reproductive tracts reach the spinal cord via the pelvic nerves; those related to abdominal viscera run in the sympathetic fibers of the hypogastric, mesenteric, and solar plexuses and the splanchnic nerves. The afferent fibers of the thoracic viscera travel via the cardiac,

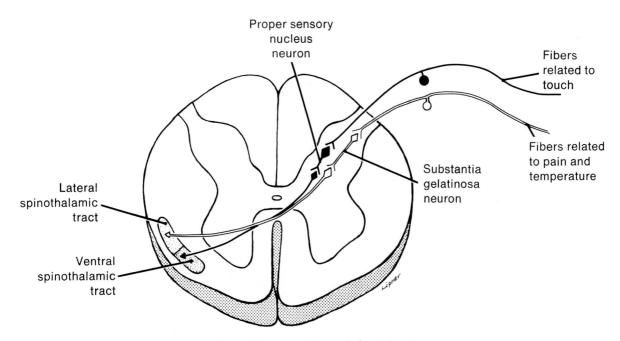

Fig. 1-10. Diagram of spinothalamic tracts.

pulmonary, and mediastinal plexuses and the cardiac nerves.[67]

Referred pain. Pain originating within the thoracic and abdominal cavities may be felt "in situ," that is, at the site of primary stimulation, or it may be "referred"[25] to a distant site on the skin segment innervated by the same spinal segment that innervates the visceral locus of origin. Fig. 1-12 shows the most accepted mechanisms by which pain is referred. The main fact is that the visceral pain fibers synapse with the same second sensory neurons that receive pain fibers from the skin.

Incoming fibers related to the cerebellar mechanisms

Dorsal spinocerebellar tract. Large dorsal root fibers from the medial division, bringing impulses from muscle, tendon, and other deep receptors or proprioceptors as well as from interoceptors, end on the large neurons of the dorsal nucleus of Clarke.[61] The axons of the latter neurons run laterally, and, approaching the surface of the lateral funiculus, they form the dorsal or direct spinocerebellar tract of Flechsig (Fig. 1-9). Fig. 1-11 shows the location and lamination or localization pattern of that tract. The dorsal spinocerebellar tract enters the inferior cerebellar tract, or corpus restiformis, and ends on the ipsilateral paleocerebellar cortex. The nucleus or column of Clarke extends from T1 to L2 or

L3. For that reason the lower lumbar and sacral fibers turn forward in the fasciculus gracilis to end above their level of entrance in the caudal part of the nucleus of Clarke. On the other hand, the cervical fibers ascend within the fasciculus cuneatus to end on the nucleus paracuneatus, which projects its fibers on the ipsilateral paleocerebellum.

Ventral spinocerebellar tract. A group of dorsal root fibers related to proprioceptors and tactile exteroceptors related to the cerebellum do not end in the nucleus of Clarke.[28] These fibers, at all levels of the cord, end on neurons of the deep layers of the dorsal horn, at the cervical, thoracic, lumbar, and sacral levels. The axons of these neurons cross the midline through the ventral white commissure, and, approaching the surface of the lateral funiculus, they form the ventral or crossed spinocerebellar tract of Gowers (Fig. 1-9).

The lamination is similar in both the ventral and the dorsal spinocerebellar tracts, showing a dorsal-to-ventral arrangement of the sacral, lumbar, and thoracic fibers (in primates including humans). After passing through the brain stem, the ventral spinocerebellar tract enters the superior cerebellar peduncle or brachium conjunctivum, crosses the midline, and ends on the contralateral paleocerebellar cortex.

Spinoreticular tract. The spinoreticular tract originates from neurons of layers V, VI, and VII, whose ax-

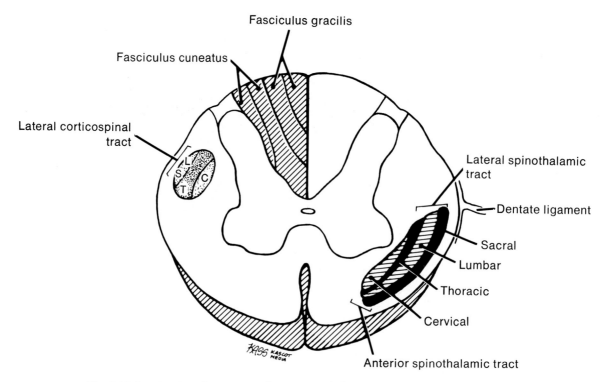

Fig. 1-11. Lamination of posterior column, spinothalamic tracts, and corticospinal tract.

ons ascend ipsilaterally and end in the lateral reticular nucleus, located behind the inferior olivary complex of the medulla oblongata. That nucleus projects on the ipsilateral paleocerebellar cortex.

Spino-olivary tract. The spino-olivary tract originates from layers V, VI, and VII. The axons of those neurons cross the midline and accumulate ventral to the ventral spinocerebellar tract as the spino-olivary tract. This tract enters the inferior olivary complex, which projects contralaterally to the paleocerebellar and neocerebellar cortices.

Spinovestibular tract. The spinovestibular tract originates from dorsal horn neurons of the upper cervical levels, which receive impulses from muscles, tendons, and joints. The tract ends in the inferior vestibular nucleus.

Incoming fibers related to the spinal cord reflex activity

Reflexes of muscle and tendon origin.* The reflex arc for the *stretch*, or *monosynaptic, reflex* responsible for the maintenance of the striated muscle tone and the realization of the deep tendon reflexes includes (1) a receptor, that is, the muscle spindle, (2) the afferent fiber I, coming from the annulospiral ending, or primary receptor, (3) the alpha motor neuron (reflex center), and (4) the efferent type A motor fiber. This is the anatomic road for the so-called *group Ia* (feedback) *control system*, or *stretch control* mechanism (Fig. 1-13).

---

*References 13, 15, 19, 22, 25, 43, 44.

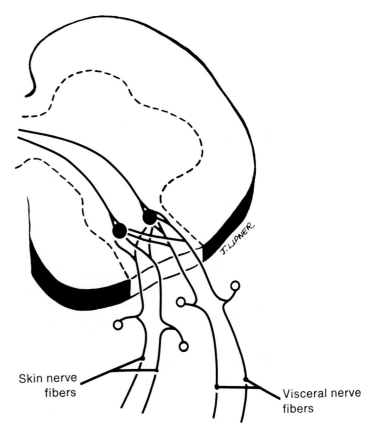

Fig. 1-12. Diagram of mechanism of referred pain and hyperalgesia.

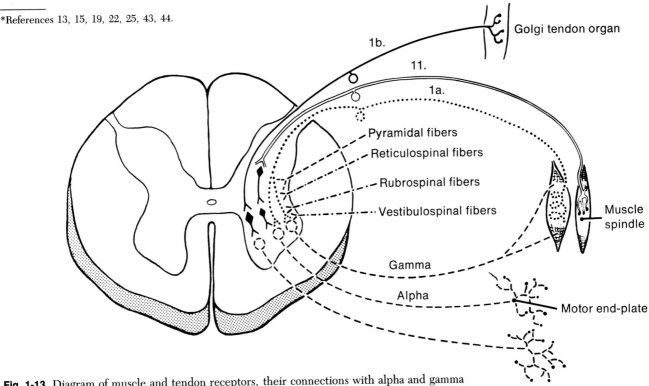

Fig. 1-13. Diagram of muscle and tendon receptors, their connections with alpha and gamma motorneurons; the monosynaptic, bisynaptic, and polysynaptic types of reflex arcs.

The *group II control system,* originating from the flower spray nerve endings of the muscle spindles, includes several interneurons in the reflex center *(polysynaptic reflex).* Its function is not yet completely understood (Fig. 1-13).

The reflex arc for the *group Ib control system,* or tension control mechanism, includes (1) a receptor, (2) the Golgi tendon organ, (3) the afferent fiber II, (4) the interneuron, and (5) the motor neuron. This *bisynaptic reflex* is responsible for the inhibitory reflex that appears when excessive tension is developed within a given muscle (Fig. 1-13).

Reflexes of cutaneous origin, or nociceptive or withdrawal reflexes, are carried out through the polysynaptic reflex. The reflexes are the ipsilateral flexor reflex, the crossed extensor reflex, and a variety of reflexes of posture and locomotion.[60]

There are *spinal cord reflexes* that cause muscle spasms: spasm resulting from broken bone, abdominal spasm in peritonitis, and spasms in muscle cramps.

Autonomic spinal cord centers and reflexes. The *reflex center* is formed by the autonomic neurons[43]: sympathetic neurons of the thoracolumbar segments (T1 to L2 or L3) and parasympathetic neurons of the sacral segments (S2 to S4 in humans).

The autonomic reflex arc includes a receptor, the afferent visceral sensory fiber, the spinal autonomic neuron, the preganglionic fibers (or white rami communicans for the thoracolumbar region), the autonomic neurons of the paravertebral sympathetic chain, the prevertebral plexuses, or the viscera, the postganglionic fibers, or gray rami communicans, and the effector smooth muscle, cardiac muscle, vessels, or glands.

The autonomic centers of the cord are the ciliospinal center of Budge (T1-2 in humans); sweating and pilomotor centers (T1 to L2 or L3); cardiovascular centers: cardioaccelerator (T1-5), vasoconstrictor (T1 to L2 or L3), adrenalinosecretor (T12-L1); gastrointestinal motility: intestine (T6-L1), colon (L2-4); vesicospinal centers: lumbar center (L2-4; hypogastric nerves), sacral center (S2-4; pelvic nerves); and genitospinal centers: erection (S2-4; pelvic nerves, or nervi erigentes), ejaculation (L2-4; hypogastric nerves).

Motor (pyramidal and extrapyramidal) and autonomic descending pathways

Pyramidal tract. The pyramidal, or corticospinal, tract[31,32,45,56] originates from the pyramidal cells of the third and fifth layers of frontoparietal areas: 31% from area 6, or the premotor area, 29% from area 4, or the primary motor cortex (2% to 3% from the giant pyramidal cells [of Betz]) and 40% from area 3-1-2, or the primary somatosensory area. Of the 1 million fibers within each bulbar pyramid, approximately 80% of

them decussate at the level of the pyramidal decussation, descending in the *lateral pyramidal tract* of the cord; 10% of the noncrossed fibers pass into the anterior part of the lateral pyramidal tract as the *anterolateral pyramidal tract of Barnes (les fibres pyramidal homolaterale superficielle de Déjerine).* The remaining 10% of the fibers pass into the *anterior* or *direct corticospinal tract,* or bundle of Türck. The majority of the fibers of this bundle cross the anterior white commissure and terminate on the spinal cord of the opposite side (Fig. 1-9).

Ninety percent of the myelinated fibers have a diameter of 1 to 4 μm. Most of the remaining 10% of the fibers are 5 to 10 μm in diameter, but about 30,000 to 34,000 fibers that originate from the cells of Betz have a diameter of 10 to 22 μm.

The pyramidal fibers end on neurons of the proper sensory nucleus (layer IV), neck (layer V), and base (layer VI) of the posterior horn; intermediate zone (layer VII); and base (layer VIII) and head (layer IX) of the anterior horn. In primates some of the corticospinal fibers end directly on the motor neurons of the anterior horn, but the vast majority form synapses with interneurons.[27,38,39]

Distribution of the pyramidal fibers is as follows: 50% to 55% go to the cervical, 20% to the thoracic, and 20% to 25% to the lumbosacral spinal segments.[66]

Extrapyramidal pathways. The *reticulospinal tract* is the most important descending motor tract after the corticospinal. Through the reticulospinal tract, the lower motor neurons receive impulses from the reticular formation itself, globus pallidus, substantia nigra, subthalamic nucleus, red nucleus, and cerebellum, that is, from the extrapyramidal and cerebellar motor control systems.[41]

Most of the reticulospinal fibers originate from pontine and medullary reticular nuclei, nucleus reticularis pontis orale, nucleus reticularis pontis caudale, nucleus reticularis magnocellularis, and nucleus reticularis.[4,48,57] The pontine reticulospinal tract is almost entirely ipsilateral and descends within the anterior funiculus (Fig. 1-9). The medullary reticulospinal tract is mainly ipsilateral with some crossed fibers and descends in the anterior part of the lateral funiculus (Fig. 1-9). The reticulospinal fibers end in layers VII and VIII, and a very few end in layer IX.[46]

The *tectospinal tract* originates in the superior colliculus, decussates (dorsal tegmental decussation of Meynert), descends within the medial longitudinal fasciculus and through the cervical levels, and ends in layers VI, VII, and VIII of the spinal gray.

The *rubrospinal tract* originates in the magnicellular and part of the parvicellular portions of the red nucleus, decussates (ventral tegmental commisure of Forel), descends anterior to the pyramidal tract, and ends in layers VI, VII, and VIII.[47]

The *interstitiospinal tract* originates in the interstitial nucleus of Cajal and descends within the medial longitudinal fasciculus.

The *vestibulospinal (Deiters') tract* originates in the lateral vestibular nucleus, or nucleus of Deiter, descends ipsilaterally, and ends in layers VII and VIII,[45] mediating impulses from the vestibulocerebellar system.

The *medial longitudinal fasciculus* descends within the anterior funiculus only through the cervical levels.

Descending autonomic pathways originate from the hypothalamus, and brain stem autonomic nuclei and descend through the dorsolateral part of the reticular formation and then through the lateral funiculus of the cord, to end in the lateral group of neurons of layer VII: sympathetic (T1 to L2-3) and parasympathetic (S2 to S4).

Spinospinal fasciculi

The spinospinal fasciculi, also known as intrinsic spinal pathways or fasciculi proprii, originate from interneurons, including ascending and descending fibers that are crossed and uncrossed, participating in the spinal reflex activity. They are located adjacent to the spinal gray in the anterior, lateral, and posterior funiculi (Fig. 1-9).

Within the posterior funiculus, descending branches of the dorsal root fibers form a tract that has a different shape, location, and name at different levels of the cord: fasciculus interfascicularis or comma field of Schultze (cervical), septomarginal tract or dorsal bundle of Hoche (thoracic), oval field of Flechsig (lumbar), and triangle of Gombault-Philippe (sacral). They also include spinospinal fibers.

MENINGES

The spinal cord is enclosed by three protective membranes: the dura mater, the arachnoid, and the pia mater (Figs. 1-1 and 1-4).

Dura mater. The spinal dura mater represents the continuation of the inner, or meningeal, layer of the cranial dura. The outer, or periosteal, layer is interrupted at the foramen magnum and is represented below this point by the periosteum of the vertebrae.

The epidural space between the spinal dura and the vertebral canal contains loose areolar tissue and a venous plexus.

The dura mater is attached to the circumference of the foramen magnum, the second and third cervical vertebrae, and the posterior longitudinal ligament. The tubular sheath of the dura ends at the level of the second sacral vertebra, at which point the dura surrounds the filum terminale and becomes the coccygeal liga-

ment, which fuses with the periosteum of the coccyx. The lower part of the dural sac, below the level of the conus medullaris, is occupied by the cauda equina. The spinal nerves on each side are covered by prolongations of the dura, which is continuous with the epineurium of the peripheral nerves.

Pia mater. The pia mater is a delicate connective tissue membrane carrying the network of blood vessels. It is composed by two layers: the intima pia and the epipial tissue. The intima pia is intimately attached to the surface of the cord by a superficial glial membrane. The cord is attached to the dura mater by two lateral series of 18 to 24 flattened bands of epipial tissue. These bands form the *denticulate ligament*, which is attached to the lateral aspect of the cord midway between the dorsal and ventral roots, along the whole length of the organ.

The perineurium of the nerves leaving the cord is reinforced by the pia mater, which blends with the dura mater at the exit of the nerves.

Arachnoid. The arachnoid together with the pia mater forms the *leptomeninges*. Between the arachnoid and the dura mater is the subdural space, and between the arachnoid and the pia mater is the subarachnoid space. The subarachnoid space is interrupted by the *longitudinal subarachnoid septum* and contains the cerebrospinal fluid.

VASCULARIZATION OF THE SPINAL CORD

The vascularization of the spinal cord* is considered below in terms of (1) the arterial supply and origin of the spinal arteries and (2) the major longitudinal arterial divisions of the spinal cord.

Arterial supply and origin of the spinal arteries

The two sources of arterial supply are the following:
1. The anterior and posterior spinal arteries, descending branches of the vertebral arteries
2. The segmental radicular arteries, branches of the segmental vessels: costocervical trunk or deep cervical artery; intercostal, lumbar, and sacral arteries (Figs. 1-14 and 1-15)

Anterior and posterior spinal arteries. The arteries supplying the upper part of the cervical spinal cord are derived from the vertebral arteries after the latter have penetrated the dura mater and entered the foramen magnum, before they unite to form the basilar artery. Two descending branches, one from each vertebral artery, unite at the level of or below the foramen magnum to form the anterior spinal artery, which lies in the pia mater in or close to the ventral spinal fissure. At a higher level each vertebral artery gives off another

---

*References 1, 5, 6, 11, 20, 21, 29, 33-37, 63, 64, 68.

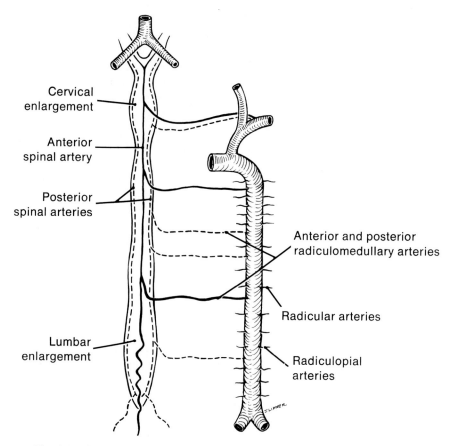

Fig. 1-14. Anterior view of anterior and posterior radiculomedullary arteries.

descending branch, the paired posterior or dorsal spinal arteries that pass along the dorsolateral aspect of the cord lateral to the entry of the dorsal root fibers.

The anterior and posterior spinal arteries usually end at the level of the fourth or fifth cervical segments, and below them the vascularization of the cord depends entirely on the segmental radicular arteries (Adamkiewicz).

Radicular arteries. The radicular arteries, or lateral spinal arteries, enter the spinal canal through the intervertebral foramina along the spinal nerves, penetrate the dura mater, and divide into ventral and dorsal branches accompanying the corresponding nerve roots. When the ventral and dorsal branches arrive close to the ventral sulcus or the posterolateral sulcus, respectively, they divide into an ascending and a descending branch, which anastomoses with homologous branches of upper and lower segments, forming longitudinal vessels of variable caliber and not always continuous. Schematically it can be said that the spinal cord presents three vertical arterial channels: one anterior, along the ventral sulcus of the cord, and two posterolateral, close to the posterolateral sulcus. A plexus of smaller arteries within the pia mater, the *arterial vasocorona* or peri-

medullary coronary arterial plexus, interconnects the larger anterior and posterolateral spinal arteries.

The number of radicular arteries that vascularize the cord varies with age. In the early stages of embryonic life, the 62 radicular arteries that arrive with 31 pairs of radicular nerves vascularize the cord. Then there is a progressive reduction and concentration of the arterial supply. In the adult only a few of the 62 radicular arteries vascularize the spinal cord: an average of eight according to Kadyi,[29] six to eight according to Lazorthes and co-workers,[36] and seven to ten according to Gillilan.[20,21] In the adult the radicular arteries, particularly in the dorsolumbar regions, can be divided into three groups according to Tanon[63]:

1. Small radicular arteries that end on the nerve roots
2. Medium-size radicular arteries, or radiculopial arteries, that arrive at the vascular network of the pia mater
3. Large radicular arteries, or radiculospinal arteries: the six to eight radicular arteries that vascularize the cord, two of which are the most constant and most important ones: the cervical radicular artery, which enters at the C5 or C6 level, and the great

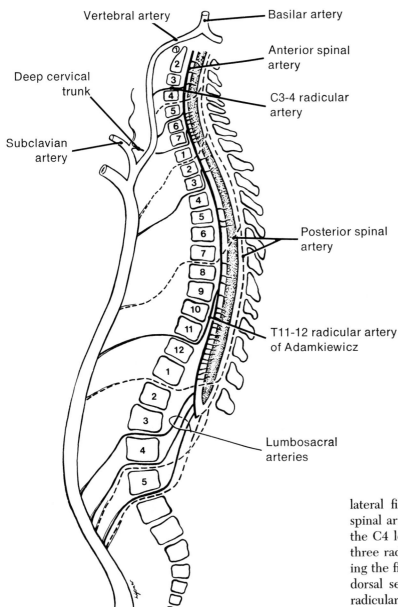

Fig. 1-15. Lateral view of anterior and posterior radiculomedullary arteries.

lateral fibers of the subclavian arteries. The anterior spinal artery reaches down only to the C4 level. From the C4 level to the C8 level, the cord receives two to three radicular arteries, and most constant accompanying the fifth or sixth cervical root. The two or three first dorsal segments receive their blood supply through a radicular artery that most frequently accompanies the first thoracic nerve and originates from the costocervical trunk.

2. The intermediate, or middorsal, arterial territory extends from T4 to T8 and has a poor vascularization. Sometimes a T7 radicular artery establishes a communication between the upper and lower territories.

3. The inferior, or dorsolumbar, arterial territory includes the lumbar enlargements and the last dorsal segments (T9 to T12). This region has a rich vascularization, but it depends on a single vessel, the great anterior radicular artery of Adamkiewicz. This artery originates on the left side in 80% of the cases. In 85% of the individuals the vessel reaches the cord with the nerve roots between T9 and L2 (middle or low variety), of which 75% are between T9 and T12 and 10% are between L1 and L2.[11] In the remaining 15% of the

anterior radicular artery (arteria radicularis anterior magna) of Adamkiewicz, or artery of the lumbar enlargement of Lazorthes, which arrives at the cord between T9 and T12

Major longitudinal arterial divisions of the spinal cord

There are three major arteries of the spinal cord according to Lazorthes[36] (Figs. 1-14 and 1-15).

1. The superior, or cervicodorsal, arterial territory extends from C1 to T2-3 and has a rich vascularization that originates from the vertebral arteries and from col-

cases the artery arises between T5 and T8 (high variety).

The great anterior radicular artery arrives at the anterior surface of the cord, where it divides into a thinner ascending and a larger descending branch. The latter is three times as large as the former and vascularizes the lumbar enlargement, the conus medullaris. Then it follows the filum terminale up to the lower end of the dural sac. At the level of the conus medullaris this artery anastomoses with two dorsal spinal arteries, forming a constant arterial loop.

Intrinsic arteries of the spinal cord

In all segments of the cord the intramedullary distribution of the arterial vessels is divided into two horizontal territories, one derived from the anterior spinal arterial system and the other from the posterior spinal system and the peripheral network (Fig. 1-16):

1. Deep territory: The central or anterior sulcal or sulcocommissural arteries, about 200 in number, reach to the depth of the anterior sulcus, divide into a left branch and a right branch, and vascularize most of the spinal gray (the anterior horn;

the intermediate zone, including the nucleus of Clarke; the base, neck, and central part of the posterior horn; and the gray commissure), and the deep portion of the white matter, including the lateral and ventral pyramidal tracts. The vessels derived from the central arteries have a centrifugal direction.

2. Peripheral territory: The peripheral territory originates from the posterolateral spinal arteries and the pial arterial network, or arterial vasocorona. These vessels have a centripetal direction (Fig. 1-16). The peripheral territory includes most of the posterior column and the superficial part of the ventral and lateral columns, including the spinothalamic and spinocerebellar tracts, as well as the tip of the posterior horn of the spinal gray.

Capillary network

All arteries penetrating the cord break up into a capillary network that is continuous throughout the organ. Thus end-arteries in a strictly anatomic sense do not exist. However, there are end-arteries from the functional viewpoint. The average diameter of the capillar-

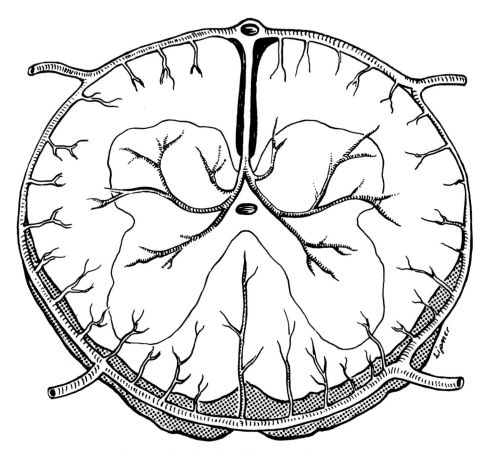

Fig. 1-16. Peripheral and deep arterial territories.

ies in the human central nervous system has been estimated by different authors as 4.5 to 6 μm and as 7.5 to 13 μm.

In the white matter the relatively large meshes of the capillary network are distributed approximately parallel with the bundles of fibers.[17]

The gray matter is much more richly vascular than is the white. In the spinal gray the meshes are smaller and less regular in disposition; nevertheless, the capillaries are arranged in definite directions related to those of the axis of the cells and their processes.[17]

Veins of the spinal cord

The intramedullary veins are scattered among the intramedullary arteries. Their areas of drainage overlap the distribution of the central arteries. The venous drainage is done through the peripheral veins. The *superficial veins* of the cord unite in an extensive venous plexus in the pia-arachnoid, which lies deep to the arterial plexus. Within the plexus are the perimedullary coronary vein, venous vasocorona, and six longitudinal channels: the ventral and the dorsal spinal veins and the two ventrolateral and the two dorsolateral spinal veins, the largest being the dorsal spinal vein. Cranially the spinal veins continue with the bulbar veins.

The drainage of the superficial veins is done through the *dorsal* and the *ventral radicular veins*. The drainage from the radicular veins is through the dorsal and the ventral *longitudinal vertebral venous sinuses* or *(plexuses)* or *epidural venous plexuses*, both connected by numerous anastomotic channels. The drainage from the epidural plexuses is through the vertebral, intercostal, lumbar, and sacral veins that emerge through the intervertebral foramina to end in the *external vertebral venous plexuses*. From there, the venous blood arrives at the veins of the abdominal and thoracic cavities and the cervical veins.

REFERENCES

1. Adamkiewicz, A.: Die Blutgefässe des menschlichen Rükenmarkesoberfläche, Sitzungsb. d.k. Akade. Wissensch. in Wien Math. Natural Kasse **85:**101, 1882.
2. Bok, S. T.: Das Rückenmark. In von Möllendorff, W., editor: Handbuch der mikroskopischen Antomie des Menshen Band 4 Teil 1, Berlin, 1927, Springer Verlag.
3. Brazier, M. A. B., editor: The interneuron, Berkeley, Calif., 1969, University of California Press.
4. Brodal, A.: The reticular formation of the brain stem. Anatomical and functional correlations, Springfield, Ill., 1957, Charles C Thomas, Publisher.
5. Carpenter, M. B.: Human anatomy, Baltimore, 1976, The Williams & Wilkins Co.
6. Craigie, H. E.: Vascular supply of the spinal cord. In Austin, G., editor: The spinal cord. Basic aspects and surgical considerations, Springfield, Ill., 1972, Charles C Thomas, Publisher.
7. Crosby, E. C., Humphrey, T., and Lauer, E. W.: Correlative anatomy of the nervous system, New York, 1962, Macmillan.
8. Déjerine, J. J.: Anatomie des centres nerveux, Paris, 1901, Rueff.
9. Déjerine, J. J.: Semiologie des affections du système nerveux, Paris, 1914, Masson & Cie Editeurs.
10. Delmas, J., and Delmas, A.: Voies et centres nerveux, Paris, 1958, Masson & Cie Editeurs.
11. Djidjian, R., Huoth, M., Houdant, R., et al.: L'angiographie de la moelle épinière, Paris, 1970, Masson & Cie Editeurs.
12. Earle, K. M.: The tract of Lissauer and its possible relation to pain pathway, J. Comp. Neurol. **96:**93, 1952.
13. Eccles, J. C.: Discussion on systems for control of movements. Tonic and phasic motoneurons and gamma loop. 1 er Congrès International des Sciences Neurologigues, Bruselles, 1957, pp. 81-87.
14. Eccles, J. C.: The physiology of nerve cells, Baltimore, 1957, The Johns Hopkins University Press.
15. Eccles, J. C.: Functional organization of the spinal cord, Anesthesiology **28:**31, 1961.
16. Erlanger, J., and Gasser, H. S.: Electrical signals of the nervous system, Philadelphia, 1937, University of Pennsylvania Press.
17. Fazio, C.: L'angioarchitettonica del midollo spinale umano e i sui rapporti con la cito-mielo-architettonica, Ric. Pat. Nerv. Ment. **52:**252, 1938.
18. Foerster, O.: Symptomatologie der Erkran Kungen des Rückenmarks und seiner Wurzeln. In Bunke, O., and Foerster, O., editors: Handbuck der Neurologie, vol. 5, Berlin, 1936, Springer Verlag, pp. 1-403.
19. Fulton, J. F.: Physiology of the nervous system, London, 1949, Oxford University Press.
20. Gillilan, L. A.: The arterial and nervous supply blood supply of the human spinal cord, Anat. Rec. **127:**466, 1957.
21. Gillilan, L. A.: The arterial blood supply of the human spinal cord, J. Comp. Neurol. **110:**75, 1958.
22. Granit, R., Holgren, B., and Menton, P. A.: The two routes for excitation of muscle and their subservience in the cerebellum, J. Physiol. **130:**213, 1955.
23. Grunner, J.: Les bases anatomiques des phénomenès douloureux. In Alajouanine, T., editor: La douleur et les douleurs, Paris, 1957, Masson & Cie Editeurs.
24. Gutman, L.: Spinal cord injury, Oxford, England, 1973, Blackwell Scientific Publications.
25. Guyton, A. C.: Structure and function of the nervous system, Philadelphia, 1974, W. B. Saunders Co.
26. Heydin, H., editor: The neuron, Amsterdam, 1967, Elsevier Publishing Co.
27. Hoff, E. C., and Hoff, H. E.: Spinal terminations of projection fibers from the motor cortex in primates, Brain **57:**454-474, 1934.
28. Hubbard, J. I., and Oscarsson, O.: Localization of the cell bodies of the ventral spinocerebellar tract in lumbar segments in the cat, J. Comp. Neurol. **118:**199, 1962.

29. Kadyi, H.: Über die Blutgefässe des menschliechen Rückenmarkes, Lemberg, U.S.S.R., 1889, Fubrynowics and Schmidt.

30. Kjellgenn, H.: Studie über der Entwicklung der Neuronen, Arch. F. Psych. Neurol., 1946, suppl. 29.

31. Lassek, A. M.: The pyramidal tract, Springfield, Ill., 1954, Charles C Thomas, Publisher.

32. Lassek, A. M., and Rasmussen, G. L.: The human pyramidal tract. A fiber numerical analysis, Arch. Neurol. Psych. 42:872, 1939.

33. Lazorthes, G.: Le système neurovasculaire, Paris, 1949, Masson & Cie Editeurs.

34. Lazorthes, G., Gouaze, A., Bastide, G., et al.: La vascularization artérielle de la moelle cervicale, Rev. Neurol. (Paris) 115:1055, 1966.

35. Lazorthes, G., Gouaze, A., Bastide, G., et al.: La vascularization artérielle du renflement lombaire, Rev. Neurol. (Paris) 144:109-122, 1966.

36. Lazorthes, G., Poulhes, J., Bastide, G., et al.: La vascularization artérielle de la moelle épinière, Neurochirurgie 4:3, 1958.

37. Lazorthes, G., Poulhes, J., Bastide, G., et al.: La vascularization de la moelle épinière (étude anatomique et physiologique), Rev. Neurol. (Paris) 106:535, 1962.

38. Liu, C. N., and Chambers, W. W.: An experimental study of corticospinal system in monkeys (Macaca mulatta), J. Comp. Neurol. 123:257, 1964.

39. Lloyd, D. P. C.: The spinal mechanisms of pyramidal system in cats, J. Neurophysiol. 4:525, 1941.

40. Magoun, H. W., and Phines, R.: An inhibitory mechanism in the bulbar reticular formation, J. Neurophysiol. 9:165, 1946.

41. Magoun, H. W., and Rhines, R.: Spasticity: the stretch reflex and extrapyramidal systems, Springfield, Ill., 1947, Charles C Thomas, Publisher.

42. Melzack, R., and Wall, P. D.: Pain mechanism: a new theory, Science 150:971, 1965.

43. Morin, G.: La moelle épinière. In Physiologie du système nerveux central, Paris, 1955, Masson & Cie Editeurs.

44. Mountcastle, V. B., editor: Medical physiology, ed 14, Saint Louis, 1974, The C.V. Mosby Co., vol. 1, part 5.

45. Nyberg-Hansen, R.: Origin and termination of fibers from the vestibular nuclei descending in the medial longitudinal fasciculus, J. Comp. Neurol. 122:355, 1964.

46. Nyberg-Hansen, R.: Site and mode of termination of reticulospinal fibers in cat, J. Comp. Neurol. 124:71-99, 1965.

47. Nyberg-Hansen, R., and Brodal, A.: Sites and mode of termination of rubrospinal fibers in the cat, J. Anat. 98:235, 1964.

48. Olsczewski, J., and Baxter, D.: Cytoarchiteatomy of human brain stem, Philadelphia, 1954, J. B. Lippincott Co.

49. Patton, H. D., and Amassion, V. E.: The pyramidal tract. In Field, J., Magoun, H. W., and Hall, V. E., editors: Handbook of physiology, vol. 2. Section 1: neurophysiology, Washington, D.C., 1960, American Physiology Society.

50. Pearson, A.A.: Role of gelatinous substance of spinal cord in conduction of pain, Arch. Neurol. Psych. 68:515, 1952.

51. Quarti, C., and Renaud, J.: Neurophysiologie de la douleur, Paris, 1972, Hermann.

52. Ramon y Cajal, S.: Histologie du système nerveux de l'homme et des vertebres, Paris, 1952, Librairie Maloine.

53. Ranson, S. W.: The structure of the spinal cord ganglia and the spinal nerves, J. Comp. Neurol. 22:159, 1912.

54. Rexed, B.: The cytoarchitectonic areas of the spinal cord of the cat, J. Comp. Neurol. 100:297, 1954.

55. Rexed, B.: Some aspects of cytoarchitectonics and synaptology of the spinal cord, In Eccles, J. C., and Shade, P., editors: Progress in brain research. Vol. 2. Organization of the spinal cord, Amsterdam, 1964, Elsevier Publisher Co., pp. 58-92.

56. Rhines, R., and Magoun, H. W.: Brain stem facilitation of cortical motor response, J. Neurophysiol. 9:219, 1946.

57. Rossi, G. F., and Zanchetti, A.: The brain stem reticular formation. Anatomy and physiology, Arch. ital. de Biologie 75:199, 1957.

58. Ruch, C. R., Patton, H. D., Woodbury, J. W., and Arnold, L. T., editors: Neurophysiology. Section 3, Philadelphia, 1965, W. B. Saunders Co.

59. Russell, J. R., and De Myer, W.: The quantitative cortical origin of pyramidal axons of Maccaca rhesus, Neurology (Minneap.) 11:96, 1961.

60. Sherrington, C. S.: The integrative action of the nervous system, ed. 2, New York, 1947, Cambridge University Press.

61. Szentagothai, J., and Albert, A.: The synaptology of Clarke's column, Acta Morphol. Acad. Sci. Hung. 5:43-51, 1955.

62. Szentagothai, J.: Neuronal and synaptic arrangement in the substantia gelatinosa Rolandi, J. Comp. Neurol. 122:219-239, 1964.

63. Tanon, L.: Les antères de la moelle dorso-lombaire [thesis], Paris, 1908, Vigot Fréres Editeurs.

64. Testut, L., and Latarjet, A.: Traitré d' anatomie humaine, vol. 2, Paris, 1948, G. Doin et Cie.

65. Truek, R. C., and Taylor, M.: Gray matter lamination of human spinal cord, Anat. Rec. 106:502, 1968.

66. Weil, A., and Lassek, A. M.: A quantitative distribution of the pyramidal tract in man, Arch. Neurol. Psychiat. 22:495, 1929.

67. White, J. C.: Conduction of pain in man: observations on its afferent pathways within the spinal cord and visceral nerves, Arch. Neurol. Psychiat. 71:1, 1954.

68. Williams, P. L., and Warurick, R.: Functional neuroanatomy of man. In Gray's anatomy, ed. 35 (Br.), Philadelphia, 1975, W. B. Saunders Co.

CHAPTER 2

Normal radiologic anatomy of the spine

MICHAEL A. MIKHAEL, M.D.

DEVELOPMENT OF THE SPINE

The vertebral elements evolve around the notochord, a medially situated rod representing the earliest evidence of the axial skeleton. The notochord itself arises from the primitive node (ectodermal) at about the twenty-third day after fertilization (gestational age) (Fig. 2-1).[3,74] Lying ventral to the neural tube, the notochord extends from the extremity of the tail to the cranial end of the midbrain. Its cephalic end passes through the basisphenoid bone into the retropharyngeal space to reenter the sphenoid bone again and terminates at the dorsum sellae (Fig. 2-2). The para-axial bar, the mesodermal column on either side of the notochord, becomes segmented into symmetrically disposed triangular primitive segments called the *somites*. Each somite is differentiated into three groups of cells: a lateral superficial group, the dermatome or the cutis plate, a middle portion, the myotome or the muscle plate, and a medial or deeper group, the sclerotome (Fig. 2-3).[3,74] Cells of the sclerotome rapidly proliferate and surround both the notochord and the neural tube with a mesodermal sheath called the membranous vertebral column. Each of these original mesoderm segments is differentiated into a cranial segment of loosely arranged cells and a caudal segment of more condensed cells. The cells from the latter group go into intervals between the myotomes to form the costal elements. Between the two portions, the caudal and the cranial, the intervertebral disc is laid down. Thus the vertebral bodies are formed of the caudal part of a segment join-

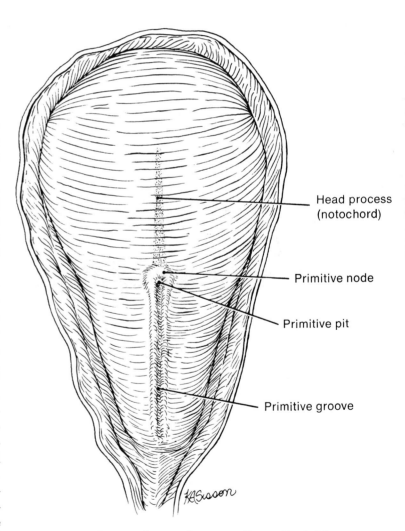

Head process (notochord)

Primitive node

Primitive pit

Primitive groove

Fig. 2-1. Embryonic disc, surface view. Stage of primitive groove and notochord.

23

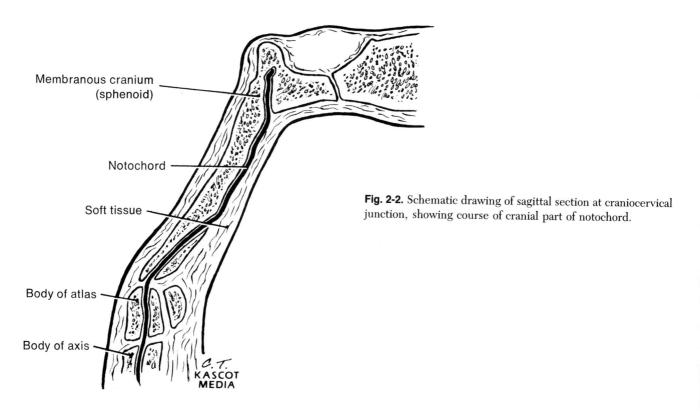

Membranous cranium
(sphenoid)

Notochord

Soft tissue

Body of atlas

Body of axis

Fig. 2-2. Schematic drawing of sagittal section at craniocervical junction, showing course of cranial part of notochord.

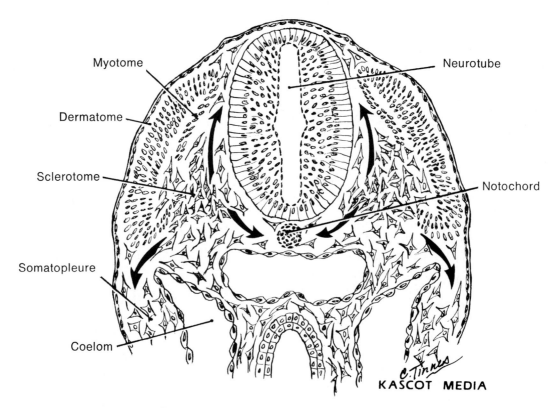

Myotome

Dermatome

Sclerotome

Somatopleure

Coelom

Neurotube

Notochord

Fig. 2-3. Separation and migration of three parts of human somite, shown in transverse section. Arrows indicate separate sclerotomic masses and direction of their spread.

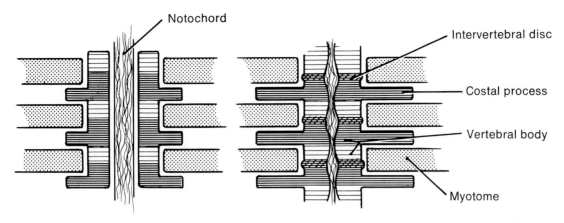

Fig. 2-4. Schematic drawing showing manner in which each vertebral centrum is developed from two adjacent segments.

ing the cranial part of the succeeding segment (Fig. 2-4). Each vertebral body is therefore a composite of two halves of two successive segments.[3,71]

This stage of growth is followed by the cartilaginous vertebral column starting in the fourth week with the appearance of two cartilaginous centers for each vertebral body, one on each side of the notochord. The early failure of some chondrification centers may be partly responsible for the development of hemivertebrae, cleft vertebrae, and certain other anomalies. A second dorsal pair of chondrification centers appears and grows to form the cartilaginous vertebral arch. The spinous process is developed from the junction of the two halves of the vertebral arch. A third pair of centers appears one for each costal process. The transverse process grows out from the vertebral arch dorsal to the costal process.[3,74]

In the cervical region a band of mesenchyme, the hypochordal bar, crosses ventral to the vertebrae at the intervertebral discs. All except the first pair disappear by fusing with the discs. In the case of the atlas it persists and develops into the ventral arch. The cartilage representing the body of the atlas fuses with the body of the axis to form the odontoid process (the dens).[27,72,74]

The notochord, the early central axis, will ultimately disappear where surrounded by the bodies of the vertebrae. However, those portions that lie in the centers of the intervertebral discs persist throughout life as part of the nucleus pulposus. The apical ligament of the dens is another remnant of the notochord. Chordomas may develop from notochordal rests that occasionally persist in the base of the skull, the sacrum, and less commonly elsewhere in the vertebral column.

At about the seventh or eighth week of fetal life, cen-ters of ossification start to appear in the vertebral arches, first in the upper cervical region and gradually extending caudally. Ossification of the bodies begins about the same time, but this occurs in the lower thoracic region and extends both caudally and cranially. At birth each vertebra consists of three main elements: the body and the two halves of the neural arch, fused with cartilaginous partitions. These bony segments will grow and fuse before puberty. At about 16 years of age, five secondary centers of ossification appear for each vertebra for the different processes and for both surfaces of the bodies. They fuse with the rest of the bone at about 25 years of age. Exceptions to this general mode of ossification occur in the first, second, and seventh cervical vertebrae, together with the lumbar region.[27,72,74]

RADIOLOGIC EXAMINATION OF THE SPINE
General anatomy

The vertebral column or back bone (columna vertebralis, spinal column) is composed of 32 to 34 segments called *vertebrae* (Fig. 2-5).[23,81,86] These segments are grouped as 7 cervical, 12 dorsal, and 5 lumbar vertebrae, as well as the sacrum and the coccyx. The vertebrae in the three cranial regions (cervical, dorsal, and lumbar) remain distinct and are known as the true, or movable, vertebrae. The sacrum consists of five fused segments and the coccyx of three to five fused segments. These segments are termed false, or fixed, vertebrae because they are united with each other in adult life to form the sacrum and the coccyx. A typical vertebra consists of two essential parts: a ventral segment (the body) and a dorsal segment (the vertebral or neural arch). The two parts together define the bony vertebral canal. The canal encases the spinal cord.

A lateral view of the vertebral column shows four

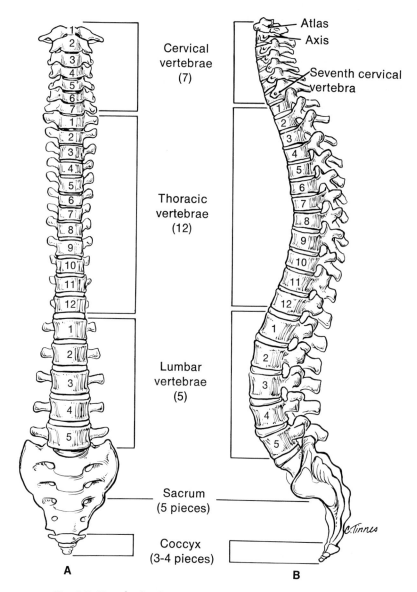

Fig. 2-5. Vertebral column. **A,** Frontal view. **B,** Lateral view.

curves: two, the cervical and the lumbar, are convex ventrally, and two, the dorsal and the sacrococcygeal (the pelvic), are concave ventrally (Fig. 2-5). The thoracic and pelvic are termed primary curves because they are present alone during fetal life. The cervical and lumbar are compensatory or secondary curves and are developed after birth. The former appears when the child is able to hold up the head (about 3 or 4 months) and to sit upright (about 9 months); the latter appears at 18 months, when the child begins to walk. The cervical curve starts from the apex of the dens to the middle of the second thoracic vertebra, where the thoracic curve begins, and ends at the middle of the twelfth thoracic vertebra. The most prominent point of the tho-

racic curve dorsally corresponds to the spinous process of the seventh thoracic vertebra. The lumbar curve, which is more marked in women than in men, begins at the middle of the twelfth thoracic vertebra and ends at the lumbosacral angle. The pelvic curve begins at the lumbosacral articulation and ends at the tip of the coccyx.

A frontal view of the vertebral column usually shows a slight lateral curvature with the convexity directed to the right side in right-handed persons and to the left in left-handed persons.

General characteristics of a vertebra. Except for the first and second cervical vertebrae the true, or movable, vertebrae have certain anatomic characteristics

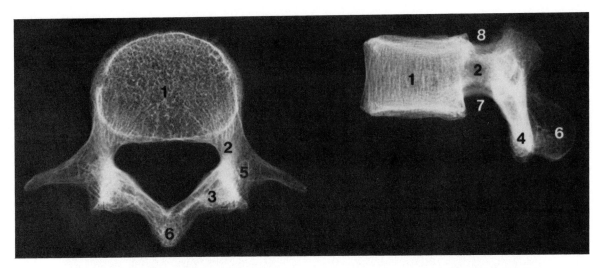

Fig. 2-6. Third lumbar vertebra. *1*, Body; *2*, pedicle; *3*, lamina; *4*, inferior articular process; *5*, transverse process; *6*, spinous process; *7*, inferior articular notch; *8*, superior articular notch.

(Fig. 2-6).[23,81,86] The body of the vertebra is the largest part and is more or less cylindric in shape with roughened cranial and caudal surfaces for the intervertebral discs. The vertebral arch consists of a pair of pedicles and a pair of laminae, which together support seven processes, that is, four articular, two transverse, and one spinous. The pedicles are two short thick processes that project dorsally—one on each side of the cranial part of the body. They connect the transverse process to the body. They are constricted in the middle to form the superior and inferior vertebral notches. The superior vertebral notch together with the inferior vertebral notch of the vertebra above forms the intervertebral foramen. The laminae are two broad plates directed dorsally and medially from the pedicles. They fuse posteriorly in the midline at the base of the spinous process to complete the neural arch.

The sacrum. The sacrum is a large triangular bone situated at the dorsal part of the pelvis. In the adult it consists of five united sacral vertebrae. The sacral canal is the continuation of the lumbar spinal canal and is incomplete distally because of the nondevelopment of the laminae and the spinous processes of the last one or two segments. Its distal end is called the *sacral hiatus*.

The coccyx. The coccyx is formed of three to five united incomplete rudimentary vertebrae fused to form the triangular bone.

Cervical spine

The cervical spine is a true movable segment of the vertebral column and contains seven vertebrae. It has the general anatomic characteristics of the other movable levels discussed before with the following exceptions: (1) C1 is a ring with no body, only an anterior and a posterior arch. Its body is attached to the body of C2 to form the odontoid process (Fig. 2-7). (2) The inferior articular surface of C1 and the superior articular facets of C2 are basically oriented in a transverse plane and are best seen in open-mouth view (Fig. 2-8). (3) The C1 transverse processes extend significantly laterally to the other cervical transverse processes. (4) The cervical transverse processes are formed of two main elements; the posterior part is the transverse element and the anterolateral part is the costal element of the embryonic vertebra. In the cervical region they join to form the foramen transversarium, or the costal transverse foramen (Fig. 2-7).

Radiologic examination of the cervical spine varies according to the information desired.[33,56,69] In spinal cord injured patients, clinical judgment should be exercised in the selection of various projections required to answer a specific question. However, a complete radiologic examination should include the open-mouth view, the anteroposterior view, the lateral view, and two oblique views together with a swimmer's view that includes the C7-T1 region. Extra views, such as the two anteroposterior pillar views of Weir and the lateral view in flexion and extension, are occasionally needed to answer a specific question.

Tomography and laminography examinations are sometimes needed for visualization of the craniocervical and the atlantoaxial articulations together with the cervicothoracic junction.

Open-mouth view. The open-mouth view is obtained with the patient's mouth slightly opened and the patient phonating (Fig. 2-8). The neck must not be hyper-

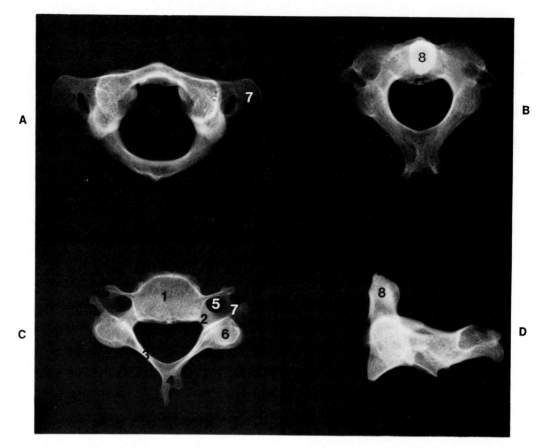

Fig. 2-7. A, Atlas. **B,** and **D,** Axis. **C,** Fourth cervical vertebra. *1,* Body; *2,* pedicle; *3,* lamina; *4,* spinous process; *5,* foramen transversarium; *6,* articular process; *7,* transverse process; *8,* odontoid process.

extended in this view or the inferior margins of the occipital bone will be superimposed over the pertinent structures. Better visualization of the atlas and axis can be obtained by keeping the mandible in motion during the roentgenographic exposure because the continued motion will eliminate the shadow of the mandible. This view is useful to study the atlanto-occipital joint, the atlantoaxial joint, the midline position of the odontoid process with equal distance to the medial margins of the atlas articular masses, the normal cortical structures and the trabecular pattern around and within the base of the odontoid, the alignment of the lateral edges of the atlas articular masses with the edges of the C2 superior articular facets, and the intact cortical margins of the transverse processes of C1.

The midline position of the odontoid and alignments of the C1-2 articulations are only reliable on straight anteroposterior films. This can be confirmed by the midline position of the C2 spinous process. Two artifacts are common in this position and may be easily misinterpreted as abnormalities. The first is caused by the vertical cleft between the two front upper incisors,

which when superimposed over the odontoid process may be misinterpreted as either a congenital persistent vertical cleft or a vertical fracture. The second artifact is the Mach effect adjacent to the inferior surface of the posterior arch of C1, which may be superimposed over the base of the odontoid. This may be misinterpreted as a fracture of the base of the odontoid. The articular surfaces of C1 and C2 are in correct anatomic position when they are parallel to each other.

Anteroposterior view. The anteroposterior view is obtained with the patient's head slightly extended, superimposing the inferior margin of the occipital bone on the mandible and leaving the cervical spine below C2 free of superimposed bony structures (Fig. 2-9). The anteroposterior projection best demonstrates and should be used to study the correct vertical alignment of the spinous processes, the smooth symmetric alignment of the lateral margins of the articular masses, the uncovertebral joints, and the bony structure of the vertebral bodies. The lamina and the articular facet joints in the cervical region are essentially en face and are poorly visualized on this projection. Likewise, the cer-

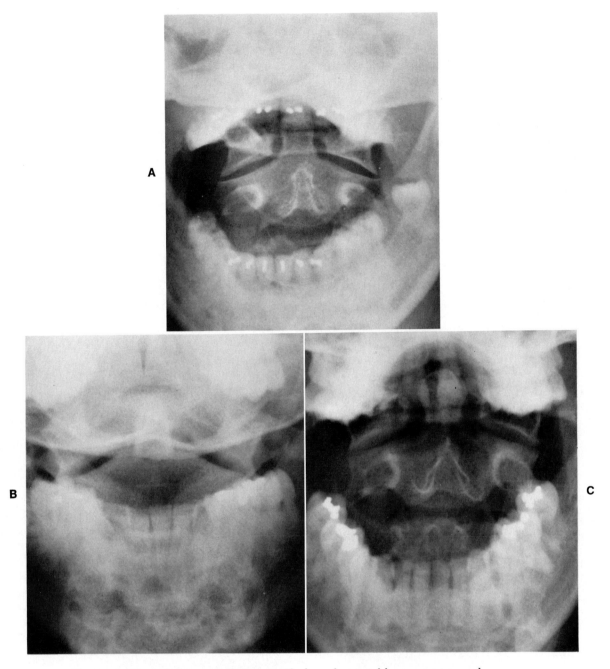

Fig. 2-8. A, Normal open-mouth view. **B,** Shadow of occipital bone superimposed over pertinent structures. **C,** Upper incisors superimposed over odontoid process.

vical pedicles are directed posterolaterally and are also poorly seen. The pedicles of the lower cervical vertebrae are directed less laterally and may be seen slightly better.

Straight lateral view. Because the film cassette is usually not close to the cervical spine but rather at the level of the shoulder region, the straight lateral view is usually taken at a 183 cm (72 in) distance to diminish as much as possible the factor of magnification. In the pa-

tient without trauma, taking this view while the patient is upright allows the patient's shoulder to drop the maximal distance from the cervical region. This view (Fig. 2-10) best demonstrates the alignment of the upper portion of the cervical spine with the foramen magnum, normal joint space between the odontoid process and the posterior surface of the anterior arch of the atlas, normal alignment of the anterior and posterior borders of the vertebral bodies, alignment of the posterior margins of the articular processes, articular facet joints, alignment of the spinal laminar lines that form the anterior margins of the spinous processes and define the posterior margin of the bony spinal canal, anteroposterior diameter of the cervical bony canal, intervertebral disc spaces, and the prevertebral soft tissues.

Correct alignment of the craniocervical junction can be studied using Chamberlain's line, McGregor's line, the bimastoid and digastric lines, McRae's line, Bull's angle, the height index, the atlanto-occipital joint angle, and the basal angle (Fig. 2-11).[11,12,64,66,68] In a straight lateral film the anterior and posterior margins of the vertebral bodies and the anterior surface of the

spinous processes should form smooth, gentle lordotic curves. The posterior margins of the articular masses should be anterior to the spinal laminar lines; if these margins are not anterior, the spinal canal may be abnormally narrowed in its anteroposterior diameter. From C3 to C7, 12 mm is the lower limit of the normal range for the anteroposterior diameter measured from the posterior border of the body to the corresponding spinal laminar line (Fig. 2-12). At C1 it is measured from the back of the odontoid process to the anterior surface of the posterior arch of the atlas, and the lower limit of the normal range is 16 mm. At the C2 level it is 14 mm (Fig. 2-13).[88] These measurements are uncor-

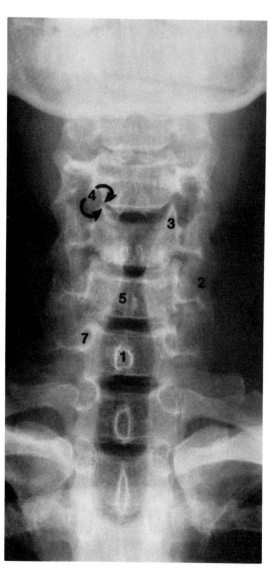

Fig. 2-9. Anteroposterior view of cervical spine. *1,* Spinous process; *2,* lateral margin of articular masses; *3,* uncinate process; *4,* uncovertebral joint; *5,* vertebral body; *6,* transverse process; *7,* pedicle.

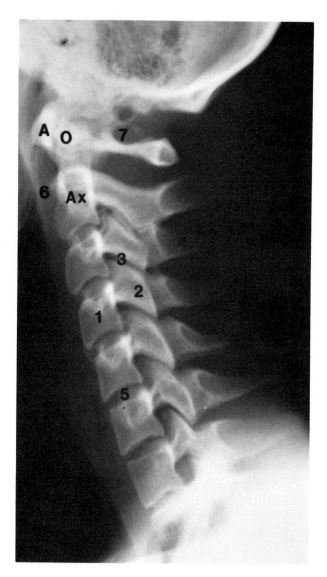

Fig. 2-10. Lateral view of cervical spine. *A,* Anterior arch of atlas; *Ax,* axis; *O,* odontoid process. *1,* Vertebral body; *2,* articular process; *3,* articular facet joints; *4,* spinal laminar line; *5,* intervertebral disc space; *6,* prevertebral soft tissue; *7,* ponticulus posticus.

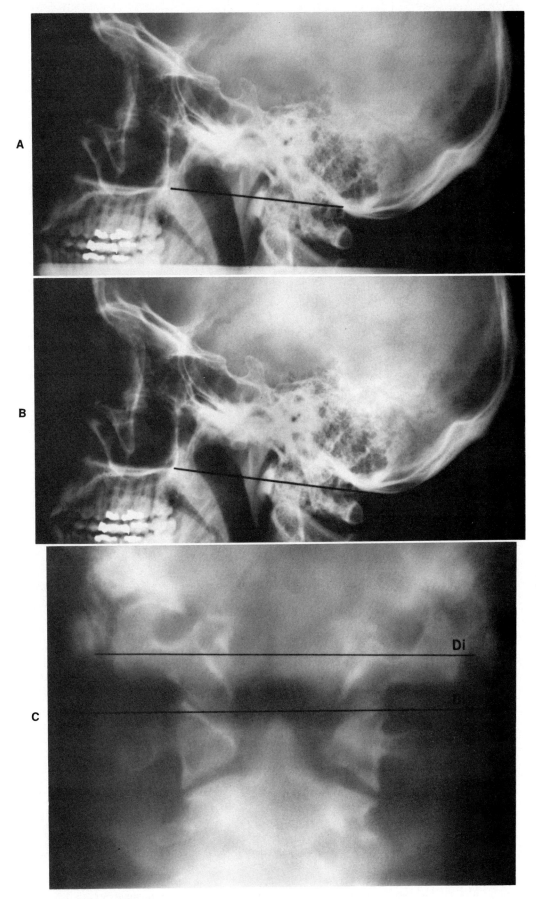

Fig. 2-11. Lines to study craniocervical junctions. **A,** Chamberlain's line: normally odontoid tip is not more than 4 to 5 mm above line. **B,** McGregor's line: normally odontoid tip is not more than 5 mm above line. **C,** Bimastoid, *Bi,* and digastric, *Di,* lines: bimastoid normally passes through atlanto-occipital joints, and digastric is normally 11 mm ± 4 mm above middle of atlanto-occipital joints.

Continued.

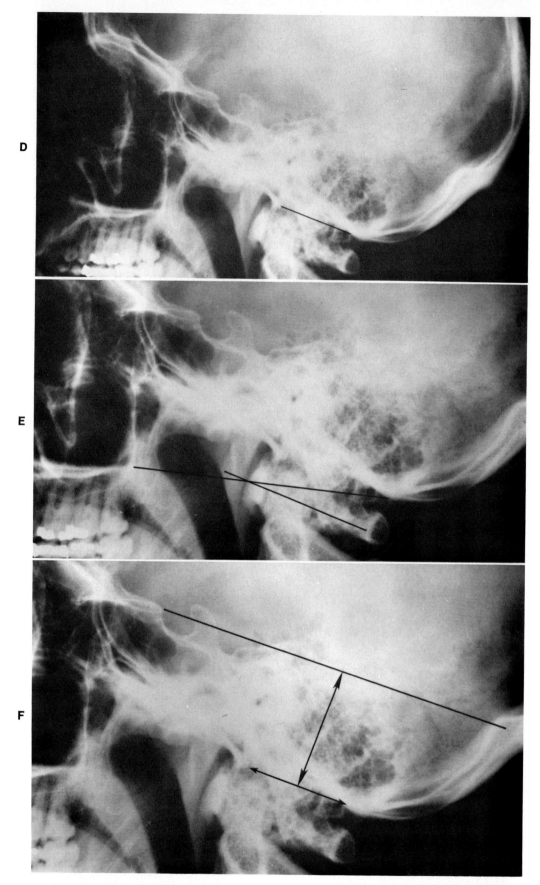

Fig. 2-11, cont'd. D, McRae's line: if line of occipital squama is convex upward or if it lies above McRae's line, basilar impression is present. **E,** Bull's angle: normal upper limit is 13°. **F,** Height index: normally not less than 30 mm.

rected for magnification. True (absolute) measurements are calculated by dividing the above-mentioned values by a factor of magnification ranging from 1.12 to 1.15.

The joint space between the anterior surface of the dens and the posterior surface of the anterior arch of the atlas should not exceed 3 mm in the adult but may normally go up to 5 mm in a young child.

In children, lateral projection films made in extension sometimes show an apparent overriding of the anterior arch of the atlas on the dens, probably because of a lack of calcification of the distal tip of the dens, rendering this structure invisible. The relationship between the tip of the odontoid process and the base of the skull is useful in the diagnosis of basilar invagination (Fig. 2-11).

In lateral views, taken with the neck flexed, the body of each vertebra is displaced slightly anteriorly with respect to the subjacent vertebra, particularly at the level of C2-3. This "step off," up to 2 or 3 mm at this interspace, should not be mistaken for a dislocation.

If the lateral projection does not include the region of the C7-T1 intervertebral space, the evaluation of the

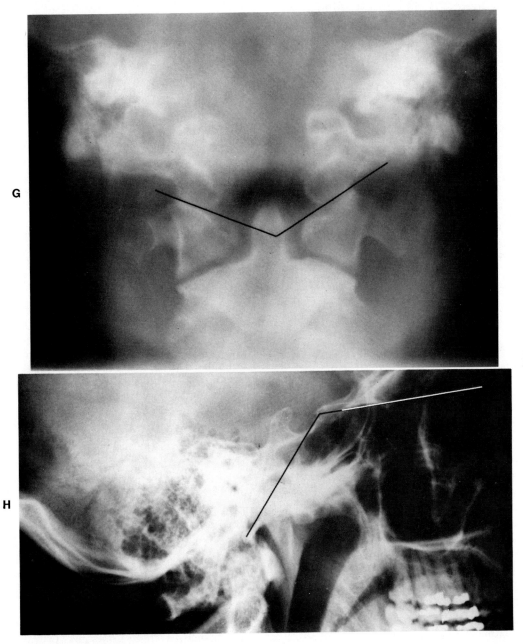

Fig. 2-11, cont'd. G, Atlanto-occipital joint angle: normally not greater than 150°. **H,** Basal angle: normal range between 122° and 143°.

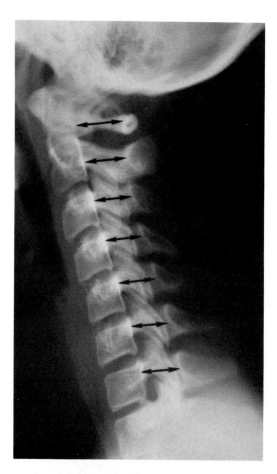

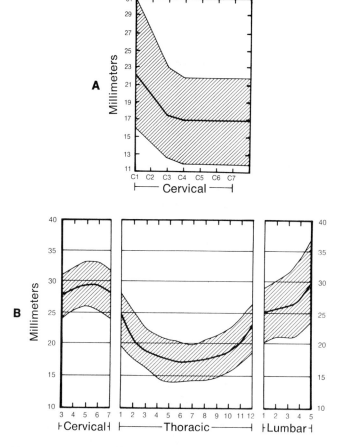

Fig. 2-12. Sagittal diameters of cervical spinal canal (*arrows*) are measured from middle of posterior surface of vertebral body to nearest point on spinal laminar line.

Fig. 2-13. A, Curves for average, maximal, and minimal measurements of normal sagittal diameters of cervical spinal canal in adults. True corrected values are about 1.5 mm less than shown above. **B,** Curves for average, maximal, and minimal measurements of normal interpedicular distances in adults. (**A** from Wolf, B. S., et al.: Mt. Sinai J. Med. (N.Y.) **23**:283, 1956. **B** from Hinck, V. C., et al.: Am. J. Roentgenol. **97**:141, 1966; © 1966, Am. Roentgen Ray Soc.)

cervical spine would be incomplete without obtaining a swimmer's view.

Oblique views. The right posterior oblique view is made in the anteroposterior direction with the film posterior to the neck and the patient's entire body turned 45° toward the right side. The left posterior oblique view is obtained by rotating the entire body 45° to the left. Some authors recommend turning the head from 15° to 45° further laterally to better show the upper cervical-intervertebral foramina. The oblique views are utilized primarily to study the intervertebral foramina and surrounding structures (Fig. 2-14). Because the axis of these foramina is directed anterolaterally, in the right posterior oblique position the left intervertebral foramina are seen and vice versa. The anteromedial margin of each foramen is formed by the uncinate process and uncovertebral joint, the superior and inferior margins are the pedicles of the two joining vertebrae, and the posterolateral margin is formed by the anteromedial surfaces of the articular facet joints and articular masses. In the right posterior oblique position the left

pedicles are parallel with the film and can be studied in their full length, while the left laminae and right pedicles are seen on end. The oblique views can also be useful to study the various portions of C1 and C2, as well as the space between the occiput and C1 where no intervertebral foramina are present.

Anteroposterior pillar (Weirs' view). Two projections are made in the anteroposterior direction with the head extended and rotated 50° to 70°: the first projection is made with the head rotated to the right and the second with the head rotated to the left.[69] The central beam is angulated 35° to 40° caudad. Because the beam is parallel to the plane of the articular facet joints and the articular masses, these projections provide an excellent view of these joints, as well as the ventral and dorsal surfaces of the laminae. The pillar views offer an addi-

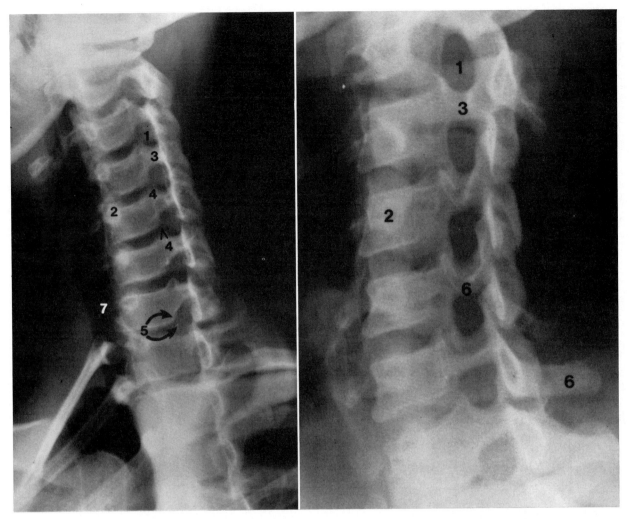

Fig. 2-14. Right posterior oblique views of cervical spine. *1,* Left intervertebral foramen; *2,* right pedicle; *3,* left pedicle; *4,* uncinate process; *5,* uncovertebral joint; *6,* left transverse process; *7,* right transverse process.

tional look to the articular masses and the alignment of their lateral margins, the articular facet joints, the laminae, and the spinous processes.

Swimmer's view. As mentioned before, if the C7-T1 intervertebral space and vertebral bodies are not demonstrated on the lateral view, a swimmer's view is a necessity to complete the study of the cervical spine (Fig. 2-15). This view can be taken by depressing the tube-side shoulder and elevating the film-side arm, that is, putting the patient in a swimming position. The film cassette is placed in the axillary region of the raised arm, and the tube is angulated 15° to 20° caudad. Through patient cooperation, minimal tube angulation can be achieved, which offers the least distortion of the cervicothoracic vertebral junction. This special view is important to study the space, and the height and configuration of the vertebral bodies at the C7-T1 level.

Flexion and extension lateral views. Flexion and extension lateral views are necessary to study the mobility of the cervical spine as a whole and the mobility of each vertebra in relation to the neighboring vertebrae. Study of mobility is important following surgical stabilization of the spine and prior to rehabilitation. The views are done with the neck in as much flexion as the patient can achieve and then in extension, in the same way the straight lateral view is obtained. To measure the angle of mobility of each vertebra a diagram of the extension view is obtained. Then by superimposing one vertebra in this diagram on the corresponding vertebra on the lateral flexion view and drawing the vertebra above, the angle of mobility of the latter vertebra can be measured (Fig. 2-16). The importance of these two views is obvious in preoperative and postoperative studies and in patients, both with trauma and without trauma, sus-

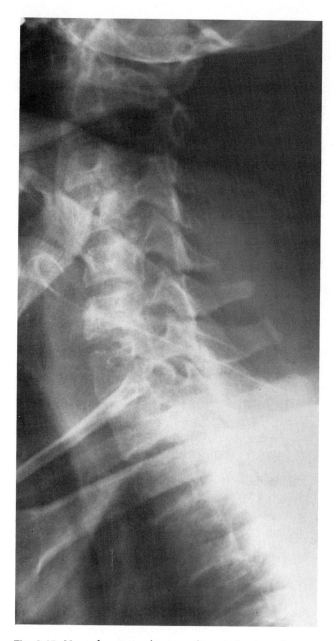

Fig. 2-15. Normal swimmer's view of cervical spine, showing lower cervical and upper dorsal levels.

pected of having subluxations of the various vertebrae.

Pediatric age group. In infants the cervical spine is examined by means of recumbent anteroposterior and lateral views. In the lateral projection it is helpful to extend the child's neck manually and to bring the arms as far dorsally as possible with the shoulders drawn down. Oblique, flexion, and extension views are not usually required.

In the newborn infant the cartilaginous odontoid process often is not visible. In later infancy and early childhood as the dens calcifies, its structures become mani-

fest as a vertically split bar at 2 to 3 years of age, sometimes demarcated from the anterosuperior aspect of the body of C2 by a thin basal line of cartilage. The tip of the dens has a small V-shaped cleft, later filled by a calcified epiphysis that fuses with the rest of the body. The vertical cleft between the two lateral masses occasionally persists into adolescence. The cartilage between the base of the dens and the subjacent body of C2 may be visible up to the age of 10 years and sometimes is mistaken for a fracture.

Thoracic spine

Twelve vertebrae are included in the thoracic spine and progressively increase in size caudally (Fig. 2-17). Other than in size they are all similar from T1 to T12. The pedicles of the thoracic vertebrae are oriented almost straight anteroposteriorly and are angled only 10° to 15° posterolaterally away from the sagittal plane with the exception of T1 and T2. The pedicles of T1 and T2 have a greater posterolateral angulation similar to that of the cervical vertebrae. Like the vertebral bodies, the pedicles also become progressively larger caudally. The thoracic transverse processes are directed posterolaterally, are posterior to the plane of both the articular facets and the spinal neural arch, and diminish in length caudally. The intervertebral foramina are directed straight laterally. With the exception of T12 all the inferior articular facets of the thoracic vertebrae face slightly anteromedially. T12 articular facets face anterolaterally to articulate with the superior facets of L1 that are oriented close to the anteroposterior plane. The thoracic transverse processes, unlike the cervical and lumbar transverse processes, are not complex because the embryonic costal element has separated from the transverse element and has formed the medial end of the corresponding rib. This is why in the thoracic region there are no transverse foramina. Each thoracic vertebral complex has eight diarthrodial joints, two superior facets, two inferior facets, and two costotransverse and two costovertebral joints.

The radiologic study of the thoracic spine should include an anteroposterior view, a lateral view, and a swimmer's view of the cervicodorsal junction (Figs. 2-15, 2-17, and 2-18).[23,69] Although oblique views have been used to study the posterior elements by rotating the patient forward and backward 15° to 20° from the lateral projection, tomography is far superior.

Anteroposterior view. The anteroposterior view (Fig. 2-17) should be taken in the anteroposterior direction; the area of the spine to be studied is close to the film, the concavity of the normal thoracic kyphosis faces the x-ray tube, and therefore the divergent rays remain slightly more perpendicular to the upper and lower thoracic vertebral bodies. Because of the increased

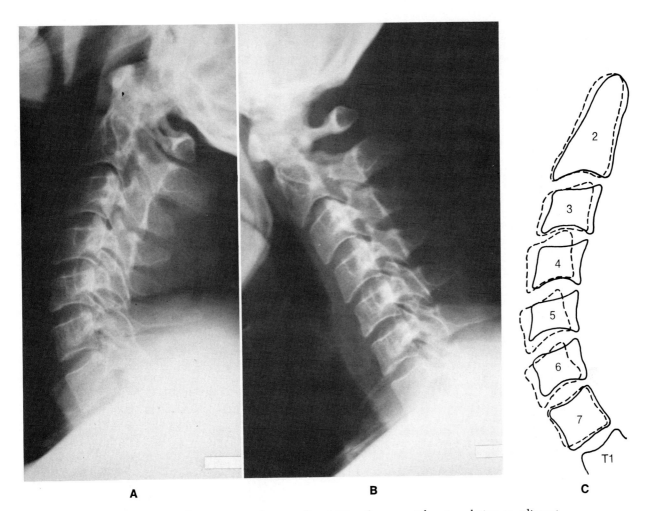

A   B   C

Fig. 2-16. Method to measure degree of mobility of any vertebra in relation to adjacent vertebrae. **A,** Lateral cervical spine in extension. **B,** Lateral cervical spine in flexion. **C,** Diagram showing degree of mobility. To make this diagram follow these steps: (1) Apply a transparent sheet on film A and draw margins of different vertebrae in solid lines. (2) Apply same sheet, with cervical spine draw in extension, on film B. (3) Superimpose margins of C7 in drawing (solid line) on margins of C7 on film B. (4) Draw margins of C6 as in film B on sheet in interrupted line. (5) Difference between margins of C6 drawn in interrupted line and that which was drawn in solid line represents degree of mobility of C6 on C7 on flexing neck. By repeating the same steps, mobility of vertebrae of interest can be studied.

thickness of the soft tissue in the lower thoracic region, this area is usually underexposed on the radiograph and the superior end of the thoracic column is overexposed. Fuchs[29] utilized the heel effect of the x-ray tube to obtain a more uniform density throughout the entire thoracic vertebral area. He positioned the tube with its long axis parallel to the sagittal plane of the body, with the anode at the upper end. This projects a greater concentration of rays toward the thicker lower thoracic region.

The anteroposterior view of the thoracic spine is used to study the trabecular structure of the vertebral bodies and pedicles, the alignment of the vertebral bodies and the spinous processes, the interpediculate distances, the transverse processes, and the paravertebral soft tissues. The measurement of the interpediculate distances is important in evaluating the transverse diameter of the spinal canal (Figs. 2-13 and 2-19). In this view the laminae are seen and their margins can be studied (Fig. 2-17).

Straight lateral view. The straight lateral view (Fig. 2-18) is made with the patient's arms straight forward and the patient in the straight lateral position. Because the bones and soft tissues of the shoulders overlie the upper two or three thoracic vertebrae, this upper area is studied better with the swimmer's view.

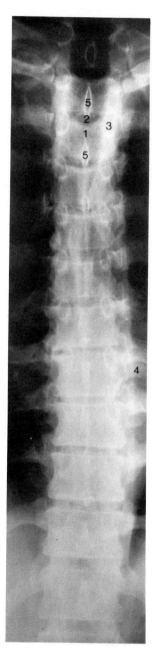

Fig. 2-17. Anteroposterior view of dorsal spine. *1*, Body of vertebra; *2*, intervertebral disc space; *3*, pedicle; *4*, transverse process; *5*, spinous process.

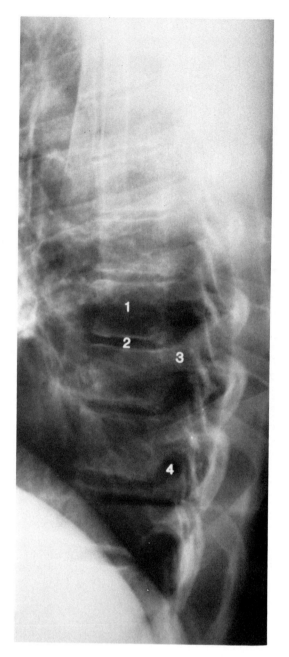

Fig. 2-18. Lateral view of dorsal spine. *1*, Body of vertebra; *2*, intervertebral disc space; *3*, pedicle; *4*, intervertebral foramen.

The lateral view is helpful in studying the alignment of the anterior and posterior margins of the vertebral bodies, the cortical margins and the trabecular structure of the vertebrae, the intervertebral disc spaces, the pedicles, the intervertebral foramina, and the spinous processes. The facet joints may be visible at some levels but they cannot be consistently studied on plain films.

In the lateral view the posterior elements of the thoracic vertebrae and the correspponding ribs are superimposed.

Specific information about the posterior bony elements of the dorsal spine is best evaluated by tomography.

Lumbar spine

The lumbar spine contains five vertebrae (Figs. 2-20 to 2-22). The lumbar vertebrae are the largest of the

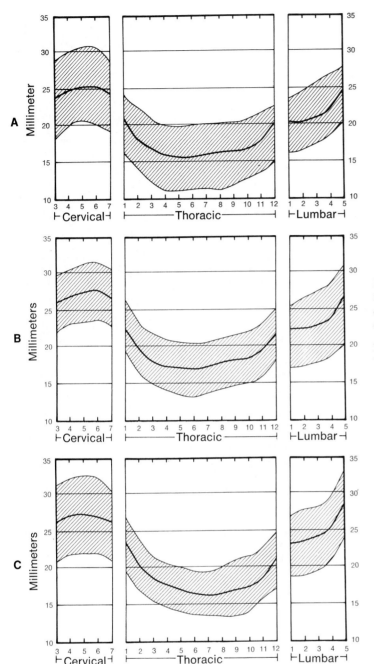

Fig. 2-19. Curves for average, maximal, and minimal measurements of normal interpedicular distances in children. **A,** Ages 3 to 5 years. **B,** Ages 6 to 8 years. **C,** Ages 9 and 10 years. (From Hinck, V. C., et al.: Am. J. Roentgenol. **97:**141, 1966; © 1966, Am. Roentgen Ray Soc.)

vertebral column, increasing slightly in size from L1 to L5. The components of the vertebrae are heavier than in any other spinal area. These features reflect both their increased weight-bearing function and the strong muscles to which they are attached. The lumbar vertebral bodies have a larger transverse than anteroposterior diameter, which in turn is larger than the vertical height. The pedicles are basically oriented in an anteroposterior plane except for L5, whose pedicles are di-

rected posterolaterally. The upper lumbar transverse processes are slightly behind the posterior plane of the spinal canal, whereas the lower lumbar transverse processes are directly lateral to the canal. The articular facet joints are basically oriented 45° posterolaterally away from the midline plane. The spinal canal is triangular with the base of the triangle formed by the posterior surface of the vertebral body and the lateral sides by the regions of the articular facet joints and the lam-

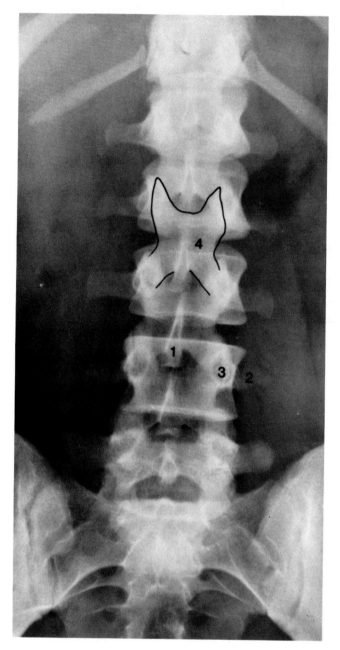

Fig. 2-20. Anteroposterior view of lumbar spine. *1,* Spinous process; *2,* transverse process; *3,* pedicle; *4,* lamina.

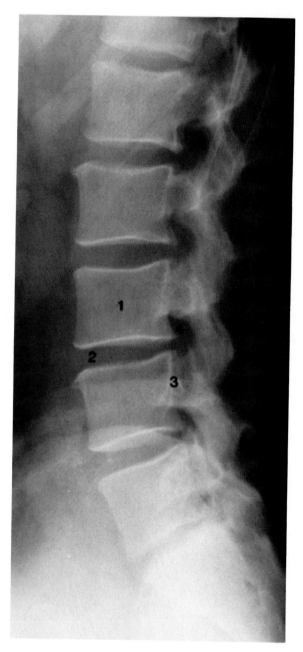

Fig. 2-21. Lateral view of lumbar spine. *1,* Vertebral body; *2,* intervertebral disc space; *3,* pedicle; *4,* intervertebral foramen.

inae. The laminae are very short and are attached to relatively broad, thick spinous processes. In the lumbar area the embryonic costal and transverse elements of the transverse process are totally fused. The costal element forms the anterior portion of the transverse process. A complete radiologic examination of the lumbar spine should include an anteroposterior view, a lateral view, two oblique views, and a cone-down lateral view for the lumbosacral junction.[23,69]

Anteroposterior view. If the anteroposterior view (Fig. 2-20) is taken with the patient supine and the legs extended, the lumbar lordosis is accentuated, and the angle between the plane of the upper and lower lumbar vertebral bodies and the divergent rays is increased. This problem is usually solved by flexing the hips of the patient or by obtaining the view in the posteroanterior direction with the patient standing. This view best shows the correct alignment of the spinous processes,

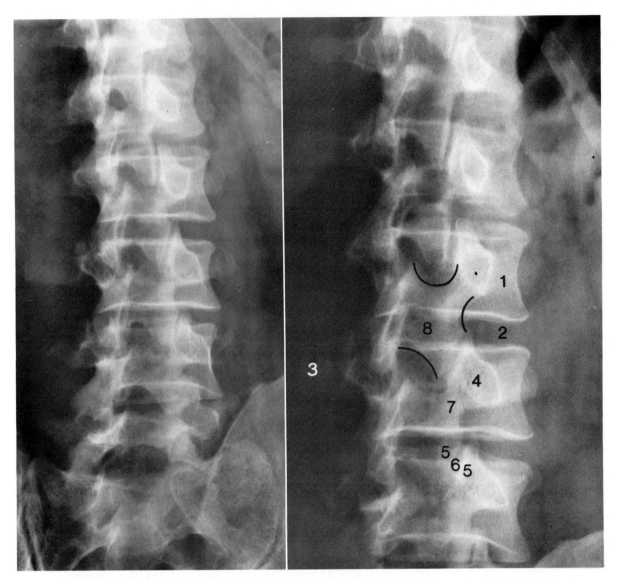

Fig. 2-22. Left posterior oblique views of lumbar spine. *1*, Vertebral body; *2*, intervertebral space; *3*, right transverse process; *4*, left pedicle; *5*, left articular facets; *6*, left articular joint; *7*, left pars interarticularis; *8*, left lamina.

the cortical margins and the trabeculation of the vertebral bodies and the transverse processes, the pedicles, and the interpediculate distances (Figs. 2-13 to 2-19). In the upper lumbar and lower thoracic regions nearly 7% of the patients have either a unilateral or a bilateral flattening of the pedicles in the vertical plane. This can be differentiated from an abnormal compression of the pedicle by the presence of intact cortical margins, convexed medial borders of the pedicle, and a normal interpediculate distance. The posterolateral plane of the L5 pedicle makes it a poorly defined structure on this view.

Lateral view. The lateral view (Fig. 2-21) is taken either in the upright or the reclining position. If the lum-

bosacral angle is to be evaluated, this view should be taken with the patient standing.[41] The lumbosacral angle is the angle between the horizontal line and the plane of the superior margin of the sacrum. The normal value in the standing position is between 25.7° and 56.5° with a mean of 41.1°. This view is used to study the slightly lordotic alignment of the anterior and posterior borders of the vertebral bodies, the intervertebral disc spaces, the cortical margins and the trabecular structure of the bodies of the vertebrae, the pedicles, the spinous processes, and the intervertebral foramina. The lumbar intervertebral spaces increase in height from L1-2 to L4-5 with L5-S1 slightly smaller than L4-5. The posterior elements of the lumbar vertebrae, in-

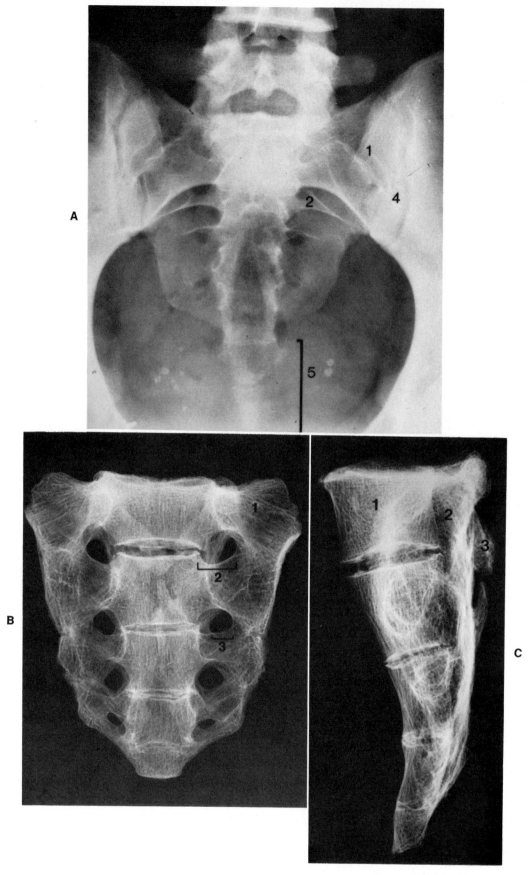

Fig. 2-23. A and **B,** Anteroposterior views of sacrum. *1,* Ala of sacrum; *2,* anterior sacral foramen; *3,* posterior sacral foramen; *4,* sacroiliac joint; *5,* coccyx. **C,** Lateral view of sacrum. *1,* Sacral vertebral body; *2,* sacral spinal canal; *3,* spinous process.

cluding the articular processes and the transverse processes and laminae, are superimposed and difficult to evaluate in this view. They are best evaluated in the oblique views and by tomography.

Oblique views. The oblique views (Fig. 2-22) are made in the anteroposterior direction with the film posterior to the patient whose body is turned 45° toward one side and then to the other. Rotating the pelvis slightly further than the rest of the body gives a slightly better look at all the lumbar facet joints, including the L5-S1 articular area. The oblique views demonstrate the structures of the neural arch on the corresponding side. They are also used to study the anterolateral vertebral body margins, the intervertebral spaces, the transverse processes, the pedicles, the articular facets and joints, the pars interarticularis, and the laminae of the corresponding side of the view. The familiar visual image of a Scotty dog is formed by the transverse process mimicking the nose, the pedicle mimicking the eye, the superior articular facet mimicking the ear, the pars interarticularis mimicking the neck, the inferior articular facet mimicking the front paw, and the lamina mimicking the body. The only opposite-sided structures seen better on the oblique views are the transverse processes because they are parallel to the film.

Lateral coned-down view of the lumbosacral junction. The lateral coned-down view of the lumbosacral junction is taken in the lateral position and centered at the plane of the L5-S1 intervertebral space. This view is important to evaluate the L5-S1 intervertebral space, the bodies and alignment of the anterior and posterior surfaces of L5 and S1 vertebrae, the S1 superior articular facets, the anterior surface of the sacrum, and the sacral bony canal.

The sacrum

The sacrum is studied with anteroposterior and lateral views (Fig. 2-23). In the anteroposterior projection the plane of the sacrum is normally directed 15° to 30° posteriorly, therefore projecting the superior sacral segments nearly on end. A true en face view may be obtained by angling the central ray 15° to 25° cephalad, placing it almost parallel to the superior surface of S1. The anteroposterior view is used to study the superior articular facets of S1, the cortical margin and the trabecular structure of the body and ala of the sacrum, the anterior and posterior sacral foramina, and the sacroiliac joints. The anterior sacral foramina are larger than the posterior foramina. They are sharply defined with medial margins and poorly defined laterally. The posterior sacral foramina are smaller and are usually slightly medial. The posterior border of the sacral bony canal is usually unfused below S3.

The coccyx

The coccyx is usually studied with the sacrum. In cases of trauma, cone-down lateral and anteroposterior views may be needed. In the coccygeal region there are no posterior elements nor is there a neural bony canal. The coccyx varies markedly in appearance.

RADIOLOGIC EXAMINATION OF THE SPINAL CANAL
The spinal canal

The spinal canal is the cylindric tunnel within the spine. It is formed of the neural arches and the back of the vertebral bodies, as well as the ligaments attaching the vertebrae. It extends from the craniocervical junction and ends in the sacral hiatus. It contains the three meningeal tubes, one within the other, the spinal cord, blood vessels, lymphatics, and supporting elements (see Fig. 1-1).[25,81,86]

The space between the spinal canal and the first soft tissue tube, the dura mater, is called the epidural space. In this space are located the spinal ligaments, connective and areolar tissues, the epidural venous plexus, the lymphatic channels, and supporting elements. The thickness of the epidural space varies considerably in different individuals, depending chiefly on the quantity of epidural fat present; it also may vary within the same individual depending on the amount of blood in the epidural plexus.

The spinal dura mater is fixed to the circumference of the foramen magnum and C2. It represents only the inner layer of the cranial dura mater. The outer or endosteal layer of the cranial dura ends at the foramen magnum and is replaced by the periosteum lining the vertebral canal. The subdural space lies between the dura and the arachnoid membrane. This compartment is a potential rather than an actual cavity, as seen at the operating table. However, after injecting contrast media into it, as occasionally happens, the subdural space can be visualized as a relatively distensible cavity. Traumatic perforation of the delicate arachnoid, such as by a needle piercing the meninges, frequently results in large subdural collections of the cerebrospinal fluid (subdural hygroma), which may persist for many days after a diagnostic lumbar puncture.

The middle meningeal layer is the arachnoid. It bonds the subarachnoid space, where the major portion of the cerebrospinal fluid is present. The arachnoid sac ends caudally as a tapering cul-de-sac usually at the level of S1 with variations as much as one vertebral segment. The subarachnoid space is partially divided by a posterior longitudinal septum that connects the arachnoid with the pia mater and forms a partition most complete in the thoracic region, where it forms a discontinuous septum (see Fig. 1-1). The dentate ligaments extend in the coronal plane on each side of the spinal cord and incompletely subdivide the subarachnoid cavity into ventral and dorsal compartments. These ligaments are a series of narrow bandlike structures that extend between the pia mater and the arachnoid and that at intervals are fixed to the inner surface of the dura mater. Their function presumably is to suspend the spinal cord in the central portion of the subarachnoid space. However, the spinal cord does move transversely as well as dorsally and ventrally with changes in position caused by the laxity of these ligaments. The arachnoid forms sheaths around the spinal roots as far as the point of exit from the vertebral canal.[60] These arachnoidal sheaths are sometimes quite loose and may show cystic dilatations commonly encountered in the lumbar region (Fig. 2-37, *E*).

The spinal pia mater is the innermost layer that covers the entire surface of the spinal cord and is intimately adherent to it. The pia mater forms sheaths for the spinal nerves, which are closely applied to the nerves and blend with their membranous investments. The pia mater is a vascular membrane between and beneath the layers of which are carried the nutrient vessels of the spinal cord.

The spinal cord is the innermost cylindric neural structure inside the vertebral canal (see Fig. 1-1). In adult life the spinal cord extends from the margin of the foramen magnum to the level of the lower part of the body of the first lumbar vertebra. On the average it is about 40 to 45 cm in length. The spinal cord is almost circular in shape, but it expands transversely to an oval contour at its cervical and lumbar enlargements, which give rise to the limbs' innervations. The cervical enlargement of the cord begins at the third cervical vertebra, it is maximal opposite C5-6, and it diminishes down to T2. The slightly smaller lumbar expansion starts at T10 and reaches its greatest size opposite T12, below which it rapidly tapers into the conus medullaris at the level of L1-2.[49] The conus medullaris terminates in a filament, the filum terminale. The filum has an intradural part consisting chiefly of pia mater. At the level of S2, it blends with the dura mater and extends caudad through the lumbosacral canal to attach to the dorsum of the first segment of the coccyx.

Until the third fetal month the spinal cord and vertebral column are equal in length. Thereafter because the spine grows more rapidly than the cord, the lower end of the cord comes to lie opposite the third lumbar vertebra at birth and opposite the L1-2 interspace (the adult position) at the age of 5 years. Occasionally because of variations in growth the conus medullaris may lie as high as T12-L1 or as low as L3.

The spinal cord is divided into 31 imaginary segments corresponding to 31 pairs of spinal nerves (see Fig. 1-2). The roots of the spinal nerves emerge from the vertebral canal at each intervertebral level starting at the occipitoatlantal articulation and extending to the first intercoccygeal articulation. The first cervical nerve

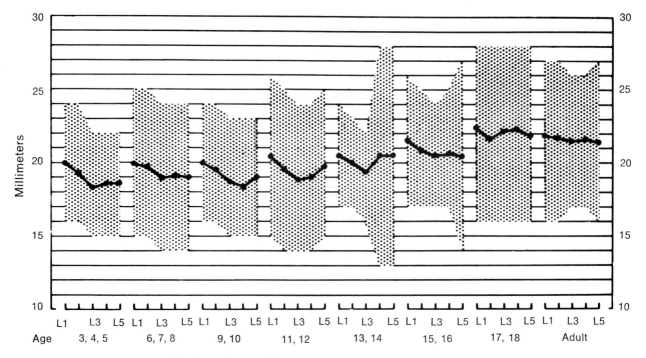

Fig. 2-24. Normal values of sagittal diameter of lumbar spinal canal in children and adults. (From Hinck, V. C.: Radiology **85:**929, 1965.)

appears between the occiput and the atlas. The second cervical nerve appears between C1 and C2, and the eighth cervical nerve appears between C7 and T1. From this level each nerve leaves the vertebral canal below the pedicle of the corresponding vertebra, for example, the third lumbar nerve appears below the pedicle of the third lumbar vertebra in the intervertebral space between L3 and L4.

Because the spinal cord ends at the level of L1, there is a special relationship between the spinal cord seg-

ments, the spinal nerve roots, and the vertebral bodies. The spinal cord segments do not correspond in anatomic level with the corresponding vertebral segments. The fourth cervical spinal cord segment lies approximately opposite the third cervical vertebra, and the twelfth thoracic spinal cord segments lie opposite the ninth thoracic vertebra. Thus between C4 and T12 the vertebral localization of lesions is approximately one to three segments higher than the neurologic localization (see Fig. 1-2).

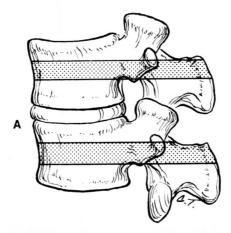

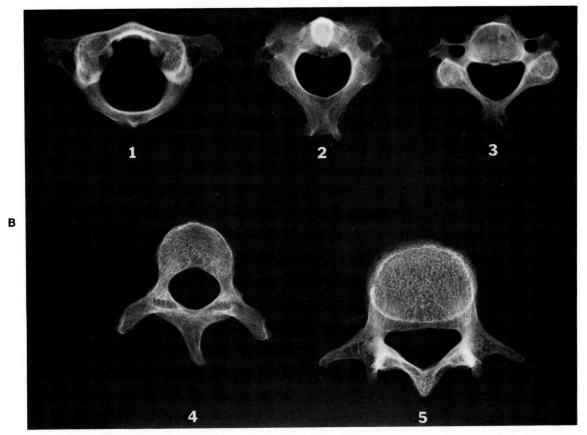

Fig. 2-25. A, Spinal canal can be divided into a series of osseous *(dotted area)* and articular segments. Osseous segments are bigger than articular ones. **B,** Radiographic pictures showing transverse plane of spinal canal at level of, *1,* atlas; *2,* axis; *3,* fourth cervical vertebra; *4,* middorsal vertebra; *5,* fifth lumbar vertebra.

There is a marked difference between the intradural courses of the nerve roots at different levels. In the cervical region the roots pass out of the dural sac at almost right angles to the cord. In the thoracic region each successive root has a slightly greater inclination caudad from the transverse plane of its origin. The lumbar and sacral nerve roots descend in almost parallel bundles to form the cauda equina surrounding the centrally located filum terminale. The fifth lumbar nerve roots emerge from the vertebral canal five vertebrae caudad to the level of their origin from the spinal cord.

The spinal canal and its measurements (Fig. 2-24) can be studied as follows: by conventional radiographs described before, by polytomography, and in a cross-sectional plane by transaxial tomography and computed tomography. The soft tissue contents can be studied by myelography, computed tomography, discography, and arteriography.

The bony vertebral canal

The vertebral canal can be divided into a series of osseous and articular segments (Fig. 2-25).[48] The osseous segment is a bony ring formed by the vertebral body anteriorly, the pedicles laterally, and the laminae, the pars interarticularis, and the dorsal spinous process posteriorly. This segment is a small rostral-caudal portion of the spinal canal. The larger articular segment is formed anteriorly by the intervertebral disc and the vertebral bodies, the intervertebral foramina and the articular facets laterally, and the laminae, spinous process, and ligamenta flava dorsally.[32,33] The regional variations in size and shape of the vertebral canal are related to the size and shape of the spinal cord described before. The cervical spinal canal is heart shaped while the dorsal is predominantly oval. The lumbar canal is usually triangular in shape, although the first lumbar vertebra could be oval like the dorsal and the last could be trefoil (Fig. 2-25).[33,39,46]

Measurements of the spinal canal can be roughly obtained from the plain films; however, they can be studied more accurately on tomography.[42,43,56,88] Tomographic studies include transaxial tomography, computed tomography, and thin-section tomography (polytomography).

Transaxial tomography. In transaxial tomography, cross sections are obtained perpendicular to the long

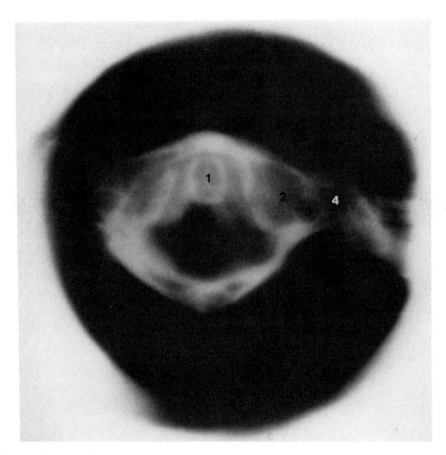

Fig. 2-26. Transaxial tomography slice at level of atlas. *1*, Odontoid process; *2*, lateral mass; *3*, foramen transversarium; *4*, transverse process.

axis of the body (Fig. 2-26).[32,33,48] Before the invention of computed tomography (CT), transverse tomography was the only method that permitted the radiographic visualization of the spinal canal in cross section. Direct measurements of the anteroposterior and transverse diameters of the spinal canal can be easily carried out taking into consideration the factor of magnification. Transaxial tomography is extremely helpful in cases of trauma and in diagnosing the different types of spinal stenosis (Fig. 2-26).

Computed tomography. The cross-sectional anatomy of the normal spine as studied by computed tomography (CT) describes a continuum of interosseous and articular segments through successive vertebral levels (Fig. 2-27).[46,48,55,82] It illustrates and emphasizes the constantly changing geometric configuration of the spinal canal.

In infants the cervical spinal canal is round to slightly oval coronally, the thoracic spinal canal is oval sagittally, and the vertebral body is relatively small in cross section. The lumbar spinal canal varies from round to oval coronally, and again the vertebral body is relatively small. In older children the cervical spine becomes more oval coronally; the thoracic spine more rounded to oval coronally; and the lumbar canal relatively smaller and rounded or triangular shaped with the apex dorsally. The vertebral body becomes relatively and absolutely larger than the canal, particularly in the lumbar region, with increasing age. The sacral canal is usually oval coronally and changes to a more triangular shape in older children.

In the adult, as mentioned before, the cervical spinal canal is heart shaped, the dorsal is oval, the lumbar is triangular to trefoil, and the sacral is triangular (Figs. 2-

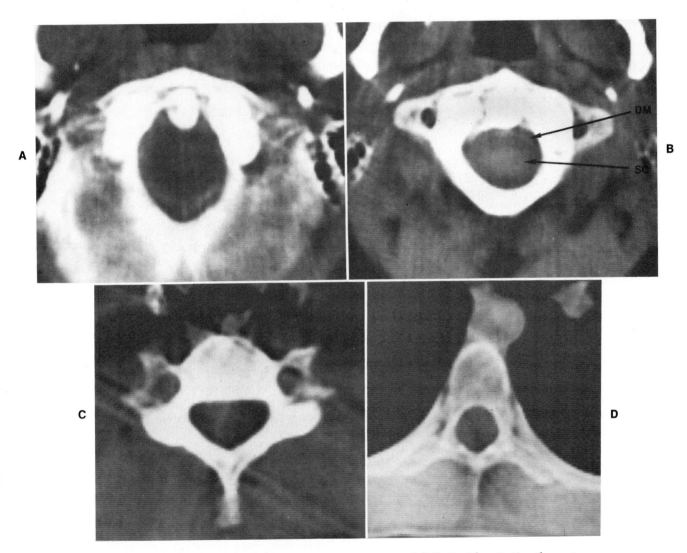

Fig. 2-27. Normal computed tomography scans. **A,** Base of skull. **B,** Atlas. **C,** Fourth cervical vertebra. **D,** Middorsal vertebra.

Continued.

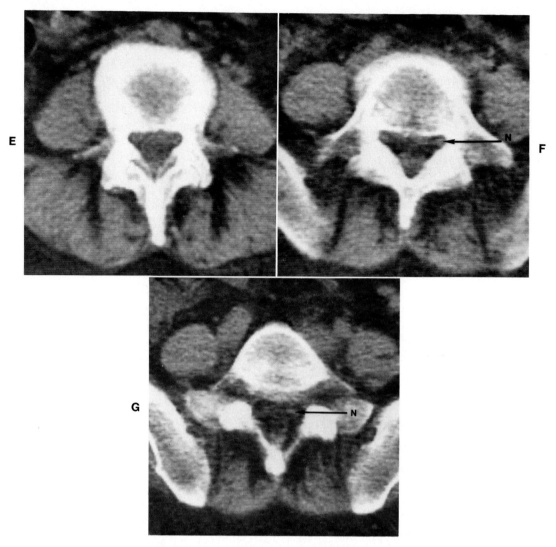

Fig. 2-27, cont'd. E, Third lumbar vertebra. **F,** Fifth lumbar vertebra. **G,** Lumbosacral junction. *Dm,* Dura mater; *N,* nerve roots inside spinal canal; *Sc,* spinal cord.

25 and 2-27). The disc spaces are seen as ill-defined, poorly corticated images.[48]

It is not as yet possible by CT machines available today to detect clearly and constantly the cord and roots within the spinal subarachnoid space without opacification of the cerebrospinal fluid.[21] However, the extradural sacral roots surrounded by fat within the lower spinal canal can be clearly seen at times (Fig. 2-27).

CT of the spine is extremely helpful to study both the bony and soft tissue portions of the spinal canal in cases of trauma.

Polytomography. Polytomography (thin-section tomography) of the spine is extremely useful in cases of trauma. It facilitates detection of fracture lines and loose fragments, particularly displaced fragments inside the spinal canal (see Fig. 4-9, *D*). It is much easier and

more accurate to measure the sagittal and the coronal diameters of the spinal canal, as well as the width of the lateral recess on polytome slices (Fig. 2-28). However, transaxial tomography is superior in measuring the different diameters of the spinal canal (Fig. 2-29).

Measurements of the spinal canal. Measuring the various diameters of the bony spinal canal is important in diagnosing both traumatic and nontraumatic spinal stenosis.[42,43,52,78,88] These diameters can be measured with transaxial tomography and with computed tomography studies. Some measurements can be made on polytomographic studies. Six measurements can be investigated in cases of suspected stenosis (Fig. 2-29): (1) the anteroposterior or sagittal diameter, that is, the greatest distance between the anterior and posterior margins of the canal in the midline; (2) the transverse

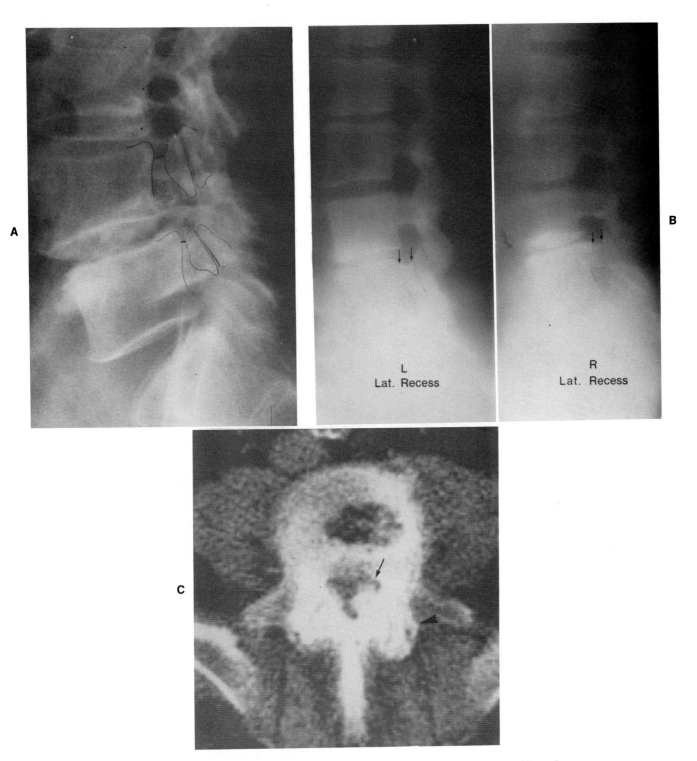

Fig. 2-28. A, Lateral radiograph (touched) of lumbar spine showing narrowing of lateral recess of L5 as compared to L4. Side of narrowing cannot be easily determined. **B,** Lateral polytomes (touched) of lumbar spine showing narrow right lateral recess at L5. **C,** Another case of narrow interfacet diameter and narrow left lateral recess at L5 shown on CT scan (*arrow*). Note extensive hypertrophy of left superior articular facet of L5 (*arrowhead*).

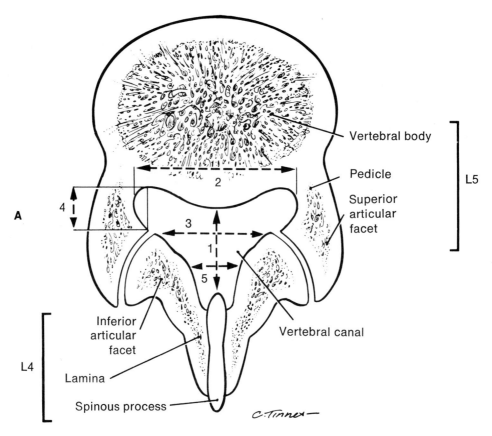

Fig. 2-29. A, Diagram showing, *1,* anteroposterior, or sagittal, diameter; *2,* transverse, or interpedicular, diameter; *3,* interfacet diameter; *4,* width of lateral recess; *5,* interlaminar diameter. **B,** Curves representing normal range of absolute width of lateral recess as measured at L3, L4, and L5 in 50 asymptomatic cases. **C,** Curve representing absolute width of lateral recess as measured on both CT and polytomes in 29 symptomatic patients with suspected narrow lateral recess at L4 and L5. All patients showed marked clinical improvement after surgery.

diameter, or the interpedicular distance, that is, the distance between the medial borders of the pedicles; (3) the interfacet diameter, that is, the distance between the anteromedial points of the facet joints; (4) the height of the pedicle, that is, the distance between the anterior margin of the canal and the anteromedial point of the facet joint, which represents the width of the lateral recess; (5) the interlaminar diameter, measured between the medial border of the laminae in a plane dorsal to the interfacet measurement, and (6) the cross-sectional area of the bony spinal canal. Spinal stenosis can be classified into five main categories (Figs. 2-29 to 2-31)[32,48,55]:

1. Anteroposterior stenosis, evaluated by the anteroposterior diameter
2. Interpedicular (lateral) stenosis, evaluated by the interpedicular diameter
3. Interfacet (posterolateral) stenosis, evaluated by the interfacet diameter
4. Lateral recess (anterolateral) stenosis, evaluated by the width of the lateral recess
5. Interlaminar stenosis, evaluated by the interlaminar diameter

This classification is both of diagnostic and therapeutic importance because surgical management differs depending on the type of stenosis.

The lateral recess is extremely important in assessing the anterolateral spinal canal stenosis.[4,24,25] It is bounded posteriorly by the medial portion of the superior articular facet, laterally by the pedicle, and ventrally by the vertebral body and the adjacent disc space. Its width equals the distance between the posterior border of the vertebral body and the anteromedial border of the corresponding superior facet. Its depth equals the distance between the facet joint and the medial border of the pedicle (Fig. 2-29, *A*). It is narrower in its upper portion and widens gradually as it approaches its lower part, where it becomes continuous

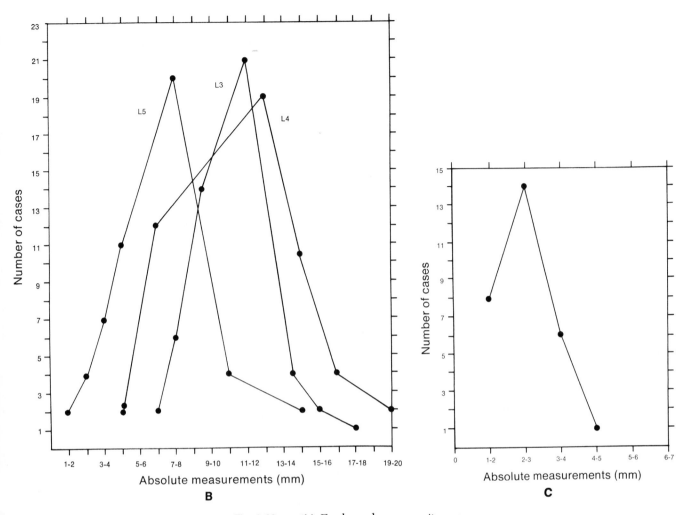

Fig. 2-29, cont'd. For legend see opposite page.

with the lateral canal (intervertebral canal) and fora-men. In the lateral recess the nerve root of the corre-sponding vertebra descends rather vertically to reach the corresponding intervertebral foramen where it leaves the spinal canal. The superior articular facet of one vertebra is anterior and lateral to the inferior facet of the vertebra above (Fig. 2-29, A).[6] Hypertrophy of the superior articular facet will compromise the corre-sponding lateral recess, particularly in its upper part, compressing the corresponding nerve root.[6,25] The com-pressed nerve root usually appears flattened especially in water-soluble myelography. With polytomography the lateral recess can be measured on the lateral and oblique slices of the lumbar spine between the upper border of the vertebral body and anterior border of the corresponding superior articular process at the level of the superior border of the pedicle (Figs. 2-28 and 2-29, A).

The diagnosis of lumbar stenosis can be readily made

by studying the configuration of the canal on axial view and obtaining the above-mentioned measurements. The interpedicular and sagittal diameters correlate poorly with nontraumatic lumbar stenosis, but their use should not be completely abandoned at least for the time being. If the sagittal or the interpedicular diameter is small on routine films, the patient probably has lumbar stenosis. However, if the sagittal or interpedicular mea-surement is normal, lumbar stenosis cannot be ex-cluded. The interfacet and the lateral recess measure-ments have been the most sensitive in cases of spinal canal narrowing. Since the primary pathology in ac-quired nontraumatic lumbar stenosis is articular process hypertrophy, the reliability of these measurements can be readily appreciated. Hypertrophy of the superior facet causes encroachment on the corresponding lateral recess, while encroachment on the posterior interfacet portion of the spinal canal is caused by hypertrophy of the inferior facets of the vertebra above. This encroach-

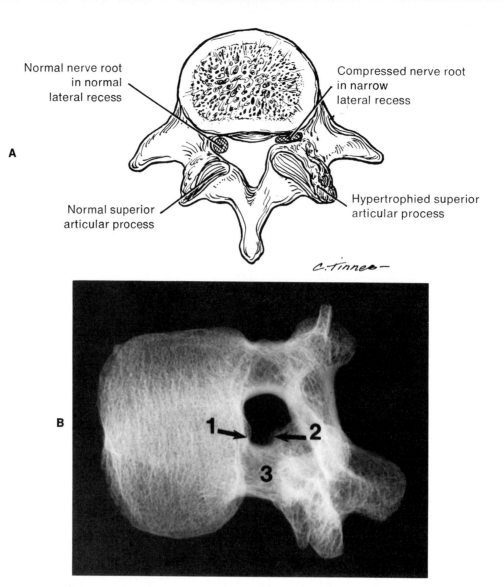

Fig. 2-30. A, Drawing showing normal lateral recess (*left*) with normal nerve and narrow lateral recess (*right*), from hypertrophied corresponding superior articular facet, with compressed flattened nerve. B, Radiograph of lumbar vertebra showing boundaries of lateral recess. Note that its upper part is narrowest portion and it widens at its lower part. *1*, Back of body of vertebra; *2*, superior articular process; *3*, pedicle.

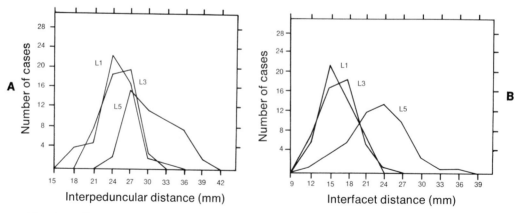

Fig. 2-31. Curves representing normal values of interpedicular, **A**, and interfacet, **B**, distances in lumbar region as measured with CT. (From Lee, C. P., et al.: Radiology **128**:95, 1978.)

ment causes the midportion of the spinal canal to be deep and narrow (trefoil configuration). Associated osteophytes from the posterior margins of the vertebral bodies, hypertrophy of the ligaments, herniated intervertebral discs, or displaced intraspinal fragments in cases of trauma will further complicate the picture and add more narrowing to the spinal canal.

Sometimes the interfacet distance is not the most narrow transverse diameter, and in these cases more pronounced narrowing is found dorsal to the interfacet plane, that is, the interlaminar diameter (Fig. 2-29).

The cross-sectional area of the spinal canal can be useful in the diagnosis of spinal stenosis.[32] The normal range has been calculated to be 4.5 to 7 sq cm and 5.2 to 9.3 sq cm at the articular segments of L4 and L5, respectively (values corrected for magnification). All patients with values less than 4.5 sq cm are considered to have lumbar stenosis. Some symptomatic cases, however, had values greater than 4.5 sq cm. In such cases the linear spinal canal measurements were abnormal (Fig. 2-29). Thus the cross-sectional area index does not help in the preoperative mapping of what segment of the spinal canal is involved nor does it enable the surgeon to plan his surgical approach accordingly.[80]

The absolute (corrected) normal values of the interpedicular, sagittal, interfacet, and lateral recess measurements of the lumbar spine are included in Figs. 2-29 and 2-31.

MYELOGRAPHY

The indications and techniques of myelography used in patients with spinal cord injury differ significantly from those usually used in nontraumatic cases and are discussed in Chapter 5. In this chapter the currently used contrast media will be discussed and the radiographic anatomy of the normal myelograms will be presented.

Contrast media currently used for myelography

Gases as contrast media. Air still is the medium of choice for myelography in particular conditions (Figs. 2-32 and 2-33).[13,47,50,63,81] Other gases, such as oxygen, are used because of their great diffusibility and more rapid elimination.[70] Gases are the least irritating contrast media and are essentially nontoxic. They are completely resorbed in a relatively short period of time with minimal changes in the cerebrospinal fluid (a transient slight increase in the protein and cells). The only contraindication to gas myelography is increased intracranial pressure.

The main disadvantages associated with pneumomyelography include the modest contrast produced by gas in the spinal canal, which can be overcome by using 125 to 130 kV(p) and thin-section tomography. Also, since gases do not freely permeate the subarachnoid space into the nerve root sheaths, the nerve roots are not visualized. As a result nerve root avulsions and small, lateral-lying disc protrusions may be completely missed. Moreover, arachnoiditis and vascular malformations may not be clearly recognized. The cerebrospinal fluid must be drained off and replaced by the gas. This makes the examination uncomfortable, particularly when it is necessary to study the entire spinal subarachnoid space. Postmyelographic headache may be quite severe and may last for several days.

Pneumomyelography is superior to positive-contrast techniques in showing intramedullary abnormalities such as atrophic and cystic lesions of the spinal cord (syringomyelia and hydromyelia). It is used as well in examining the craniocervical junction especially when combined with thin-section tomography (Fig. 2-33).

One useful application for air myelography is the demonstration of congenital malformations, particularly in the lumbar area in infants and children (Fig. 2-32). A cervical or suboccipital approach has been recommended because of a possible low distal end of the cord as well as local cutaneous conditions such as may exist with meningoceles. Air myelography is far preferable to positive-contrast studies especially when done with polytomography. In such cases, if Pantopaque is used via a cisternal puncture, it is difficult to remove and its density may obscure some of the fine details.

On satisfactory air myelogram the cord appears as a tubular structure of increased density with the negative gas shadows on both sides. The dorsal subarachnoid space usually is less distinctly demonstrated, since the cord lies closer to the dorsal wall of the subarachnoid sac, especially in the lower thoracic region. The ventral outline of the cord is directed in a mild curve toward the ventral wall of the subarachnoid sac with which it finally blends at about the level of T12.

The spinal cord is cylindric in shape with a slight flattening dorsoventrally. The average sagittal diameters of the cord in the cervical, midthoracic and the L1 regions are 10 mm, 8 mm, and 10.5 mm, respectively (Fig. 2-42).

Several techniques are available for pneumomyelography.* A lumbar puncture is done while the patient is on his side with the head of the table tilted up 15° to 20° and the head of the patient bent down over his shoulder to trap air in the upper cervical region and rest of the spinal canal. The cerebrospinal fluid is then removed from the subarachnoid space with air injected in fractional doses to replace the fluid until no more fluid can be aspirated and instilled air starts to come

---

*References 10, 12, 37, 40, 49, 57, 79.

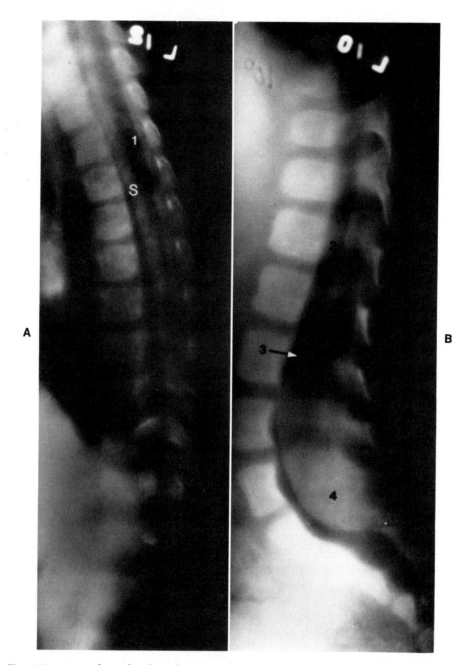

Fig. 2-32. Air myelography, lateral tomographic slices. **A,** Lower cervical and dorsal levels. **B,** Lower dorsal and lumbar levels. *1,* Dorsal subarachnoid space; *2,* ventral subarachnoid space; *3,* distal end of spinal cord; *4,* fibrolipoma; *5,* spinal cord. Note that distal spinal cord is adherent to ventral surface of mass (fibrolipoma) at about L4 level.

Fig. 2-33. Air myelography of craniocervical junction. **A,** Plain film showing wide cervical canal at C1 and C2 levels. **B,** Lateral tomogram showing wide upper cervical canal. **C,** Left vertebral angiogram showing low posterior inferior cerebellar arteries *(arrow).* **D,** Pneumomyelogram: lateral tomogram slice showing herniated tonsils, *T,* and buckled upper cervical spinal cord, *S.* Note very shallow cisterna magna.

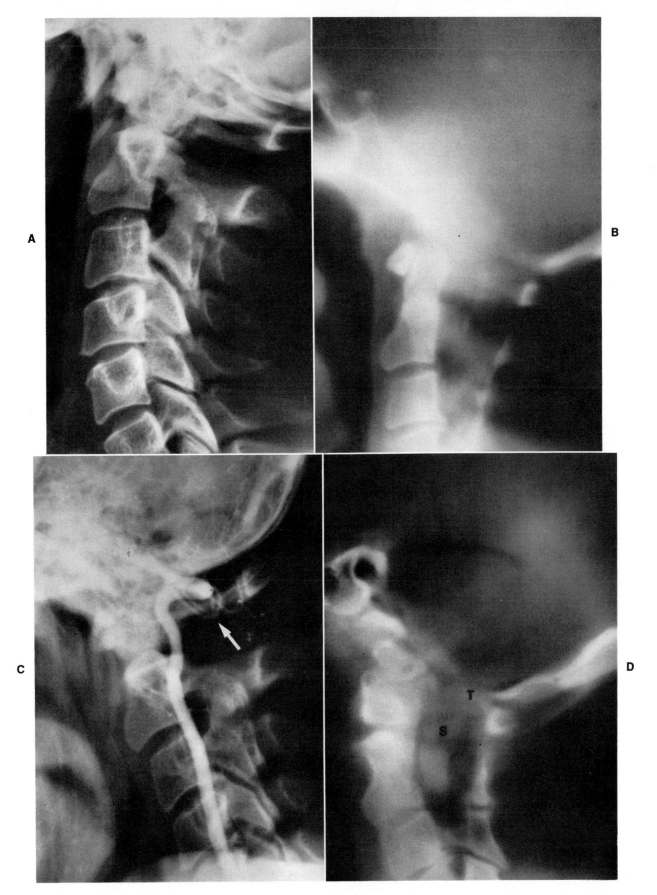

Fig. 2-33. For legend see opposite page.

through the needle. Then the patient is examined by ordinary lateral films followed by thin-section tomography (polytomography) for better evaluation of the subarachnoid space and the spinal cord. The patient could be examined in the supine position with the same techniques of plain films and polytomography. The rate of insufflation seems to influence the reaction of the patient to the examination. To minimize unpleasant sensations gas should be relatively slowly injected into the subarachnoid space.

Metrizamide. Metrizamide (Amipaque) is a water-soluble, triiodinated contrast medium. It does not dissociate in solution (nonionic) because it is not a salt but a substituted amide. Its solution therefore has a much lower osmolarity than other water-soluble contrast media used before.[2,9,23,31,38] It is supplied as lyophilized powder that is freshly dissolved just before its use in a bicarbonate buffer solution to form the desired concentration.

There are several advantages to using water-soluble contrast agents. These include better visualization of the nerve roots and nerve root sleeves, no need for withdrawal of contrast material after the study, and the ability to inject these water-soluble agents using a smaller spinal needle (Fig. 2-34).

With metrizamide, adequate and consistent visualization of the cervical and dorsal canal is possible.[83] In the case of cervical examination, it is preferable to use the higher concentration (250 to 300 mgI/ml) in a dose of 10 ml and injected through lumbar puncture or puncture at the C1-2 interspace. In cases injected through a lumbar puncture, injection should proceed slowly to minimize turbulence and mixing of the contrast agent with the spinal fluid. Then contrast medium is carried quickly to the cervical region by lowering the head of the table. Postexamination care should include keeping the patient's head elevated 45° for at least 6 to 8 hours. Painful spasm in the legs can be controlled by slow intravenous injection of 5 to 10 mg diazepam (Valium). Headache is by far the most frequent and significant adverse reaction, with an incidence ranging from 21% to 57%. It is more severe and more frequently accompanied by nausea and vomiting in females, and it is more common after cervical myelography. The incidence of headache following Pantopaque myelography is about 32%, and following simple lumbar puncture with 22-gauge spinal needle it is 36%.[34,45,53,77]

In our experience, metrizamide myelography is very informative in cases of suspected lumbar and lower thoracic pathology. It should be used particularly in old or obese patients since removal of Pantopaque could be both difficult and painful. Metrizamide also proved to be helpful in investigating cases of suspected arachnoiditis (Fig. 2-35). As in all water-soluble myelo-

graphic studies, the radiographic views should be taken using 75 to 80 kV and a high milliamperage.

Pantopaque. Pantopaque is a mixture of ethyl esters of isomeric iodophenylundecylic acids containing 30.5% of bound organic iodine. It flows more freely, has a lesser tendency to form globules, and can be more readily removed from the spinal canal than iodized oil (Lipiodol). It is available as a 30% viscous, clear, colorless liquid.

There has been much argument as to whether Pantopaque should be removed routinely from the subarachnoid space after myelography.[20,44,65,81] In England it had been customary to use about 6 ml and to leave it in the spinal canal. Pantopaque in these relatively small quantities appears to be well tolerated, with no significant reaction to its presence. However, larger quantities of Pantopaque are needed for more informative studies, especially for the thoracic and cervical regions, and must be removed at the end of the study. The main objections to removing Pantopaque are difficulty of aspiration and pain associated with aspiration.

Pantopaque, when left in the subarachnoid space, is absorbed very slowly, at a rate of about 1 ml/yr.[8,67] Gradual disappearance of epidural Pantopaque usually is more rapid than in the subarachnoid space. Pantopaque also has a tendency to become encysted, probably as a result of local arachnoiditis.[7] Following Pantopaque myelography serum protein–bound iodine levels may remain elevated for many years when the oil is not completely removed. However, Pantopaque is still a satisfactory medium for most problems in the spinal canal, with a reasonably low incidence of complications.

Subdural injection of Pantopaque occurs when the needle bevel penetrates the dura mater but only pushes the arachnoid forward or when part of the bevel is in the subarachnoid space and part in the subdural (Fig. 2-36).[5,51] While injecting the contrast material, all or part of it may accumulate in the subdural space. To overcome this difficulty we recommend introducing the needle under fluoroscopic control and advancing it in jerky, short forward movements (1 to 2 mm) in order to puncture the arachnoid efficiently rather than to push the membrane by a gradually advancing tip of the needle. Once cerebrospinal fluid is obtained, another 2 mm forward push of the needle is done to ensure that the whole bevel is inside the subarachnoid space. If all of the Pantopaque is injected in the subdural space, the opaque column may resemble the subarachnoid injection in the frontal projection. A lateral film made with the horizontal beam will demonstrate the more peripheral location of the injected contrast material either dorsally or, less often, ventrally.

Pantopaque in the subdural space moves slowly and requires a greater table tilt to produce its movement. It

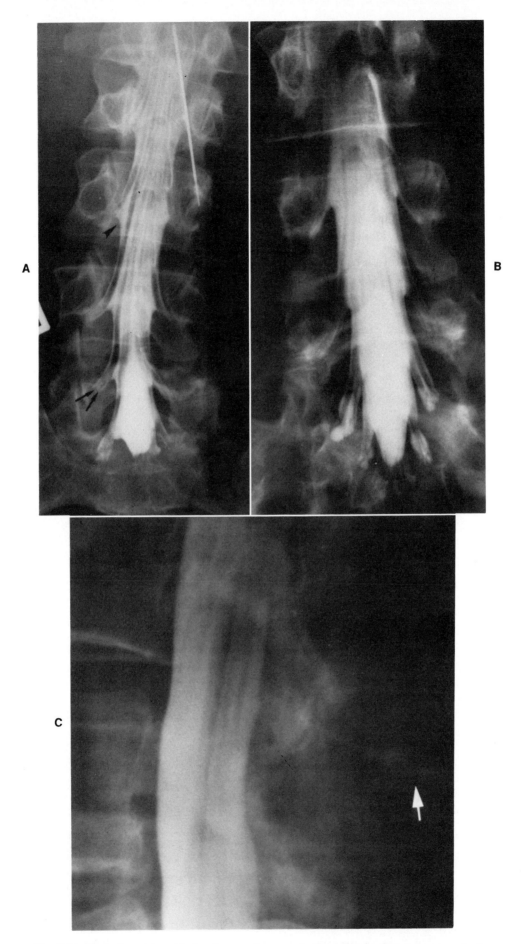

Fig. 2-34. Normal metrizamide lumbar myelogram. **A,** Note clearly shown nerve roots *(arrow)* inside arachnoid sac and axilla *(arrowhead)* of nerve root sheath. **B,** Smaller caliber needle should be used and could be removed once contrast medium is injected. **C,** Contrast medium occasionally leaks along needle tract if bigger caliber needle is used. Arrow points to nerve roots before uniting to form nerve trunk.

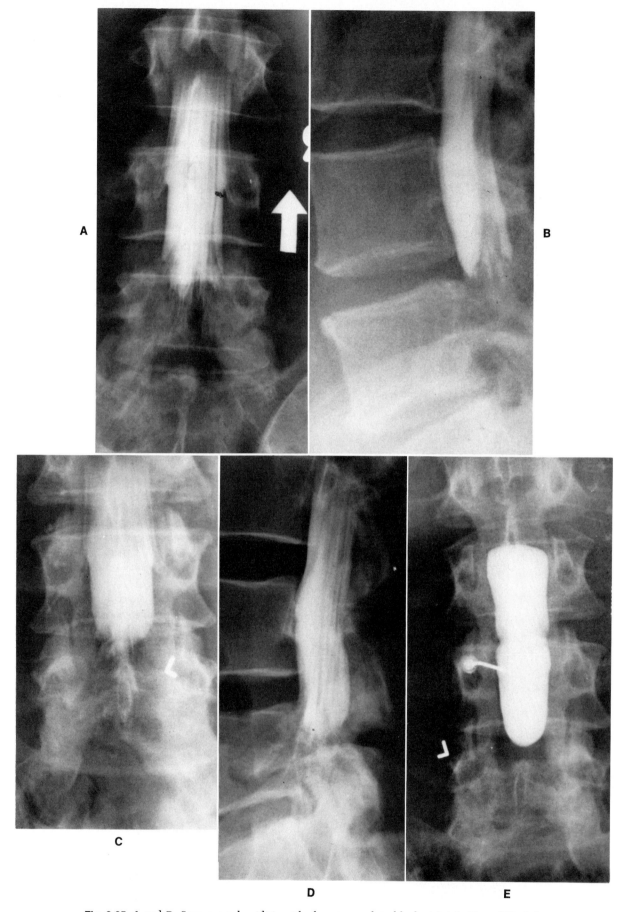

Fig. 2-35. A and **B,** Severe arachnoiditis with almost complete block at L4-5. Note diffusibility of metrizamide along arachnoidal adhesions, giving lower end of thecal sac a brushlike appearance. **C** and **D,** Severe arachnoiditis in another patient with block at L5. **E,** Same case studied with Pantopaque. Note distal end of thecal sac with false appearance of smooth, blunt end.

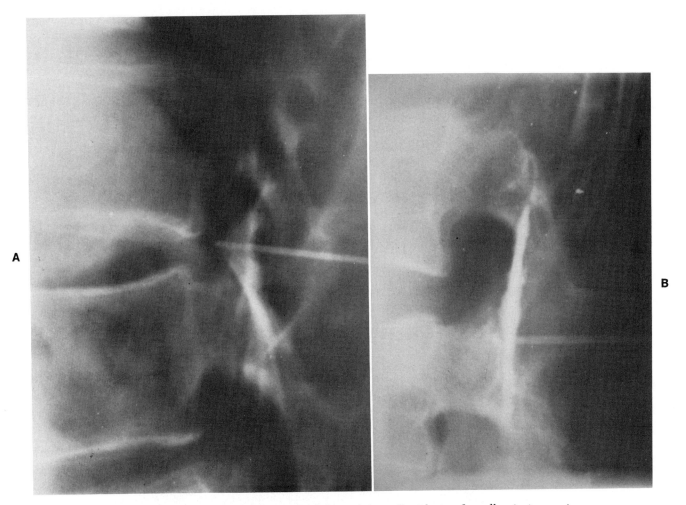

Fig. 2-36. A, Arachnoid mater is pushed forward (tented) with tip of needle. Amipaque is being injected into subdural space. **B,** Very small amount of subdural Pantopaque is injected. It is very helpful to check position of needle by cross-table lateral film, whenever needed, before injecting total amount of contrast medium.

is difficult to remove, although at times it is possible to recover varying amounts by manipulating the needle.

Epidural injection of Pantopaque occurs when the needle tip lies in the epidural space, is partly in the epidural and partly in the subarachnoid space, or traverses the sac penetrating the ventral aspect vertically. The epidural Pantopaque spreads along and coats the nerve roots in a characteristic bizarre streaking pattern, described by some authors as a Christmas tree pattern, often beyond the intervertebral foramina. It does not flow for any distance when the table is tilted. It usually is absorbed slowly, with significant quantities being absorbed only over a number of years.

Intravenous injection of Pantopaque occurs when a needle tip enters an epidural vein either during the instillation of Pantopaque or later in the examination.[30,35,54] It results in transient venous opacification and fairly

rapid disappearance of the droplets of oil seen under fluoroscopic examination running in the vascular channel toward the heart. Rarely the patient may complain of a chest pain and cough caused by multiple small pulmonary emboli. Chest pain may also occur when the patient strains violently or coughs during the examination in such a manner that a vessel is torn by a displaced needle tip.

Normal lumbar myelogram

The subarachnoidal sac, filled with the injected contrast material, tapers caudally and ends in most cases at about the second sacral segment (Figs. 2-34 and 2-37).[71] The width of the Pantopaque column in the frontal projection varies with the size of the thecal sac. When the sac is wide, it may be necessary to use a larger volume of Pantopaque to obtain a completely satisfactory study.

Occasionally there may be a short caudal sac that terminates at the lumbosacral interspace. In the latter instance a herniated lumbosacral disc can be missed since it is not covered by Pantopaque. The caudal end of the sac varies in shape from a pointed to a rounded extremity and rarely to a bifid fork. The depth of the subarachnoid space in the lateral views also varies. This variation in depth influences the density of the contrast column and the volume needed to fill the sac up to the middle of the body of the fourth lumbar vertebra in the erect position. Normally about 8 to 12 ml is required. If less than 6 ml fills the canal to that level, the column of Pantopaque is slender and the subarachnoid space is considered narrow. Differentiation must be made between a narrow thecal sac and a narrow spinal canal. If

a wide, lucent space exists between the walls of the spinal canal and the Pantopaque-filled thecal sac in the erect position, the sac is considered narrow. The size of the sac, however, varies with various physiologic conditions, such as strain, and the amount of cerebrospinal fluid drained. A narrow thecal sac does not necessarily mean a narrow spinal canal. The configuration of the sac is important because when the sac is narrow, laterally placed disc herniations may exist without producing visible defects on the Pantopaque column. In these instances even a slight deformity of an axillary pouch becomes significant. Anteriorly the column is separated from the posterior surface of the vertebral bodies only by the longitudinal ligament and the dura mater. At the level of the lumbosacral interspace the sac has a ten-

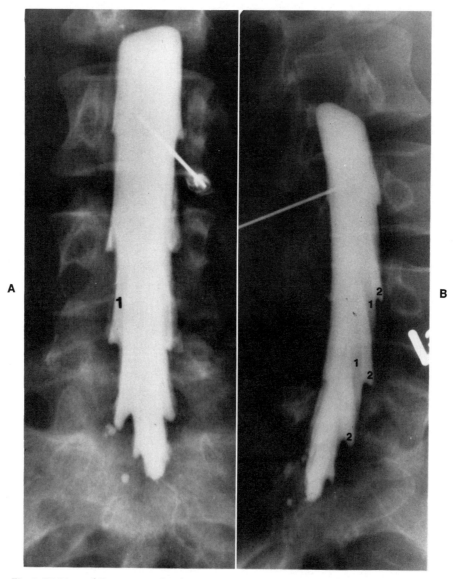

Fig. 2-37. Normal Pantopaque lumbar myelogram. **A,** Frontal view. **B,** Oblique view.

dency to be separated from the floor of the canal. That is why in some cases no definite myelographic defects can be seen at the L5-S1 level, although the clinical picture points to a herniated disc.

The roots of the normal cauda equina appear as parallel or slightly divergent radiolucent linear markings on frontal views and as obliquely downward-directed sheaths on oblique views (Figs. 2-34 and 2-37). Displacement of cauda equina roots by the lumbar puncture needle is seen frequently and is associated with pain on syringe aspiration. The patient usually complains of sharply localized pain as soon as the nerve is brought into the needle tip while the contrast medium is being aspirated.

As each root courses downward to leave the thecal sac, it lies against the lateral wall of the sac, in the lateral recess, medial to the pedicle of the corresponding vertebra (Figs. 2-30 and 2-34). At the site of exit of each root from the thecal sac there is a downward and lateral outpouching of the dura and the arachnoid, referred to as the *axillary pouch,* which is well visualized in the oblique projections. The prolongation of the subarachnoid space over each nerve root can be opacified with Pantopaque to a varying degree, but it can be more consistently opacified with aqueous contrast media. In these circumstances the nerve root itself may be visualized as a radiolucent streak within the opaque contrast medium filling the sheath (Fig. 2-34). The lateral tri-

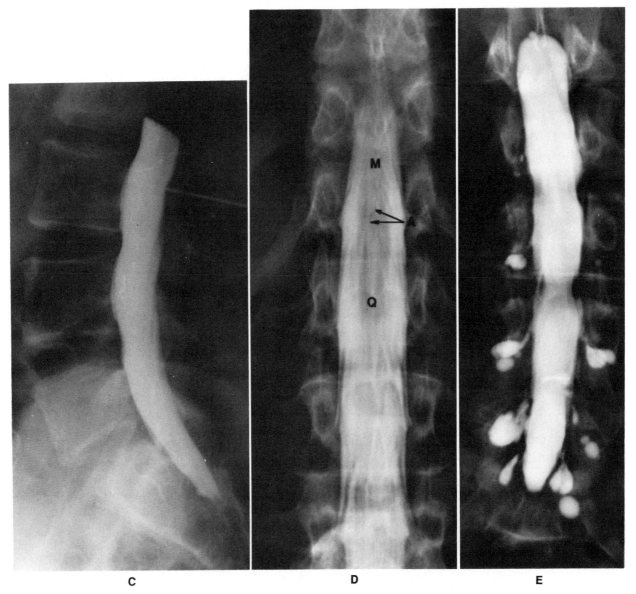

C   D   E

Fig. 2-37, cont'd. C, Cross-table lateral view. **D,** Normal conus medullaris, *M,* and cauda equina, *Q.* Note anterior cerebral artery, *A.* **E,** Multiple large arachnoidal diverticula in lumbar region. *1,* Nerve root; *2,* axilla of nerve root sheath.

angular outpouching of the meninges below the exit point of the nerve root, referred to as the *axilla of the nerve sheath*, contains no anatomic structures and therefore fills with contrast medium. The apex of the axillary pouch corresponds to the point where the root leaves the thecal sac.

Normally at about the intervertebral foramen the anterior and posterior roots unite just distal to the posterior ganglion to form the spinal nerve. Flattening of the nerve root proximal to this union and the prominence of the nerve root inside the sac are abnormal findings and might indicate a laterally inclined small herniated disc or stenosis of the lateral recess (Fig. 2-30). The changes are more apparent in water-soluble myelography than in Pantopaque studies.

The axillary pouches at a given level tend to be symmetric, although filling of these pouches may vary. In general the sacral pouches fill more completely than do the lumbar pouches. An asymmetric filling of the axillary pouches at a single level is not abnormal per se. The pathologic pouch is usually characterized by amputation, deformity, widening, deviation medially or laterally, or by a combination of two or more of these changes.

Lumbar myelography is not complete without examination of the lower dorsal levels. It is important in lumbar myelography to examine the conus medullaris and the cauda equina and to carry the Pantopaque column to at least the level of T10 to rule out lesions high in the conus responsible for radicular pains.

Normal thoracic myelogram

The thoracic myelogram examination includes frontal views taken as the patient is gradually tilted head-downward in the prone position (Fig. 2-38). The Pantopaque passes along the anterior and lateral aspects of the canal, outlining the spinal cord as a central radiolucent shadow. The anterior spinal artery is identified as a relatively straight line in the middle of the cord ending in a tortuous way in the region of the conus medullaris (Fig. 2-38, A). Occasionally, especially in films with good penetration, the artery of Adamkiewicz, as well as some radicular arteries, can be identified on myelography.[1,22] The thoracic nerves are seen as obliquely placed radiolucent linear shadows of variable length. The thoracic axillary pouches are less prominent than those in the lumbar region and project only slightly laterally. Irregularities of the Pantopaque column in the dorsal region are frequently seen in frontal projections and may take the form of round or oval radiolucencies as the column passes over normal bulging intervertebral discs. These defects may be constant or inconstant. Because they occur so commonly in normal patients, a diagnosis of a herniated thoracic disc based

on these findings alone usually is erroneous. A defect is more significant if it produces some obstruction to the flow of Pantopaque as shown by fluoroscopy, if it can be constantly demonstrated in the running lateral view, if it can be demonstrated on the decubitus films, and if it correlates well with the clinical findings. These inconstant defects can be minimized by using larger volumes of Pantopaque.

A running cross-table lateral view of the thoracic region taken with the horizontal beam can be obtained by the following method. After pooling the Pantopaque in the cervical canal the head side of the table is tilted upward until the contrast medium starts to move downward under fluoroscopy. While readying the overhead x-ray tube, the head of the table is raised another 15° upward. The Pantopaque column starts to run downward across the dorsal surface of the thoracic vertebrae. A cross-table lateral view of the dorsal spine taken 10 to 15 seconds after raising the table the extra 15° usually demonstrates a Pantopaque column crossing the back of the dorsal vertebrae and the intervertebral spaces comparable to the lateral view of the lumbar myelogram taken in the erect position. This view is very helpful in diagnosing midline disc protrusions or herniations. In cases where a large amount of Pantopaque was used (40 to 45 cc), the running cross-table lateral view is usually not needed.[36]

As the patient is tilted head upward, the thoracic arachnoidal diverticula often become evident. Those sacs that communicate freely with the subarachnoid space are not clinically significant.

The upper thoracic part is usually best examined with the Pantopaque in the cervical region since it is usually possible to keep the Pantopaque column intact down to the third or fourth upper thoracic segment.

The oblique and decubitus films are very helpful to study the lateral portions of the thoracic spinal canal and to confirm the presence of a mass shown on prone views.

When the study is designed to rule out arteriovenous malformation, in patients with posttraumatic subarachnoid bleed, the needle should be taken out and the patient should be examined in the supine position. The arteriovenous malformations are more commonly seen on the dorsal surface of the spinal cord. It is important to use a relatively large amount of contrast material and to examine the entire spinal canal in the supine as well as the prone position. Pulsations or changes in the size and shape of a defect at fluoroscopy following Valsalva's maneuver should be considered as diagnostic clues for vascular lesions. Pantopaque myelography is useful in a significant number of cases in suggesting the possibility of the vascular abnormality and in recommending an angiographic study. A negative Pantopaque my-

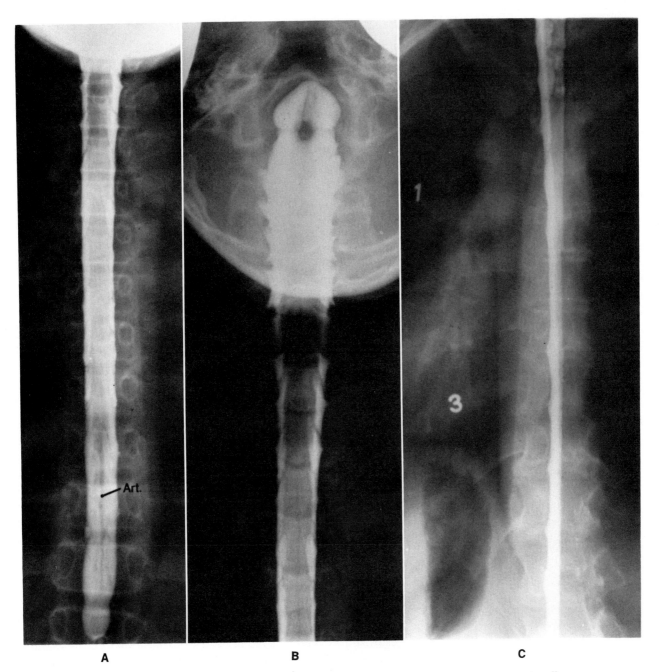

A   **B**   **C**

Fig. 2-38. Normal dorsal myelogram. **A,** By using 35 to 40 cc of Pantopaque it is occasionally possible to cover most of thoracic area with intact column of contrast agent. **B,** Upper thoracic area is always examined with cervical region. **C,** Decubitus views are sometimes helpful to study lateral portions of spinal canal.

elogram does not exclude an arteriovenous malformation.

Normal cervical myelogram

Views for the cervical myelogram include frontal, oblique, and lateral projections, as well as views for the foramen magnum (Figs. 2-39 and 2-40). Under fluoroscopic control the cervical subarachnoid space is filled

by tilting the head of the table downward, permitting Pantopaque to pass through the lumbar and thoracic canals. The neck of the patient should be in hyperextension and his head raised above the level of his body to prevent spilling of Pantopaque into the head. The column of Pantopaque should be maintained as intact as possible. On entering the lower cervical canal a momentary delay in passage often occurs as the head of

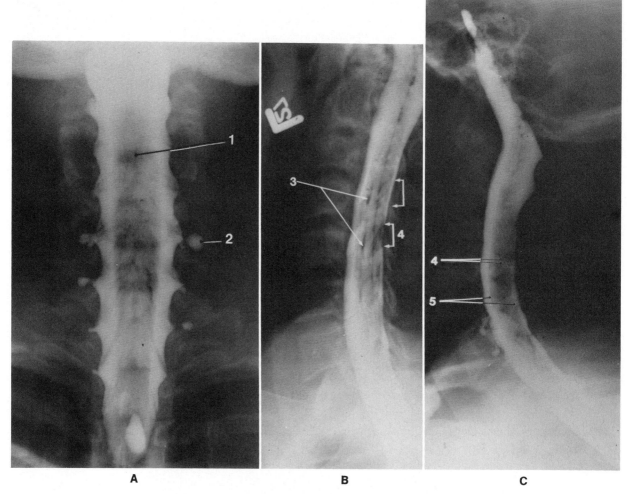

Fig. 2-39. Normal cervical myelogram. **A,** Anteroposterior prone view. **B,** Lateral view. **C,** Overexposed cross-table lateral view, showing lower cervical and upper dorsal areas. *1,* Anterior spinal vessels; *2,* arachnoid pouch; *3,* dentate ligament; *4,* posterior nerve rootlets; *5,* anterior and posterior borders of spinal cord.

the column assumes a ∪-shaped configuration corresponding to the cervicothoracic bulge of the cord. The cervical spinal cord is seen as a central radiolucent bar (Figs. 2-39 and 2-40). On both sides are indentations caused by emerging nerve trunks. The cervical enlargement of the spinal cord involves primarily the transverse diameter and therefore can be appreciated mainly in the frontal projection. The lateral projection reveals a fairly uniform sagittal diameter of the cervical cord from C2 to C7 (Fig. 2-39, *B*). The dorsal margin of the posterior subarachnoid space has a straight or slightly concave margin. At its cranial end it expands at the level of the atlas where it merges imperceptibly with the cisterna magna.

The transverse diameters of the spinal cord measured directly from spot films made in the frontal projections should be corrected for magnification in order to deter-

mine the absolute (true) measurements.[52,73,76] Using a target-tabletop distance of 50 cm (20 in), a maximum film-tabletop distance of 45 cm (18 in), and an estimated 20 cm (8 in) distance of the midcervical spine above the tabletop, magnification of the cervical cord was estimated to be between 1.30 and 1.35. The ratio of the transverse diameter of the cervical spinal cord to the subarachnoid space measured just below the nerve root pouches varies between 0.52 and 0.73 with a mean of 0.63 according to Paul and Chandler[75]; Khilnani and Wolf[52] report that it varies between 0.53 and 0.78 with a mean of 0.87. A cord:subarachnoid ratio greater than 80% or less than 50% should be considered highly suspicious. The normal sagittal and transverse diameters of the cord for various age groups are shown in Figs. 2-41 and 2-42.

In the frontal prone views (Fig. 2-39, *A*) within the

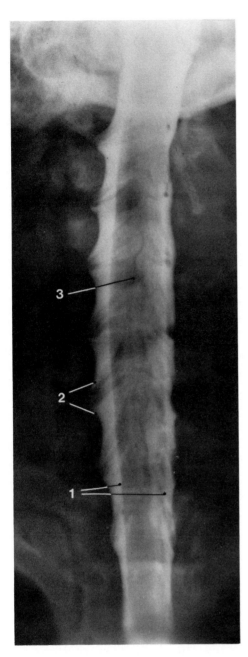

Fig. 2-40. Right oblique view of normal cervical myelogram. Note converging nerve rootlets in their course before they unite to form nerve root. Lower nerve rootlets have a greater inclination caudad from transverse plane when compared to upper cervical levels. *1*, Spinal cord; *2*, nerve root sheath; *3*, anterior spinal vessels.

contrast-filled axillary pouch, it is possible to see the anterior nerve rootlets before they fuse more laterally to form the root. The subarachnoid space is continuous over each root for a varying distance lateral to the ganglion and the intervertebral foramen. The normal axillary pouches usually are symmetrically filled. The pathologic pouch is characterized by deformity, dis-

placement, and incomplete filling or lack of filling. The anterior spinal artery usually is demonstrable as a midline linear radiolucency in the Pantopaque column. Anterior arterial radicular branches are often seen accompanying the anterior roots at various segmental levels. They join the anterior spinal artery in the midline.

In the cross-table lateral view (Fig. 2-39, *C*), the anterior surface of the cervical subarachnoid space normally lines the posterior surface of the vertebrae and intervertebral spaces, forming a fairly straight line in normal individuals. The Pantopaque column may be indented by the posterior bulges of the intervertebral discs and bony spurs in older age group. The dense radiopacity of the Pantopaque column frequently makes it difficult to distinguish the anterior surface of the spinal cord except after taking overexposed lateral views. When the anterior surface is visualized it usually lies approximately 3 mm posterior to the anterior aspect of the Pantopaque column. The dentate ligaments are visualized through the Pantopaque column as thin vertical radiolucencies ventral to the radiolucent streaks of the posterior nerve roots. This appearance is more striking in the cervical region where the ligaments are thickest. In patients with a narrow sagittal diameter of the cervical bony canal or spondylosis, prominent indentations occasionally are seen on the posterior aspect of the Pantopaque column particularly in hyperextension. They are caused by the forward bulging of the hypertrophied ligamentum flavum.

It is important to include views of the foramen magnum with cervical myelography in order to rule out a lesion at the craniocervical junction.

DISCOGRAPHY

Discography is the diagnostic procedure by which radiopaque medium is injected into an intervertebral disc in order to demonstrate the functional status of the disc. Lindblom[59] reported the first case of discography in 1948. He first used red lead injected into cadavers. Then he injected Per-Abrodil (Diodrast) directly into the disc space in the living through a long fine needle and succeeded not only in visualizing the internal architecture of the discs but also in correlating pathologic findings with clinical symptoms and signs. In 1951 Wise and Weiford[87] reported the first case of discography performed in the United States. Cervical discography was introduced by Smith in 1952 and was advocated by Cloward in 1958 and 1959 but has not gained widespread acceptance.[14,15,16,84,85]

Lumbar discography

Lumbar discography is not a substitute for myelography in patients with trauma to the spine and should not be performed as a primary procedure. However, in

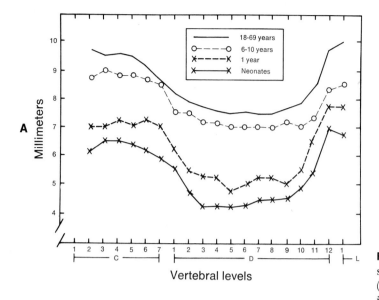

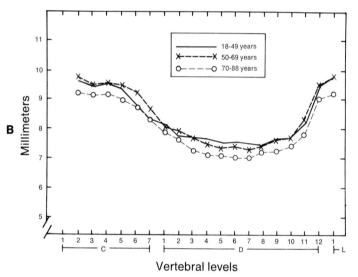

Fig. 2-41. A, Normal mean values of sagittal diameters of spinal cord at various vertebral levels in children and adults (obtained from myelograms). **B,** Normal mean values of sagittal diameters of spinal cord in various adult age groups (obtained from myelograms). (From Nordqvist, L.: Acta Radiol. [Suppl.] [Stockh.] **227:**1-86, 1964.)

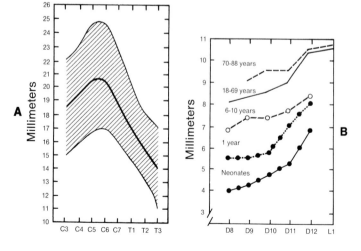

Fig. 2-42. A, Normal average, maximal, and minimal transverse diameters of spinal cord (obtained from myelograms). **B,** Normal mean values of frontal diameters of lower part of spinal cord (obtained from myelograms). (**A** from Khilnani, M. J., and Wolf, B. S.: J. Neurosurg. **20:**660, 1963. **B** from Nordqvist, L.: Acta Radiol. [Suppl.] [Stockh.] **227:**1-86, 1964.)

cases of posttraumatic persistent spinal or radicular pains and a negative myelogram examination, discography might show a ruptured disc (Fig. 2-43). It is a limited specialized procedure to study the state of the lumbar intervertebral discs. The reasons for this limitation are as follows:

1. Other lesions, such as tumors, may clinically present as herniated discs and cannot be detected by discography.
2. A second interspinal lesion may coexist with a herniated disc at a different level and could be missed by discography.
3. The abnormal disc may be in the thoracic or upper lumbar region where discography cannot safely be performed.

The patient is usually given a sedative (pentobarbital [Nembutal], 100 mg) 1 hour before the examination.

With the patient in a prone position and under fluoroscopic control the skin is infiltrated with 1% lidocaine (Xylocaine) over the proposed sites of injection. A 21-gauge long spinal needle is inserted through the interspinous ligament in the midline and is gently pushed through the ligamentum flavum and the posterior dura mater into the spinal canal, where a specimen of the cerebrospinal fluid may be collected if needed. The needle then is advanced through the anterior dura mater into the disc space. There may be transient pain as the needle punctures the anterior dura. When the needle enters the anulus fibrosus there is a definite slight resistance followed by a give, as the nucleus pulposus is punctured. Then 1.5 to 2 ml of diluted metrizamide is injected into each interspace to be examined. After each injection lateral and frontal roentgenograms are made. The posterolateral extradural approach for dis-

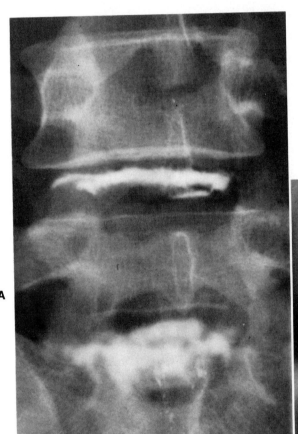

A

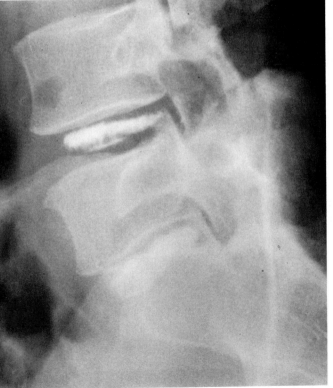

B

Fig. 2-43. Disc injection. **A** and **B**, Degenerative changes with fissured discs at L4-5 and L5-S1.

Continued.

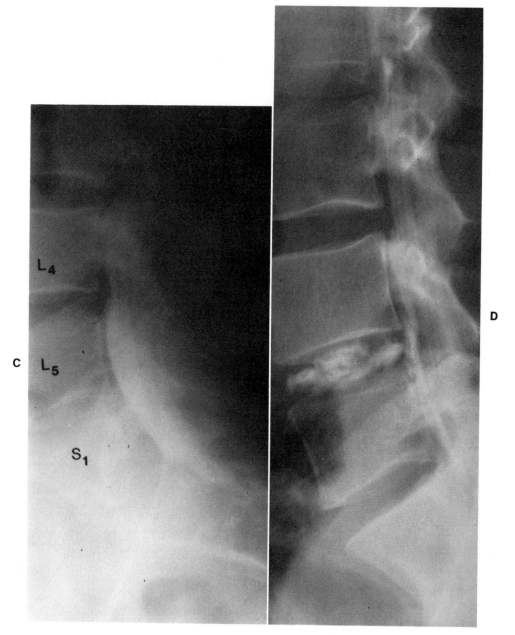

Fig. 2-43, cont'd. C, Amipaque myelogram of case of spinal trauma and lumbar radicular pain showing no evidence of herniated disc. **D,** L4-5 disc injection (same case as in **C**) showing degenerative changes and extravasation of injected contrast medium under anterior longitudinal ligament, indicating herniation of disc.

cography was reported by Erlacher in 1952.[26] This technique has the advantage of avoiding the transdural puncture.

Normal discogram

The accuracy of interpretations of lumbar discograms depends on assessment of three major findings: (1) the amount of contrast medium injected, (2) the reproduction of symptoms by the injection, and (3) the

radiologic appearance of the nucleus pulposus. Usually a normal disc accepts about 1 ml but occasionally up to 3 ml has been observed. The reproduction of the patient's pain may be caused by an escape of the contrast medium into the extradural space through a tear in the anulus or by compression of a nerve root by the ruptured disc as a result of distention of the intervertebral space with contrast material. The young adult nucleus pulposus varies in size from 1 to 2.5 cm with no apparent relationship to body habitus. In general the smaller nucleus tends to be round or oval in shape whereas the larger nucleus usually is somewhat more rectangular. Following the injection, the normal nucleus appears as a single transverse homogeneous density or as a bilocular density with a radiolucent band passing transversely through its center. The horizontal parallel densities are usually connected posteriorly but may be connected anteriorly as well. A decrease in the vertical height or fissuring of the nucleus and anterior or bilateral extension confined to the disc space without bulging of the nucleus probably indicates early degenerative changes, but is not, for clinical purposes, regarded as pathologic.

Discograms are classified as normal findings, discal degeneration, protrusion, or extrusion with epidural extension of the contrast material.[17,18,19,62] Disc extrusion is regarded as consistent with disc herniation. Pain reaction is considered important in evaluation of discal degeneration and protrusion. In evaluating discograms it should be noted that many patients with discal degenerations and others with discal protrusions are asymptomatic and best left alone. Moreover, many patients with multiple disc changes present myelographic evidence of but a single protrusion and respond well to surgery for that lesion alone.[58,59,61] In our opinion the main objection against discography as a primary diagnostic method is that the procedure is painful to the patient, requires much in the way of manipulation, and has a limited diagnostic capability.

REFERENCES

1. Adamkiewicz, A.: Die Blutgefässe der menschlichen Rückenmarksoberfläche, Sitz. Akad. Wiss. Wien, math. natur. Klasse **85**:101, 1882.
2. Almen, T.: Contrast agent design. Some aspects on the synthesis of water-soluble contrast agents of low osmolarity, J. Theor. Biol. **24**:216-226, Aug. 1969.
3. Arey, L. B.: Developmental anatomy, ed. 7, Philadelphia, 1974, W.B. Saunders Co.
4. Arnoldi, C. C., Brodsky, A. E., Cauchiox, J., et al.: Lumbar spinal stenosis and nerve root entrapment syndrome. Definition and classification, Clin. Orthop. **115**:4-5, 1976.
5. Azar-Kia, B., Batnitzky, S., Liebeskind, A., and Schecter, M. M.: Subdural Pantopaque: a radiologist's dilemma, Radiology **112**:623, 1974.
6. Badgley, C.: The articular facets in relation to low-back pain and sciatic radiation, J. Bone Joint Surg. **12**:481, 1941.
7. Bergeron, R. T., Rumbaugh, C. L., Fang, H., and Cravioto, H.: Experimental Pantopaque arachnoiditis in the monkey, Radiology **99**:95, 1971.
8. Bering, E. A., Jr.: Notes on retention of Pantopaque in subarachnoid space, Am. J. Surg. **80**:455, 1950.
9. Boyd, W. R., and Gardiner, G. A., Jr.: Metrizamide myelography, Am. J. Roentgenol. **129**:481-484, 1977.
10. Bradac, G. B., and Simon, R. S.: Cervical air myelography—an improved technique, Fortschr. Geb. Röntgenstrahlen **115**:73, 1971.
11. Bull, J. W. D., Nixon, W. L. B., and Pratt, R. T. C.: The radiological criteria and familial occurrence of primary basilar impression, Brain **78**:229, 1939.
12. Chamberlain, W. E.: Basilar impression (platybasia), Yale J. Biol. Med. **11**:487, 1939.
13. Chamberlain, W. E., and Young, B. R.: Air myelography in the diagnosis of intraspinal lesions producing low back and sciatic pain, Radiology **33**:695, 1939.
14. Cloward, R. B.: Cervical diskography, Am. J. Roentgenol. **79**:563, 1958.
15. Cloward, R. B.: Cervical discography, Acta Radiol. **1**:675, 1963.
16. Cloward, R. B., and Buzaid, L. L.: Discography; technic, indications and evaluation of normal and abnormal disk, Am. J. Roentgenol. **68**:552, 1952.
17. Collis, J. S.: Lumbar discography, Springfield, Ill., 1963, Charles C Thomas, Publisher.
18. Collis, J. S., Jr., and Gardner, W. J.: Lumbar discography. An analysis of 1000 cases, J. Neurosurg. **19**:452, 1952.
19. Collis, J. S., Jr., and Gardner, W. J.: Lumbar discography: analysis of 600 degenerated disks and diagnosis of degenerative disc disease, J.A.M.A. **178**:67, 1961.
20. Davis, D. O., and Rumbaugh, C. L.: Pantopaque myelography, Semin. Roentgenol. **7**:197, 1972.
21. Di Chiro, G., and Schellinger, D.: Computed tomography of spinal cord after lumbar intrathecal introduction of metrizamide (computer-assisted myelography), Radiology **120**:101-104, 1976.
22. Epstein, B. S.: The myelographic demonstration of the anterior spinal and radicular arteries, Am. J. Roentgenol. **91**:427, 1964.
23. Epstein, B. S.: The spine, a radiological text and atlas, ed. 4, Philadelphia, 1976, Lea & Febiger.
24. Epstein, B. S., Epstein J. A., and Jones, M. A.: Lumbar spinal stenosis, Radiol. Clin. North Am. **15**:227-239, 1977.
25. Epstein, J. A., Epstein, B. S., Rosenthal, A., et al.: Sciatica caused by nerve root entrapment in the lateral recess: the superior facet syndrome, J. Neurosurg. **36**:584, 1972.
26. Erlacher, P. R.: Nucleography, J. Bone Joint Surg. [Br.] **34**:204, 1952.
27. Francis, C. C., Werle, P. P., and Behm, A.: The appearance of centers of ossification from birth to 5 years, Am. J. Phys. Anthropol. **24**:273-299, 1939.
28. Friedmann, E.: Narrowing of the spinal canal due to thickened lamina, a cause of low-back pain and sciatica, Clin. Orthop. **21**:190, 1959.
29. Fuchs, A. W.: Thoracic vertebrae, Radiographic Clin. Photog. **17**:2-13, 1941.
30. Fullenlove, T. M.: Venous intravasation during myelography, Radiology **53**:410, 1949.
31. Funkquist, B., and Obel, N.: Effect on the spinal cord of

subarachnoid injection of water-soluble contrast medium. An experimental study in dogs, Acta Radiol. **56**:449, 1961.

32. Gargano, F. P.: Transverse axial tomography of the spine, Crit. Rev. Clin. Radiol. Nuc. Med. Dec. 1976.
33. Gargano, F. P., Jacobson, R. E., and Rosomoff, H.: Transverse axial tomography of the spine, Neuroradiology **6**:254, 1974.
34. Gass, H., Goldstein, A. S., Ruskin, R., and Leopold, N. A.: Chronic postmyelogram headache. Isotopic demonstration of dural leak and surgical cure, Arch. Neurol. **25**:168, 1971.
35. Ginsburg, L. B., and Skorneck, A. B.: Pantopaque pulmonary embolism, Am. J. Roentgenol. **73**:27, 1955.
36. Gold, L. H. A., Leach, C. G., Kieffer, S. A., et al.: Large volume myelography: an aid in evaluation of curvatures of the spine, Radiology **97**:531, 1970.
37. Goldman, R. L., and Heinz, E. R.: Gas myelography, Semin. Roentgenol. **7**:216, 1972.
38. Grainger, R. G., Kendall, B. E., and Wylie, I. G.: Lumbar myelography with metrizamide—a new non-ionic contrast medium, Br. J. Radiol. **49**:996-1003, 1976.
39. Hammerschlag, S. B., Wolpert, S. M., and Carter, B. L.: Computed tomography of the spinal canal, Radiology **121**:361-367, 1976.
40. Heinz, E. R., and Goldman, R. L.: The role of gas myelography in neurologic diagnosis, Radiology **102**:269, 1972.
41. Hellems, H. K., Jr., and Keats, T. E.: Measurement of the normal lumbosacral angle, Am. J. Roentgenol. **113**:642, 1971.
42. Hinck, V. C., Clark, W. M., and Hopkins, C. E.: Normal interpedicular distances (minimum and maximum) in children and adults, Am. J. Roentgenol. **97**:141, 1966.
43. Hinck, V. C., Hopkins, C. E., and Clark, W. M.: Sagittal diameter of the lumbar spinal canal in children and adults, Radiology **85**:929, 1965.
44. Howland, W. J., and Curry, J. L.: Experimental studies of Pantopaque arachnoiditis, Radiology **87**:253, 1966.
45. Irstam, L., and Rosencrantz, M.: Water-soluble contrast media and adhesive arachnoiditis. I. Reinvestigation of nonoperated cases, Acta Radiol. **14**:497, 1973.
46. Isherwood, I., Fawcitt, R. A., Nettle, J. R. L., et al.: Computed tomography of the spine. In Du Boulay, G. H., and Moseley, I. F., editors: The first seminar on computerized axial tomography in clinical practice, Berlin, 1977, Springer-Verlag.
47. Jacobaeus, H.: On insufflation of air into the spinal canal for diagnostic purposes in cases of tumors in the spinal cord, Acta Med. Scand. **55**:555, 1921.
48. Jacobson, R. E., Gargano, F. P., and Rosomoff, H. L.: Transverse axial tomography of the spine. I. Axial anatomy of the normal lumbar spine, J. Neurosurg. **42**:406-411, 1975.
49. Jirout, J.: Position of the lumbar intumescence of the spinal cord, Acta Radiol. [Diagn.] (Stockh.) **7**:509, 1968.
50. Jirout, J.: Pneumomyelography, Springfield, Ill., 1969, Charles C Thomas, Publisher.
51. Jones, M. D., and Newton, T. H.: Inadvertent extra-arachnoid injections in myelography, Radiology **80**:818, 1963.
52. Khilnani, M. T., and Wolf, B. S.: Transverse diameter of the cervical spinal cord on Pantopaque myelography, J. Neurosurg. **20**:660, 1963.
53. Kieffer, S. A., Binet, E. F., Esquerra, J. V., et al.: Contrast agents for myelography: clinical and radiological evaluation of amipaque and pantopaque, Radiology **129**:695-705, 1978.
54. Kinkel C. L.: Entrance of Pantopaque into the venous system during myelography, Am. J. Roentgenol. **54**:230, 1945.
55. Lee, C. P., Kazam, E., and Newman, A. D.: Computed tomography of the spine and spinal cord, Radiology **128**:95-102, July 1978.
56. Leeds, N. E., and Jacobson, H. G.: Plain film examination of the spinal canal, Semin. Roentgenol. **7**:179, 1972.
57. Liliequist, B.: Gas myelography in the cervical region, Acta Radiol. **4**:79, 1966.
58. Lindblom, K.: Protrusions of disks and nerve compression in lumbar region, Acta Radiol. **25**:195-212, 1944.
59. Lindblom, K.: Diagnostic puncture of intervertebral disks in sciatica, Acta Orthop. Scand. **17**:231-239, 1948; Nord. Med. **38**:1256, 1948.
60. Lindblom, K.: The subarachnoid spaces of the root sheaths in the lumbar region, Acta Radiol. **30**:419, 1948.
61. Lindblom, K.: Technique and results in myelography and disc puncture, Acta Radiol. **34**:321-330, 1950.
62. Lindblom, K.: Technique and results of diagnostic disc puncture and injection (discography) in lumbar region, Acta Orthop. Scand. **20**:315-326, 1951.
63. Lindgren, E.: Myelography with air, Acta Psychiatr. Scand. **14**:385, 1939.
64. Lusted, L., and Keats, T.: Atlas of roentgenographic measurement, ed. 3, Chicago, 1973, Year Book Medical Publishers.
65. Mason, M. S., and Raaf, J.: Complications of Pantopaque myelography. Case report and review, J. Neurosurg. **19**:302, 1962.
66. McGregor, M.: The significance of certain measurements of the skull in the diagnosis of basilar impression, Br. J. Radiol. **21**:171, 1948.
67. McKee, B. W., Ethier, R., Vezina, J. L., and Melancon, D.: The disappearance of a large intracranial deposit of Pantopaque twenty years after myelography, Am. J. Roentgenol. **107**:612, 1969.
68. McRae, D. L.: Craniovertebral junction. In Newton, T. H., and Potts, D. G., editors: Radiology of the skull and brain, vol. 1, St. Louis, 1971, The C. V. Mosby Co., p. 262.
69. Merrill, V.: Atlas of roentgenographic positions and standard radiologic procedures ed. 4, vol. 1, St. Louis, 1975, The C. V. Mosby Co.
70. Munro, D., and Elkins, C. W.: Two-needle oxygen myelography, new technic for visualization of subarachnoidal space, Surg. Gynecol. Obstet. **75**:729, 1942.
71. Narimatsu, K.: Form and height of normal dural sac as observed in myelography, Fukuoka Igaku Zasshi **26**:111, 1933.

72. Noback, C. R., and Robertson, G. C.: Sequence of appearance of ossification centers in the human skeleton during the first five prenatal months, Am. J. Anat. **89**:1, 1951.

73. Nordqvist, L.: The sagittal diameter of the spinal cord and subarachnoid space in different age groups, Acta Radiol. [Diagn.] (Stockh.) Suppl. **227**:1-96, 1964.

74. Patten, B. M.: Human Embryology, ed. 3, New York, 1968, McGraw-Hill Book Co.

75. Paul, L. W., and Chandler, A.: Myelography in expanding lesions of the cervical spinal cord. Exhibit at 45th Annual Meeting of the Radiological Society of North America, Chicago, Nov. 15-20, 1959.

76. Porter, E. C.: Measurement of the cervical spinal cord in Pantopaque myglography, Am. J. Roentgenol. **76**:270, 1956.

77. Radberg, C.,, and Wennberg, E.: Late sequelae following lumbar myelography with water-soluble contrast media, Acta Radiol. **14**:507, 1973.

78. Roberson, G. H., Llewellyn, H. J., and Taveras, J. M.: The narrow lumbar spinal canal syndrome, Radiology **107**:89, 1973.

79. Roth, M.: Gas myelography by the lumbar route, Acta Radiol. **1**:53, 1963.

80. Schlesinger, P.: Low lumbar nerve-root compression and adequate operative exposure, J. Bone Joint Surg. [Am.] **39**:541, 1957.

81. Shapiro, R.: Myelography, Chicago, 1975, Year Book Medical Publishers.

82. Sheldon, J. J., Sersland, T., and Leborgne, J.: Computed tomography of the lower lumbar vertebral column, Radiology **124**:113-118, July 1977.

83. Skalpe, I. O., and Amundsen, P.: Thoracic and cervical myelography with metrazamide, Radiology **116**:101-106, 1975.

84. Smith, G. W.: The normal cervical diskogram, Am. J. Roentgenol. **81**:1006, 1959.

85. Smith, G. W., and Nichols, P., Jr.: The technic of cervical discography, Radiology **68**:718, 1957.

86. Tavaras, J., and Wood, E.: Diagnostic neuroradiology, Baltimore, 1976, The Williams & Wilkins Co.

87. Wise, R. E., and Weiford, E. C.: X-ray visualization of intervertebral disc; report of case, Cleve. Clin. Q.**18**:127-130, 1951.

88. Wolf, B. S., Khilnani, M., and Malis, L. I.: The sagittal diameter of the bony cervical spinal canal and its significance in cervical spondylosis, Mt. Sinai J. Med. (N.Y.) **23**:283, 1956.

PART II

Acute phase of spinal cord injury

CHAPTER 3

Emergency care of spinal cord injury

PAUL R. MEYER, Jr., M.D.

Possibly the most important aspect of patient care in the suspected spinal cord injured victim is the suspicion that such an injury is present. Once that question has arisen, the victim must be treated as though a spine injury were present. The initial effort, therefore, becomes one of preservation of what neurologic function remains and the prevention of any further neurologic deterioration through mismanagement.

In 1972 more than 72% of the patients admitted to the Acute Spine Injury Service of the Midwest Regional Spinal Cord Injury Care System were neurologically complete[6]; that is, they had irreversible neurologic loss below the level of injury. Such a finding implied that the remaining 28% of patients had incomplete neurologic injuries with some degree of preserved neurologic function below the level of injury. In 1979 this statistic had significantly improved, with 45% of acute spinal cord injured patients arriving with incomplete neurologic injuries. It is believed that improved accident scene care and early retrieval have been responsible for this statistical improvement.[7]

EMERGENCE OF SPECIALTY CARE FACILITIES

Emergency care implies injury recognition first, followed by protection, splinting, appropriate extrication, and expeditious transfer proceedings. It also implies that after each of the above factors has been dealt with, the victim will be referred to the appropriate previously designated care facility for his particular injury. Based on federal guidelines, *predesignation* implies special

centers categorized to receive certain specific types of trauma cases. These "centers" of special competence include facilities for spinal cord injuries, burns, general trauma, poisonings, and cardiac emergencies. When such facilities are not available at the local level, referral to an existing institution may require the patient to be displaced from his community in order to ensure these types of care capabilities.[8]

Roadside or accident scene care requires both the rapid arrival of identified, experienced paraprofessionals, trained in emergency care and treatment, as well as early injury identification. For such to occur, there must be *access* to a patient care system (i.e., 911 metropolitan/urban/rural central dispatch system). Personnel responding to calls through such a system should have reached certified training levels (1) as emergency medical technicians (EMT)/ambulance and (2) in basic or advanced life support. These individuals must be able to demonstrate capabilities in patient injury identification, spine and fracture splinting, and extrication techniques. Implied is an understanding that prior to moving the patient, assessment of the injury will include patient evaluation for the presence of head injury,[10] extremity fractures, and neurologic dysfunction secondary to either cervical, thoracic, or lumbar spine injury.[8]

A cardinal rule in the assessment of a motor vehicle accident victim where sudden positive deceleration injuries to the head or face have occurred, with resulting lacerations or altered states of consciousness (irrespec-

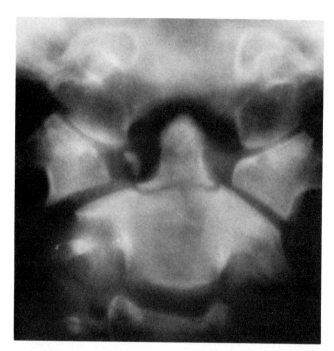

Fig. 3-1. Fracture of ring of C1 (Jefferson fracture). Polytomographic view also reveals a fracture of odontoid process. Neurologic finding: normal.

tive to other associated injuries), is that the presence of a spine injury must be suspected and treated as such until it is either confirmed or found not to be present by neurologic and radiologic examination. The same applies to the marginally conscious head trauma victim who by reason of mechanism of injury should be suspected of having sustained spinal trauma.

CERVICAL SPINE INJURIES

Injury to the upper cervical spine may result in fractures of the ring of C1 (Jefferson fracture) (Fig. 3-1), fracture of the odontoid process of C2 (Figs. 3-1 and 3-2), or posterior element fracture of C2 (hangman's fracture) (Fig. 3-3). Both the Jefferson and the hangman's

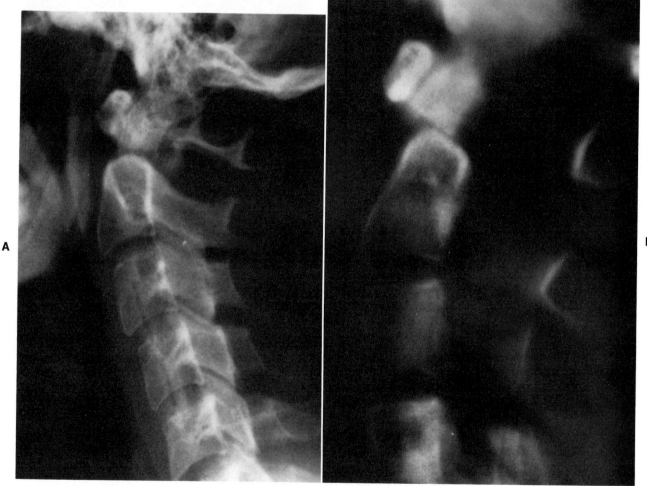

Fig. 3-2. A, Lateral radiograph and, **B,** polytomogram revealing fracture at base of odontoid process. Mechanical force: extension. Neurologic finding: normal.

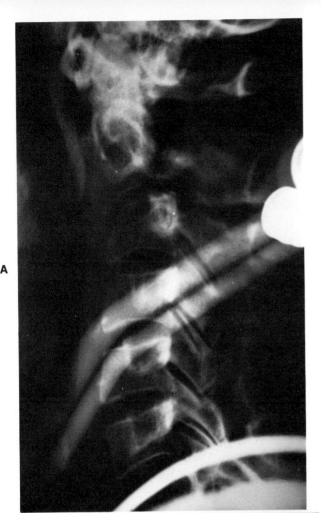

fractures are associated with an excessively applied axial load to the spine, with the hangman's fracture probably resulting from an applied hyperextension moment to the cervical spine. Fracture of the odontoid portion of C2 results from acute cervical spine extension. Neurologic injury with either of these fractures is infrequent, but the adage that a patient with a fracture of C1 or C2 either arrives in a hospital dead or neurologically normal is not completely correct. Obviously, variations do exist. Another interesting finding occasionally noted with high spine injuries is an associated injury to the brain stem. This is caused by the brain stem's proximity to the ring of C1 and the odontoid process of C2. The result may be abnormal mental or motor behavior or alterations in respiration caused by brain stem or upper cervical spinal cord neurologic involvement.

It should be appreciated that injury to the cervical or thoracic spine can result in an initial contusion-type injury to the spinal cord, with no immediately recognizable neurologic injury. During the early hours after

Fig. 3-3. Hangman's fracture secondary to excessive axial load, extension moment. **A,** Plain radiograph and, **B** and **C,** polytomograms show fracture through pedicle of C2. Neurologic finding: C5 complete.

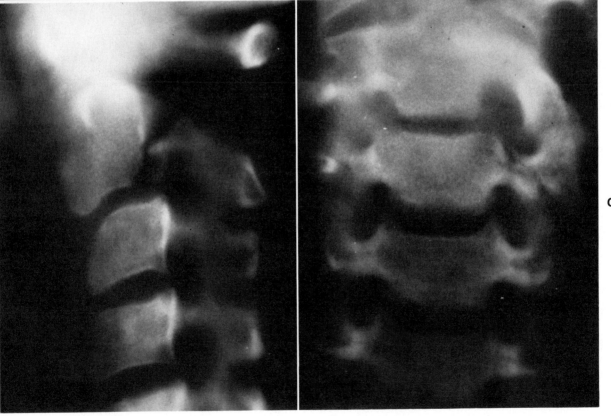

Table 3-1. Neurologic level and completeness of lesion at admission of MRSCICS* patients injured in 1979

Level	Early entry			Delayed entry			Total		
	Patients†	Patients with complete lesions	%‡	Patients†	Patients with complete lesions	%‡	Patients†	Patients with complete lesions	%‡
C1	0	—	—	0	—	—	0	—	—
C2	2	1	50	1	0	0	3	1	33
C3	1	1	100	0	—	—	1	1	100
C4	11	6	55	7	2	29	18	8	44
C5	25	16	64	19	11	58	44	27	61
C6	8	2	25	10	4	40	18	6	33
C7	7	4	57	5	2	40	12	6	50
C8	0	—	—	2	0	0	2	0	0
T1	1	0	0	2	2	100	3	2	67
T2	1	1	100	2	2	100	3	3	100
T3	0	—	—	1	1	100	1	1	100
T4	3	3	100	0	—	—	3	3	100
T5	2	2	100	1	1	100	3	3	100
T6	0	—	—	0	—	—	0	—	—
T7	0	—	—	1	0	0	1	0	0
T8	3	3	100	3	2	67	6	5	83
T9	2	2	100	1	1	100	3	3	100
T10	1	1	100	2	2	100	3	3	100
T11	4	2	50	2	2	100	6	4	67
T12	4	1	25	10	7	70	14	8	57
L1	8	4	50	3	2	67	11	6	55
L2	4	1	25	0	—	—	4	1	25
L3	0	—	—	0	—	—	0	—	—
L4	4	0	0	2	0	0	6	0	0
L5	1	0	0	0	—	—	1	0	0
S1	0	—	—	0	—	—	0	—	—
Unknown	2	1	50	0	—	—	2	1	50
TOTAL	94	51	54	74	41	55	168	92	55

*Midwest Regional Spinal Cord Injury Care System.
†Patients with normal neurologic function excluded. "Early entry" patients are those admitted less than 72 hours after injury. "Delayed entry" patients are those admitted more than 72 hours after injury.
‡Percentage with complete lesions.

trauma, depending on the unknown quantity of force that produced the initial injury, either of the following pathologic alterations in the spinal cord may occur: spinal cord edema or occasional central cord hemorrhage. The result may be either the early or late presentation of a changing neurologic pattern or, in the presence of an obvious neurologic injury, extension (proximally) of the neurologic level. This becomes a major consideration in injuries within the cervical spinal cord, not only because of loss of function in the upper extremities (which may have been initially present) but also because of the loss of voluntary, spontaneous respiratory function. These patients require mechanical ventilatory assistance and thus require intubation (nasotracheal or endotracheal) or tracheostomy.

Trauma to the neck usually results in fractures of vertebral bodies and/or neurologic injury in the midportion of the cervical spine. The mechanism of injury is almost always (90%) the result of acute flexion with some associated rotation. Extension injuries are relatively rare (10%). This fact is unfortunate because the associated neurologic injury with an extension injury is usually much less severe than that which occurs with flexion injuries. With flexion injuries the neurologic injury generally results in extensive paralysis. The vertebral level (Table 3-1) most often injured is C5, followed by C6 and C4. The reason for the high concentration of injuries to this area of the neck is that this is the area of maximal motion in flexion (C5-6) and extension (C4). Likewise, the least available space (neurocanal)[5] for the cervical spinal cord coincides with the area of maximal motion. This fact, probably more than anything else, accounts for the high incidence of neurologic injuries.

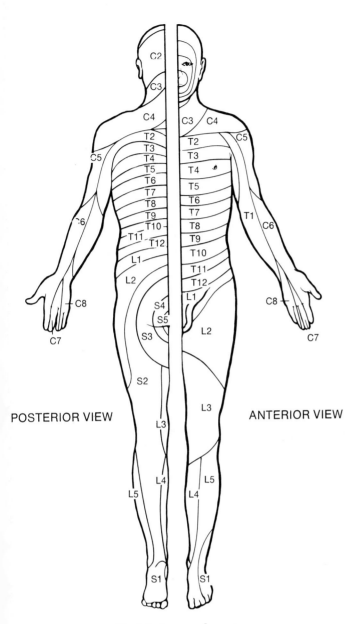

Fig. 3-4. Sensory dermatomes.

C8: able to adduct and abduct fingers but no function below

Sensory dermatome function varies slightly from individual to individual (Fig. 3-4) yet is consistent enough to also be used as a measure of determining neurologic injury level: between the thumb and index finger indicates sensory preservation in the C6 dermatome; sensation over the medial (ulnar) side of the hand indicates sensory preservation in the C7 dermatome; and sensation along the medial aspect of the upper arm and axilla usually reveals residual sensory function in the T1 and T2 dermatomes. Such motor and sensor findings should be recorded by each examiner, including the initial respondent (EMT or paramedic).

THORACIC SPINE INJURIES

Injuries to the thoracic spine and the thoracic spinal cord are more difficult to assess than those to the cervical spine. This is because loss of neurologic function over the chest is an upper motor neuron injury and more subtle, while loss of function in the lower extremities is a lower motor neuron injury and more gross. Nonetheless, there is a fixed pattern of function in the lower extremities and perineum:

L2: hip flexion

L3-4: knee extension

L5-S1: ankle dorsiflexion, plantar flexion

S2-5: voluntary perianal muscle contraction or voluntary urination

Because the rib cage provides some measure of protection to the vital structures contained within, it also serves to protect the thoracic spine. This is particularly so for translatory forces. However, when axial load to the thoracic spine is associated with flexion and rotational moments, permanent neurologic injury (paraplegia) usually results. The reason is twofold: vertebral element fractures with spine displacement (Fig. 3-5) and interruption of the blood supply to the thoracic cord.[4] It should be appreciated that the blood supply to the thoracic spinal cord has a very narrow margin of safety even with injuries of moderate intensity. This is true even when there is no spine displacement. It is important to recognize that the actual extent of the injury (at the time of initial trauma) is never known and frequently will not correlate exactly with initial radiologic findings when the patient is first examined in the emergency ward.

Neurologic interpretation

For the physician or paramedic performing the initial neurologic examination on the cervical spine injured patient, the most likely identifiable neurologic change will be the loss of sensation below a line across the chest, approximately 3 cm above the nipples (Fig. 3-4).

Neurologic assessment

Motor neuroanatomic areas of the cervical spinal cord relate directly to function in the upper extremities and indirectly to function in the lower extremities. In order to assess the level of the neurologic injury, the presence or absence of upper extremity function is determined:

C4: able to shrug shoulders but no function below

C5: able to flex elbow but no function below

C6: able to dorsiflex wrist but no function below

C7: able to extend fingers and elbow but no function below

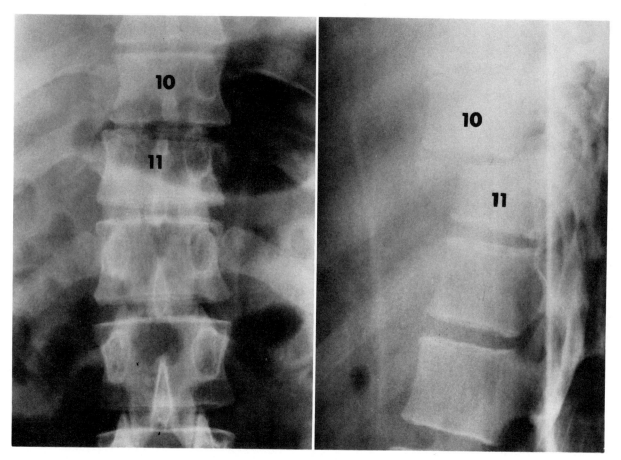

Fig. 3-5. Fracture-dislocation of thoracic spine, T10-11. Injury was secondary to acute flexion moment with axial load, resulting in fractures of facet and pedicle of T10, forward translation of T10 vertebra on T11, and wedge compression fracture of T11. Neurologic finding: incomplete L2.

As revealed by Last,[3] as the limb buds extend out laterally during the development of the human embryo between the sixth and twelfth weeks of fetal life, the nerve roots of C5, C6, C7, and T1 exiting the developing nervous system pass laterally into the developing limb. Thus the C5 nerve root finds its terminal innervation in the upper lateral arm; the C6 dermatome, to the thumbs and index fingers; the C7 dermatome, to the long finger and the radial side of the ring finger; the C8 dermatome, to the ulnar border of the ring finger and the ulnar border of the hand and forearm; and the T1 dermatome, to the ulnar border of the upper arm to meet the T2 dermatome in the axilla. This indicates that the nerve roots of C2, C3, and C4 (which compose the supraclavicular nerve of the cervical plexus) provide sensation to the skin dermatomes over the anterior, superior, and posterior aspects of the neck and chest and the superior lateral aspects of the shoulders. This "cervically" oriented sensation extends down to within 2 to 3 cm above the nipple line. At this point,

the C4 dermatome meets the T3 dermatome. This finding may be confusing to the inexperienced examiner and often leads to an erroneous identification of the level of injury. To avoid this occurrence, sensation in the arm must be carefully examined and recorded. Remembering the dermatomes of C2 through T2, one will be able to differentiate between an injury to the cervical cord and one to the thoracic cord. Two other major thoracic spinal cord dermatome landmarks to remember are the umbilicus (T10) and the inguinal ligament crease (T12). The principal sacral dermatomes to remember are the S2-5 segments, which are found on neurologic examination to be in the perianal area. Sensation in the perianal area is the most important neurologic finding in the cervical spine injured victim.

A peculiarity of injuries to the thoracolumbar region of the spine and spinal cord is the occurrence of *root escape*. Root escape implies the avoidance of nerve root injury in the presence of significant vertebral column injury. As an example, injury to the thoracolumbar vertebral column at the T12-L1 level normally produces injury to the conus medullaris segment of the spinal cord (L5-S5) and either a flaccid or spastic paralysis from the level of L5 distally. Anatomically, however, the L1 nerve root exits the spinal cord at the vertebral body level of T10. Thus, within the vertebral column interval between T10 and T12-L1, the nerve roots of L1, L2, L3, and L4 exit the spinal cord; with spinal trauma these roots may escape with either no injury or partial (incomplete) nerve root injury, thus the term *root escape*.

ACCIDENT SCENE MANAGEMENT

Once the presence of a vertebral column injury is either suspected or apparent, due to the distribution of the associated neurologic loss, splinting of the spine for protection from further injury becomes paramount. Management of the cervical spine requires that one member of the retrieval team assume total position control of the head and neck in order to prevent inadvertent flexion, rotation, or extension. Mild cervical traction with each hand clasping either side of the head, about the ear, is applied in order to maintain traction and alignment during the application of a spine board with sandbags (Fig. 3-6) or a cervical immobilizing orthosis (Fig. 3-7) with a head halter. After head-neck-thorax immobilization has been attained, the patient is extricated.

For thoracic or lumbar spine trauma, following the injury identification, the patient is usually placed horizontally on an automobile seat or spine board before extrication. Other splints such as "scoop" stretchers or Styrofoam dilatancy (air evacuation) mattress splints may also be used for the spine splinting and extraction.

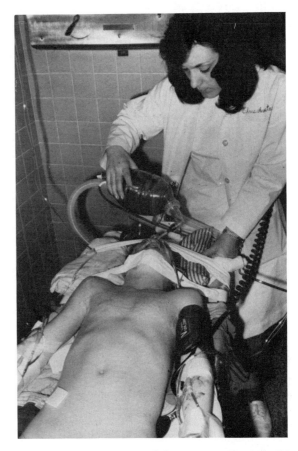

Fig. 3-6. Acute cervical spine dislocation at C3-4 with C5 incomplete neurologic injury. Admission examination revealed need for cardiopulmonary resuscitation. Patient was managed on spine board, head was sandbagged and taped for stability during resuscitation efforts.

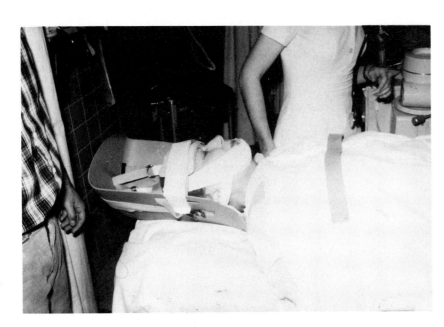

Fig. 3-7. Meyer cervical orthosis (Zimmer) applied to patient with odontoid fracture. Patient had other associated injuries, including femur fracture. Note harness supporting chin and occiput and maintenance of traction by elastic straps. Band across forehead allows patient to be turned on side without loss of head-neck-thorax relationship.

Rolled towels or blankets can be carefully placed beneath the neck or lumbar spine. Although such objects may tend to preserve the normally present cervical and lumbar lordotic curve, the benefit more likely derived is unweighting of the head and thoracolumbar spine from the spine board or splint. Caution must be taken to ensure that there is padding between bony prominences and a firm or hard splint, since the splint is likely to be in place for a prolonged period of time. If allowed to develop, skin pressure areas may result within only a matter of hours.

Once a patient has been extricated and can adequately be examined, resuscitation needs may be expanded: the airway suctioned; vital signs obtained and recorded; associated injuries such as fractures and lacerations identified, splinted, and dressed; and intravenous fluids (Ringer's lactate) administered. After administration of the recommended protocol, which is expanded later in this chapter, the patient should be carefully and expeditiously evacuated to a predesignated primary care trauma facility[8] for immediate appropriate resuscitation and evaluation. Once stabilized, the patient should then be referred to a higher level of care, if indicated.

TRANSFER MODES AND PROTOCOLS

One example of transfer of spinal cord injured patients involves the Midwest Regional Spinal Cord Injury Care System,[7] currently one of 14 federally sponsored (Rehabilitation Services Administration, Department of Health and Human Services) regional model spinal cord injury centers; this system functions well as a component of the Illinois Trauma Program, begun in 1971 for the identification, retrieval, transport, and care of the critically injured patient. Spinal injury care has been dramatically enhanced through development of this program and the subsequent development and adherence to established protocols for triage, transfer, and treatment of the spinal cord injured patient. The Midwest Regional Spinal Cord Injury Care System, in conjunction with the Illinois Emergency Medical Service, has established guideline criteria for air/ground transport of spinal cord injured patients, depending on the severity of the injury and the distance required for transfer (Fig. 3-8). Patients requiring transfer within a 45-mile radius of the Spinal Injury Center most often are transported by overland critical care vans; between 45 and 75 miles, by helicopter; and for distances greater than 75 miles, by fixed-wing aircraft. On occasion, the patient may be transported over shorter distances by helicopter, but this would depend on individual circumstances.

In the area of prehospital patient care, emphasis should be placed on identification, extrication, and

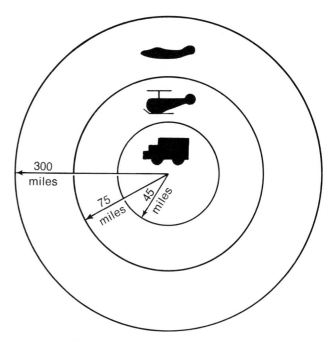

Fig. 3-8. Mode of transportation scheme for acute trauma victims: 0 to 45 miles, by overland critical care van, depending on critical care and support requirements and accessible trained paramedics or nursing attendants; 45 to 75 miles, by helicopter; 75 to 300 miles, by fixed-wing aircraft. The latter two allow rapid transport of marginally stable trauma victim with minimal support capabilities.

transfer. A number of questions, such as the following should be answered and the information made available to the receiving institution to which the patient is being referred:

1. Who is doing the patient identification (fireman, policeman, paramedic)?
2. What is the level of expertise of the person doing the patient identification?
3. What drugs and equipment should be available for use during the prehospital patient management phase?
4. Who assumes administrative and legal responsibility for patient transfer and in-transit care?

This will ensure continuity of care between prehospital and hospital phases of management. Regional, comprehensive (category I as established by the American College of Surgeons[2]) trauma facilities, including spinal cord injury centers, usually assume responsibility for pretransfer arrangements and prehospital management and may lend assistance in the initial retrieval of the victim at the site of the injury.

A major component of the Illinois Trauma System is the *trauma coordinator*, who is responsible for ensuring transfer arrangements and who, with physician direction, determines whether the patient is medically capable of surviving the transfer. The trauma coordinator also arranges for referring-physician and receiving-physician communication prior to the transfer, if any doubt should exist. Once the patient has been accepted for transfer, both the receiving physician and the trauma coordinator are responsible for notifying the emergency room and the Spinal Injury Center, as well as the attending consultants, of the patient's time of arrival. Here, too, there are questions that must be asked of the referring physician or institution in order to ensure a safe transfer:

1. What are any associated injuries?
2. Are there any open fractures? If there are open fractures and the patient is not able to arrive at the Spinal Cord Center within 6 hours of trauma, the wound should be debrided at the hospital of origin.
3. Is the patient in shock, and if so, why? Request a pretransfer surgical evaluation and clearance.
4. What are the baseline results of blood gas measurements, hematocrit and hemoglobin, and urinalysis? If shock does exist and is due to blood loss, loss must be replaced prior to transfer. If blood gas levels are abnormal, radiologic, anesthesiologic, or chest physician evaluations must be recorded prior to transfer along with the institution of appropriate corrective measures: intubation, chest tube, and so on.

Although prehospital management of the spinal cord injured patient primarily relates to resuscitation and stabilization of the fractured spine and vital signs, two drugs are recommended for administration, in the absence of contraindications, as soon after trauma as possible: mannitol, 20%, 500 ml, and dexamethasone, 50 mg, by intravenous push. The rationale behind their use is the following[9,11,12]: mannitol has been considered to be the most efficacious and the safest diuretic for use in brain trauma victims under controlled situations. In relation to the spinal cord injured victim and assuming that vascular autoregulative reflexes are of the same origin or influenced by those of the brain,[1] mannitol may be effective in reducing cord edema and thereby be effective in reducing the vascular compromise that already exists with swelling and hemorrhage about and within the spinal cord of the victim. Steroid therapy has similarly been used in the head injured patient and has been shown to effectively reduce brain edema and provide a protective influence on the traumatized neuron, enhancing cell membrane integrity and protecting the contained lysosomes. This, in turn, enhances the survival of the traumatized, but not yet destroyed, neural cell. It has been our practice to administer both mannitol and steroids in the overt spinal cord injured victim only when the patient is referred to the Spinal Injury Center within the very early hours after injury. It has also been our rule *not* to administer mannitol and steroids to patients with sustained spine trauma *without* neurologic injury. Of complete neurologically injured patients admitted to the Midwest Regional Spinal Cord Injury Care System between 1972 and 1979,[8] a definite decrease in the number of complete injuries has occurred. What remains a question is whether this occurrence is the result of improved prehospital care (which undoubtedly has been a significant factor) or the use of one or both of these drugs.

The prehospital (trauma center) medical orders recommended to the referring physician and institution therefore are the following:

1. Mannitol, 20%, 500 ml—3- to 4-hour run-in
2. Dexamethasone, 50 mg, by intravenous push: and 10 mg every 6 hours the first day and reduced on a graduated scale over the next 5 days
3. Nasogastric tube to reduce gastric dilation and the possibility of emesis
4. Appropriate cervical splint, such as the Meyer Cervical Orthosis (Fig. 3-7), if available, or appropriate backboard or emergency stretcher with sandbags, adhesive tape, etc.
5. Indwelling catheter to monitor renal function, the need for fluid replacement, or trauma to the urogenital system
6. Nasal oxygen to maintain a high arterial P_{O_2}, particularly in the quadriplegic patient with loss of chest function who is relying only on diaphragmatic function
7. Appropriate antibiotics (intravenously) and human tetanus antisera (Hyper-Tet) prior to transfer if open wounds exist

In the event that respiratory compromise is either present or anticipated, a registered respiratory therapist, emergency room nurse, intensive care unit nurse, physician, or experienced paramedic should accompany the transfer of a high cervical spine injured (C5 and above) patient.

A trauma care facility must have available and in place all of the emergency room services required for managing the most critically injured trauma victim. There must be specific physicians (neurosurgeons, orthopedic surgeons, general surgeons, and anesthesiologist or his delegate) in the emergency room at the time of the patient's arrival. The support services that may be required for immediate injury assessment and patient evaluation include computed tomography (CT); polytomography; somatosensory cortical evoked potential monitor (and operator); surgical suite available on a 24-hour basis; blood capture and readministration capabilities; acute spinal cord injury unit capable of providing acute nursing care (ratio of 1:1 or 1:2) and patient monitoring during the course of the patient's acute hospitalization.

Emergency care of the spinal cord injured victim in actuality is often care of the multitrauma patient, that is, one who has sustained multiple organ system injury. It becomes incumbent therefore for the early management of this kind of patient to be disciplined, rehearsed, and standardized and to be performed by competent and well-trained emergency personnel. To enhance this care process, triage, transfer, and treatment protocols should be developed and in place; specific care facilities should be predesigned in order to expedite early management of the patient with acute trauma.

Once the patient's vital signs have been assessed and airway and vascular resuscitation is ongoing, it becomes paramount to evaluate and record the findings of a carefully executed neurologic examination. Irrespective of the individual performing the examination, it must be exacting because the future care this patient will receive relative to the neurologic injury found will be based on the first (field) neurologic assessment and the emergency room neurologic assessment. If there is no change in the neurologic findings, the patient's care will likely be conservative. On the other hand, in the face of a changing neurologic picture, aggressive care, including surgery, may be indicated.

REFERENCES

1. Fahmy, N. R., Mossad, B., and Milad, M.: Effects of blood pressure on spinal cord blood flow in dogs, Anesthesiology **51**:879, 1979.
2. Hospital resources for optimal care of the injured patient, Bull. Am. Coll. Surgeons **64**(8):43-48, Aug. 1979.
3. Last, R. J.: Innervation of the limbs, J. Bone J. Surg. [Br.] **31**:452, 1949.
4. Lazorthes, G., Gouaze, A., Zadek, J. D., et al.: Arterial vascularization of the spinal cord, J. Neurosurg. **35**:253, 1971.
5. Lusted, L., and Keats, T.: Atlas of roentgenographic measure/variance, ed. 4, Chicago, 1978, Year Book Medical Publishers, pp. 121-122.
6. Meyer, P., Rosen, J., and Hamilton, B.: Annual Progress Report I (1972), Midwest Regional Spinal Cord Injury Care System, OHD-RSA-DHEW Grant no. 13P-55864.
7. Meyer, P., Rosen, J., and Hamilton, B.: Annual Progress Report VII (1978), Midwest Regional Spinal Cord Injury Care System, OHD-RSA-DHEW Grant no. 13P-55864 .
8. Meyer, P. R.: Specialty care units. C. Spinal cord injury. In Manual of the trauma systems development workshops, HRA Contract 232-78-0170, Oct. 1979.
9. Meyer, P. R., Rosen, J. S., Hamilton, B. B., and Hall, W. J.: Fracture-dislocation of the cervical spine: transportation, assessment, and immediate management. In American Academy of Orthopaedic Surgeons: Instructional course lectures, vol. XXV, St. Louis, 1976, The C. V. Mosby Co., pp. 171-183.
10. Teasdale, G., and Jennett, B.: Assessment and prognosis of coma after head injury, Acta Neurochir. (Wien) **34**:45, 1976.
11. White, R. J.: Advances in the treatment of cervical cord injuries, Clin. Neurosurg. **26**(23):556-569, 1979.
12. White, R. J.: Intracranial injuries, New methodology in diagnosis and treatment. In Nykus, L. M., editor: Surgical annual, 1979, Appleton-Century-Crofts, pp. 295-311.

CHAPTER 4

Fractures and dislocations of the spine

LEE F. ROGERS, M.D.

The pattern, frequency, and distribution of spinal injury vary with the age of the patient, with the nature of the patient population served by the reporting institution, and to some extent with the inclusive dates of the injuries reported. It is generally recognized that the distribution of spinal fractures and dislocations varies throughout the entire length of the spine, indicating a variance in susceptibility to injury from segment to segment.[4] There are three peaks of incidence: C1-2, C5-7, and T12-L2[15] (Fig. 4-1). These peaks were first recognized by Jefferson.[54] In children fractures of the cervical spine are less frequent and an appreciable incidence is found in the midthoracic spine and in the upper lumbar spine.[42,49] Formerly the majority of spinal fractures and spinal cord injuries were caused by industrial accidents, particularly mining.[34,45,46,69] These injuries have decreased as safety precautions have been instituted. However, there has been a definite rise in the number of spinal fractures and associated spinal cord injuries,[30] which is attributable to an increase in automobile and other traffic accidents.

Fractures involving adjacent vertebrae are relatively common, particularly in children,[42,43,47] but fractures of widely dispersed segments of the spinal column are generally rare and when found are a manifestation of severe trauma and are often accompanied by spinal cord injury.[15,59,86] Approximately 20% of spinal fractures are associated with fractures elsewhere.[98]

Spinal cord injuries occur in 10% to 14% of spinal fractures and dislocations.[78] The distribution of spinal fractures in those patients who sustain cord injury var-

ies to some extent from the general distribution of spinal fractures given above. There are three peaks of incidence: the lower cervical spine, the thoracolumbar junction, and the midthoracic spine (Fig. 4-2).[15] Injuries of the cervical spine produce neurologic damage in approximately 40% of cases,[17] whereas injuries to the thoracolumbar junction have an incidence of 4%, and those to the thoracic spine have an incidence of approximately 10%. However, in patients sustaining fractures of the vertebral bodies and posterior elements with some degree of malalignment of the spine, the incidence of neurologic deficit is approximately 60%.[14]

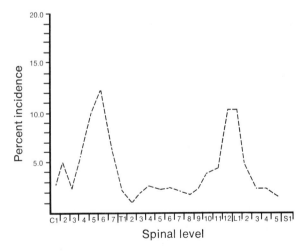

Fig. 4-1. Distribution of nonselected spinal injuries according to Jefferson's series of 2006 cases.[54] Peaks of injury in cervical, thoracolumbar, and craniovertebral junctions.

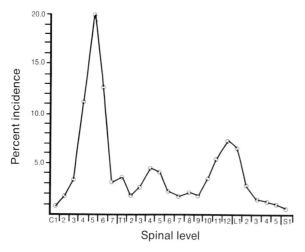

Fig. 4-2. Distribution of spinal injury in 710 patients admitted to the Midwest Regional Spinal Cord Injury Care System. Peaks of injury in cervical, midthoracic, and thoracolumbar junction.

Eighty-five percent of spinal cord injuries occur immediately at the time of trauma, 5% to 10% are late complications, and an alarming 5% to 10% occur in the immediate postinjury period.[83] The last figure is quite likely the result of mishandling of the patient, a very important consideration for all concerned in the care of patients with suspected or proven spinal injury. Ten percent of traumatic cord injuries have no overt radiographic evidence of vertebral injury.[78,88,101] Generally these are older patients with degenerative arthritic changes of the spine who have sustained hyperextension injuries.[72] The spinal cord becomes compressed between the osteophytic spurs on the posterior margin of the vertebral bodies and the hypertrophied ligamentum flavum, resulting in a hematomyelia and an associated neurologic deficit. On occasion, young individuals may sustain a hyperextension injury resulting in a spinal cord injury without an associated fracture or dislocation even in the absence of degenerative changes of the spine.[14]

MECHANISM OF INJURY

Injuries to the spine are the result of indirect forces generated by movement of the head and trunk and are only rarely the result of direct blows to the vertebra. An appreciation of the forces involved in the creation of spinal fractures is a great aid in the assessment of patients who have sustained an injury of the spine. The forces involved are frequently multiple and therefore complex. The combination of flexion, compression, and rotational shearing is particularly common.[45,46,48,80] However, it is of value to consider the potential forces separately since each is associated with a relatively spe-

cific pattern of injury. In general, it can be said that compression forces create fractures, whereas rotational shearing forces disrupt ligaments.

Flexion

Flexion is the most common force operative in spinal injury.[45,46] The fulcrum of flexion movements of the spine is at the anterior portion of the vertebral bodies. Thus the maximal forces are focused here and result in anterior wedging of the vertebral body. As the vertebral bodies are compressed anteriorly, the posterior elements, particularly the spinous processes, laminae, and the intervening ligaments, are placed in tension. These tensile forces may produce ligamentous injuries and fractures of the posterior elements. As the head is flexed on the trunk, the maximal force is focused in the cervical spine on the vertebral bodies of C4 through C7. As the trunk is flexed on itself, the force is focused at the thoracolumbar junction, which accounts for the high percentage of fractures occurring at T12 to L2. The force may be directed either anteriorly or laterally. The anterior flexion forces are directed toward the anterior superior margin and the lateral flexion forces toward the lateral superior margin of the vertebral bodies.

Compression

It is difficult to separate compression forces from flexion forces. It is helpful to think of the vertebrae in a neutral position sustaining a vertical or axial load. The intact vertebrae and intervertebral discs serve as a shock-absorbing mechanism. As the spine is compressed, the major distortion is a bulge of the vertebral end-plate. This bulging causes blood to be squeezed out of the cancellous bone of the vertebral body. As the pressure increases, the end-plate bulges more. If the resilience of the end-plate is exceeded, a concave fracture of the end-plate results. If the compressive forces are even greater, the disc virtually explodes into the vertebral body, creating a comminuted fracture and displacing the fragments centripetally. These have been designated *explosion* or *bursting fractures*.[45,46] In the cervical spine a special variety of this type has been termed a teardrop fracture because of the characteristic appearance of the anterior inferior fragment of the vertebral body.[87] The longitudinal ligaments remain intact, and therefore the fracture is considered stable. However, one of the posterior vertebral body fragments may be displaced into the spinal canal, resulting in cord injury.

Extension

Extension of the head on the trunk creates tension in the anterior longitudinal ligament, which may tear either at the intervertebral disc space or at the margin of a cervical vertebral body avulsing a small fragment from either the anterior superior or anterior inferior margin of the vertebral body.[13,63,65] The posterior elements of the cervical spine are simultaneously compressed, resulting in fractures of the spinous processes, laminae, and facets. Extension plays a very minor role in thoracolumbar fractures. It probably accounts for the fractures of the pars interarticularis and articular processes of the lower lumbar spine that are occasionally encountered.

Rotation

Rotational forces disrupt the interspinous ligaments and fracture the posterior elements, particularly the articular facets, and laminae. The spinal ligaments withstand tensile and compression forces rather well but are very susceptible to disruption by rotation and shearing forces. Rotational forces play a major role in fracture-dislocations of the spine.[45,46]

Shearing

Shearing refers to a horizontal force applied to one portion of the spine relative to the other. The horizontal force may be directed in any direction: anterior, posterior, lateral, or in-between. Shearing forces tend to disrupt ligaments and are frequently operative in fracture-dislocation of the thoracic or lumbar spine. Shearing and rotational forces are frequently combined.

Distraction

Distraction refers to forces that are pulling in opposite directions, the opposite of compression. These tensile forces are operative in cervical and thoracolumbar injuries. The head weighs 4.5 kg (10 lb) and is therefore capable of creating a significant degree of inertia and momentum of force. The momentum of the head is translated into tensile forces within the cervical spine. The direction of the tensile force is directly dependent on the direction of the movement of the head. If the head is moving away from the trunk, this tends to counter or lessen the severity of the compression generated by other simultaneously operating forces, such as flexion or extension, and allows an injury of the interspinous ligaments and displacement of the vertebral body elements without a significant degree of bony injury. Distraction is also operative in transverse fractures and fracture-dislocations of the thoracolumbar spine: injuries that may occur in the absence of vertebral body compression.

RADIOLOGIC INTERPRETATION

The stability of the spinal column is maintained by a combination of bony elements, the vertebrae, and the

ligaments, apophyseal joint capsules, and intervertebral discs.[102] The degree of instability depends on the extent of the disruption and the relative strength of the structures that remain intact.[8,45,46]

The spine is commonly described as consisting of two columns. The anterior column is composed of the vertebral bodies, intervertebral discs, and the anterior and posterior longitudinal ligaments. The posterior column is formed by the facets, apophyseal joints, pedicles, laminae, spinous processes, and all intervening ligaments. If one of the two columns remains intact, the injury is considered stable, if both columns are disrupted, the injury is unstable.

Disruption through bone or soft tissue is equally important in this determination. Since there is no direct radiologic evidence of soft tissue injury, the presence of such injuries must be implied by variations in the alignment of or distance between the bony elements joined by the soft tissue structures in question.[73,74,90,109] It is important to appreciate that at the time of the radiologic examination only the residual displacement between vertebral elements is visualized. At the time of injury there may have been gross displacements that have spontaneously reduced partially or completely, leaving minimal deformities.

Radiologic examination of a potential spinal injury must be tailored to the patient's clinical signs and symptoms. The patient with an obvious neurologic deficit may require only anterioposterior and lateral views of the area in question to sufficiently define a fracture or fracture-dislocation. On the other hand, an acutely injured patient without localizing signs or symptoms will probably require a more complete examination, including oblique projections, in order to identify or exclude a fracture or dislocation. If these examinations should suggest the presence of an injury, it might be necessary to obtain either additional special projections or tomograms in order to clarify or substantiate the lesion in question. On occasion, particularly in the cervical spine, stress views may be necessary; these are lateral views of the cervical spine obtained in flexion and extension. They should never be obtained as a matter of routine. When these are deemed necessary in the acutely injured patient, they should be performed under the immediate supervision of a physician in order to avoid the creation or extension of a neurologic injury.

Tomography

Tomography is used chiefly to verify the presence or absence of fractures and to determine their position; to visualize otherwise obscured areas of the spine, particularly at the craniovertebral and cervicothoracic junction and the upper thoracic spine; and to clarify the status of posterior elements.[16] It is of value in the evaluation of bursting fractures of the vertebral bodies to locate the position of fragments displaced into the spinal canal. Although polytomography with complex motion is preferred,[16,84] standard linear tomography is frequently sufficient. Tomography can be accomplished in all patients including those with spinal injury by judicious handling. Careful transfer to the examining table is accomplished by a minimum of three assistants. Examinations may be obtained while the patient remains in cervical traction by attaching a pulley to the examination table.[19] All life-support systems can be maintained during the examination.

Because of the cross-sectional display, computed tomography (CT) offers a unique opportunity to evaluate fractures by precisely localizing fracture fragments in relation to the spinal canal and demonstrating otherwise obscure fractures of the posterior elements.[18,21,93,100] Although CT affords an exceptional and, in many ways, a better view of any given vertebra, the important relationship between adjacent vertebrae is better demonstrated and more easily appreciated with standard tomography. Reconstruction of images in the sagittal and coronal planes is becoming more available and should improve the information obtainable by computed tomography.

THE CERVICAL SPINE

The initial radiograph of a patient seriously suspected of an injury to the cervical spine should be a horizontal-beam lateral view. *Be certain that this includes all*

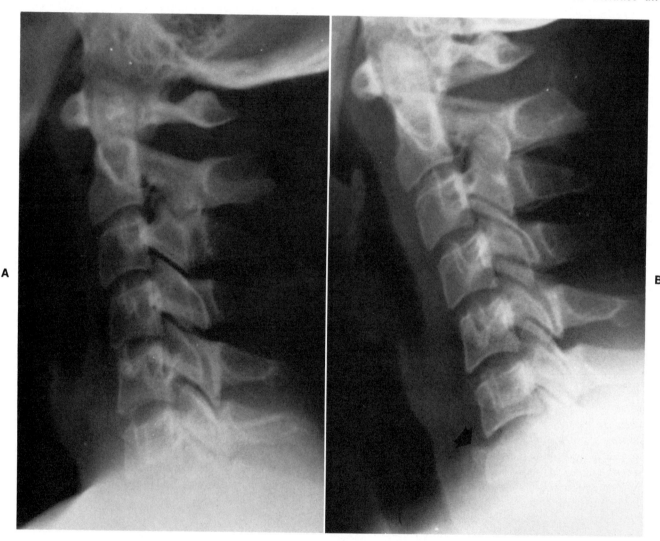

Fig. 4-3. Twenty-one-year-old man who dove into a shallow pool. **A,** Note that on this lateral radiograph only six cervical vertebrae are visualized and there is no apparent injury. **B,** Repeat examination was obtained with traction on arms, and compression fracture of seventh cervical vertebra is now demonstrated. Note small triangular fragment (*arrow*) at its anterosuperior margin.

seven cervical vertebrae.[31,39,40,50] Injuries of C6 and C7 are quite common but are easily overlooked if these vertebrae are not included on the lateral radiograph (Fig. 4-3). They are frequently obscured by the overlying shoulders. Pulling down on the arms by holding the wrists improves the visualization. If this should fail, the swimmer's projection should be obtained. To do so, one arm of the patient is extended over the head while the other arm remains by the side. This places the upper torso in a slightly oblique projection and allows visualization of the cervicothoracic junction. Ultimately it may prove necessary to resort to tomography to demonstrate the lower cervical vertebral bodies. Next, an anteroposterior view of the spine and an open-mouth view of the atlas and axis (C1 and C2) should be obtained. All of these radiographs must be reviewed in sequence to exclude an overt injury before the decision is made to move the patient for the purposes of obtaining oblique projections or other additional radiographs. It is possible to obtain oblique radiographs of the patient while in the supine projection.[1] These are obtained by angling the tube 30° from the horizontal plane and placing a nongrid cassette flat on the table adjacent to the patient's neck on the side opposite the tube. Flexion and extension views in the acutely injured patient should only be taken under the immediate supervision of the physician. The standard cervical spine series consist of five projections: lateral, anteroposterior (AP), open-mouth, and right and left oblique.

Radiologic interpretation

Changes in the retropharyngeal soft tissue represent important clues to underlying hemorrhage or edema and are therefore indirect signs of cervical spinal injury.[31,36] The width of the retropharyngeal soft tissues anterior to the spine at C3-4 should not exceed 4 mm (Fig. 4-4, *A*). The width of the soft tissue anterior to C6, the retrotracheal space, should not exceed 14 mm in children and 22 mm in adults. Swelling of the nasopharyngeal soft tissues is an important clue to injuries of C1 and C2.[25] There are no normal measurements established for the width of the soft tissue in the nasopharynx. The presence of adenoidal tissue in the child makes this determination more difficult in the younger population than in the adult.

Very serious injuries may be manifested by seemingly minor degrees of malalignment (Fig. 4-4). On the lateral view four separate gentle anteriorly convex lines are formed by joining the anterior margins of the vertebral bodies, the posterior margins of the vertebral bodies, and the anterior margin of the spinous processes at their junction with the laminae and finally at their junction with the posterior tips of the spinous processes.[31,39,40] Any abrupt reversal in angulation or disruption of these lines should alert the observer to the possibility of an underlying injury.

It is particularly important to evaluate the width of the intervertebral disc spaces. Trauma to the intervertebral disc is manifested by a decrease in the height of the disc space. This may be subtle. Recognition depends on the observation that the involved disc space is narrower than the adjacent intervertebral disc spaces above and below the space in question. Disruption of the disc is often associated with a minimal degree of subluxation, on the order of 1 to 2 mm.

The distance between the spinous processes, the interspinous distance, of the cervical spine is an important clue to injuries of the interspinous ligaments and therefore the posterior column. Widening of the interspinous distance can be demonstrated on either the lateral or frontal view. At times the spinous processes are not well visualized on the initial lateral radiograph. Rotational displacement is demonstrated by lateral displacements of the spinal processes to the affected side as visualized on the anteroposterior projection.

Craniovertebral junction (C1-2)

The atlas and axis are structurally and functionally distinct from the remaining cervical vertebrae.[44] The atlas, or C1, is a ring structure consisting of two lateral articular masses joined by thin anterior and posterior arches. The lateral articular masses contain the superior and inferior facets. A thin transverse process extends from each lateral articular mass and contains a foramen through which passes the vertebral artery. The superior facets of the atlas articulate with the occipital condyles and the inferior articular facets articulate with the superior articular facets of the axis. The axis, or C2, consists of a vertebral body on which is situated a bony protrusion, the dens. The dens articulates with the anterior arch of the axis. The superior articular facets of the axis are broad, sloping surfaces on the superior surface of the pedicles and vertebral body just lateral to the dens. The pedicles of the axis are pierced by the foramina transversaria traversing superiorly and posterolaterally. The foramina divide the pedicles into two short segments, one thin and more variable segment located anteriorly and inferiorly and a more substantial segment located posteriorly and superiorly. The posterior segments form broad bases with the laminae. The laminae are broadened on their inferior margins to form the inferior articular facets.

The peculiar bony structure at the craniovertebral junction is associated with its own unique ligamentous structure. Broad ligamentous structures extend from the anteroposterior surfaces of the spinal canal to the margins of the foramen magnum. The dens is attached to the anterior margin of the foramen magnum by three

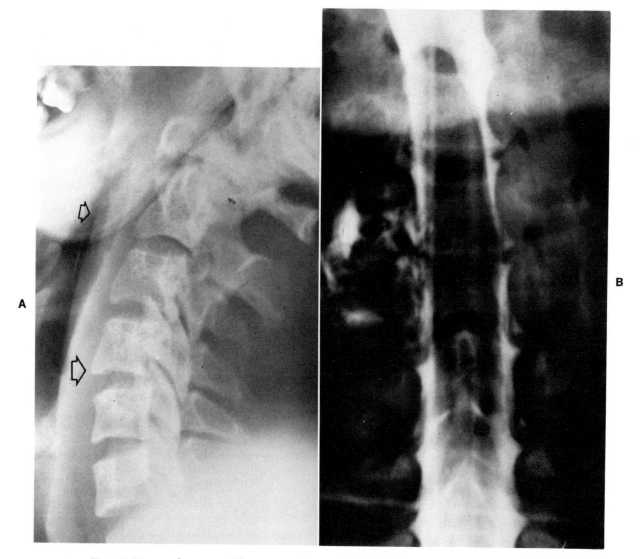

Fig. 4-4. Twenty-three-year-old man injured in an auto accident with resultant quadriplegia. **A,** Initial lateral radiograph demonstrates retropharyngeal soft tissue swelling anterior to upper cervical vertebral body *(top arrow).* Note very subtle degree of subluxation at C4-5 interspace. The fourth vertebral body *(bottom arrow)* is slightly anterior to the fifth. **B,** Myelogram demonstrates widening of cord indicative of hematomyelia, and there is extravasation of Pantopaque into soft tissues of right side of neck, indicative of dural tear.

separate ligaments, one apical and two alar ligaments, each extending from the right and left lateral surfaces of the dens. A tough ligament, the transverse ligament or ligamentum transversarium, extends between the lateral articular masses of C1. The dens lies between this ligament and the anterior arch of the atlas.

These peculiar structural arrangements confer a great range of rotation, flexion, and extension on the cranium relative to the cervical spine.[25] The fulcrum of flexion and extension of the cranium on the neck lies at the second cervical vertebra. The weight of the cranium is transmitted through the occipital condyles and atlas to the superior articular facets of the axis. It is then divided into three portions and transmitted inferiorly: anteriorly through the vertebral bodies and intervertebral discs and posteriorly through the pedicles onto the inferior articular facet and from there to the other apophyseal joints. In a properly positioned radiograph, in the neutral position, C1 sits squarely on C2 without offset; that is, the lateral margin of the lateral articular mass of C1 lies exactly opposite the opposing lateral margin of C2.[31,40,52,53] The distance between the medial margin of the lateral articular mass of C1 and the dens is symmetric. With rotation or abduction of the head

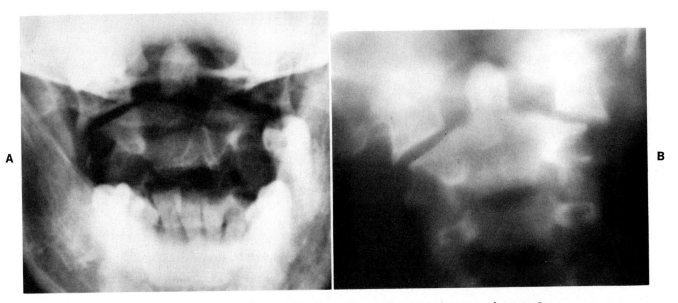

Fig. 4-5. Forty-four-year-old woman who sustained an injury in a diving accident. **A,** Open-mouth view demonstrates lateral displacement of both lateral masses of C1 that overhang body of C2. Distance between medial margin of articular mass of C1 and dens is considerably increased. **B,** Tomogram demonstrates radiologic findings to excellent advantage. Note lateral displacement of articular masses at C1 bilaterally such that they project beyond lateral border of C2.

C1 moves as a unit toward the side to which the head is rotated or abducted. The lateral articular mass of C1 is then offet laterally toward the side of this motion, and the distance between the medial margin and the lateral mass and the dens increases on this side. On the opposite side there is a corresponding medial offset of the lateral articular mass of C1 and an abbreviation of the distance between the medial borders of the lateral mass of the dens. This produces a unilateral offset. Usually this is of the magnitude of 1 to 2 mm, rarely up to 4 mm.

Fractures of the craniovertebral junction are rarely the result of direct trauma. They usually occur as the result of forces transmitted through the cranium and its contents. The nature of the resultant injury depends on the amount and direction of the force and the relative position of the head and neck. From the clinical standpoint fractures and dislocations at the craniovertebral junction are rarely associatd with permanent neurologic deficits. Transient paresis may occur. However, postmortem examinations of individuals who died in automobile and other traffic accidents have demonstrated an appreciable incidence of such injuries.[2] There is no discrepancy between these two statements since a neurologic deficit at this level, in most situations, would lead to immediate death. With immediate rescucitation it is possible that an occasional patient with a high spinal cord transection may survive.

The important radiographs in the evaluation of craniovertebral injuries are the anteroposterior open-mouth projection and the lateral view of the cervical spine. Tomography is frequently required for a full clarification of the abnormalities (Figs. 4-5, 4-7, and 4-8). Before all injuries can be safely excluded it may be necessary to obtain tomograms in both the anteroposterior and lateral projections. Many injuries at the craniovertebral junction are only minimally displaced and therefore may be overlooked if the examination is not done in both projections. These injuries are frequently associated with soft tissue swelling in the retropharynx and nasopharynx.

The atlas (C1). The most common fracture of C1 is a bilateral vertical fracture through the neural arch.[92,94] It is caused by hyperextension of the head on the neck, which compresses the neural arch of C1 between the occiput and the neural arch of C2. It is best demonstrated on the lateral view. Characteristically, because of the ligamentous attachments, there is minimal displacement but there may be some angulation at the fracture site. It carries no risk of neurologic deficit. This fracture must be distinguished from developmental defects. These vary from a complete absence of the posterior neural arch to short segmental defects located laterally, which might be mistaken for fractures. The margins of these defects are rounded and consist of cortical bone. In addition, the opposing portions of the neural arch at the defect are often slightly tapered.

Horizontal fractures of the anterior arch of the atlas have been described. These are characteristically minimally displaced, are best visualized on the frontal view, and are often associated with fractures of the ends. Horizontal fractures are caused by an avulsion mediated through the tendinous ligamentous insertion on the anterior tubercle by the anterior longitudinal ligament and the longus colli muscle.

A Jefferson fracture[71,92] is a comminuted fracture of the ring, involving both the anterior and posterior arches (Figs. 4-5 and 4-7). This allows centripetal displacement of the fragments. Bursting fractures of the ring of the atlas have been designated *Jefferson fractures* in recognition of Sir Geoffrey Jefferson,[54] a British neurosurgeon who in 1919 first described the mechanism of injury. The Jefferson fracture is created by blows on the vertex. The force is transmitted from the cranium to the cervical spine through the occipital condyles. The lateral articular masses of the atlas become compressed between the occipital condyles and the superior articular facets of the axis. The lateral articular masses of C1 are wedge-shaped. The superior articular facets of the atlas slope inward and the inferior articular facets slope outward. Therefore, as the occipital condyles are driven toward the axis, the lateral articular masses of the atlas are displaced laterally. The weaker segments of the atlas, the anterior and posterior arches, are stressed and finally broken, disrupting the ring and forcing the lateral articular masses of the atlas to spread apart. Most Jefferson fractures are the result of automobile accidents. Blows to the vertex and falls in which the individual strikes his head account for the remainder. The most significant findings are on the frontal projections of the atlas and axis. The crucial observation is the bilateral offset or spreading of the lateral articular masses of C1 in relation to the opposing articular surfaces of C2 (Fig. 4-5, *A*). Frontal tomograms may aid in this demonstration (Fig. 4-5, *B*). It is difficult to visualize the lines of fracture, but their presence may be implied by lateral displacement of the lateral masses relative to the peripheral margins of the superior facet of C2, as visualized on the frontal projection. Occasionally the fractures are demonstrated on the lateral projection. The demonstration of these fractures is not an absolute necessity. Bilateral offset or spreading of the lateral articular masses is sufficient for the diagnosis. At times fracture lines may not even be demonstrated by tomography. Computed tomography has been shown to demonstrate the fracture quite well.[100] (See Fig. 5-1, *A*.)

The axis (C2). Fractures of the neural arch of the axis are among the most common injuries of the cervical spine. They are the result of acute hyperextension of the head on the neck.

The full force of an acute hyperextension of the head on the neck is transmitted through the pedicles of C2 onto the apophyseal joints. The weakest points in this chain are the interarticular segments of the pedicle. Thus the arch of C2 is fractured anterior to the inferior facet. The anterior longitudinal ligament is placed under tension and is disrupted. These injuries are commonly sustained in an automobile accident as the chin or forehead encounters the steering wheel or dashboard, forcing the head into hyperextension.[25] This injury is identical to that created by judicial hanging, thus the designation *hangman's fracture*.[25,91] The fracture is usually associated with an anterior subluxation of C2 on C3. This may be difficult to identify or recognize on the radiograph.[56,99] It is difficult to visualize the fracture on the anteroposterior view. The injury is best demonstrated on the lateral view (Fig. 4-6). The atlantoaxial joint and dens are intact. The fractures of the neural arch of the axis are often anterior to the inferior facets (Fig. 4-6, *A*). They are oblique, extending from superior posteriorly to inferior anteriorly. The fractures may be symmetric but usually vary slightly in obliqueness and relative anteroposterior position. When the bilateral fractures of the neural arch are symmetric, they are easily visualized because of the resultant overlap, but they may be difficult to see when they are in different portions of the arch on each side (Fig. 4-6, *B*). Oblique views may demonstrate the fracture of the neural arch to good advantage. Tomograms are of definite value in questionable cases. An avulsion fracture of the anterior inferior margin of the axis or anterior superior margin at C3 is often present and identifies the site of rupture of the anterior longitudinal ligament. The ligament may rupture at the level of the C2-4 interspace, and therefore no avulsion fracture occurs. At times these may be an associated fracture of the neural arch of C1. There is a surprising paucity of neurologic findings in these fractures when encountered in the clinical situation. However, in a postmortem study of head and neck injuries in fatal traffic accidents, Alker and co-workers[2] did find that this was the most frequent fracture of the cervical spine. A transient hyperextension may result in fracture without neurologic deficit. If the force is sustained following the creation of the fracture the cord is susceptible to transection as is seen in judicial hanging.

Fractures of the odontoid process[3,5,85] are often difficult to visualize because of minimal displacement (Figs. 4-7 and 4-8). The fracture is most frequently transverse and located at the base of the dens at its junction with the body (Fig. 4-7). On occasion fractures of the tip of the odontoid process occur. These are avulsion fractures mediated through the attached apical or alar liga-

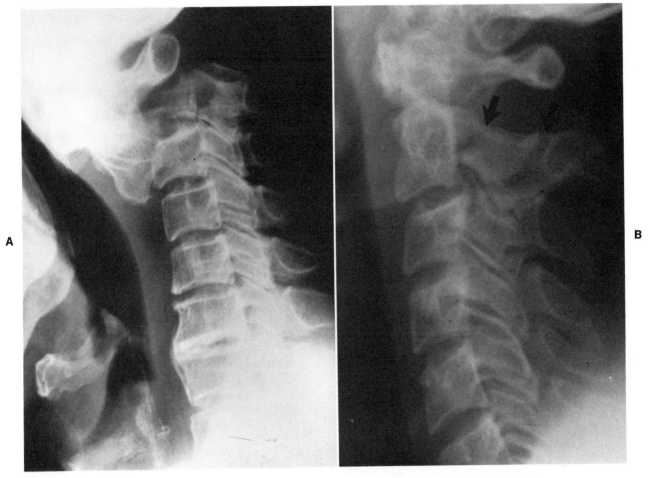

Fig. 4-6. Hangman's fractures. **A,** Seventy-seven-year-old alcoholic was first seen in emergency room without neurologic deficit despite marked displacement of bilateral fractures of neural arch of axis. **B,** Thirty-five-year-old man who sustained a neck injury in an automobile accident. Bilateral fractures (*arrows*) of neural arch of axis are asymmetric and not easily visualized. Note subtle nature of subluxation of C2 on C3.

ments. Oblique fractures extending into the body of the axis either anteriorly or posteriorly are also encountered (Fig. 4-8). The dens is most frequently displaced anteriorly but may be displaced in any direction. The fragments are rarely distracted more than 2 or 3 mm. The diagnosis depends primarily on the radiographic findings in the anteroposterior projection. On the lateral projections, soft tissue swelling will be seen anterior in the nasopharynx and retropharyngeal tissues (Fig. 4-8, *A*), but minimal displacement usually precludes demonstration of the fracture line in this projection. Tomography may have to be performed (Figs. 4-7 *C*, and 4-8, *B* and *C*) in both the anteroposterior and lateral projections in order to demonstrate the fracture. The lateral projection is utilized to demonstrate the oblique fractures of the base of the odontoid process that extend into the body of the vertebra (Fig. 4-8, *C*).

The transverse fracture at the base of the dens must

be differentiated from a developmental abnormality termed an *os odontoideum*. The latter is rounded, has a cortical margin around its entire surface, and is usually more widely separated from the base of the odontoid process than is a fracture. Admittedly at times this distinction may be difficult. This is further complicated by the fact that nonunion of this type of fracture is rather frequent in the adult and when the ossicle is closely approximated with the base of the odontoid process and is normal in shape with a smooth inferior cortical margin, it may be impossible to distinguish this categorically from an old ununited fracture. Dens fractures are infrequent in children,[89] but occasionally an apophyseal separation is encountered. This involves the synchondrosis between the ossification centers of the dens and the body.

Fractures of the dens are occasionally associated with atlantoaxial dislocations[24] and fractures of C1[62] (Fig. 4-

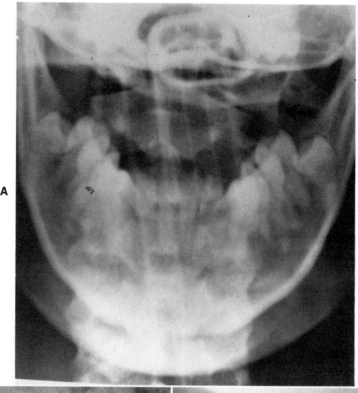

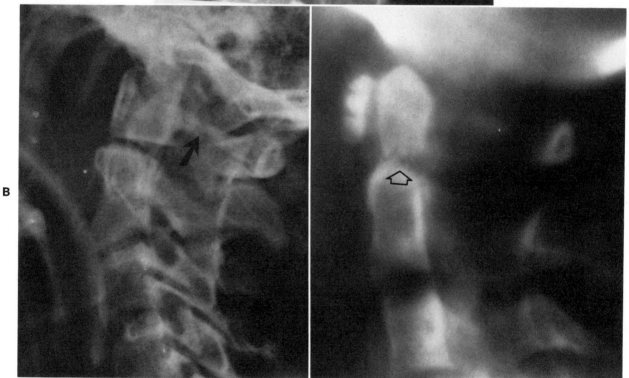

Fig. 4-7. Twenty-year-old man who was injured in an automobile accident and became immediately quadriplegic. There is a Jefferson fracture of C1 and a fracture at base of odontoid process. **A,** Frontal view of cervical spine demonstrates lateral displacement of left articular mass of C1 *(arrow)*. Base of odontoid process is not visualized. **B,** Lateral view demonstrates soft tissue swelling anterior to cervical spine, and there is a suggestion of transverse fracture at base of odontoid process. Fracture of neural arch of C1 is also demonstrated *(arrow)*. **C,** Lateral tomogram demonstrates fracture at base of odontoid process *(arrow)*.

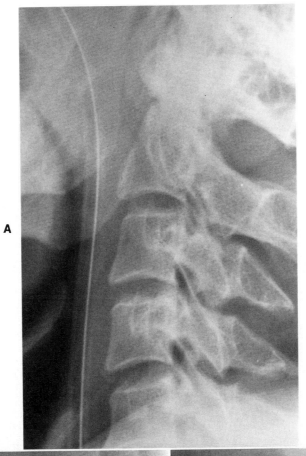

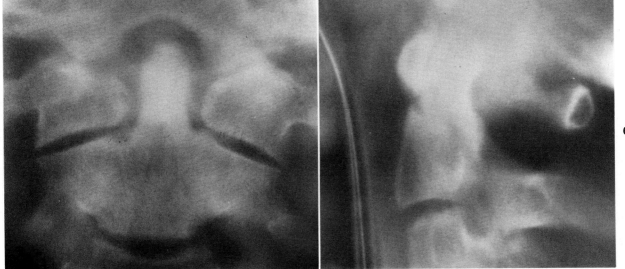

Fig. 4-8. Fifty-two-year-old man who became immediately quadriplegic after an automobile accident. He sustained an oblique fracture to base of odontoid process, which extended into body of second cervical vertebra. **A,** Lateral view of cervical spine demonstrates no definite abnormality. Soft tissue swelling is present in nasopharynx. **B,** Frontal tomogram fails to demonstrate any evidence of fracture. **C,** Lateral tomogram demonstrates oblique fracture across base of dens extending into vertebral body posteriorly. There is slight posterior displacement of odontoid fragment.

7), are usually fractures of the posterior neural arch, but may also be associated with fractures of the anterior arch and Jefferson fractures. Since fractures of the dens are often not readily apparent, it is important to specifically look for an associated fracture of the dens when faced with a fracture of C1 or an atlantoaxial dislocation.

Isolated fractures of the anterior inferior margin of C2 occur. The avulsion is mediated through tension in the anterior longitudinal ligament. At times, a similar lesion occurs at C3 or in any of the other cervical vertebral bodies. The injury is caused by hyperextension, and the resultant fracture has been termed the *hyper-*

extension teardrop. Since this fracture is frequently a component of a hangman's fracture, it is important to determine that the neural arch of C2 is intact before making the definitive diagnosis of a hyperextension teardrop fracture.

Dislocations and subluxations involving the craniovertebral junction. The anterior atlantoaxial dislocation is the most common. This is usually associated with rheumatoid arthritis or its variants and is rarely caused by trauma. Traumatic dislocations do occur, however. In the arthritides the dislocation or subluxation is caused by laxity of the transverse ligament of the atlas. In traumatic subluxation or dislocation the ligament is

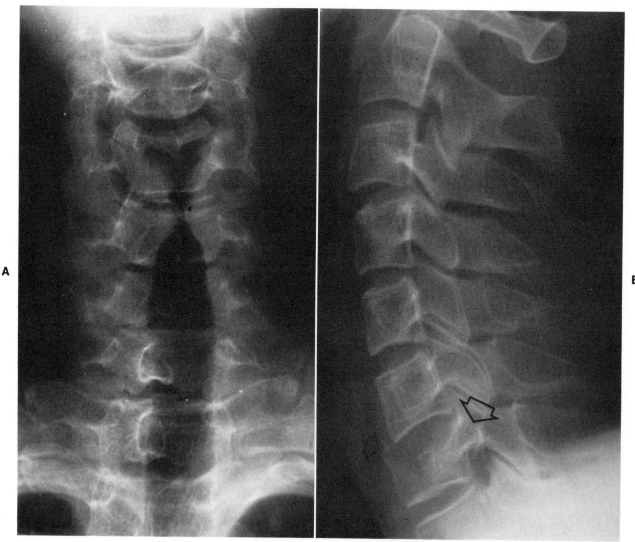

Fig. 4-9. Seventeen-year-old adolescent injured in an automobile accident. There was no neurologic deficit, but there was a bursting fracture of C7. **A,** Frontal view of cervical spine. There is no obvious fracture demonstrated. **B,** Lateral view of cervical spine. There is obvious compression fracture involving superior end-plate of seventh vertebral body. Note very small anterior fragment *(small arrow)* and questionable fragment *(large arrow)* at posterior margin of compressed vertebral body.

disrupted. This is presumed to be caused by a combination of hyperflexion and shearing. The normal measurement between the anterior cortex of the dens and the posterior cortex of the anterior arch of the atlas is 2.5 mm in adults and 5 mm in children. Measurements in excess of these dimensions are indicative of an atlantoaxial subluxation. The injury is demonstrated on the lateral projection and may not be evident with the spine in neutral position or in extension. Flexion may be necessary to disclose the subluxation.

Atlanto-occipital dislocations occur but are almost invariably fatal.[2] The spine is usually displaced posteriorly. This results in a disruption of the medulla oblongata and immediate death. A posterior atlanto-occipital dislocation with survival has been reported.[28] Posterior dislocation of the atlas on the axis, C1 on C2, has been reported.[38] In this injury the anterior arch of the atlas comes to rest against the posterior surface of the dens. These abnormalities are easily demonstrated on the lateral view of the spine.

It is reasonable to ask how anyone could sustain any of the various fractures and dislocations of the craniovertebral junction without sustaining a neurologic injury. The spinal cord occupies only 50% of the spinal canal at this level. This in itself affords some margin of safety. It is then possible to reduce the dimensions of the spinal canal by 50% without necessarily injuring the spinal cord. At C1 approximately one third of the ring is occupied by the dens and its associated ligaments, one third by the spinal cord, and the remaining third by the subarachnoid space, meninges, and epidural fat. In spite of the presence of the dens there still is a 50% margin of safety at C1. Therefore when a dislocation occurs, provided there is no more than a 50% reduction in the dimension of the spinal canal, no neurologic injury need occur. Fractures of the ring of the atlas, either the posterior arch or Jefferson fractures or hangman's fractures of C2 actually increase the width of the spinal canal by displacement of the fragments. In the Jefferson fracture the fragments are centripetally displaced, and in fractures of the posterior arch of C1 and of the neural arch of C2 as encountered in hangman's fractures, the fragments are posteriorly displaced to some extent; this in effect increases the dimensions of the spinal canal, and thus neurologic injury is avoided.

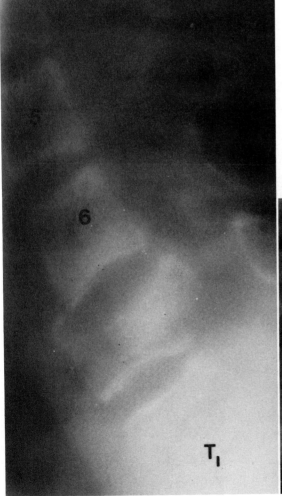

C

Fig. 4-9, cont'd. C, Lateral tomogram demonstrates bursting fracture of vertebral body. Note posteriorly displaced fragment within spinal canal. **D,** Computed tomography also demonstrates to excellent advantage the compromise of spinal canal by posteriorly displaced vertebral body fragment. (Courtesy Michael A. Mikhael, M.D., Evanston Hospital.)

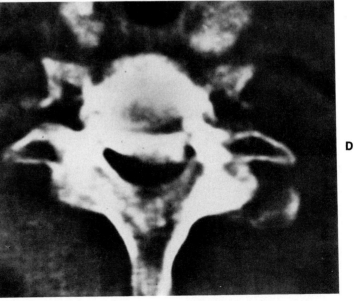

D

Vertebral body fractures of the cervical spine

Variations in vertebral body height consist of varying degrees of anterior wedging with or without comminution of the vertebral body.[6,22] The height of the fourth or fifth vertebral body or both may be less than that of the adjacent third and sixth vertebral bodies. This decrease is generalized without associated wedging and is a normal variant. If the anterior height of a vertebral body is 3 or more mm less than the posterior vertebral body height, a fracture of the vertebral body can be assumed. Anterior wedging of the vertebra results from varying combinations of flexion and axial compression. The wedge is formed predominantly by a depression of the superior end-plate (Figs. 4-3 and 4-9). If a pure flexion force is operative, a simple wedge fracture occurs. At times this may be accompanied by a small triangular fragment from the anterior superior surface of the vertebral body (Figs. 4-3 *B*, and 4-9, *B* and *C*). When axial compression forces predominate, the intervertebral disc is driven into the vertebral body below and the vertebral body explodes into several fragments.

This is termed a *bursting fracture* (Fig. 4-9). It is important to realize that these fragments are driven centripetally and quite frequently a fragment from the posterior superior surface of the involved vertebra is driven into the spinal canal (Fig. 4-9, *C* and *D*). This frequently results in spinal cord injury. It may be difficult, if not impossible, to visualize this posteriorly displaced fragment on the plain radiograph. When faced with a severely comminuted or markedly compressed vertebra, tomography should be done to exclude or identify the commonly associated posteriorly displaced fragment in the spinal canal (Fig. 4-9, *C* and *D*).

The teardrop fracture is a specific form of the bursting fracture described by Schneider and Kahn.[8] The injury is a fracture-dislocation consisting of a comminuted fracture of a vertebral body with a characteristic triangular or quadrilateral fragment from the anterior inferior margin of the vertebral body, the teardrop (Fig. 4-10). The fracture is usually accompanied by a spinal cord injury and was thus termed the *teardrop fracture*. The posterior portion of the vertebral body is displaced

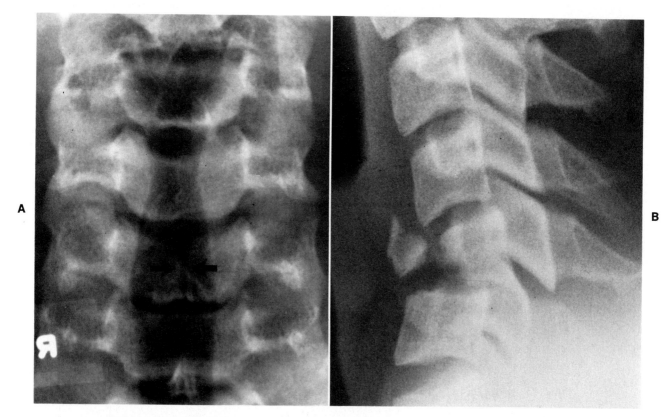

Fig. 4-10. Teardrop fracture in 17-year-old adolescent with quadriplegia. **A,** Anteroposterior projection of cervical spine, which demonstrates vertical sagittal fracture of C5 *(arrows)*. **B,** Lateral view of cervical spine demonstrates classic teardrop fracture with anterior fragment and posterior displacement of C5 on C6 with compromise of canal. Note also widened interspinous distance between C5 and C6 and associated disruption of apophyseal joints at same level.

into the spinal canal. Often there are associated fractures of the spinous processes or disruptions of the interspinous ligaments. On the anteroposterior projection there is frequently a vertical sagittal split in the affected vertebra (Fig. 4-10, A), and at times there is a similar fracture in the superiorly adjacent vertebral body.

On occasion a vertical split of the vertebral body may be seen without other associated abnormalities.[66,77,95] This is caused by predominantly compressive forces in the sagittal plane. It is thought to be created by an acute herniation of the intervertebral disc into the vertebral body below. The fracture line is only apparent on the frontal projection and may easily be mistaken for air in the larynx. The vertebra is split in the sagittal plane into almost equal halves. The slight separation of these fragments widens the interpedicular distance in the involved vertebra.

Isolated avulsion fractures of the anterior inferior margins of the vertebral bodies may occur. These are caused by hyperextension and most commonly affect C2. Small avulsion fractures of the anterior inferior surface of the vertebral body or of an osteophytic spur often accompany spinal cord injuries resulting from hyperextension. Indeed, such fractures may be the only radiologic evidence of injury in these patients.

Dislocation and fracture-dislocation of the cervical spine

When a vertebral body is displaced anteriorly such that 50% or more of the vertebral body overrides the vertebral body below, there is practically always an associated bilateral locking of the facets.[7,41] This injury is caused by flexion combined with distraction forces, which results in ligamentous disruption. The apophyseal joints at the affected level are completely disrupted, allowing the superiorly located vertebra to displace anteriorly to such a degree that the facets become locked in a position anterior to the facets of the vertebral body below. This requires at least a 50% displacement of one vertebral body on the other (Fig. 4-11, A). The spinal canal is, of course, severely compromised by this displacement, and spinal cord injuries are frequent.

A displacement of 50% or less of one vertebra on the other is usually caused by a unilateral locking of the facets (Figs. 4-11, B, and 4-12, B):[7,12,41] This injury is caused by a combination of flexion, distraction, and rotation, resulting in a unilateral displacement and locking of the facet joints.[103] The radiologic clue to this injury on the lateral view rests with the recognition that the articular pillars are visualized in the true lateral profile above the injury but are in the oblique profile below the injury or vice versa.[39,53] On the anteroposterior view the spinous processes are displaced toward the affected side at the level of injury (Fig. 4-12, A).

Because the spinal canal is much less compromised by a unilateral rotational displacement, spinal cord injuries are less frequent. The degree of anterior displacement may be decreased by an associated fracture of the affected facet. Such fractures usually involve the posterior margin of the anteriorly displaced facet. The fragment does not displace with the remainder of the articular pillar, and therefore there is less rotational displacement.

The facet joints may be disrupted and subluxated with minimal displacement. On the lateral view the articular pillars are not properly seated, but the displacement is insufficient for facet locking. It is usually accompanied by an anterior angulation of the spine at the involved interspace and widening of the interspinous distance between the affected vertebrae. The affected intervertebral disc is often wedge shaped, being slightly decreased in height anteriorly and increased in height posteriorly. This is often accompanied by a minimal anterior subluxation of the vertebral body at the affected interspace. Abel[1] has referred to this displacement as *sagging* and has found it to be highly suggestive of instability of the posterior elements.

The phrase *delayed traumatic dislocation of the cervical spine* has been utilized to describe cases wherein the initial radiographs are normal but some degree of subluxation is identified on a subsequent examination.[58] These are actually nothing more than ligamentous disruptions of the cervical spine that were either not demonstrated or not recognized on the initial radiographs but that later are accentuated when the spine is either intentionally or inadvertently placed in some displacement degree of flexion.

All of the ligamentous structures between two adjacent vertebrae may be disrupted without associated bony injury. The radiologic manifestation of these severe injuries may be alarmingly subtle and easily overlooked despite the severity of the injury and its resultant instability (Fig. 4-4). Gross instability is often first demonstrated after the patient is placed in cranial tongs and the vertebrae become widely separated despite the use of only 4.5 to 6.8 kg (10 to 15 lb) of traction. The only way to avoid error is to be suspicious of seemingly minor variations in alignment.

Fractures of the posterior elements. Isolated fractures of the spinous processes of the lower cervical and upper thoracic spine[68] occur as a result of rotation of the trunk relative to the head and neck. These are known as *clay shoveler's fractures*, having been first described in men involved in that activity. Fractures of the spinous process may also occur as a result of extension. In extension the neural arches of the spinous processes are compressed against each other and may fracture.[27]

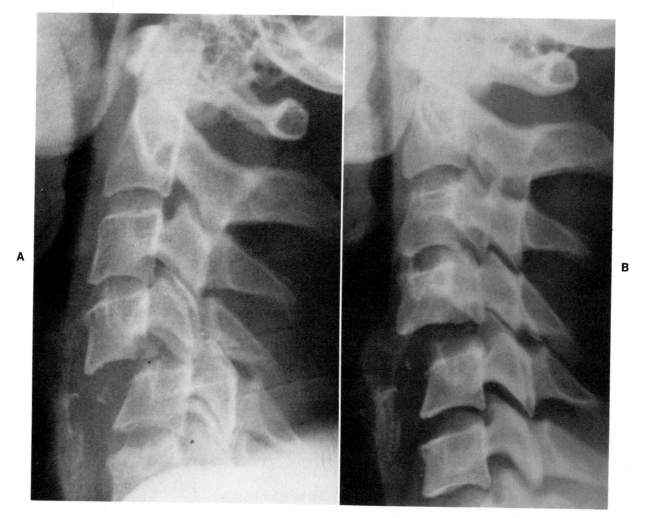

Fig. 4-11. Thirty-one-year-old man who sustained a fracture-dislocation of C4-5 in an automobile accident. He was immediately paraplegic. There is bilateral locking of facets. **A,** Initial lateral radiograph demonstrates marked anterior displacement of C4 on C5. Inferior facet lies anterior to superior facet of C5. Note associated fracture of inferior posterior aspect of fourth vertebral body. **B,** After application of cranial traction, bilateral facet locking was converted to unilateral facet lock. Vertebral body of C4 remains anteriorly dislocated approximately 25% the width of the vertebral body, which is characteristic of a unilateral facet lock. Note that vertebral bodies at C5 and below are seen in true lateral profile whereas those at C4 and above are seen in oblique profile. This is characteristic of unilateral facet lock.

Fractures of the articular pillars and facets[6] occur as a result of the compressive forces associated with hyperextension (Fig. 4-13, *C*). Unilateral fractures result from lateral bending. These are frequently difficult to visualize.[68] On both the anteroposterior and oblique projections the lateral margin of the articular pillars presents a smooth, undulating surface. Any cortical disruption or break in this line may indicate a fracture. The articular pillars normally lay at a 25° to 30° angle with the horizontal plane, and therefore when normally situated, the articular surfaces of the facets cannot be visualized in profile on any radiograph utilizing a perpendicular central ray. The fractured articular pillar or facet is frequently rotated such that it becomes horizontal and its articular surface is readily visualized on the standard frontal projection (Fig. 4-13, *C*). The articular pillars and facets of C3 through C7 are best demonstrated by anteroposterior views obtained with 20° to 30° of caudad angulation of the central ray. These are known as *pillar views*. This allows a profile view of the articular pillars, and laminae and fractures involving these structures can be more easily visualized. The fractures are variable in appearance. There may be a vertical or horizontal fracture line, compression with

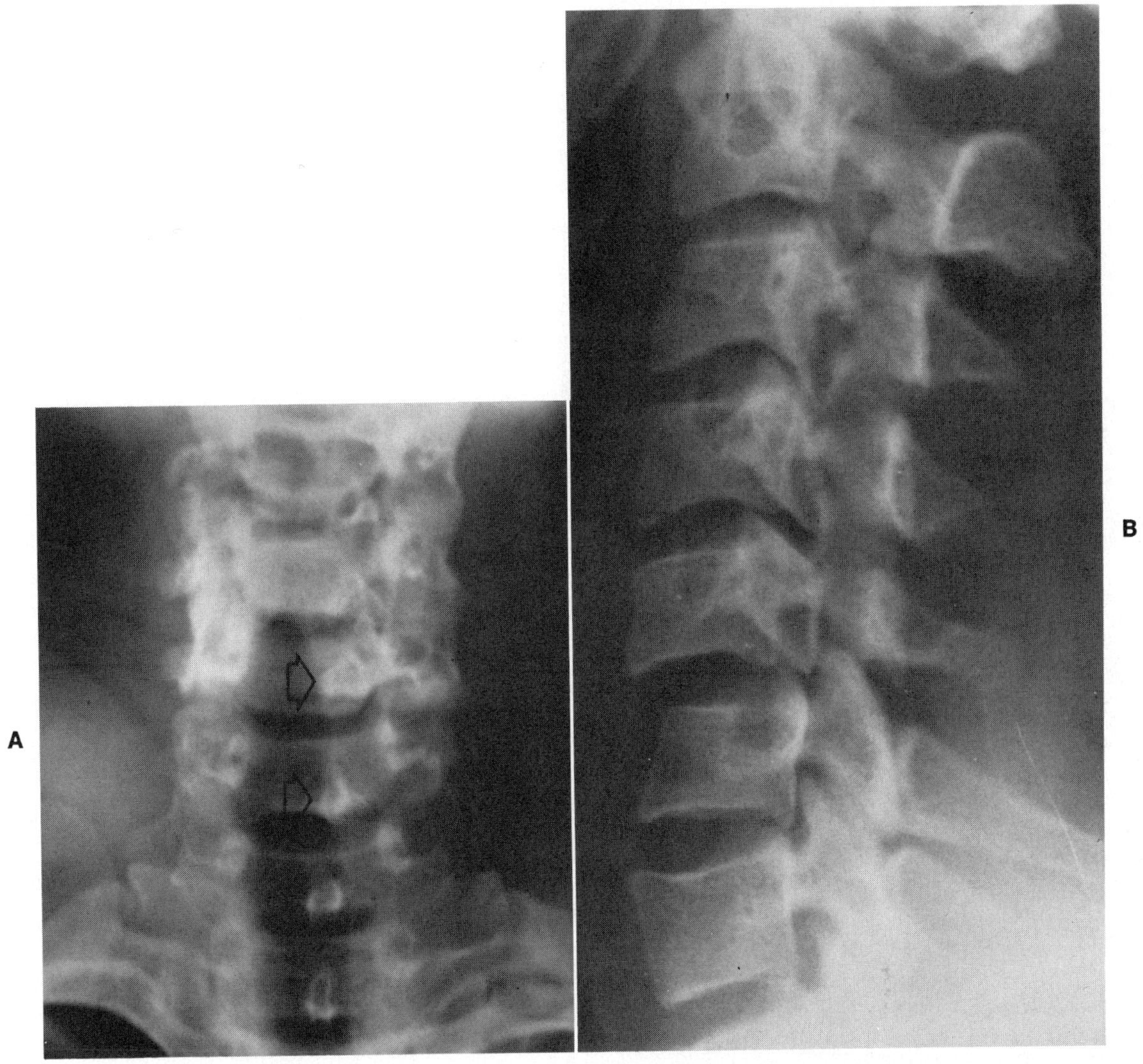

Fig. 4-12. Twenty-six-year-old man who fell from a second-floor window and sustained a unilateral rotary dislocation of facet at C5-6. There was no neurologic deficit. **A,** AP projection of cervical spine demonstrates displacement of spinous processes *(arrows)* to left of midline in keeping with rotation. It is left facet that is dislocated at C5-6 level. **B,** Lateral radiograph demonstrates typical findings of unilateral facet lock. Anterior displacement of C5 on C6 is less than 25%. Vertebrae below dislocation are seen in lateral profile and those proximal to location are seen in oblique profile.

flattening or wedging of the articular pillar, or even circular or elliptic lucencies within the cancellous portion of the pillar. These lucencies are the result of compression or crushing of the pillar with subsequent reexpansion or distraction of the fracture by apposing forces, for instance, a crush or compression of the pillar by hyperextension and distraction by hyperflexion. Such a combination of forces is operative in whiplash injuries. Horizontal shearing and rotational forces with significant compression create horizontal fractures through the articular pillar. One of the articular surfaces or facets may then become displaced anteriorly or posteriorly, depending on the direction of the forces involved. Fractures of the articular pillar may extend into the adjacent pedicle or lamina.

Fractures of the laminae may either be vertical or horizontal. Occasionally they occur in isolation, but usually they are components of a more complex fracture involving the vertebral body and other posterior elements.

The healing of fractures involving the posterior elements is quite variable and frequently delayed. Because of this it is very difficult to accurately date such injuries.

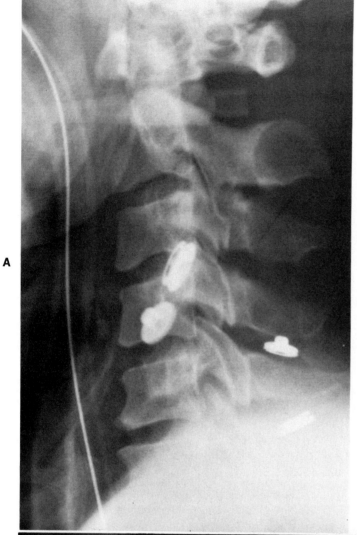

Fig. 4-13. Forty-four-year-old man who sustained an injury of the cervical spine in an automobile accident. He was immediately quadriplegic and was found to have central cord compression syndrome. There was no evidence of dislocation. Spondylosis of cervical spine was identified with fracture of posterior elements of C6 and C7. **A,** Initial lateral radiograph demonstrates no obvious abnormalities of cervical spine. Only six vertebrae are demonstrated. Minimal spur formation is present on vertebral bodies at C5-6. **B,** Lateral tomogram demonstrates narrowing of C6-7 interspace with osteophytic spur formation at its apposing margins. There is faint visualization of fracture of spinous process at C7 *(large arrow)*. Spur formation is also present at C7-T1 *(small arrow)*. **C,** Frontal tomogram demonstrates fracture of inferior facet of C6 *(arrow)* on left. Fragment is rotated and now lies horizontal.

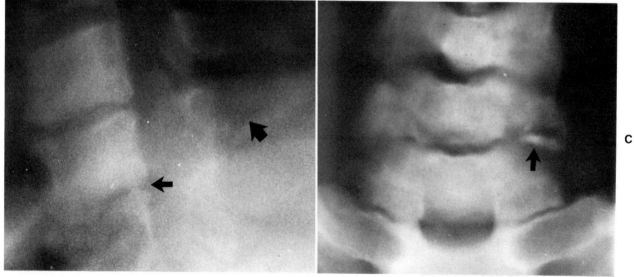

Associated neurologic injury. Spinal cord injuries are usually associated with fracture-dislocation of the spine.[33,60,64,78,98] Spinal cord injury accompanies 85% of bilateral facet locks, 75% of teardrop and severe crush fractures, and 30% of unilateral facet locks. Approximately 10% of spinal cord injuries have no evidence of fracture or dislocation (Figs. 4-13 and 4-14).[78,101] These are usually in older individuals with spondylosis of the cervical spine (Fig. 4-13), and at times they may be accompanied only by a fracture of the anterior inferior margin of the vertebral body or of an associated osteophytic spur. The mechanism of injury is a compression of the spinal cord between the hypertrophied ligamentum flavum and the osteophytic spur formation on the posterior margin of the vertebral body. Approximately 4% of fracture-dislocations of the cervical spine, with a

spinal cord injury, will have a second level of fracture at the thoracolumbar junction.[15]

To some extent it is possible to predict the type of underlying bony injury of the spine on the basis of the neurologic deficit.[60,64] Total motor and sensory loss below the level of injury is usually associated with a bilateral facet lock or severe bursting fractures of the vertebral body. The central spinal cord injury syndrome consists of disproportionately more motor impairment of the upper than of the lower extremity, bladder dysfunction, and usually urinary retention and varying degrees of sensory loss below the level of the lesion. This syndrome is associated with hyperextension injuries including those without obvious fractures. The anterior spinal cord injury syndrome is characterized by immediate, complete paralysis, with hypoesthesia and hypal-

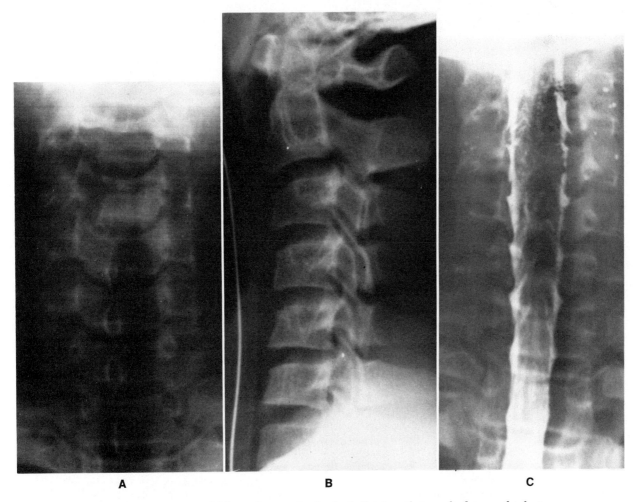

A   **B**   **C**

Fig. 4-14. Sixteen-year-old boy who sustained a football injury that resulted in quadriplegia. **A,** Frontal projection of cervical spine demonstrates no evidence of abnormalities. **B,** Lateral radiograph of cervical spine reveals no evidence of fracture or dislocation. There is a slight reversal of normal lordotic curve. **C,** Myelogram demonstrates enlargement of cord consistent with hematomyelia.

gesia to the level of the lesion and with the preservation of motion, position, and vibratory sense. This syndrome is usually associated with bursting and teardrop fractures of the vertebral body. Motor weakness or paresis either in all four limbs or combined to the upper extremity without sensory loss is particularly associated with fractures of the axis, C2, either a hangman's fracture or a fracture of the dens, or unilateral facet lock of the lower cervical spine. The deficit is usually transient. The Brown-Séquard syndrome consists of unilateral motor paralysis and contralateral loss of pain and temperature sense. It is commonly associated with unilateral facet locks or bursting fractures and may occasionally be seen as the result of a hyperextension injury.

FRACTURES OF THE THORACOLUMBAR SPINE
Incidence and distribution

Two thirds of all fractures involving the thoracolumbar spine occur at T12, L1, and L2. Ninety percent occur between T11 and L4. Fractures of the mid and upper dorsal spine are relatively uncommon in adults except for those resulting from convulsions caused by

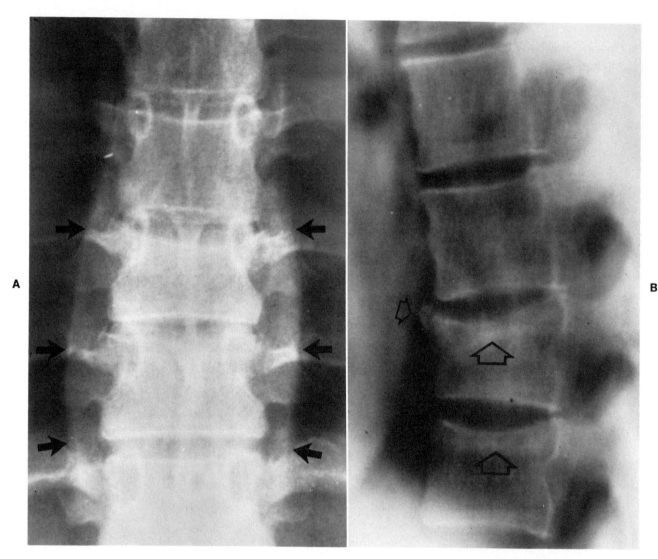

Fig. 4-15. Twenty-year-old woman who sustained a compression fracture of eighth and ninth thoracic vertebrae in a fall. There was no neurologic deficit. **A,** AP radiograph of lower thoracic spine demonstrates a paraspinous mass bilaterally *(arrows)*. There is decrease in height of eighth and ninth vertebrae. Superior end-plates are distorted. **B,** Lateral tomogram demonstrates depression of superior end-plate of both eighth and ninth thoracic vertebrae. There is small triangular fragment at anterior superior margin of T8 *(small arrow).* Beneath both depressed end-plates there is a line of sclerosis indicative of impaction *(large arrows).*

either electroshock therapy or tetany. On the other hand, in children the peaks of incidence of spinal fractures are T4-5[42,47] and L2.[42] Fractures involving adjacent vertebrae are relatively common, particularly in children because multiple contiguous fractures are the rule rather than the exception.[42,47] Approximately 20% of thoracolumbar fractures are associated with other skeletal injuries.[45,69,98] The frequent association of compression fractures of the thoracolumbar junction with fractures of the calcaneus is particularly noteworthy.

Radiologic interpretation

The examination begins with properly exposed and positioned anteroposterior and lateral views of the lumbar and dorsal spine. In view of the distribution of spinal fractures it is very important that the lower thoracic vertebrae be included on examinations for suspected lumbar spine trauma. A swimmer's view is required to adequately visualize the upper thoracic spine. Oblique views of the dorsal spine are rarely informative and can be safely omitted. The patient's condition may not permit the performance of oblique projections of the lumbar spine, and for the same reason the lateral views of the lumbar or dorsal spine may have to be obtained utilizing a horizontal, cross-table beam.

The only indirect clue to fracture is the presence of a paraspinous mass. These can only be demonstrated in the thoracic spine. These paraspinous masses represent hematomas that have accumulated beneath and dissected along the paraspinous ligaments (Fig. 4-15, A). They are bilateral but are usually asymmetric and may extend considerably beyond the site of fracture.

It is more difficult to identify fractures of the posterior elements and even the vertebral bodies themselves in the thoracic spine. On the lateral projection the vertebral bodies and particularly the posterior elements are obscured by the overlying pectoral girdle. A modified swimmer's view is helpful in this regard. While the patient lies supine, one arm is held fully extended over the head and the other is held at 90° flexion. It is helpful to have the patient grasp an IV pole with the flexed arm in order to maintain the position.

Tomography is used chiefly to clarify the status of the posterior elements and to verify the presence or absence of suspected fractures and determine their position. It is very useful in the evaluation of bursting fractures of the vertebral bodies to locate the position of fragments displaced into the spinal canal and for the clarification of the abnormalities associated with fracture-dislocations. Computed tomography is also helpful in the precise localization of fracture fragments in relation to the spinal canal and the demonstration of fractures of the posterior elements.

Classification

Approximately 75% of thoracolumbar fractures are compression fractures with the posterior elements intact; 20% are fracture-dislocations, usually fractures of both the posterior elements and the vertebral bodies; and 5%, which are of variable stability, involve only the posterior elements.[45,69,96]

Compression fracture

Compression fractures are by far the most common. The dominant features are anterior wedging or depression of the superior end-plate of the vertebral body (Fig. 4-15). Occasionally the force of compression is focused at the inferior instead of the superior end-plate. This is much less frequent but has no pathologic significance. These fractures are the result of a combination of truncal flexion and axial compression. The extent of the vertebral compression and degree of comminution depends on the severity of the force applied and the relative strength of the vertebra. In older individuals the osteoporosis fractures may occur during the course of normal activities. These are, in a sense, insufficiency fractures. In children the bone is resilient, and frequently toruslike fractures of the vertebral bodies occur that give rise to a breaklike projection on the anterior margins of the vertebra. These are usually in the superior margin but may be found inferiorly, in the middle, or both superiorly and inferiorly.

Compression fractures are best identified in the lateral projection. The vertebral body is wedge shaped with most of the compression being focused anteriorly. The height of the posterior portion of the vertebral body may not be affected. The superior end-plate is depressed and forms a concavity in the superior portion of the vertebra (Figs. 4-15 and 4-16). Beneath the concave depression there is a band of poorly marginated sclerosis indicative of the impaction of bony trabeculae (Figs. 4-15 and 4-16). The anterior superior margin of the wedged vertebra usually forms an irregular beak projecting beyond the anterior border of the vertebral body (Fig. 4-16, B). This beak has a sharp point projecting inferiorly. At times the anterior superior margin of the vertebral body may be displaced anteriorly as a separate small triangular fragment (Fig. 4-18, C). If the inferior end-plate should be affected, these same findings are seen except that they involve the inferior end-plate with the beak pointing superiorly. In children the vertebral compression is more of a torus fracture, and therefore the beak that is formed is contiguous with the wedged vertebra.[42,47]

More severe compressive forces drive the nucleus pulposus into the vertebral body, resulting in a virtual explosion of the vertebral body displacing the resultant bony fragments centripetally.[45,96] These are termed

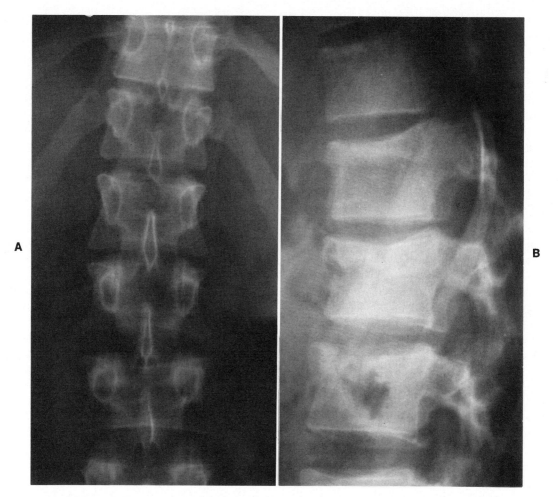

Fig. 4-16. Thirty-year-old man who sustained a compression fracture of T12, L1, L2, and L3 in an automobile accident without associated neurologic deficit. **A,** AP view demonstrates distortion and lack of definition of superior end-plate of involved vertebrae. **B,** Lateral view demonstrates variety of compression fracture of superior end-plates. Note characteristic beak at anterior superior margin of each involved vertebral body.

bursting fractures (Fig. 4-17). Frequently the posterior superior fragment is driven into the spinal canal. This may result in a spinal cord or nerve root injury. Such fragments may not be identified on the standard projections, and tomography (Fig. 4-17, *A*) or computed tomography (Fig. 4-17, *B*) should be done to exclude their presence when faced with a severely comminuted fracture of the vertebral body.

The importance of identifying a dislocation or a loss of vertebral body height indicating the presence of a compression fracture is universally appreciated. However, it is also important to determine the status of the posterior elements.[96] Their disruption represents an important clue to the possibility of an unstable fracture. In the frontal projection there are two clues to the recognition of disruption of the posterior elements. With either a transverse fracture of the posterior elements or

a disruption of the ligaments there may be sufficient angulation of the superior fragment or vertebrae so that a portion of the vertebral body is no longer overlaid by the posterior elements. This separation and elevation of the posterior elements give rise to an empty or vacant appearance of the vertebral body involved. Another key is the recognition of a break in the continuity of the oval-shaped cortex of the pedicles and/or the tear-shaped cortex of the spinous process (Fig. 4-18, *A* and *B*). A fracture line may be visualized within the lamina or articular processes. Confirmation rests with an adequately exposed lateral view of the spine (Fig. 4-18, *C*).

Fractures of the posterior elements often accompany the more severe compression fractures of the vertebral bodies (Fig. 4-18). These consist of either vertical or horizontal fractures involving the lamina, spinal processes, and pedicles.[96] It is quite likely that a greater

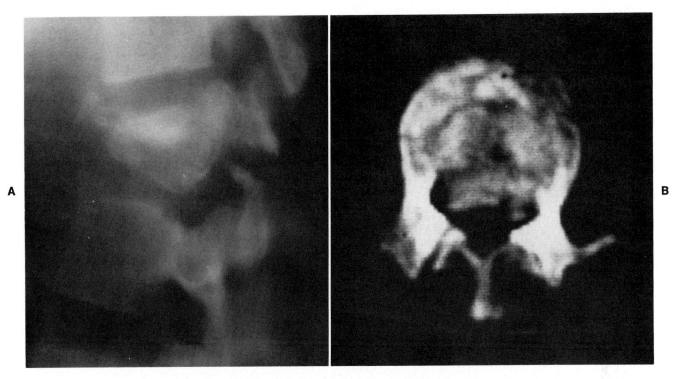

Fig. 4-17. Twenty-five-year-old woman who was injured in an automobile accident and sustained a bursting fracture of L1 with compression of cauda equina; treatment is shown in Fig. 7-39. **A,** Lateral tomogram demonstrates severe compression of vertebral body of L1 with posterior displacement of superoposterior portion of vertebral body into spinal canal. There is also a subluxation of facet joint at T12-L1 and transverse fracture involving pedicle of L1. **B,** Computed tomogram clearly demonstrates comminuted fracture of L1 with posterior displacement of vertebral fragments that lie within and compromise the spinal canal.

number of fractures of the posterior elements would be demonstrated by obtaining routine tomographic examination of the spine in the presence of compression fractures of the vertebra.[16] The fractures of the posterior elements are frequently obscure because of the complexity of the overlapping shadows and the lack of displacement of the fracture fragment.[82] It is quite likely that the number of posterior element fractures is directly related to the severity of the compression fracture. It would seem judicious to obtain a tomographic examination to evaluate the posterior elements when presented with a severe or markedly compressed vertebral body. Tomography is therefore justified in the presence of a severe compression fracture for two reasons: first, to demonstrate associated fractures of the posterior elements, and second, to disclose a posteriorly displaced fragment of the vertebral body.

The Kümmell phenomenon: posttraumatic collapse

In 1891 Kümmell described a delayed posttraumatic collapse of the vertebral body leading to a gibbous deformity. Since then others[79] have noted a delayed pro-

gressive angular deformity following either roentgenographically inapparent or minimal fractures. Such progression is occasionally encountered after an otherwise routine compression fracture. This is more likely to occur in the thoracolumbar spine. It is not to be construed as an indication of a pathologic fracture. The etiology is presumed to be secondary to vascular damage, although this has not been proven. The collapse generally occurs within 8 weeks of the initial injury.

Fracture-dislocation of the thoracolumbar spine

Fracture-dislocations are the result of a combination of flexion, axial compression, and rotational shearing forces.[23] The dominant features are fractures of both the posterior elements and vertebral bodies with anterior displacement of the vertebral bodies above the level of the dislocation.[55] Most are grossly unstable because of disruption through both the anterior and posterior columns. They are partially reduced by simply placing the patient's shoulder in line with the pelvis. Because of this, it is quite likely that the amount of displacement demonstrated on the radiologic examination is considerably less than that which was created at the time of

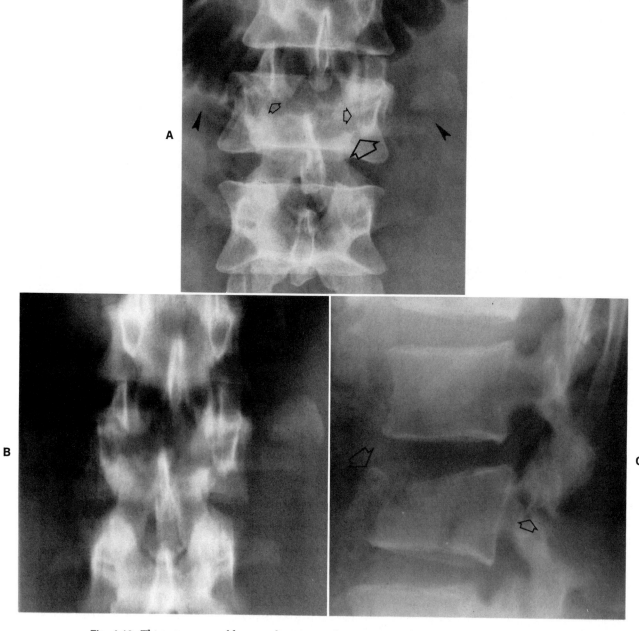

Fig. 4-18. Thirty-two-year-old man who sustained compression fracture of L3 with comminution of posterior elements of L3. There was no neurologic deficit. **A,** AP projection demonstrates loss of vertebral body height and disruption of cortical margins of both pedicles *(small arrows)* and left lamina of L3 *(large arrow)*. There are also horizontal fractures of transverse processes *(arrowheads)*. **B,** Linear tomography demonstrates fractures of posterior elements to good advantage. **C,** Lateral radiograph demonstrates fracture of vertebral body with typical triangular body *(large arrow)*. There is.a fracture involving pedicles and base of superior facet *(small arrow)*.

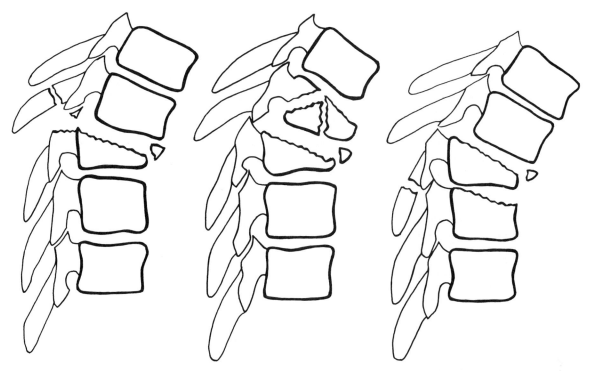

Fig. 4-19. Diagrammatic representation of typical fractures of thoracic spine associated with paraplegia. On left is a fracture-dislocation with compression of vertebral body below and a typical small triangular fragment displaced anteriorly from compressed vertebra. In the middle the vertebral body above the dislocation has sustained a burst fracture with a large posterior superior fragment that is attached to pedicle. To the right is a fracture-dislocation associated with additional compression fracture below level of dislocation. There are a variety of fractures of posterior elements and dislocation of apophyseal joints demonstrated in this diagram about the level of dislocation. These are highly variable and not characteristic of any particular pattern of injury.

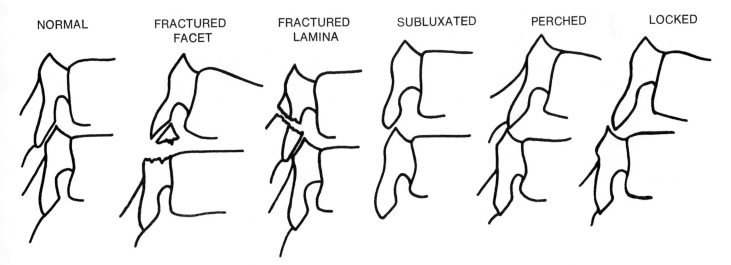

NORMAL   FRACTURED FACET   FRACTURED LAMINA   SUBLUXATED   PERCHED   LOCKED

Fig. 4-20. Variety of abnormalities found in apophyseal joints in association with fracture-dislocations of thoracolumbar spine. Note perched facets wherein inferior tip of superior facet becomes perched on superior aspect of inferior facet following disruption of apophyseal joint. Facets may also become locked, as is more typical of cervical spine. (From Rogers, L. F., et al.: Am. J. Roentgenol. **134:**67, 1980. © 1980, Am. Roentgen Ray Soc.)

injury.[45,57] The displacement may be so minimal that it is difficult to appreciate. Fracture-dislocations of the first through the eighth thoracic vertebrae are almost invariably associated with neurologic deficit, most commonly a complete motor and sensory deficit. Sixty to seventy percent of fracture-dislocations of the thoracolumbar junction of the lumbar spine are associated with a neurologic deficit.[57,69] The most common site for a fracture-dislocation of the upper thoracic spine is at the level of T4-5 and T5-6.[15] The most frequent site of a dislocation of the thoracolumbar junction is at T12-L1.

The typical fracture-dislocation of the upper dorsal spine[61] consists of an anteriorly displaced vertebra associated with a wedged compression fracture of the subjacent vertebral body (Figs. 4-19 and 4-20). A small triangular fragment of bone is found anterior to the wedged vertebra (Figs. 4-18 and 4-21). The facet joints are disrupted frequently with a fracture of the superior facet of the vertebra below the dislocation or a fracture through the lamina beneath the superior facet of the vertebra above the dislocation. Alternatively there may be locking or perching of the facets of the two affected vertebrae (Fig. 4-20). Frequently there is a bursting fracture of the anteriorly displaced vertebral body in addition to the compression fracture of the vertebral body below the dislocation (Figs. 4-19 and 4-22). Characteristically a large posterior superior fragment of the crushed vertebral body remains attached to the pedicles (Figs. 4-19 and 4-22). At times there are additional compression fractures of the vertebrae below the wedged vertebra adjacent to the dislocation (Figs. 4-19 and 4-21, B). Mid and upper dorsal fracture-dislocations may be difficult to visualize because of the minimal lateral displacement or rotation at the fracture site (Fig. 4-21, A).

Minimal anterior or posterior subluxations may occur without associated fractures but with spinal cord injury (Fig. 4-23). Traumatic paraplegia with injury levels in the upper dorsal spine may occur in the absence of frac-

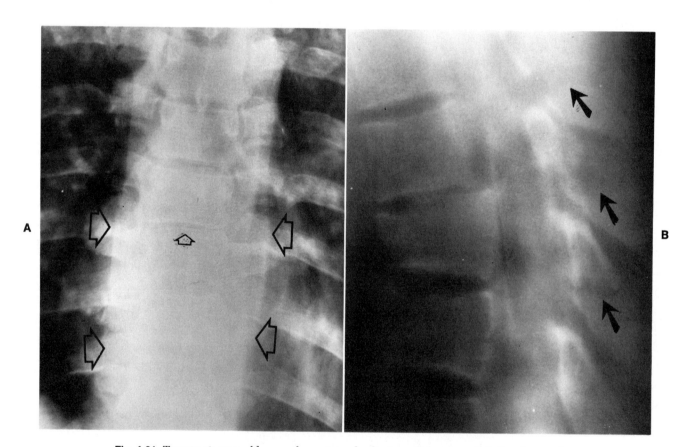

Fig. 4-21. Twenty-six-year-old man who sustained a fracture-dislocation of T6-7 with paraplegia. **A,** AP view of spine demonstrates bilateral paraspinous hematoma *(large arrows)*. T6-7 interspace *(small arrow)* is slightly narrowed with T6 offset slightly to right of T7. **B,** Lateral tomogram demonstrating anterior dislocation of vertebral body of T6 on T7. There is additional compression fracture of superior end-plate at T8. Note variety of fractures of lamina and spinous processes T5, T6, and T7 *(arrows)*.

tures or dislocations. The mechanism is similar to that encountered in the cervical spine: a hyperextension injury resulting in compression of the cord between the ligamentum flavum posteriorly and apposing margins of the vertebral bodies and intervertebral disc anteriorly producing a hematomyelia.

Complex fracture-dislocations with either anterior or posterior dislocation also occur and may be difficult to classify (Fig. 4-24). The basic components are combined fractures of both the posterior elements and vertebral bodies in association with a dislocation.

The typical fracture-dislocation at the thoracolumbar junction is similar in appearance to that described for the thoracic spine; however, there is usually less compression of the vertebral body below the level of dislocation.[57,61] Holdsworth[45,46] described a peculiar fracture of the vertebral end-plate associated with a disruption of the intervertebral disc; he termed this fracture a *slice fracture*. It consists of a large, thin fragment of the anterior portion of the superior end-plate of the compressed

vertebral body below the level of the dislocation (Fig. 4-25). Although occasionally such slice fractures from the superior margin of the vertebra may be encountered more commonly, a small triangular fragment is seen as has been described above (Figs. 4-26 and 4-27). The intervening facet joints are disrupted with fractures of the superior facets of the vertebral body below the dislocation or locking (Fig. 4-28) or perching of the facets[57,69] similar to that fracture-dislocation described above.

At times the facets on one side are disrupted whereas the fracture line on the opposite side proceeds through the pedicle or pars interarticularis and then forward through a portion of the vertebral body.

On occasion there may be bilateral fractures of either the pedicles or pars interarticularis, anterior displacement of the vertebra associated with a disruption of the intervertebral disc, and either no or a very minimal compression fracture of the vertebral body below the level of dislocation.[76] Rarely dislocation may be associated with ligamentous disruption posteriorly and disc disruption anteriorly

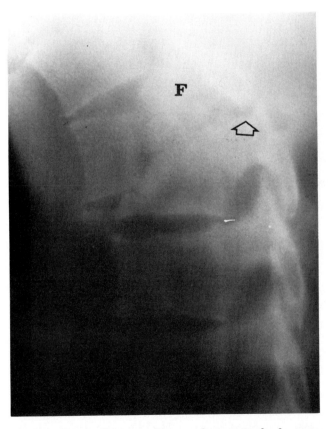

Fig. 4-22. Twenty-four-year-old man who sustained a fracture-dislocation at T4-5 with paraplegia. Lateral tomogram demonstrates comminution of anteriorly displaced fracture of vertebral body above level of dislocation. Large posterior fragment remains attached to pedicle, *F*. Vertebral body below dislocation is compressed. Note locking of facets *(arrow)*.

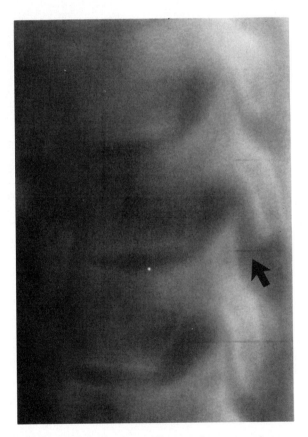

Fig. 4-23. Twenty-seven-year-old man who sustained a posterior subluxation of T7 on T8 in a motorcycle accident, which resulted in complete paraplegia. Lateral tomogram shows approximately 4 mm of posterior subluxation of facet joints *(arrow)*.

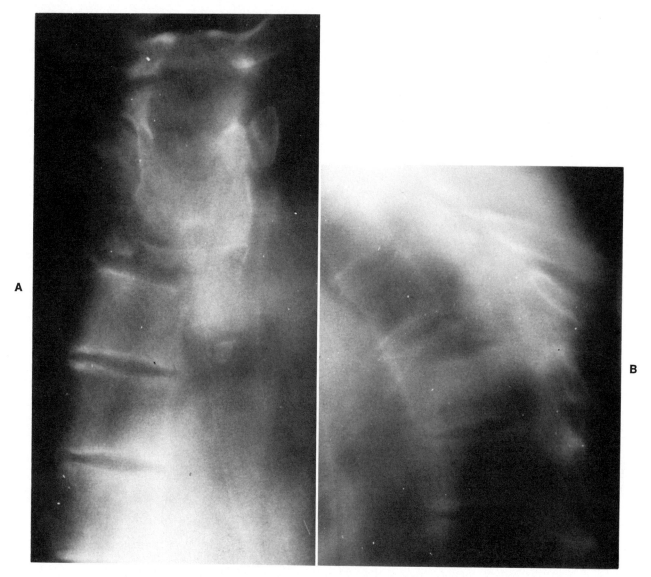

Fig. 4-24. Sixty-five-year-old man who sustained a complex fracture-dislocation at T4-5 with marked lateral displacement, resulting in complete paraplegia. **A,** Frontal tomogram demonstrates comminution on lateral displacement of fourth thoracic vertebra with considerable overriding of vertebral body. **B,** Lateral tomogram demonstrates overriding of vertebral bodies with approximately 5 mm anterior dislocation of T4 on T5. There is an acute anterior angulation at level of dislocation.

without any accompanying fracture. The mechanism for these injuries is more fully described below.

Transverse fractures of the spine

In 1948, Chance[69,82] described an unusual fracture of the vertebral body consisting of a "horizontal splitting of the spine and neural arch, ending in an upward curve which usually reaches the upper surface of the body just in front of the neural foramen." In his three cases there was little wedging of the vertebral body. With the advent of the automobile lap-type seat belt in

the 1950s and its general acceptance and common usage in the 1960s, the Chance fracture has been found with increasing frequency as a result of injuries sustained while wearing the lap-type seat belt.[20,26] Howland and co-workers[82] in 1965 reported a case of a complete transverse fracture of the third lumbar vertebra in a 19-year-old man injured in an automobile accident while wearing a seat belt. The authors theorized that "this injury was produced by the seat belt acting as a fulcrum over which the vertebral body was split transversely into two parts." The fracture was termed a *fulcrum*

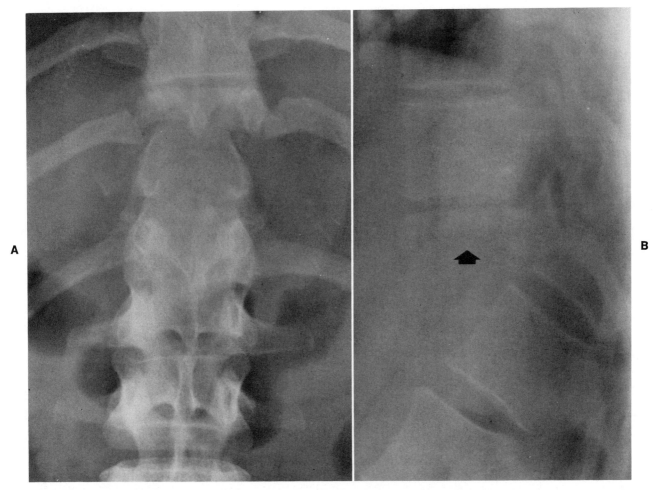

Fig. 4-25. Slice fracture of T11 in 26-year-old woman involved in an airplane crash, resulting in complete paraplegia. **A,** AP radiograph of spine demonstrating peculiar vacant or absent appearance of inferior portion of eleventh vertebral body with wide separation of eleventh and twelfth ribs. **B,** Lateral radiograph demonstrating marked anterior displacement of spine above level of dislocation. Note sliced fragment consisting of superior end-plate and facet of T11 *(arrow)*.

fracture of the lumbar spine. This theory was refined by Smith and Kaufer.[97] In the usual hyperflexion injury of the spine, the compression forces generated are sustained by the anterior half of the vertebral body, thus resulting in a wedge or compression fracture of the vertebral body. With the wearing of a seat belt the fulcrum of the force is displaced anteriorly and lies at the seat belt. The entire spine is therefore posterior to the flexion axis and all of its components are subjected to tension stress. This results in a disruption of the ligaments of the posterior elements of the spine, or should the ligaments remain intact, a transverse or fission-type fracture of the posterior elements and, at times, the vertebral body. This same pattern has been seen without the use of a seat belt as a result of injuries in which the individual either fell or was thrown forward so that

the anterior abdominal wall came in contact with some object, such as a tree limb or a fence railing. This object serves as a fulcrum in a manner similar to a seat belt and forces the body into acute flexion.

The fulcrum-type force creates either ruptures of the posterior ligaments and facet joints or fractures of the posterior elements and vertebral body or varying combinations of ligamentous rupture and fracture. There are three basic patterns resulting from fulcrum-type injuries of the spine.[82] The first pattern involves disruption of the posterior spinous ligaments, articular facets, and the intervertebral disc. There may be an associated avulsion of an articular facet or posterior inferior aspect of the vertebral body. The pedicles and spinous and transverse processes remain intact. The second pattern is one of a transverse fracture involving the posterior

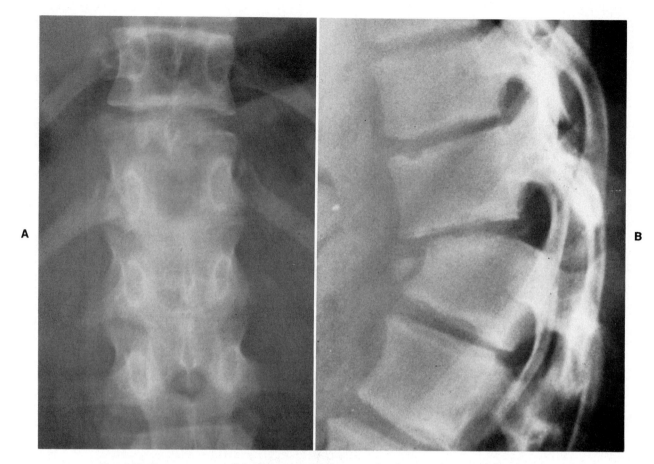

Fig. 4-26. Seventeen-year-old adolescent who sustained a fracture-dislocation at T11-12 in motorcycle accident. **A,** AP view demonstrates disruption of facet joints bilaterally with distraction of posterior elements. This peculiar vacant appearance of T12 is result of absence of overlying posterior elements of T11. **B,** Lateral radiograph demonstrates anterior dislocation of T11 on T12 with minimal compression of anterosuperior margin of T12 and typical triangular fragment lying anterior to body of T12. This configuration is typical of fracture-dislocations at thoracolumbar junction.

Fig. 4-27. Forty-three-year-old man who sustained a fracture-dislocation in industrial accident. **A,** AP view demonstrates severe compression of vertebral body at T12 with minimal compression of superior end-plate of L1. **B,** Lateral radiograph demonstrates T11-12 dislocation and compression of T12 and L1 without clarifying status of posterior elements. **C,** Lateral tomogram clearly demonstrates disruption of facet joints with locking of facets at T11-12 *(arrow)*. In addition, comminution of twelfth thoracic vertebra with posterior displacement of fracture fragment is demonstrated. Note also slight anterior wedging of first lumbar vertebral body.

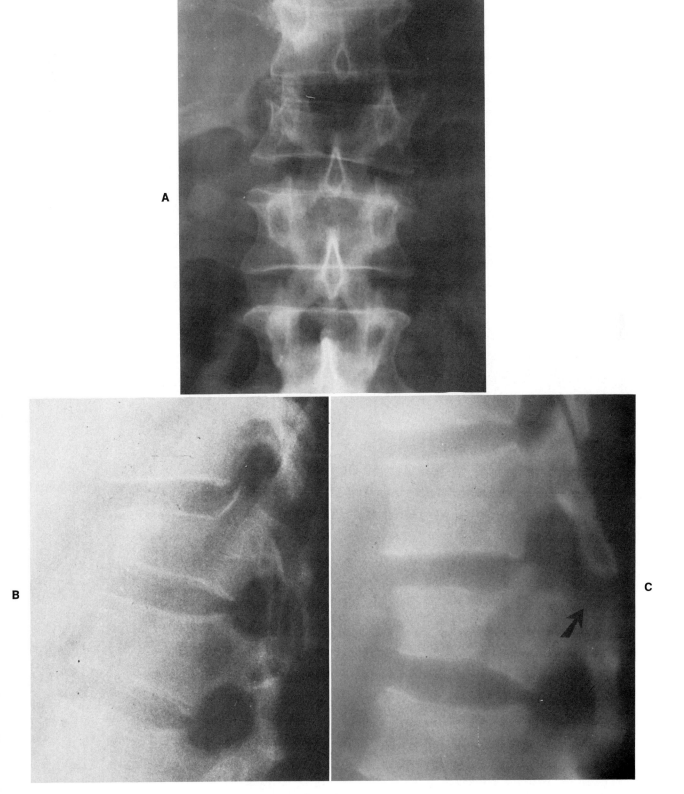

Fig. 4-27. For legend see opposite page.

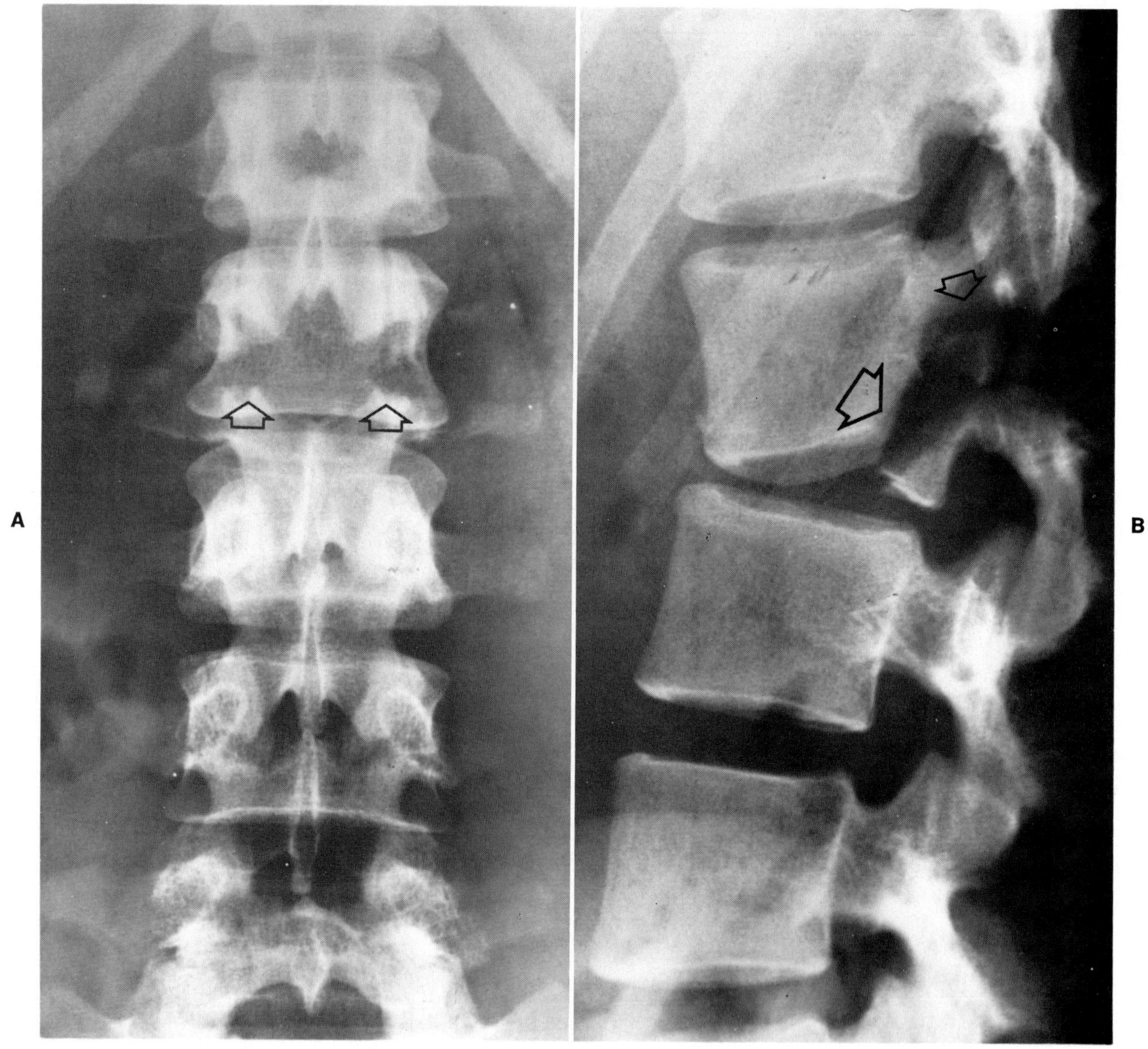

Fig. 4-28. Twenty-year-old woman who sustained a Chance fracture of spine in an automobile accident. She was wearing a seat belt. There was no neurologic deficit. Laparotomy disclosed presence of a transection of pancreas. **A,** AP projection of lumbar spine reveals peculiar vacant appearance of second lumbar vertebra secondary to distraction of posterior elements. There is a horizontal fracture through pedicles *(arrows)* and transverse process of L2 and a horizontal fracture of transverse process of L1 on right. On frontal projection, vertebral body appears intact. **B,** Lateral projection clearly demonstrates transverse or horizontal fracture of pedicles *(small arrow)*, which extends anteriorly through inferior and posterior portion of vertebral body *(large arrow)*. There is an acute angulation of spine at L2-3 disc space. Note that vertebral body height of L2 is normal. This is in keeping with absence of compression that is typical of distraction injuries.

elements with or without extension into the posterior superior or posterior inferior aspect of the vertebral body. The fracture line may involve one or both pedicles, transverse processes, and articular facets, as well as the lamina and spinous process. This is the classic Chance fracture (Fig. 4-28). The third pattern involves a transverse fracture of the posterior elements with an associated transverse fracture of the vertebral body. This fracture involves the spinous process, lamina, pedicles, and usually the transverse processes.

Characteristically, there is minimal compression of the vertebral body. When present, it involves the anterior superior aspect. Neither is there any degree of lateral displacement or rotation of the fracture fragments. Anterior displacement of the superior vertebral body or the superior fragment is unusual. When present, it is commonly associated with an injury of the spinal cord or cauda equina. Transverse fractures of the lumbar vertebrae are often associated with significant visceral injuries. The phrase *seat belt syndrome* was first coined by Garrett and Braunstein in 1962.[20] It designates those injuries frequently encountered in individuals injured while wearing a lap-type seat belt. Typically, the individual affected is a passenger, either in the front or back seat, and is involved in a head-on collision resulting in sudden deceleration at impact. The impact speed frequently exceeds 50 miles per hour. The syndrome consists of one or more of the following injuries[20,82]: transverse abrasions of the lower anterior abdominal wall outlining the position of the seat belt at the time of impact; ruptures of the anterior abdominal wall musculature; longitudinal lacerations of the small bowel, particularly on the antimesenteric border of the jejunum and ileum; tears of the mesentery; ruptures of the second or third portion of the duodenum, spleen, or pancreas (Fig. 4-28); injuries to the cauda equina or spinal cord; and transverse fractures of the lumbar spine. These injuries may be both clinically and radiologically obscure. When a transverse fracture is identified, everyone should be alerted to the potential for associated abdominal visceral injury.[21] Neurologic deficits occur in approximately 15% of cases.[82]

Fractures of the posterior elements

Fractures limited to the posterior elements are rarely associated with neurologic deficits. Fractures of the transverse processes are quite common. These result from pulls of the paraspinous muscles or occasionally from direct blows. They are frequently multiple. The line of fracture is usually vertically or obliquely oriented. The vertebrae are otherwise intact. Occasionally the ossification center for the transverse process fails to unite with the vertebral body. This results in a vertical line of lucency between the vertebral body and the

transverse process. The bony margins of this line are sharply defined by cortical bone and should not be mistaken for a fracture.

Isolated fractures of the remaining posterior elements are unusual, and associated neurologic deficits are rare. Fractures of the pars interarticularis[29,51,67,105] or articular facets are occasionally encountered. Characteristically there is very little displacement and the fracture line is obscure. The injury is most likely caused by acute hyperextension. Isolated fractures of the spinous process of lamina may be seen occasionally.[16] These are at times difficult to visualize. Tomography may be required.[16] These isolated fractures are usually identified when tomography is obtained in a patient who complaints of persistent pain in the face of a normal plain film radiologic examination.

MULTIPLE-LEVEL SPINAL INJURIES

Multiple, noncontiguous vertebral injuries are defined as "injuries to the vertebral column at more than one site, with these sites being separated by an area of normal spine."[59] Although uncommon, multiple, noncontiguous vertebral fractures are clinically important in those patients with spinal injury. An unrecognized second level of injuries may lead to extension of the neurologic deficit or subsequently cause pain, instability, or deformity. Only a few investigations of this problem have been published. Kewalramani and Taylor[59] reviewed 120 cases of spinal cord injury and found five patients (4.2%) with multiple noncontiguous vertebral injuries. Bentley and McSweeney[9] reported three cases of simultaneous cervical and thoracic injury and one case of cervical and thoracolumbar junction injury. Griffith and co-workers[34] reported five cases (3.2%) with multiple noncontiguous fractures in a review of 155 cases of thoracic or lumbar injury. Roberts and Curtis[81] reported one case of noncontiguous fracture in a review of 25 cases of paraplegia secondary to fracture or fracture-dislocation in the thoracic or lumbar spine. Calenoff and co-workers[15] noted a 4.5% incidence in a series of 710 patients admitted to the Midwest Regional Spinal Cord Injury Care System.

In Calenoff and co-workers' series[15] 80% of the patients had sustained fractures at two levels whereas 20% had three or more levels of injury. The initial injury that was thought to account for the spinal cord deficit was termed the *primary injury* and additional fractures were termed *secondary* or *tertiary*. Eighty-three percent of the primary injuries were fracture-dislocations, and 5% were compression fractures. Of the nonprimary lesions, 64% were compression fractures, and 17% were fracture-dislocations. Thirteen percent were isolated neural arch fractures, and isolated vertebral body avulsion fractures occurred in 4%. One nonprimary lesion was a fracture of the odontoid process. Of the secondary lesions, 40% occurred above and 60% below the primary lesion.

An analysis of the vertebral levels at which primary and nonprimary injuries occurred yields definite patterns of injury in the series by Calenoff and co-workers (Fig. 4-29): pattern A—six of seven primary injuries at C5-7 were associated with secondary injuries at T12 or in the lumbar spine (Fig. 4-30); pattern B—six of eight primary injuries at T2-4 were associated with secondary injuries in the cervical spine (Fig. 4-31); and pattern C—five of seven primary injuries at T12-L2 were associated with secondary injuries at L4-5 (Fig. 4-32).

There was a cluster of six primary injuries at T5-7 in which the pattern of secondary involvement was not clearly defined: three secondary lesions were proximal

(in the cervical spine) and three were distal (T10-L1). The three major patterns and the one subpattern account for 23 (77%) of the total number of patients.

There is a significant peak incidence of primary fractures at T2-7 in patients with multiple-level injuries (Fig. 4-33, *A*). Although these levels account for 46.7% of all primary fractures in this group, they account for only 16% of the vertebral injuries in the Midwest Regional Spinal Cord Injury Care System patients with spinal cord injuries.[15] There was no incidence peak at T2-7 in Jefferson's unselected spinal fracture population.[54] Thus in patients with multiple-level, noncontiguous fractures, there is a disproportionate number of primary vertebral injuries in the middle and upper dorsal regions (Fig. 4-33, *B*); a primary injury at this level

PRIMARY LESION   SECONDARY LESION

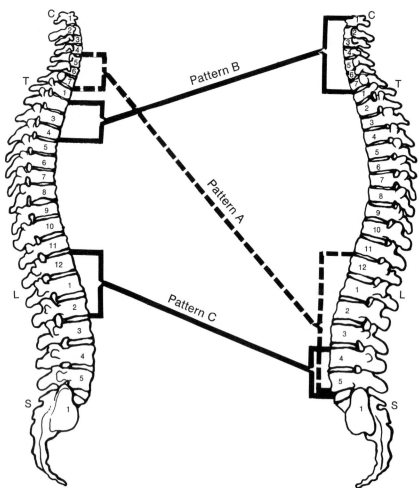

Fig. 4-29. Three major patterns of multiple level injury. *Pattern A* corresponds to primary lesion at C5-7 with secondary lesion at T12 or lumbar spine. *Pattern B* corresponds to primary lesion at T2-4 with secondary lesion in cervical spine. *Pattern C* corresponds to primary lesion in thoracolumbar junction with secondary lesion at L4-5. (From Calenoff, L., et al.: Am. J. Roentgenol. **130**:665, 1978. © 1978 Am. Roentgen Ray Soc.)

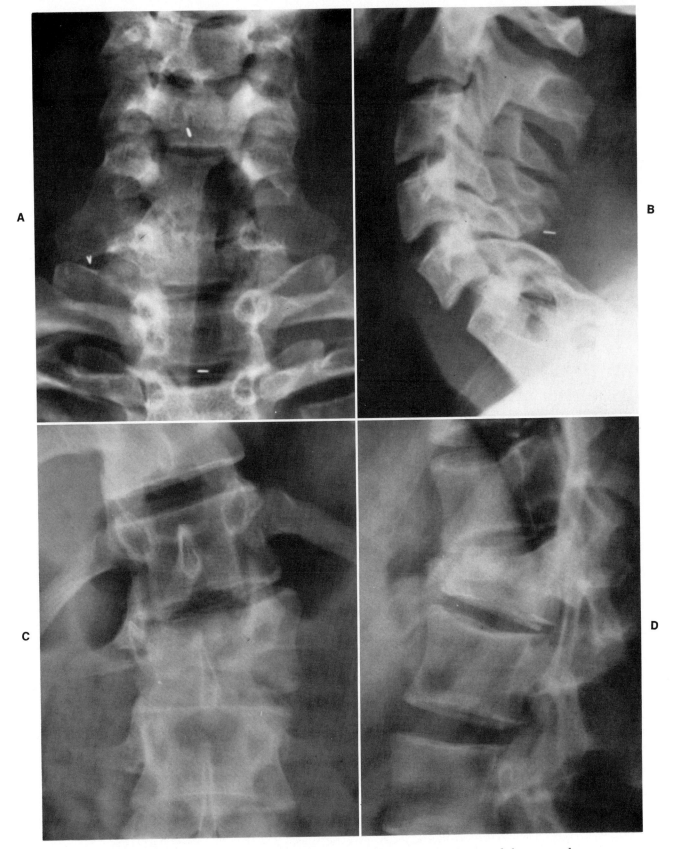

Fig. 4-30. Example of pattern A in Fig. 4-29. **A** and **B,** Primary C7 fracture-dislocation and posterior element fractures were treated by laminectomy and anterior spinal fusion. **C** and **D,** Anteroposterior and lateral views of lumbar spine 108 days later show unrecognized healing fracture of L1 with resulting kyphosis and levoscoliosis of lumbar spine. (From Calenoff, L., et al.: Am. J. Roentgenol. **130:**665, 1978. © 1978 Am. Roentgen Ray Soc.)

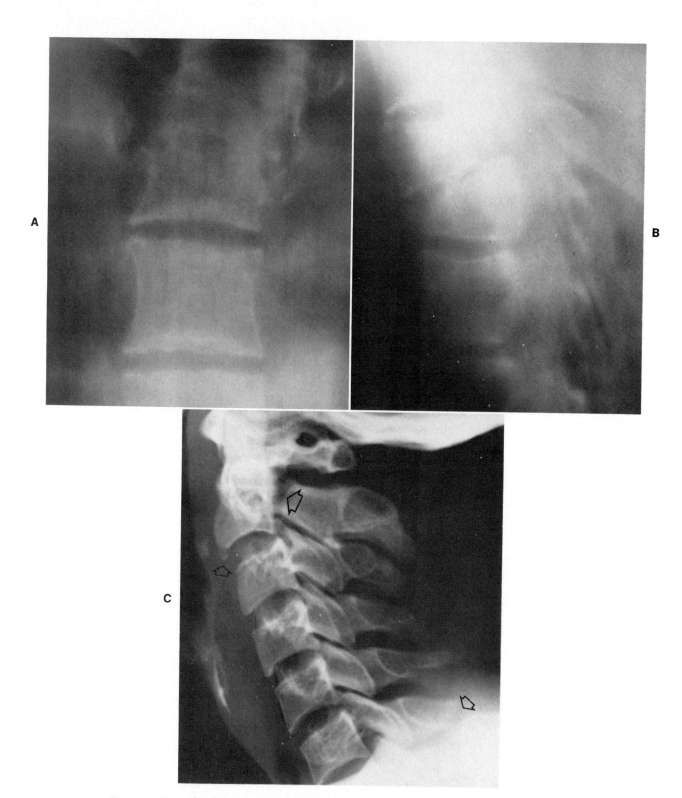

Fig. 4-31. Example of pattern B in Fig. 4-29. **A** and **B,** Primary fracture-dislocation involved bodies of T4-5. **C,** Second-level injury, diagnosed simultaneously with primary lesion, was a hangman's fracture *(large arrow)*. There is small avulsion fracture in anterior inferior surface of body of C2 *(small arrow)* and fracture of spinous process of C6 *(small arrow)*. This, in effect, is a three-level spinal injury. (From Calenoff, L., et al.: Am. J. Roentgenol. **130:**665, 1978. © 1978 Am. Roentgen Ray Soc.)

should alert the physician to the possibility of a second vertebral injury elsewhere.[15,86] Similarly, in the study of Griffith and co-workers[34] upper and middle dorsal fracture correlated with multiple noncontiguous vertebral fracture.

In multiple-level, noncontiguous fractures, secondary injuries are disproportionately numerous at L4 and L5. These two levels account for 28.6% of secondary injuries. There was also a peak of secondary injuries (14.3%) at C1 and C2. Thus 42.9% of secondary injuries in multiple-level spinal fracture occurred at the ex-

tremes of the spine (Fig. 4-33, *A*). These areas might escape radiologic evaluation because of the probable lack of neurologic findings and the difficulty of obtaining radiographs of these portions of the spine in the immobilized patient suspected of spinal cord injury.

The three identifiable patterns of noncontiguous fractures should be an aid in directing attention to the probable area of secondary fracture and in insisting that radiographs be obtained of these areas as soon as possible. Early recognition of second and third levels of fracture is important because of their clinical signifi-

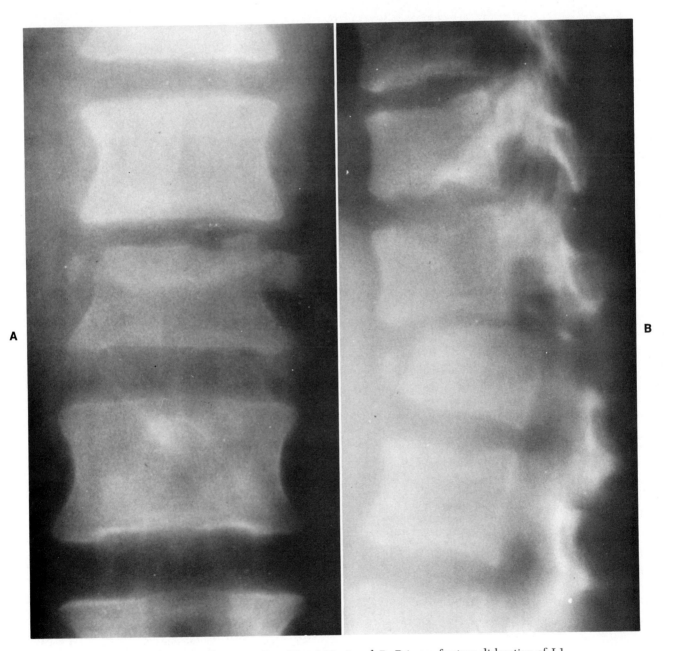

Fig. 4-32. Example of pattern C in Fig. 4-29. **A** and **B**, Primary fracture-dislocation of L1 well demonstrated by polytomography was treated by Harrington rod and bone graft.

Continued.

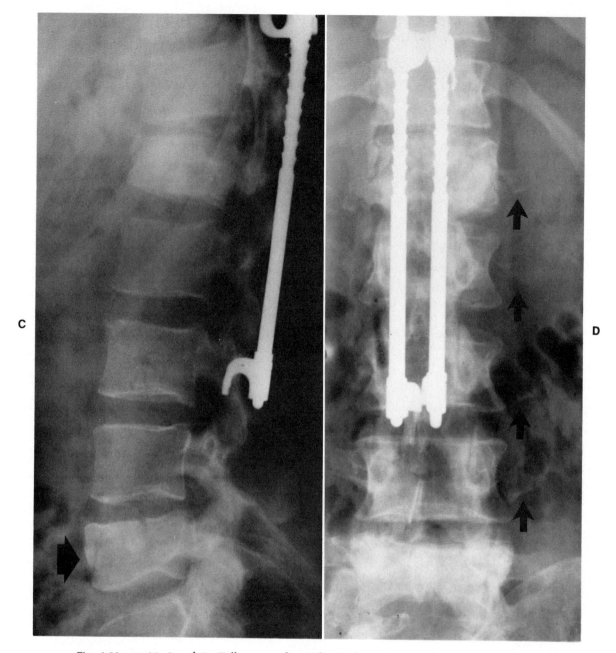

Fig. 4-32, cont'd. C and **D,** Follow-up radiographs 37 days after initial injury revealed an associated compression fracture of L5 *(arrow* in **C).** Note fractures of transverse process *(arrows* in **D).** (From Calenoff, L., et al.: Am. J. Roentgenol. **130:**665, 1978. © 1978 Am. Roentgen Ray Soc.)

cance. An unrecognized secondary lesion proximal to a primary lesion may result in pain or extension of the neurologic deficit proximally. Distal secondary lesions can result in instability, progressive scoliosis, and problems with skin maintenance caused by abnormal stress from altered body mechanics. Local infection can lead to sepsis and death. In an apparent upper motor neuron paraplegic or quadriplegic, conversion of bladder,

bowel, and sexual functions to those associated with a lower motor neuron lesion may result from a distal secondary fracture. Decisions regarding bowel and bladder care, sexual counseling, and possible surgical intervention may be influenced.

In multiple-level, noncontiguous vertebral fractures, early recognition of the secondary or tertiary level of injury is essential for appropriate therapy and to mini-

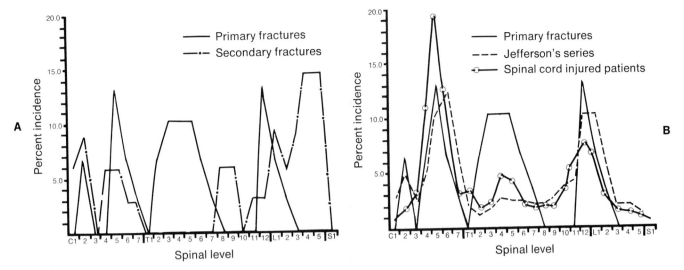

Fig. 4-33. A, Distribution of primary and secondary lesions in patients with multiple noncontiguous fractures. Note high incidence of secondary lesions at extremes of spinal column. **B,** Comparison of site of injury in primary lesions in multiple noncontiguous level fracture group: Jefferson's series of 2006 unselected spinal fractures, and 493 patients with symptomatic spinal cord injuries admitted to Midwest Regional Spinal Cord Injury Care System. Note disproportionate incidence of primary lesions in upper and midthoracic spine in multiple-level fracture group. (From Calenoff, L., et al.: Am. J. Roentgenol. **130**:665, 1978. © 1978 Am. Roentgen Ray Soc.)

mize the extent of neurologic deficit. Since in severely injured patients conventional neurologic examination may be impossible because of shock, unconsciousness, or associated injury, it is recommended that total spine radiography be performed as soon as possible on all patients sustaining a significant degree of spinal trauma.[15,86] Care should be taken to include the craniovertebral and lumbosarcral junctions. Any suspicious areas should be clarified by additional projections, including tomography.

OPEN OR PENETRATING INJURIES: MISSILE AND STAB WOUNDS OF SPINE AND SPINAL CORD

The nature of the spinal fracture and spinal cord injury is dependent on the caliber and velocity of the missile.[11,107] Civilian injuries tend to be of a lower velocity and smaller caliber, whereas military injuries are of a higher velocity and larger caliber. Approximately 15% of civilian spinal cord injuries are caused by open or penetrating injuries by bullets or knife wounds.[70] The bullet may penetrate and remain within the spinal canal. It is then identified within the canal on both the anteroposterior and lateral projections. Occasionally it may penetrate and traverse the canal and come to rest in another portion of the body or pass out of the body through a wound of exit. In this instance small bullet fragments may be identified within the spinal canal

along the course of the missile. Frequently the missiles ricochet after encountering some portion of the spine and come to rest elsewhere. The site of impact is identifiable by multiple small fragments of the bullet and fragmentation of the underlying bone (Fig. 4-34). The degree of fragmentation depends on the velocity and caliber of the missile. It is possible to sustain a spinal cord injury without an associated fracture of the spine. The nearby passage of a high-velocity missile may cause sufficient blast and concussive forces to result in a spinal cord injury without radiographically identifiable fractures.

Penetrating injuries from stab wounds are usually located in the dorsal spine and may be associated with fractures of the lamina and other posterior elements at the site of injury.[11] Whereas missile injuries are usually associated with a complete neurologic deficit, those associated with stab wounds are often incomplete. The Brown-Séquard syndrome is particularly common.

PATHOLOGIC FRACTURES OF THE SPINE

Metastatic disease of the spine commonly is indicated by a pathologic fracture, almost invariably a compression fracture of the vertebral body. The radiologic feature that distinguishes a pathologic fracture is the presence of associated bony destruction, particularly involving the cortex (Fig. 4-35). Although the cortex of pedicle always comes to mind in this context, the

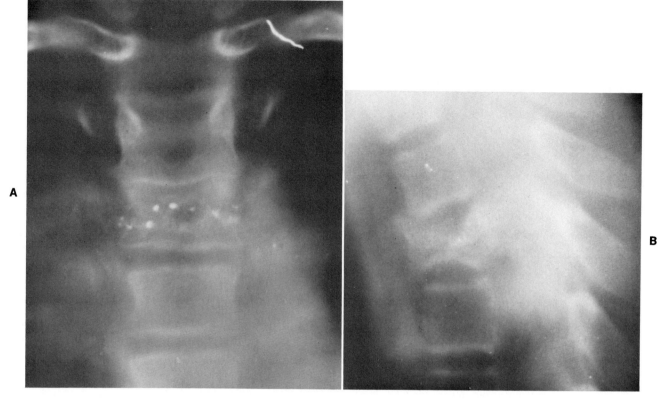

Fig. 4-34. Twelve-year-old boy who sustained an accidental gunshot wound of T3, which resulted in paraplegia. **A,** AP tomogram demonstrating multiple metallic fragments traversing body of T3. There is an associated paraspinous hematoma and a compression fracture of vertebral body. **B,** Lateral tomogram demonstrates severity of compression fracture of vertebral body and location of multiple metallic fragments within fracture site.

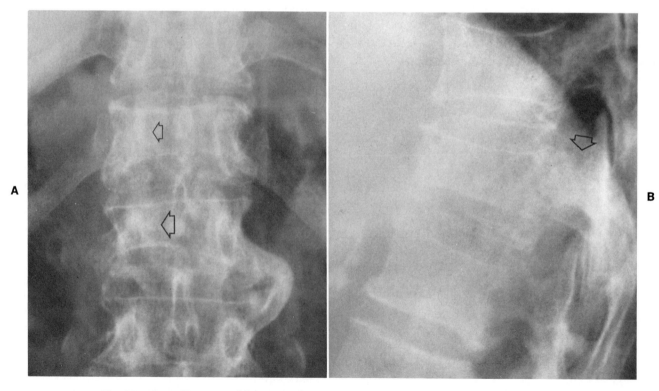

Fig. 4-35. Sixty-three-year-old woman who was known to have carcinoma of breast. She had a recent onset of back pain. There was no neurologic deficit. **A,** There is compression of vertebral bodies of T12 and L1. Right pedicle is absent on T12 *(upper arrow)* and is poorly defined on L1 *(lower arrow).* **B,** Lateral radiograph demonstrates minimal compression of L1 and moderate compression of T12. There is destruction of posterior cortex and pedicle of T12 *(arrow).*

recognition of cortical destruction of any component of the vertebra is equally important and diagnostic. The pedicles may not be involved by the malignant process and furthermore are frequently spared in multiple myeloma. The history, of course, may be helpful in that the injury or inciting episode may have been trivial, but this does not allow any discrimination between an insufficiency fracture of osteoporosis and a pathologic fracture associated with metastatic disease. The presence of a surrounding soft tissue mass is further evidence to suggest metastatic disease, but it could be caused by a hematoma alone, particularly if the mass is small. It is important, then, to search for evidence of bone destruction when faced with any spinal fracture in older individuals and particularly so when the fractures are multiple or discontiguous in order to exclude the possibility of a pathologic fracture.

The spinal cord injury or deficit associated with metastatic deposits in the spine may occur abruptly from a sudden fracture and the formation of hematoma with compression of the spinal cord or cauda equina, or it may occur more gradually by growth of the tumor within the spinal canal. The degree and exact site of

the extradural compression can be identified by myelography.

Other forms of pathologic fracture occur but are rare. Vertebrae plana is a distinctive form of compression associated with eosinophilic granuloma. Primary tumors occur in the vertebral body and posterior elements, but these are rare and usually are indicated by pain without pathologic fractures or spinal cord injury. The most common primary tumors are osteoblastoma, aneurysmal bone cyst, giant cell tumors, and chondrosarcoma.

SPINAL FRACTURES IN ANKYLOSING SPONDYLITIS

Fractures of the spine in ankylosing spondylitis have a peculiar pattern because of the rigidity of the ankyloses and an associated osteoporosis of the underlying vertebral bodies.[10,104,106,108] The fractures are particularly common in the cervical spine (Fig. 4-36), are often related to trivial trauma, and are usually caused by hyperextension forces.[32,75,106] The fractures characteristically involve the posterior elements and an associated intervertebral disc space of the lower cervical spine.

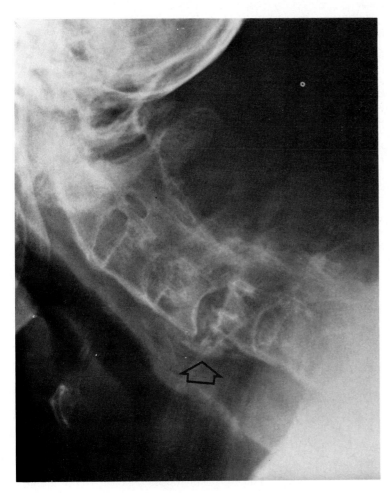

Fig. 4-36. Thirty-two-year-old man with ankylosing spondylitis sustained a fracture of C4-5 after a minor car accident 3 weeks prior to this radiograph. There is already callus formation (*arrow*).

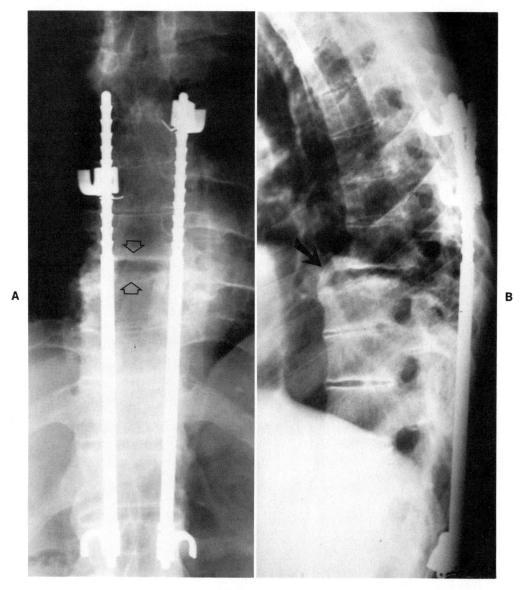

Fig. 4-37. Forty-three-year-old man with ankylosing spondylitis sustained a fracture-dislocation of T8-9 in an automobile accident, which was treated by Harrington rod stabilization. **A,** Frontal view shows fracture at level of interspace *(arrows)*. **B,** Lateral view shows early callus formation *(arrow)*.

Similar fractures may occur any place within the spinal column, however (Fig. 4-37). The fracture traverses the syndesmophytes at the involved interspace and characteristically spares the vertebral body. Healing occurs quickly after the application of a brace or body cast as appropriate.

Fracture-dislocations occur with the fracture line located in the same position as that described above.[32,35,37] The degree of displacement and resultant spinal cord injury are variable and in part depend on the severity of the forces involved and the degree of compromise of the spinal canal. In Woodruff and Dewing's review[106] the initial mortality from this fracture was 45%.

REFERENCES

1. Abel, M. S.: Occult traumatic lesions of the cervical vertebrae, St. Louis, 1970, Warren H. Green.
2. Alker, G. J., Young, S. O., Leslie, E. V., et al.: Postmortem radiology of head and neck injuries in fatal traffic accidents, Radiology **114:**611, 1975.
3. Anderson, L. D., and d'Alonzo, R. T.: Fractures of the odontoid process of the axis, J. Bone Joint Surg. [Am.] **56:**1663, 1974.
4. Anderson, P. T., and Horlyck, E.: Fracture of the spine, Acta Orthop. Scand. **40:**653, 1969.
5. Apuzzo, M. L. J., Heiden, J. S., Weiss, M. H., et al.: Acute fractures of the odontoid process, J. Neurosurg. **48:**85, 1978.

6. Babcock, J. L.: Cervical spine injuries: diagnosis and classification, Arch. Surg. 3:646, 1976.
7. Beatson, T. R.: Fractures and dislocations of the cervical spine, J. Bone Joint Surg. [Br.] 45:21, 1963.
8. Bedbrook, G. M.: Stability of spinal fractures and fracture-dislocations, Paraplegia 9:23, 1971.
9. Bentley, G., and McSweeney, T.: Multiple spinal injuries, Br. J. Surg. 55:565, 1968.
10. Bergmann, E. W.: Fractures of the ankylosed spine, J. Bone Joint Surg. [Am.] 31:669, 1949.
11. Black, P.: Injuries of the vertebral column and spinal cord: mechanisms and management in the acute phase. In Ballinger, W. F., Rutherford, R. B., and Zuidema, G. D., editors: The management of trauma, chap. 6, Philadelphia, 1973, W. B. Saunders Co.
12. Braakman, R., and Vinken, P. J.: Unilateral facet interlocking in the lower cervical spine, J. Bone Joint Surg. [Br.] 49:249, 1967.
13. Burke, D. C.: Hyperextension injuries of the spine, J. Bone Joint Surg. [Br.] 53:3, 1971.
14. Burke, D. C.: Spinal cord trauma in children, Paraplegia 9:1, 1971.
15. Calenoff, L., Chessare, J. W., Rogers, L. F., et al.: Multiple level spinal injuries: importance of early recognition, Am. J. Roentgenol. 130:665, 1978.
16. Casey, B. M., Eaton, S. B., Du Bois, J. J., et al.: Thoracolumbar neural arch fractures, J.A.M.A. 224:1263, 1973.
17. Castellano, V., and Bocconi, F. L.: Injuries of the cervical spine with spinal cord involvement (myelinic fractures): statistical considerations, Bull. Hosp. Joint Dis. 31:188, 1970.
18. Colley, D. P., and Dunsker, S. B.: Traumatic narrowing of the dorsolumbar spinal canal demonstrated by computed tomography, Radiology 129:95, 1978.
19. Deeb, Z. L., Martin, T. A., and Kerber, C. W.: Traction device for use with polytome table, Am. J. Roentgenol. 131:732, 1978.
20. Dehner, J. R.: Seatbelt injuries of the spine and abdomen, Am. J. Roentgenol. 111:833, 1971.
21. Dershner, M. S., Goodman, G. A., and Perlmutter, G. S.: Computed tomography in the diagnosis of an atlas fracture, Am. J. Roentgenol. 128:688, 1977.
22. Dolan, K. D.: Cervical spine injuries below the axis, Radiol. Clin. North Am. 15:247, 1977.
23. Drew, R., McClelland, R. R., and Fischer, R. F.: The dominance of vertebral column fractures associated with neurologic deficits among survivors of light-plane accidents, J. Trauma 17:574, 1977.
24. Eismont, F. J., and Bohlman, H. H.: Posterior atlanto-occipital dislocation with fractures of the atlas and odontoid process, J. Bone Joint Surg. [Am.] 60:397, 1978.
25. Elliott, J. M., Rogers, L. F., Wissinger, J. P., and Lee, J. F.: The hangman's fracture, Radiology 104:303, 1972.
26. Fletcher, B., and Brogdon, B. G.: Seat-belt fractures of the spine and sternum, J.A.M.A. 200:167, 1967.
27. Forsyth, H. F.: Extension injuries of the cervical spine, J. Bone Joint Surg. [Am.] 46:1792, 1964.
28. Fox, J. L., and Jerez, A.: An unusual atlanto-axial dislocation: case report, J. Neurosurg. 47:115, 1977.

29. Fullenlove, T. M., and Wilson, J. G.: Traumatic defects of the pars interacticularis of the lumbar vertebrae, Am. J. Roentgenol. 122:634, 1974.
30. Gehrig, R., and Michaelis, L. S.: Statistics of acute paraplegia and tetraplegia on a national scale: Switzerland 1960-77, Paraplegia 6:93, 1968.
31. Gerlock, A. J., Kischner, S. G., Heller, R. M., and Kay, J. J.: The cervical spine in trauma, Philadelphia, 1978, W.B. Saunders Co.
32. Good, A. E.: Nontraumatic fracture of the thoracic spine in ankylosing spondylitis, Arthritis Rheum. 10:467, 1967.
33. Gosch, H. H., Gooking, E., and Schneider, R. C.: An experimental study of cervical spine and cord injuries, J. Trauma 12:570, 1972.
34. Griffith, H. B., Gleave, J. R. W., and Taylor, R. G.: Changing patterns of fracture in the dorsal and lumbar spine, Br. Med. J. 1:891, 1966.
35. Grisolia, A., Bell, R. L., and Peltier, L. F.: Fractures and dislocations of the spine complicating ankylosing spondylitis, J. Bone Joint Surg. [Am.] 49:339, 1967.
36. Hanafee, W., and Crandall, P.: Trauma of the spine and its contents, Radiol. Clin. North Am. 4:365, 1966.
37. Hansen, S. T., Taylor, T. K. F., Honet, J. C., and Lewis, F. R.: Fracture-dislocations of the ankylosed thoracic spine in rheumatoid spondylitis, J. Trauma 7:827, 1967.
38. Haralson, R. H., III, and Boyd, H. B.: Posterior dislocation of the atlas on the axis without fracture, J. Bone Joint Surg. [Am.] 51:561, 1969.
39. Harris, J. H., Jr. Acute injuries of the spine, Semin. Roentgenol. 13:53, 1978.
40. Harris, J. H., Jr.: The radiology of acute cervical spine trauma, Baltimore, 1978, The Williams & Wilkins Co.
41. Harviainen, S., Lahti, P., and Davidsson, L.: On cervical spine injuries, Acta Chir. Scand. 138:349, 1972.
42. Hegenbarth, R., and Ebel, Kl.-D.: Roentgen findings in fractures of the vertebral column in childhood: examination of 35 patients and its results, Pediatr. Radiol. 5:34, 1976.
43. Henrys, P., Lyne, E. D., Lifton, C., and Scalciccioli, G.: Clinical review of cervical spine injuries in children, Clin. Orthop. 129:172, 1977.
44. Hohl, M., and Baker, H. R.: The atlanto-axial joint, J. Bone Joint Surg. [Am.] 46:1739, 1964.
45. Holdsworth, F.: Fractures, dislocations, and fracture-dislocations of the spine, J. Bone Joint Surg. [Am.] 52:1534, 1970.
46. Holdsworth, F. W.: Fractures, dislocations, and fracture-dislocations of the spine, J. Bone Joint Surg. [Br.] 45:6, 1963.
47. Horal, J., Nachemson, A., and Scjeller, S.: Clinical and radiological long term follow-up vertebral fractures in children, Acta Orthop. Scand. 43:491, 1972.
48. Howorth, M. B.: Fracture of the spine, Am. J. Surg. 92:573, 1956.
49. Hubbard, D. D.: Injuries of the spine in children and adolescents, Clin. Orthop. 100:56, 1974.
50. Jacobs, B.: Cervical fracture and dislocation (C3-7), Clin. Orthop. 109:18, 1975.

51. Jacobs, R. R.: Bilateral fracture of the pedicles through the fourth and fifth lumbar vertebrae with anterior displacement of the vertebral bodies; case report, J. Bone Joint Surg. [Am.] 59:409, 1977.

52. Jacobson, G., and Adler, D. C.: An evaluation of lateral atlanto-axial displacement in injuries of the cervical spine, Radiology 61:355, 1953.

53. Jacobson, G., and Adler, D. C.: Examination of the atlanto-axial joint following injury, Am. J. Roentgenol. 76:1081, 1956.

54. Jefferson, G.: Discussion on spinal injuries, Proc. R. Soc. Med. 21:625, 1927-28.

55. Jonas, J. G.: Fracture-dislocation of the dorsal spine, South. Med. J. 69:1502, 1976.

56. Kattan, K. R.: Backward "displacement" of the spino-laminal line at C₂: normal variation, Am. J. Roentgenol. 129:289, 1977.

57. Kaufer, H., and Hayes, J. T.: Lumbar fracture-dislocation, J. Bone Joint Surg. [Am.] 48:712, 1966.

58. Kessler, L. A.: Delayed, traumatic dislocation of the cervical spine, J.A.M.A. 224:124, 1973.

59. Kewalramani, L. S., and Taylor, R. G.: Multiple noncontiguous injuries to the spine, Acta Orthop. Scand. 47:52, 1976.

60. King, D. M.: Fractures and dislocations of the cervical part of the spine, Aust. N.Z. J. Surg. 37:57, 1967.

61. Laasonen, E. M., and Riska, E. B.: Preoperative radiological assessment of fractures of the thoracolumbar spine causing traumatic paraplegia, Skeletal Radiol. 1:231, 1977.

62. Lipson, S. J.: Fractures of the atlas associated with fractures of the odontoid process and transverse ligament ruptures, J. Bone Joint Surg. [Am.] 59:940, 1977.

63. Macnab, I.: Acceleration injuries of the cervical spine, J. Bone Joint Surg. [Am.] 56:1797, 1964.

64. Marar, B. C.: The pattern of neurological damage as an aid to the diagnosis of the mechanism in cervical-spine injuries, J. Bone Joint Surg. [Am.] 56:1648, 1974.

65. Marar, B. C.: Hyperextension injuries of the cervical spine, J. Bone Joint Surg. [Am.] 56:1655, 1974.

66. McCoy, S. H., and Johnson, K. A.: Sagittal fracture of the cervical spine, J. Trauma 16:310, 1976.

67. Melamed, A.: Fracture of pars interarticularis of lumbar vertebra, Am. J. Roentgenol. 94:584, 1965.

68. Miller, M. D., Gehweiler, J. A., Martinez, S., et al.: Significant new observations on cervical spine trauma, Am. J. Roentgenol. 130:659, 1978.

69. Nicoll, E. A.: Fractures of the dorso-lumbar spine, J. Bone Joint Surg. [Br.] 31:376, 1949.

70. Norrell, H. A.: Fractures and dislocations of the spine. In Rothman, R. H., and Simeone, F. A., editors: The spine, vol. II, Philadelphia, 1975, W. B. Saunders Co.

71. O'Brien, J. J., Butterfield, W. L., and Gossling, H. R.: Jefferson fracture with disruption of the transverse ligament, Clin. Orthop. 126:135, 1977.

72. Olsson, O.: Fractures of the upper thoracic and cervical vertebral bodies, Acta Chir. Scand. 102:87, 1951.

73. Penning, L.: Diagnostic clues by x-ray injuries of the lower cervical spine, Acta Neurochir. (Wien) 22:234, 1970.

74. Quesada, R. S., Greenbaum, E. I., Hertl, A., and Zoda, F.: Widened interpedicular distance secondary to trauma, J. Trauma 15:167, 1975.

75. Rapp, G. G., and Kernek, C. B.: Spontaneous fracture of the lumbar spine with correction of deformity in ankylosing spondylitis, J. Bone Joint Surg. [Am.] 56:1277, 1974.

76. Rennie, W., and Mitchell, N.: Flexion distraction fractures of the thoracolumbar spine, J. Bone Joint Surg. [Am.] 55:386, 1973.

77. Richman, S., and Friedman, R. L.: Vertical fracture of cervical vertebral bodies, Radiology 62:536, 1954.

78. Riggins, R. S., and Kraus, J. F.: The risk of neurologic damage with fractures of the vertebrae, J. Trauma 17:126, 1977.

79. Rigler, L. G.: Kummell's disease with report of a roentgenologically proved case, Am. J. Roentgenol. 15:749, 1931.

80. Roaf, R.: A study of the mechanics of spinal injuries, J. Bone Joint Surg. [Br.] 42:810, 1960.

81. Roberts, J. B., and Curtiss, P. H.: Stability of the thoracic and lumbar spine in traumatic paraplegia following fracture or fracture-dislocation, J. Bone Joint Surg. [Am.] 52:1115, 1970.

82. Rogers, L. F.: The roentgenographic appearance of transverse or Chance fractures of the spine: the seat belt fracture, Am. J. Roentgenol. 111:844, 1971.

83. Rogers, W. A.: Fractures and dislocations of the cervical spine: and end-result study, J. Bone Joint Surg. [Am.] 39:341, 1957.

84. Russin, L. D., Guinto, F. C., Jr.: Multidirectional tomography in cervical spine injury, J. Neurosurg. 45:9, 1976.

85. Schatzker, J.: Fractures of the dens (odontoid process): an analysis of thirty-seven cases, J. Bone Joint Surg. [Br.] 53:392, 1971.

86. Scher, A. T.: Double fractures of the spine—an indication for routine radiographic examination of the entire spine after injury, S. Afr. Med. J. 53:411, 1978.

87. Schneider, R. C.: The syndrome of acute anterior spinal cord injury, J. Neurosurg. 12:95, 1955.

88. Schneider, R. C., Cherry, G., and Pantek, H.: The syndrome of acute central cervical spinal cord injury, J. Neurosurg. 11:546, 1954.

89. Seimon, L. P.: Fracture of the odontoid process in young children, J. Bone Joint Surg. [Am.] 59:943, 1977.

90. Selecki, B. R.: Cervical spine and cord injuries: mechanisms and surgical implications, Med. J. Aust. 1:838, 1970.

91. Seljeskog, E. L., and Chou, S. N.: Spectrum of the hangman's fracture, J. Neurosurg. 45:3, 1976.

92. Shapiro, R., Youngberg, A. S., and Rothman, S. L.: The differential diagnosis of traumatic lesions of the occipito-atlanto-axial segment, Radiol. Clin. North Am. 11:505, 1973.

93. Sheldon, J. J., Sersland, T., and Leborgne, J.: Computed tomography of the lower lumbar vertebral column, Radiology 124:113, 1977.

94. Sherk, H. H., and Nicholson, J. T.: Fractures of the atlas, J. Bone Joint Surg. [Am.] 52:1017, 1970.

95. Skold, G.: Sagittal fractures of the cervical spine, Injury **9**:294, 1978.

96. Smith, G. R., Northrop, C. H., and Loop, J. W.: Jumper's fractures: patterns of thoracolumbar spine injuries associated with vertical plunges, Radiology **122**:657, 1977.

97. Smith, W. S., and Kaufer, H.: Patterns and mechanisms of lumbar injuries associated with lap seat belts, J. Bone Joint Surg. [Am.] **51**:239, 1969.

98. Stauffer, E. S., and Kaufer, H.: Fractures and dislocations of the spine. In Rockwood, C. A., Jr., and Green, D. P., editors: Fractures, vol. 2, Philadelphia, 1975, J. B. Lippincott Co.

99. Swischuk, L. E.: Anterior displacement of C2 in children: physiologic or pathologic? Radiology **122**:759, 1977.

100. Tadmor, R., Davis, K. R., Roberson, G. H., et al.: Computed tomographic evaluation of traumatic spinal injuries, Radiology **127**:825, 1978.

101. Taylor, A. R., and Blackwood, W.: Paraplegia in hyperextension cervical injuries with normal radiographic appearances, J. Bone Joint Surg. [Br.] **30**:245, 1948.

102. White, A. A., and Hirsch, C.: The significance of the vertebral posterior elements in the mechanics of the thoracic spine, Clin. Orthop. **81**:2, 1971.

103. Whitley, J. E., and Forsyth, H. F.: The classification of cervical spine injuries, Am. J. Roentgenol. **83**:633, 1960.

104. Wilkinson, M., and Bywaters, E. G. L.: Clinical features and course of ankylosing spondylitis, Ann. Rheum. Dis. **17**:209, 1958.

105. Wiltse, L. L., Widell, E. H., and Jackson, D. W.: Fatigue fracture: the basic lesion in isthmic spondylolisthesis, J. Bone Joint Surg. [Am.] **57**:17, 1975.

106. Woodruff, F., and Dewing, S. B.: Fractures of the cervical spine in patients with ankylosing spondylitis, Radiology **80**:17, 1963.

107. Yashon, D., Jane, J. A., and White, R. J.: Prognosis and management of spinal cord and cauda equina bullet injuries in sixty-five civilians, J. Neurosurg. **32**:163, 1979.

108. Yau, A. C. M. C., and Chan, R. N. W.: Stress fracture of the fused lumbo-dorsal spine in ankylosing spondylitis, J. Bone Joint Surg. [Br.] **56**:681, 1974.

109. Zatzkin, H. R., and Kveton, F. W.: Evaluation of the cervical spine in whiplash injuries, Radiology **75**:577, 1960.

CHAPTER 5

Neuroradiologic assessment of spinal cord injuries

MICHAEL A. MIKHAEL, M.D., and MASOUD HEMMATI, M.D.

It is generally accepted that acute compromise of the spinal cord by a posttraumatic extramedullary or intramedullary lesion is a clinical emergency. An accurate knowledge of both the nature and the level of the compromising factor is valuable in deciding the therapeutic plan. The extramedullary factors include bony fragments, herniated intervertebral discs, hematomas, and foreign bodies. The intramedullary factors include cord swelling from edema or hematoma and cord infarction.*

Clinical examination is not usually conclusive in the differentiation between extramedullary and intramedullary compromising factors. The neurologic evaluation may localize the lesion within one or two segments above or below the actual anatomic level. Plain films and polytomographic studies may demonstrate the posttraumatic changes in the bony structures. However, these changes do not necessarily indicate the site or the degree of cord injury. There are cases in which the cord damage is irreversible without evidence of bony injury, whereas other cases may have severe fracture or dislocation of the spine with minor neurologic deficit.

In addition to plain films, polytomography and disc injection, computed tomography, myelography, and angiographic studies can be used to evaluate the anatomic structure of the bony spinal canal, spinal cord, and re-

lated soft tissues including the gross vascularity to the damaged segment.[9,12,15,25,48] To obtain the most beneficial information, with reliability and safety, the chosen radiologic procedures should be weighed for each individual case according to the presenting clinical status. Some authors have found a special procedure to be of limited value and at times not indicative because of possible complications.[2,34] Others advocate following a standard diagnostic protocol for spinal cord injury cases.[40] In a brief review of the literature one will find much debate over the risks and benefits of performing angiography and myelography and whether or not and when they can be done.

It is our belief that the diagnostic procedures needed for each individual patient should be determined according to the type and site of the trauma, the clinical findings, and the ability of the patient to withstand the procedure. Careful evaluation of the plain films and polytomographic studies is usually necessary before considering any other radiologic procedures. This evaluation often helps to determine the type and mechanism of injury and along with the patient's clinical conditions will help the radiologist to choose the most appropriate diagnostic study.

BIOMECHANICS OF THE SPINE

A review of the biomechanics of the spine may help in understanding the traumatic changes in the spine

---

*References 2, 4-6, 13, 14, 19, 24, 27, 34, 40, 41, 43, 46, 47.

130

and the choice of radiologic procedure. Biomechanical studies of the physical properties of the spine and the spinal cord have shown that the spinal canal changes in length as a result of physiologic flexion, extension, and lateral bending.[5,6] It is lengthened during flexion and is shortened during extension. These changes in the length of the bony canal are always followed by similar changes in the spinal cord. The effective cross-sectional area of the canal also undergoes changes with physiologic axial rotation and horizontal displacement.

The spinal cord (cord and pia mater) is a structure with a special biomechanical characteristic. When removed from the spinal canal and suspended in a vertical position, the spinal cord lengthens because of its own weight by more than 10%. This extreme flexibility suddenly changes into stiff resistance when the cord is stretched to produce any further deformation. The load-displacement curve of the spinal cord is similar to that of ligaments and has two distinct phases: an initial phase in which large displacement is obtained with very small forces and a second phase in which a relatively larger force is required to produce relatively smaller changes.[5,6] The extreme flexibility of the cord in the initial phase is achieved by folding and unfolding the specially designed structure of the cord, such as an accordion. Beyond these normal limits of folding and unfolding, the tissue is subjected to a direct tension force that is counteracted by its inherent elastic properties.

In flexion the length of the spinal canal is increased, however, the maximal increase is that for the posterior quarter of the canal. In extension the canal is shortened with the maximal decrease on the concave side, its posterior part. The spinal cord folds like an accordion during extension. These folds, which are more distinct on its posterior surface, where the maximal decrease in length occurs, can be visualized as a series of posterior bulges during myelography. The ligamenta flava encroachment may also contribute to these folds, especially in older people, since these ligaments become hypertrophied and less elastic with age. During full flexion the cord, its nerve roots, and dentate ligaments are under physiologic tension. The dentate ligaments are inclined inferiorly. The tensile force in the ligaments thus has two components with respect to the axis of the spinal cord. The axial component balances the tension in the cord, probably reducing its magnitude. The transverse component balances each other in pairs and anchors the cord near the center of the canal. The central position of the spinal cord provides maximal protection from bony impingement or shock during trauma.

Compression loading of the discs does not usually produce disc herniation.[8] The disc only bulges in a horizontal plane under such physiologic loading. However, when the disc is degenerated, such compression loading may result in relatively high stress on the disc. The bending and rotational loads are probably more dangerous to the disc than is axial compression. During bending the disc bulges on the concave side of the curve and collapses on the convex side. In flexion of the spine the intact disc protrudes anteriorly and is depressed posteriorly. An injury to the posterior stretched part of the disc's annulus results in herniation of the nucleus into the canal.

Hyperflexion injuries can result in severe neurologic damage without visible bone disruption. Hyperextension injuries usually are more difficult to diagnose because of the inherent stability of the spine that remains. The possibility of damage to the cord by compression from a displaced herniated disc anteriorly and enfolding of the ligamenta flava posteriorly is important. Patients may develop acute spinal cord syndromes with or without evidence of injury to the bony spinal canal. Transient cord compression from spinal cord contusions with edema or hematoma may progress to complete transverse cord necrosis. Hyperextension injuries are more liable to occur in the presence of chronic spinal stenosis.[4,14] During the movement of extreme hyperextension the combination of wrinkling of the ligamenta flava and increased dorsal bulging of the intervertebral discs results in further narrowing of the spinal canal.[7,8] With the presence of hypertrophied degenerative posterior bony osteophytes the possibility for damage is further increased.[14] Hyperextension injury can also produce severe damage in the newborn infant during breech delivery. Kaplan[32] postulated that hyperextension injuries may cause thrombosis of the anterior spinal artery with consequent cord damage. Angiography is sometimes needed for the evaluation of the vascular damage to the cord.

COMPUTED TOMOGRAPHY

The principle of transaxial tomography was described as early as 1947 by Vallebona.[58] The studies of Takahashi,[53] Gargano and co-workers,[15] and Jacobson and co-workers[30,31] have provided comprehensive data for evaluation of the spinal canal by axial tomography. Although axial tomography is a noninvasive diagnostic technique and can be used to study the cross-sectional anatomy of the spine, it has not received much popularity. The reasons include the fact that proper equipment is not available in many institutions, the lack of expertise in this field, and the recent utilization of computed tomography (CT).* CT is more popular and is available in many centers dealing with spinal trauma. It enables the cross-sectional study of not only the bony

---

*References 10, 11, 17, 18, 30, 48.

spine, such as in the case of axial tomography, but also the soft tissue elements.[11,18,36] The study does not require excessive patient manipulation, and it is widely utilized in many institutions. With high-resolution CT scanners there has been marked improvement in the delineation of the spinal fractures and the visualization of the posttraumatic abnormalities of the spinal cord. It is possible with CT to examine the spine in the standard transaxial, as well as the sagittal and coronal, planes, either by direct or by computer-reconstructed images. Widely separated fractures are more easily visualized but even hairline fractures may be successfully demonstrated with the perpendicular reconstructed scans.[10,11,36] To minimize distortion resulting from exaggerated or normal lordosis of the spine in the cervical and lumbar regions the gantry can be angled to such a degree that the x-ray beam will become perpendicular to the vertical axis of the vertebrae at each level.

Indications

Initially CT studies for the spine were regarded as an adjunct examination to polytomography and had poor clinical acceptance. Polytomography was present before CT and was more popular; also, with polytomography the pictures are magnified and easily interpreted. However, with individuals gaining increased experience in both performing and interpreting CT scans, these scans have now been accepted and their usefulness realized. Polytomography is superior to CT in delineating horizontal fractures. CT is superior to polytomography in the following ways:

1. Imaging the spinal canal itself in a cross-sectional plane, demonstrating any posttraumatic spinal stenosis, and delineating the exact relationship of fracture fragments or foreign bodies to the spinal canal
2. Imaging the multiple radiating fractures within compressed vertebral bodies
3. Examining the intraspinal and extraspinal soft tissues[10,18,36,48]
4. Showing the axial, coronal, and sagittal sectional anatomy of the bony and soft tissues of the spinal and paraspinal regions
5. Examining the patient in supine position (one position) without need to move him to lateral position

Patients with spinal trauma must be evaluated initially by routine plain radiographs to determine areas of gross abnormalities. After this initial evaluation, polytomography may be used to study in detail the areas of special interest as determined by the findings on radiographs or by clinical examination.[34] The polytomography study usually shows in detail the fractures, the displacements, and other acute bony changes. CT should be done on all patients with suspected spinal trauma when they are symptomatic and both the plain films and polytomograms are normal or show findings that cannot explain the clinical status. Compromise to the spinal canal is best evaluated in the cross-sectional plane where CT provides this information with minimal patient discomfort. The normal diameters of the canal are discussed in Chapter 2.[17,22,36,48] In many cases CT must follow polytomography even if the latter is abnormal in order to examine the spinal canal and the soft tissues both inside and outside the canal, especially when the clinical status is not stable.

In summary, in spinal injury, the main indications for CT are the following:

1. Normal plain films and polytomographic studies in patients with suspected spinal injury and acute neurologic deficit
2. Abnormalities on the plain films or polytomograms of the spine that cannot explain completely the clinical picture (the neurologic deficit)

In a few institutions CT is gradually replacing polytomography and is done in every case of spinal trauma (more informative with high-resolution scanners).

Radiologic findings

CT adds a third dimension to the radiologic examination of the spine and to the correct interpretation of the pathologic changes. It clearly demonstrates the relationship of the fracture fragments, loose fragments, or foreign bodies to the bony spinal canal and spinal cord.[10,18,22,36,48] High-resolution scanners may be useful in detecting intraspinal and extraspinal hematomas, spinal cord abnormalities, and sometimes herniated discs.

The possible pathologic features that can be seen on CT studies of the spine in cases of trauma include the following:

1. Detection of fractures (Figs. 5-1 to 5-9)
   a. Vertically oriented sagittal and coronal fractures of the vertebral bodies, the laminae, the spinous processes, the lateral masses, and the articular pillars; widely separated fractures; hairline fractures when oriented perpendicular to the CT section
   b. Horizontal fractures in coronal and sagittal reconstruction images
   c. Radiating fractures within compressed vertebral bodies
2. Displacement of fragments and spinal compromise (Figs. 5-4 to 5-9)
   a. Fragment displacement (bony and foreign bodies) at the site of fracture, especially in relation to the spinal canal
   b. Disruption of the normal relation between the

Text continued on p. 138.

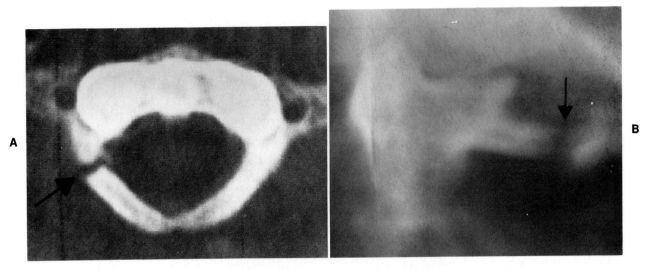

Fig. 5-1. Seventeen-year-old adolescent involved in a motorcycle accident had a fracture at C1-2 level, neurologically intact. Fracture of posterior arch of C1 *(arrow)* is shown on CT scan, **A,** and conventional polytomogram, **B.** Relation of fracture to cross-sectional anatomy of bony spinal canal is clearly demonstrated on CT scan (no bony encroachment).

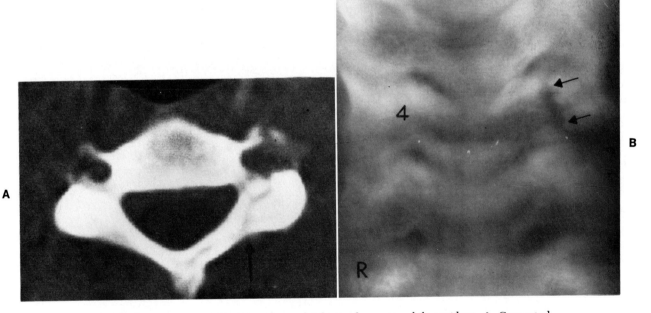

Fig. 5-2. Nineteen-year-old man with quadriplegia after automobile accident. **A,** Computed tomography of spine at C4 level demonstrates fracture through lateral mass and base of lamina of left side *(arrow)*. No bony encroachment on spinal canal. **B,** AP tomogram of cervical spine demonstrates fracture of base of lamina and lateral mass of left side *(arrows)*. It is difficult to evaluate spinal canal as clearly as in **A.**

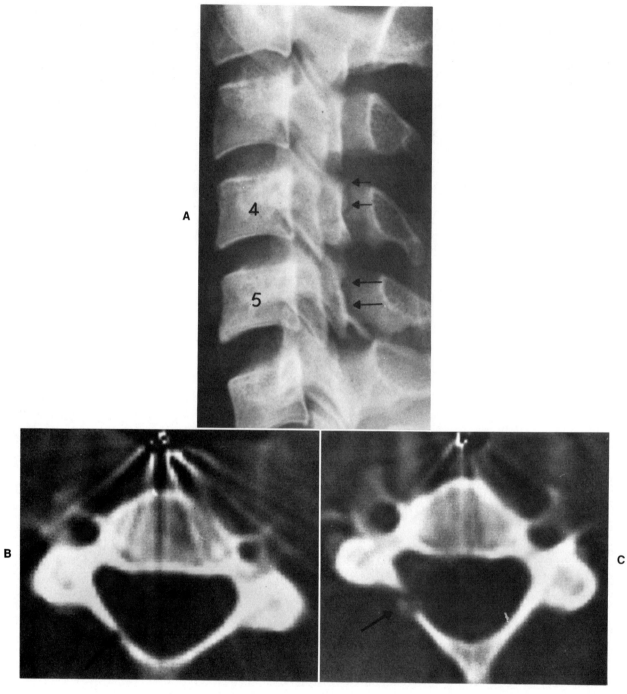

Fig. 5-3. Twenty-five-year-old man involved in automobile accident became quadriplegic. **A,** Lateral view of cervical spine demonstrates fractures through posterior arches at C4 and C5 levels *(arrows)*. **B** and **C,** CT scans of spine at C4 and C5 levels, respectively, showing fractures of laminae of both vertebrae on right side *(arrows)*. Note clear relation of fracture to cross-sectional anatomy of spinal canal. No bony encroachment.

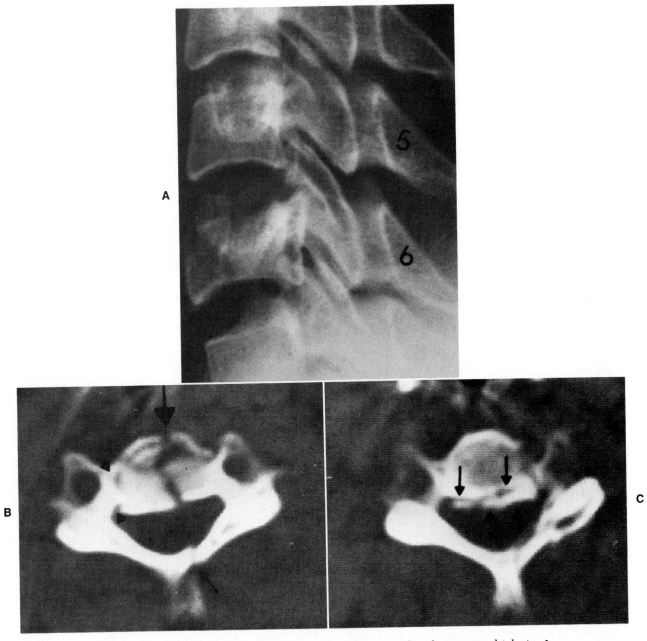

Fig. 5-4. Twenty-four-year-old woman involved in diving accident became quadriplegic. **A,** Lateral view of cervical spine shows fracture-dislocation at C6 level. **B,** CT scan of spine at C6 level showing comminuted fracture of body of C6 *(large arrow)*. There is a fracture of base of right pedicle with posterior displacement of a fragment of body into spinal canal on right side *(arrowheads)*. Note fracture of lamina of left side *(small arrow)*. **C,** CT scan of C5 showing posterior displacement of body of C6 with encroachment on spinal canal *(arrowheads)*. Posterior margin of body of C5 is seen more anteriorly *(arrows)*.

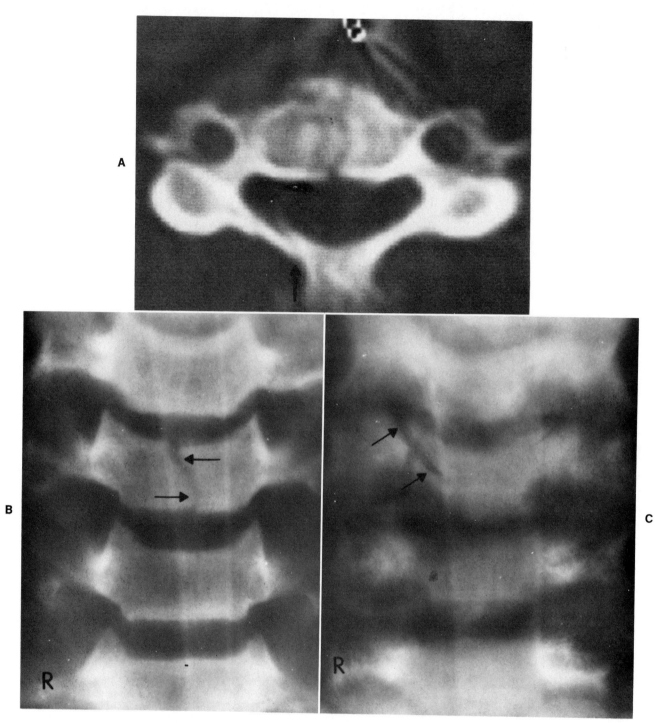

Fig. 5-5. Fifteen-year-old boy involved in diving accident became quadriplegic. **A,** CT scan at C5 demonstrating comminuted fracture of body of C5 and oblique fracture through lamina on right side *(arrow)*, with encroachment on neural canal. **B** and **C,** AP polytomograms of cervical spine showing fracture of body and right lamina of C5 *(arrows)*. Relation of fractures to spinal canal is not as clearly demonstrated as on CT scan, **A.**

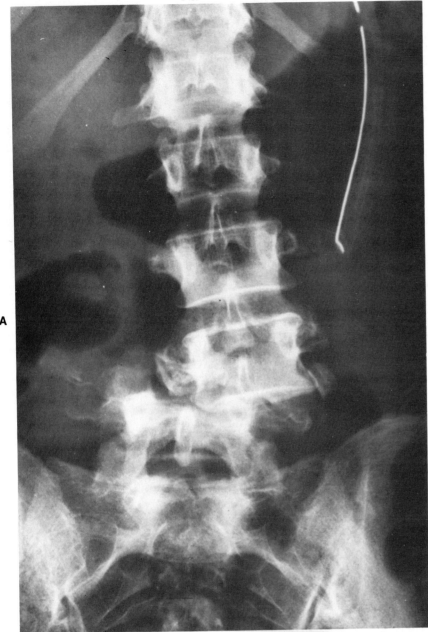

A

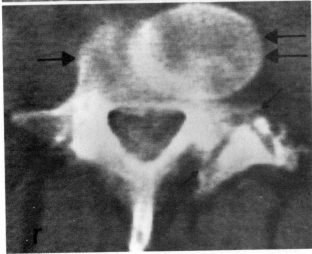

B

Fig. 5-6. Thirty-eight-year-old woman run over by a car. **A,** Plain film of lumbosacral spine showing fracture-dislocation at L4-5 level. **B,** CT scan showing comminuted fracture of lateral mass of L5 on left side *(small arrows)*. There is visualization of bodies of L4 *(double arrows)* and L5 *(single arrow)* in same plane, which indicates impaction of both bodies. Note displacement of body of L4 to left when compared to body of L5. No bony encroachment on spinal canal. (See also Fig. 5-31.)

odontoid process and the anterior arch of the atlas; the widening of the space, the posterior displacement of the odontoid process and its magnitude, and the asymmetric position of the dens between the lateral masses

   c. Malalignment of the spine (Fig. 5-6)

   d. Cross-sectional image of posttraumatic spinal stenosis and the specific spinal diameter or diameters compromised by the fracture (Figs. 5-4 and 5-5)

3. Soft tissue abnormalities (high-resolution scanners)

   a. Paravertebral hematomas and vascular injuries, such as rupture of posttraumatic aortic or other large vessels or true or false aneurysms

   b. Intraspinal hematomas

   c. Spinal cord swelling or hematomas

   d. Herniated intervetebral discs

The high-resolution, fourth-generation CT scanners achieve superb definition of the spinal neural canal, the subarachnoid space, and the spinal cord. In addition, their ability in reconstruction of the coronal and sagittal planes enables the radiologist to diagnose the variety of spinal malalignments, horizontal and vertical fractures, and in some cases herniating discs.

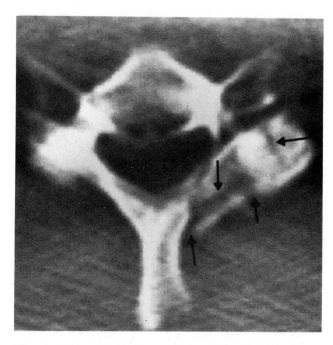

Fig. 5-7. Twenty-seven-year-old man involved in an automobile accident became quadriplegic. CT scan of C6 shows comminuted fracture of lamina and lateral mass on left side (*arrows*). There is no bony encroachment on spinal canal. Myelography or angiography or both may be necessary for further evaluation.

Fig. 5-8. Thirty-two-year-old woman sustained a gunshot wound to lower thoracic spine and became paraplegic. **A,** Plain film of lower thoracic spine showing bullet in profile with inferior aspect of T10 on right side. **B,** AP and **C,** lateral polytomograms of lower thoracic spine demonstrate that bullet is inside spinal canal located in sagittal axis of spine. **D,** CT scan of lower T10 showing bullet and its relation to cross-sectional anatomy of spinal canal. Note trajectory of bullet (*arrows*).

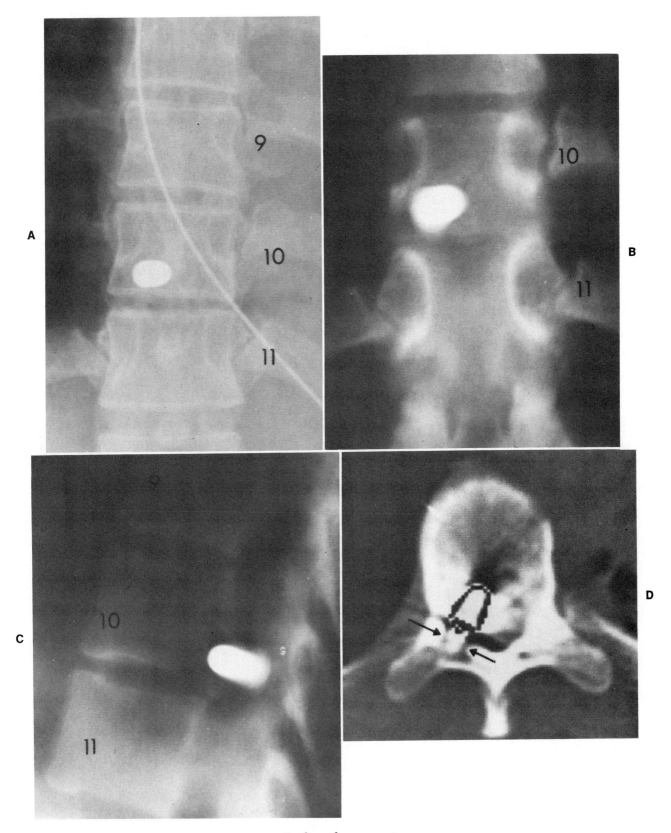

Fig. 5-8. For legend see opposite page.

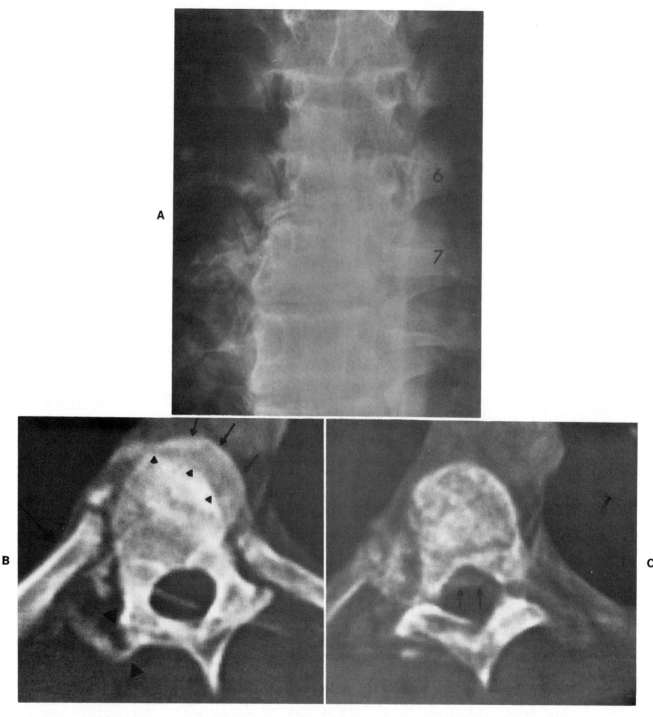

Fig. 5-9. Seventeen-year-old boy involved in motorcycle accident had fractures at T6 and T7 levels. **A,** AP view of midthoracic spine demonstrating compression fractures of T6 and T7. Note lateral displacement to left of T6 in relation to T7. **B,** CT scan of thoracic spine at T6-7 level shows comminuted fracture of lateral mass of T7 on right side *(large arrowheads)*. There is dislocation of right rib *(large arrow)* caused by impaction of T6 and T7. Note visualized portion of body of T6 *(small arrows)* to left side of body of T7 *(small arrowheads)*. **C,** CT scan at T6 level showing that, in addition to compression fracture of body, there is a protrusion of some loose bone fragments into neural canal *(arrows)*.

MYELOGRAPHY IN SPINAL TRAUMA

Hinkel and Nichols (1946)[27] and Barnes (1948)[3] were among the pioneers in performing myelography for spinal cord injuries. They have stressed the value of the procedure and how the results can direct the neurosurgeon in planning the surgical therapy. In their studies they used Pantopaque and iodized oil (Lipiodol) as contrast media. With the advancement of radiographic techniques and equipment, as well as the use of gas and water-soluble contrast agents, the previously reported complications occur less frequently.*

*References 23, 27, 37, 40, 44, 50, 52.

In acute spinal cord injury, myelography can be regarded as a second insult to an already insulted cord. It is generally accepted that immobilization plays an important role in the management of cord injuries. In some patients the damage to the cord is incomplete at the initial stage of injury. They may have a good potential for recovery. Since performing myelography requires transportation and manipulation, the improper handling of the patient may diminish his potential of recovery. Moreover, it is conceivable that the physical and chemical effects of the contrast material may add to the problem.

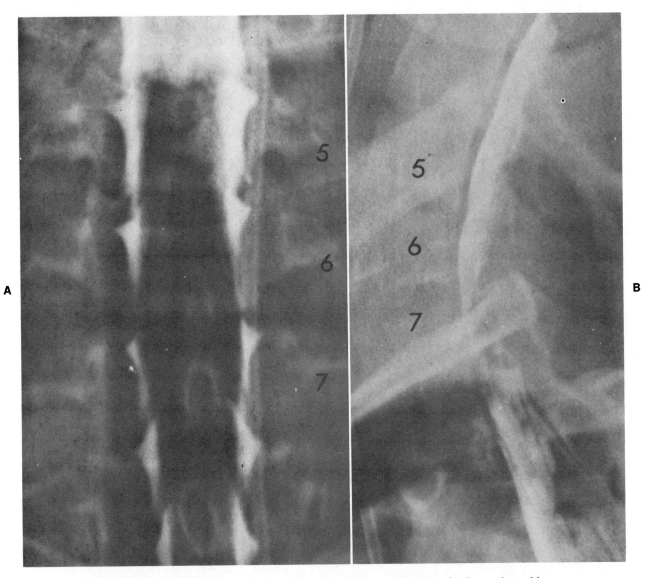

Fig. 5-10. Traumatic cord swelling. Twenty-year-old man became quadriplegic after a blow on back of head by a heavy object. Plain cervical spine films and polytomography failed to demonstrate any fracture or dislocation. Myelography was indicated for further evaluation. **A,** AP and, **B,** lateral views of cervical Pantopaque myelogram in prone position via lumbar route. Note widening of spinal cord in both dimensions, without evidence of extradural defect, presumably from cord swelling.

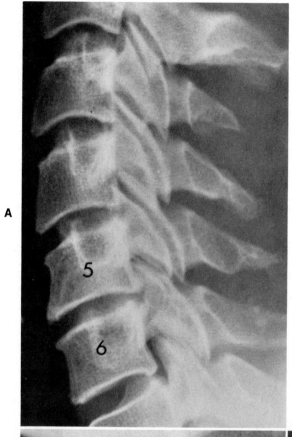

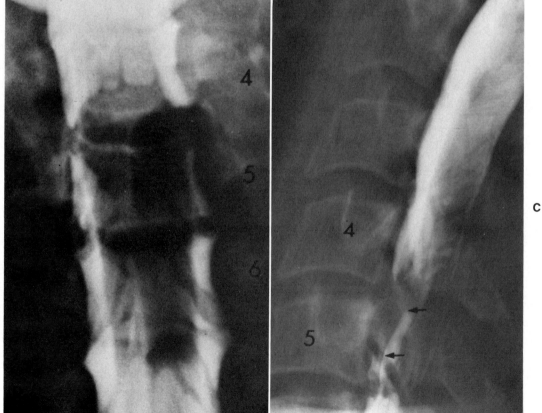

Fig. 5-11. Traumatic epidural hematoma. Thirty-four-year-old man who experienced trauma to neck 2 weeks before being seen with left cervical radiculopathy. **A,** Lateral cervical spine shows no evidence of fracture or dislocation. Myelography is indicated. **B,** AP and **C,** lateral views of cervical Pantopaque myelogram via lumbar route show widening of spinal cord at C4-5 level, compression on C5 nerve root sleeve of left side, and anterior epidural defect at C4-5 level (*arrows* on lateral view) compressing cord. At surgery, anterior epidural hematoma was removed at C4-5 level.

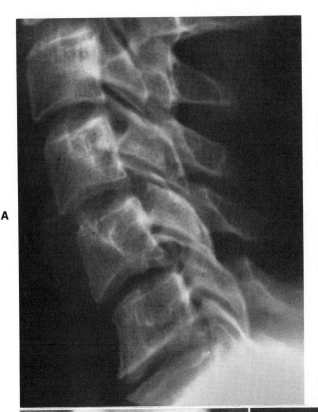

A

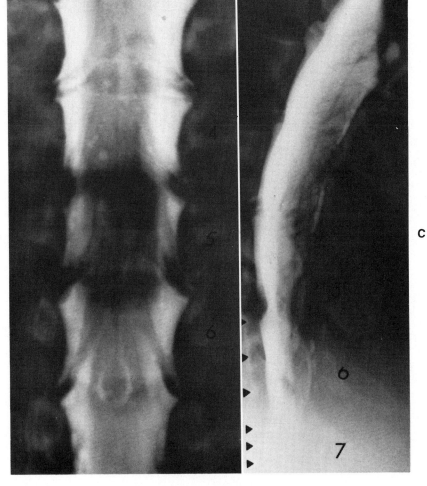

B

C

Fig. 5-12. Traumatic epidural hematoma. Forty-year-old man sustained a diving injury and became quadriplegic. **A,** Lateral cervical spine film shows no fracture or dislocations, with only minor degenerative changes in lower cervical spine. **B,** AP view of cervical Pantopaque myelogram via lumbar route shows normal-appearing spinal cord. There is mild compression on nerve root sleeves at C4-5 and C5-6 levels on left side, which is probably caused by degenerative osteophytes. **C,** Lateral view of cervical myelogram shows posterior displacement of subarachnoid space from posterior margin of body of C6 *(arrowheads)* without evidence of cord compression. This is probably caused by a small epidural hematoma. Findings cannot explain neurologic deficit. Angiography, indicated for further evaluation, was not done because of unstable clinical status of patient.

Indications

Myelography is indicated, in cases of suspected spinal injury, to look for an operable lesion. Emergency myelography should be performed after the patient has been clinically evaluated, his condition becomes stable, and surgery is considered as a possible method of treatment.

The main indications for myelography are the following:

1. Cord compression syndromes, with normal polytomograms and CT scans, looking for intramedullary and/or extramedullary soft tissue changes (cord swelling, hematoma, disc herniation) (Figs. 5-10 to 5-15)

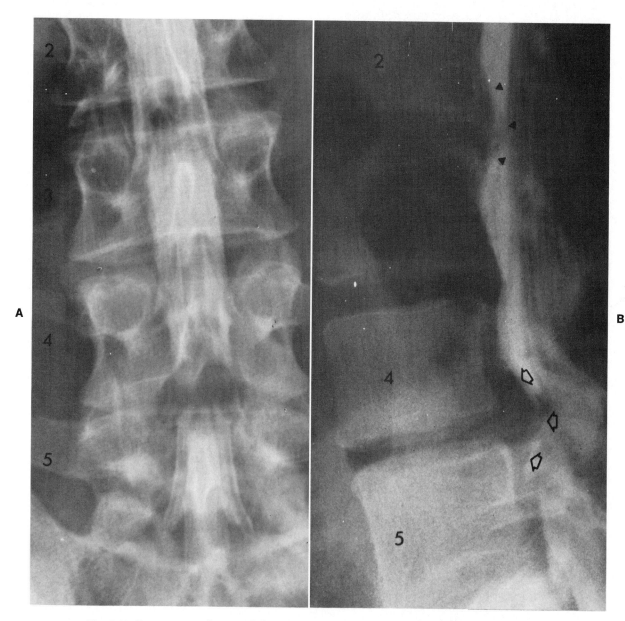

Fig. 5-13. Posttraumatic herniated disc. Twenty-six-year-old man involved in an automobile accident was first seen with lumbar radiculopathy. Plain radiographs of lumbar spine (not shown) demonstrated no evidence of fractures or dislocations. Lumbar Amipaque myelography was indicated and was performed. **A,** AP view. **B,** Lateral view.

2. Neurologic deficit that cannot be explained by the abnormal findings on polytomograms and CT scans (cord enlargement, hematoma, disc herniation, nerve avulsion) (Figs. 5-15 to 5-20)
3. Abrupt change in the neurologic status, such as acute deterioration after being stable or arrest of improvement, which cannot be explained by findings on CT scans or polytomograms or both (partial block progressing to a complete block) (Figs. 5-21 to 5-26)
4. Penetrating wounds (Figs. 5-27 and 5-28)
5. Preexisting spinal stenosis (Fig. 5-29)

Text continued on p. 160.

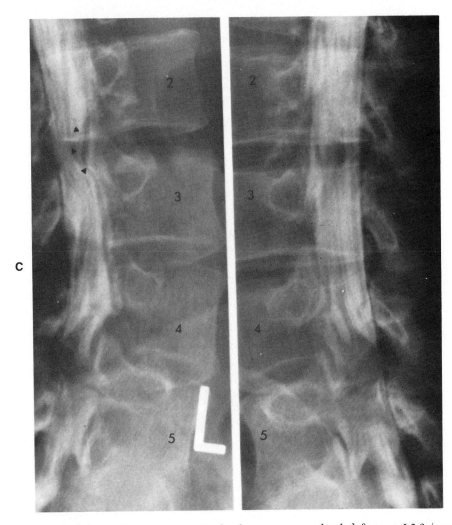

Fig. 5-13, cont'd. C, Oblique views. Study shows two extradural defects at L2-3 (*arrowheads* in **B**) and L4-5 (*arrows* in **B**). Note that extradural defect at L2-3 level is unilateral (*arrowheads* in **C**). At surgery, two herniated discs were found and removed (L2-3 and L4-5 levels).

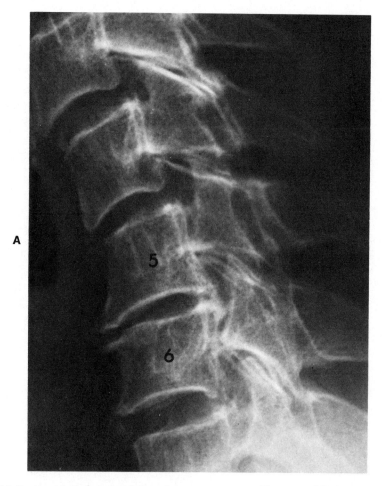

Fig. 5-14. Posttraumatic herniated disc. Seventy-one-year-old woman fell down the stairs. **A,** Lateral view of cervical spine shows mild degenerative osteophyte at C5-6 level but no fracture or dislocation.

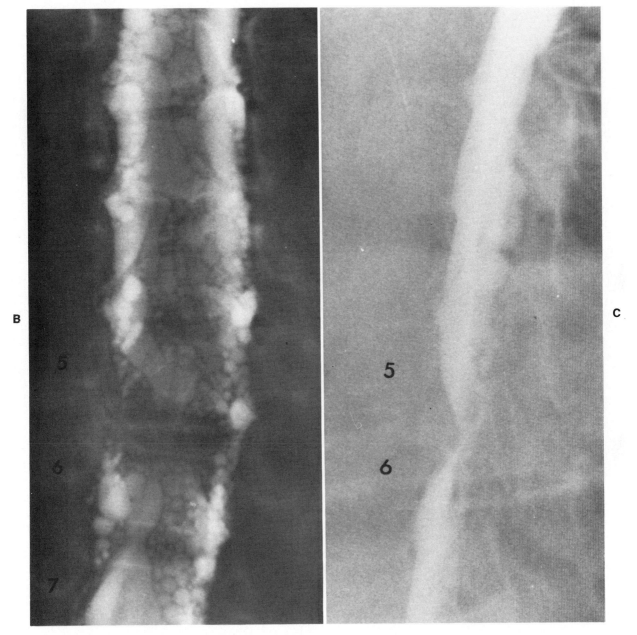

Fig. 5-14, cont'd. B, AP and **C,** lateral views of cervical Pantopaque myelogram via lumbar route show a ventral extradural defect at C5-6 level with widening of spinal cord at same level. At surgery a herniated disc was found.

Fig. 5-15. Posttraumatic herniated disc and rupture of dura mater. Twenty-three-year-old man involved in automobile accident. Plain cervical spine film (not shown) demonstrated no evidence of fracture. There was minimal subluxation at C4-5 level. Pantopaque myelogram via lumbar route in prone position. **A,** AP view shows widening of spinal cord at C4 and C5 levels. **B,** Lateral view shows ventral extradural defect at C4-5 level compressing on spinal cord at this level *(arrowheads)*. Note leakage of contrast material caused by a dural tear at C4-5 level laterally and posteriorly *(arrows* in **A** and **B**). At surgery, a herniated intervertebral disc was found at C4-5 level.

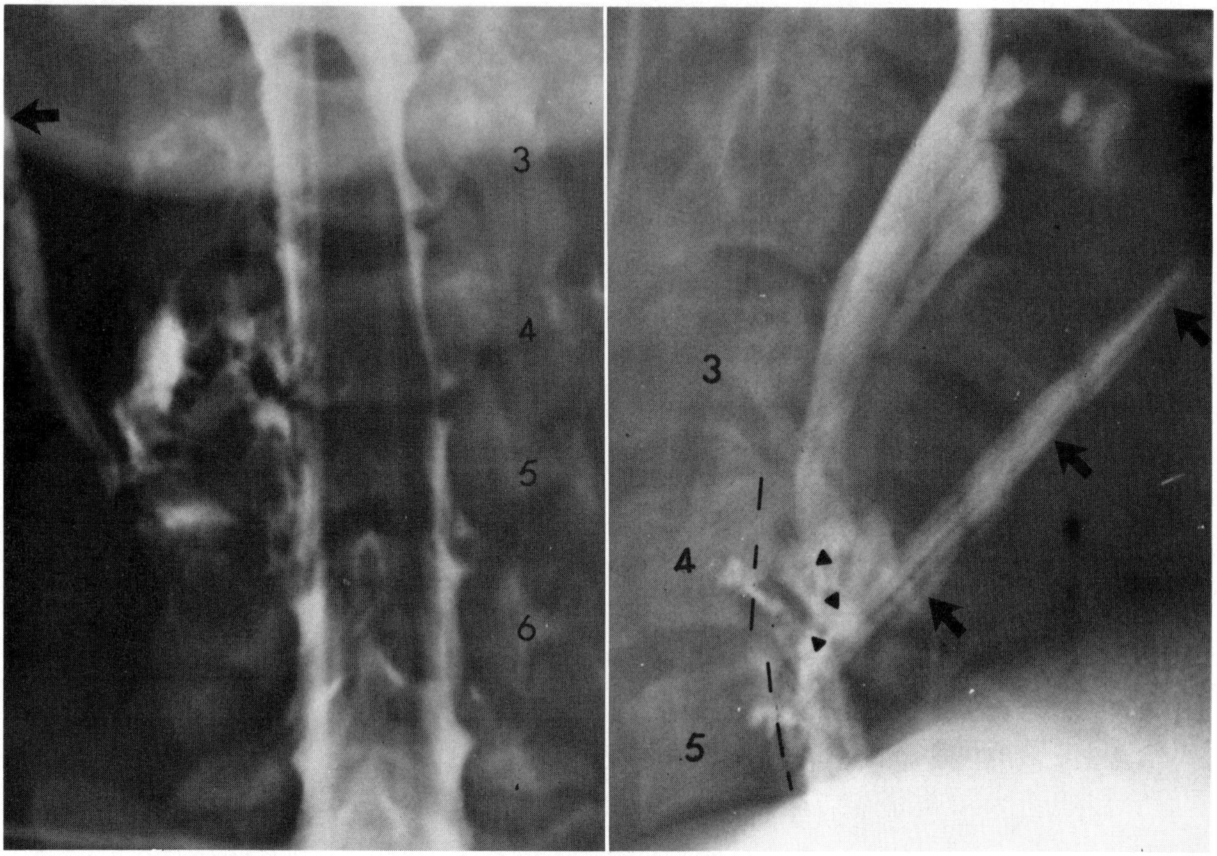

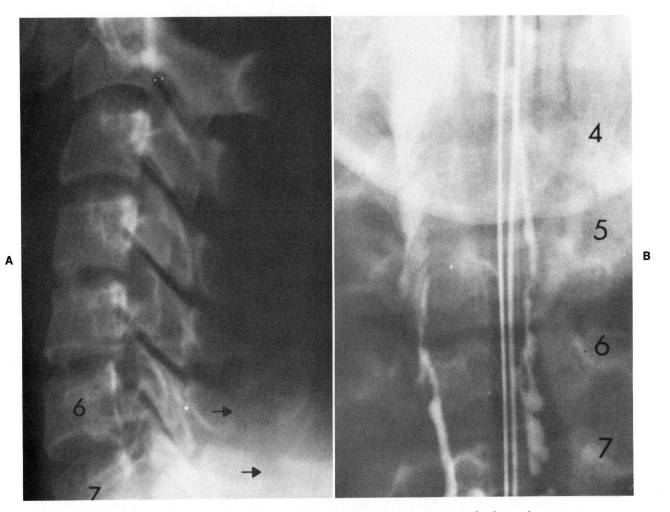

Fig. 5-16. Traumatic cord swelling. Twenty-four-year-old woman was quadriplegic after an automobile accident. **A,** Lateral view of cervical spine shows fractures of posterior elements of C6 and C7 *(arrows).* These fractures cannot explain neurologic deficit. **B,** AP cervical Pantopaque myelogram via lateral C1-2 cervical puncture shows no evidence of blockage or extradural defect. Note widening of cervical cord from C4 through C7 level, presumably from cord swelling.

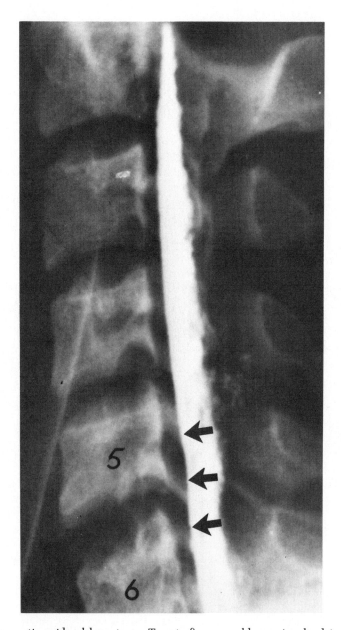

Fig. 5-17. Traumatic epidural hematoma. Twenty-five-year-old man involved in an automobile accident experienced weakness of the legs. Radiograph of cervical spine (not shown) demonstrated a fracture of lateral masses of C5-6. Lateral view of cervical Pantopaque myelogram via lateral C1-2 puncture shows no evidence of blockage. There is a smooth slight posterior displacement of anterior margin of subarachnoid space from posterior margin of bodies of C5 and C6 probably caused by small focal, epidural hematoma *(arrows)*. No evidence of compromise to spinal cord. No surgery was done, and patient improved with conservative treatment.

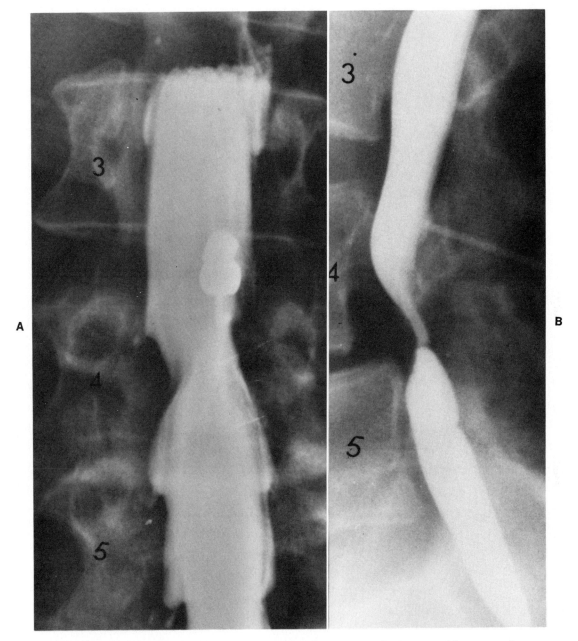

Fig. 5-18. Posttraumatic spondylolisthesis and herniated disc. This 48-year-old woman who fell down the stairs was first seen with low back pain. **A,** AP and **B,** lateral views of lumbar Pantopaque myelogram. There is spondylolisthesis at the L4-5 level and a ventral extradural defect at this level. At surgery a herniated disc was removed.

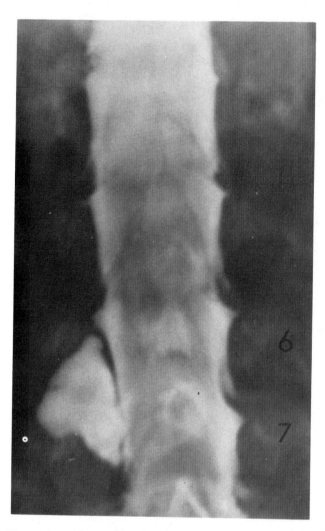

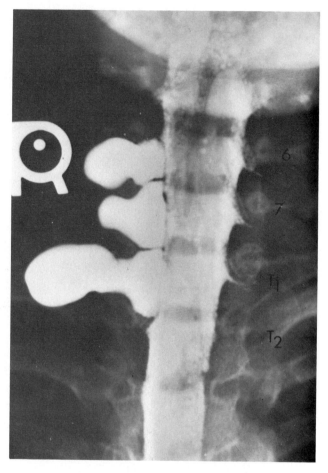

Fig. 5-19. Avulsion of brachial plexus. This 46-year-old man sustained a traction injury to his right shoulder. Pantopaque myelography via lumbar route disclosed extraluminal collection of contrast material at C6-7 level on right side. There is a traumatic meningocele caused by avulsion of C7 nerve root.

Fig. 5-20. Avulsion of brachial plexus. This 9-year-old boy fell off his bicycle and sustained a traction injury to his right arm and shoulder with a fracture of right scapula. Right upper limb was anesthetic. Pantopaque cervical myelography via lumbar route demonstrates avulsion of right brachial plexus. There is collection of considerable amount of contrast material in extraluminal pockets caused by avulsion of C7, C8, and T1 nerve roots.

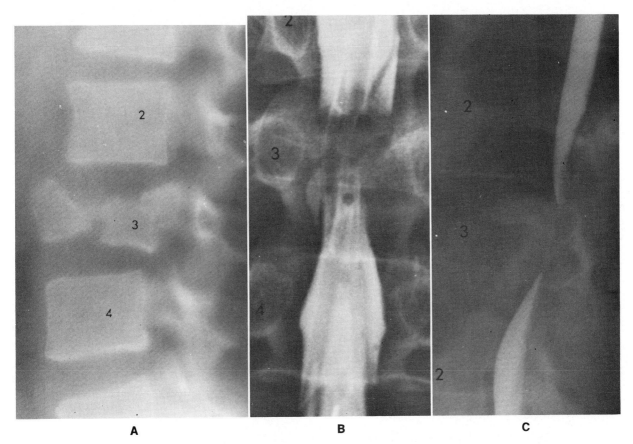

A   B   C

Fig. 5-21. Partial block caused by comminuted fracture. This 36-year-old man was involved in an automobile accident. **A,** Lateral polytomogram of lumbar spine shows comminuted fracture of body of L3. There is displacement of posterior fragment of body of L3 into spinal canal, causing more than 50% compromise. **B,** AP and, **C,** lateral Amipaque lumbar myelograms in prone position show partial block to flow of Amipaque at L3 level (high-grade posttraumatic spinal stenosis).

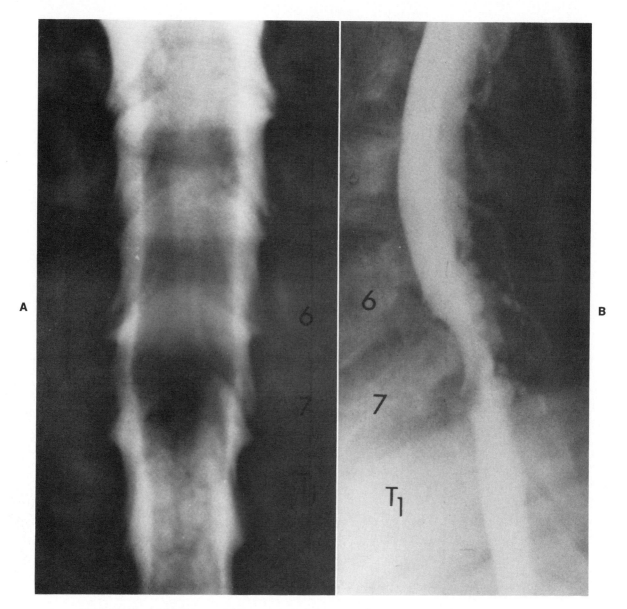

Fig. 5-22. Partial block caused by comminuted fracture. This 20-year-old man had a history of fracture-dislocation of C7 and quadriparesis. Cervical Pantopaque myelogram via lumbar route shows widening of spinal cord at C7 level from posterior displacement of fractured body of C7 into spinal cord.

Fig. 5-23. Partial block from vertebral subluxation. This 50-year-old woman was first seen with slight pain and weakness in left upper limb following an automobile accident. **A,** AP tomograph of cervical spine shows oblique fracture through lamina and pedicle of C6 on left side. **B,** Lateral tomogram of cervical spine shows subluxation at C6-7 level. **C** and **D,** Cervical Pantopaque myelogram via lumbar route in prone position shows, on left side, a ventral extradural defect at C6-7 level with compression of nerve root sleeve. Note that although ventral defect is prominent, there is no evidence of widening of cervical cord, which explains relatively minor clinical symptoms.

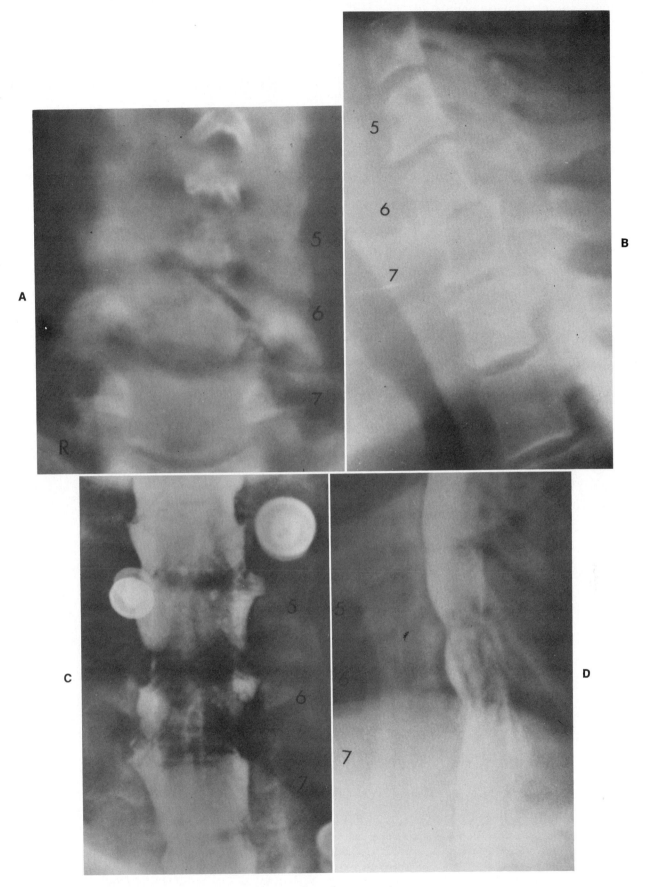

Fig. 5-23. For legend see opposite page.

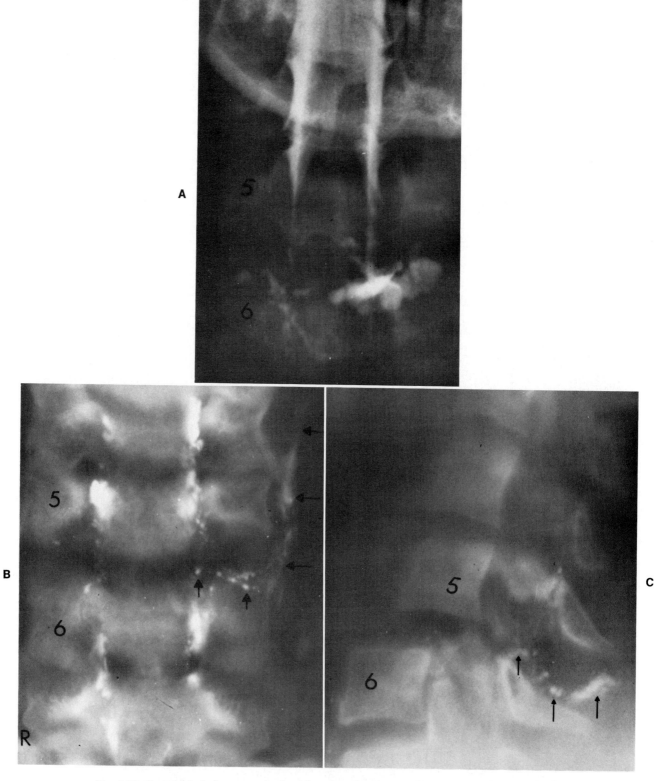

Fig. 5-24. Partial block from vertebral subluxation: dural tear. This 21-year-old woman was involved in an automobile accident. Cervical radiographs (not shown) revealed a fracture-dislocation at C5-6 level. **A,** Pantopaque myelogram via lateral C1-2 puncture shows widening of spinal cord at C5 level with high-grade block to flow of Pantopaque at C5-6 level. **B,** AP and, **C,** lateral polytomograms of cervical spine following myelography show extent of fracture-dislocation and point of dural tear, which is posteriorly and laterally at C5-6 level (*arrows*).

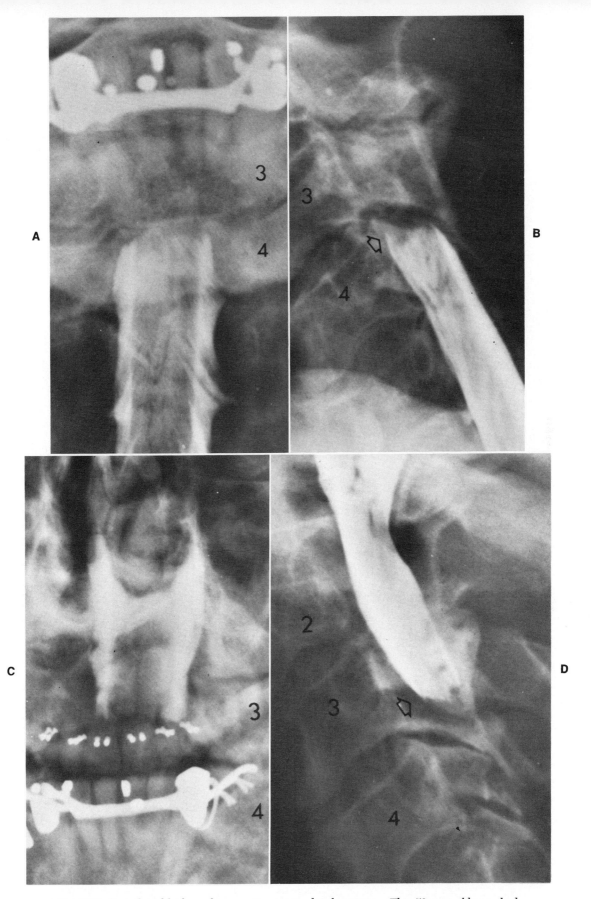

Fig. 5-25. Complete blockage from posttraumatic disc herniation. This 53-year-old man had been in an automobile accident. Cervical spine radiographs (not shown) revealed severe degenerative changes with no evidence of fracture. **A** and **B,** Pantopaque cervical myelograms via lumbar route in prone position show complete blockage at C3-4 level caused by a ventral extradural defect at this level. Note posterior displacement of ventral aspect of subarachnoid space *(arrow).* **C** and **D,** Pantopaque myelograms via lateral C1-2 cervical puncture in prone position again show complete blockage at C3-4 level. Note posterior displacement of ventral aspect of subarachnoid space *(arrow).* At surgery a herniated disc and degenerative osteophytes were found.

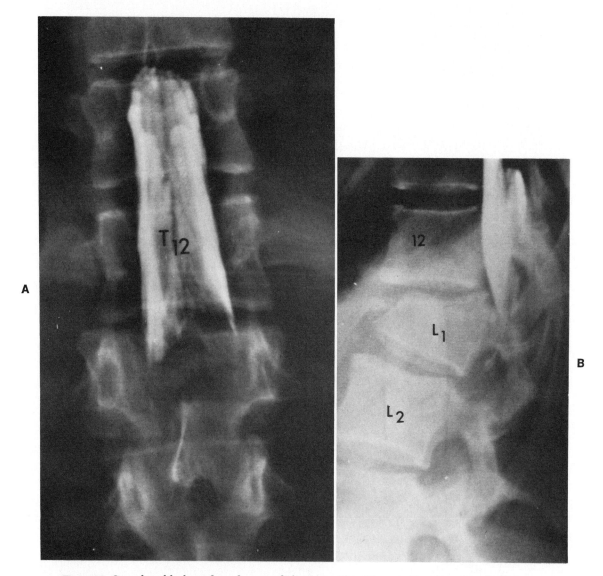

Fig. 5-26. Complete blockage from fracture-dislocation. This 15-year-old girl was involved in an automobile accident and suffered fracture displacement of L1. **A,** AP and, **B,** lateral Pantopaque myelograms in prone, semiupright position via lateral C1-2 cervical puncture show complete block of flow of Pantopaque at T12-L1 level. Note posterior displacement of L1 in lateral view and compression and widening of conus medullaris in AP view.

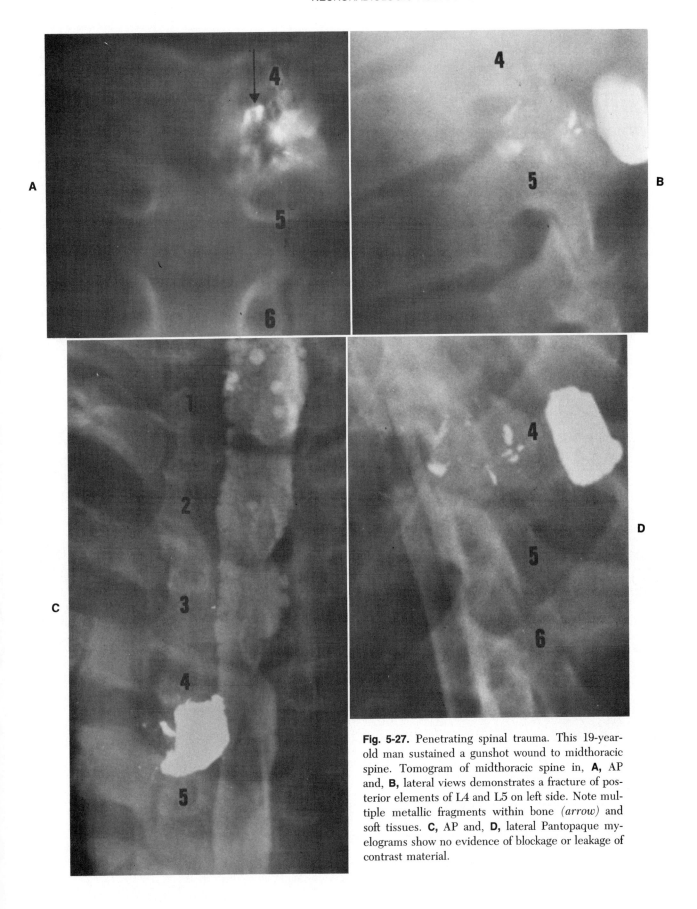

Fig. 5-27. Penetrating spinal trauma. This 19-year-old man sustained a gunshot wound to midthoracic spine. Tomogram of midthoracic spine in, **A,** AP and, **B,** lateral views demonstrates a fracture of posterior elements of L4 and L5 on left side. Note multiple metallic fragments within bone *(arrow)* and soft tissues. **C,** AP and, **D,** lateral Pantopaque myelograms show no evidence of blockage or leakage of contrast material.

Penetrating wounds. Penetrating wounds of the spine are mostly caused by gunshot wounds (Figs. 5-27 and 5-28). They are commonly associated with some sort of fracture, with the spine usually remaining in stable condition.[24,46,61] Depending on the relation between the trajectory of the bullet and the spinal cord, the symptoms may vary from a complete transection of the cord and quadriplegia (in the case of cervical injury) to Brown-Séquard syndrome, anterior spinal syndrome, or central cord syndrome.[24,47,61] The bullet may pass through the spinal cord to be stationed in the soft tissues or may stay in the spinal canal or within the cord.

Hinkel and Nichols[27] stated that ideally every patient exhibiting neurologic signs after a penetrating spinal wound should have a myelogram. However, this has been challenged by several authors.[24] Myelography is indicated for patients with penetrating spinal wound when they are neurologically unstable or show a deteriorating course.

Plain films, polytomograms, and CT scans may demonstrate the fragments of the bullet and the fractured bones about the spinal canal.[34] If the bullet has not pierced the dura mater (Fig. 5-27), extradural defects are either caused by the bullet, a bony fragment, a hematoma, or any combination of the preceding factors. When the dura mater is pierced by the bullet fragments, myelography may show intradural as well as extradural defects and occasionally cerebrospinal fluid leakage (Fig. 5-28).

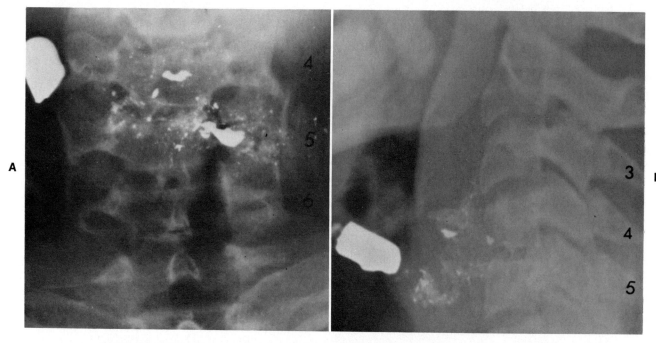

Fig. 5-28. Penetrating wound to cervical spine. This 18-year-old man suffered a gunshot wound to spine at C4-5 level and was found to be quadriparetic. **A,** AP and, **B,** lateral views of cervical spine demonstrate comminuted fractures of C4 and C5. Multiple bullet fragments are seen in spinal canal, bony structures, and soft tissues. **C** and **D,** Cervical Pantopaque myelography in prone position via lumbar route demonstrates widening of spinal cord at C4-5 level. Note posterior displacement of spinal cord in lateral view, **D,** from presence of bullet fragments and possible hematoma in ventral portion of neural canal *(arrows)*. **E,** Lateral view of the cervical spine obtained 2 days after myelography demonstrates contrast material in paravertebral soft tissues *(arrow)*. (See also Fig. 5-40.)

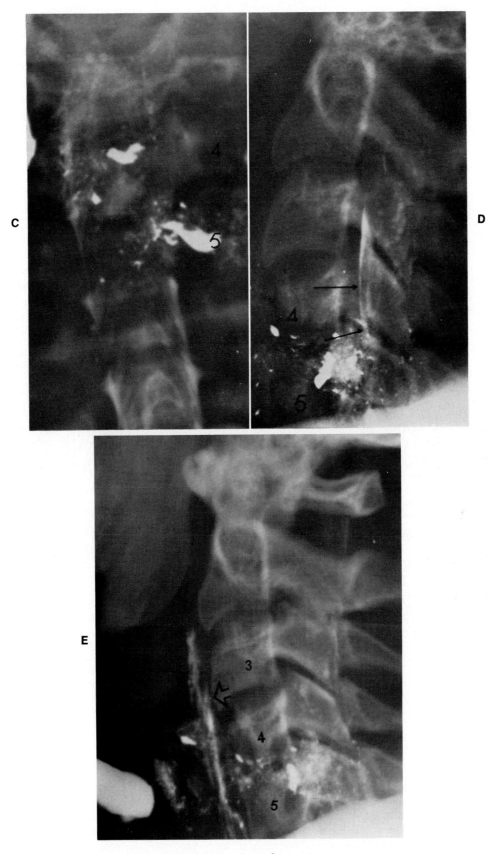

Fig. 5-28, cont'd. For legend see opposite page.

Spinal stenosis. Myelography is indicated in patients with preexisting spinal stenosis (primary or secondary) who have sustained spinal trauma, with or without fracture, in order to evaluate the already borderline relationship between the spinal canal and the cord (Fig. 5-29).[4,22,26,39]

In these patients even a minor injury not producing a fracture may result in significant neurologic deficit that may progress rapidly. The myelographic signs may vary from incomplete to complete blockage to the flow of the contrast material. The traumatic compression of the cord may be caused by either degenerative osteophytes or disc herniations in a hyperflexion injury or by the rigid and thickened ligamentum flavum in a hyperextension injury. In patients with spinal stenosis, mild swelling of the cord, a bulging or herniated disc, or a small epidural hematoma can produce severe symptoms, whereas in a normal canal the same lesions may not produce any symptoms.

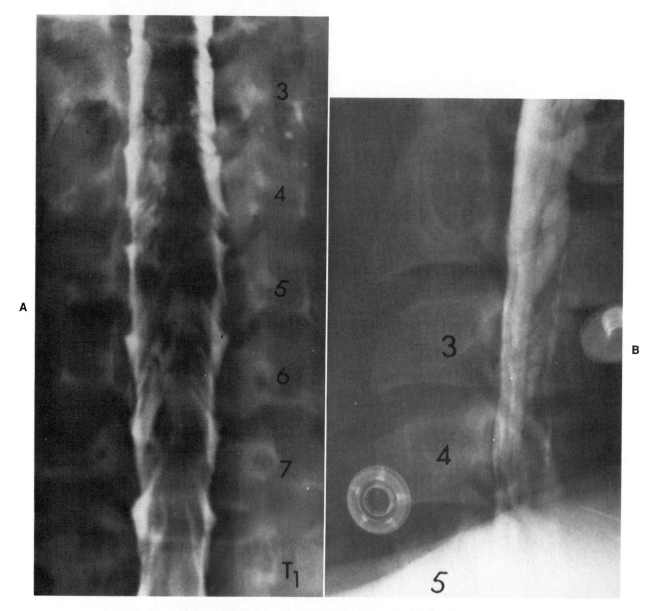

Fig. 5-29. Congenital spinal stenosis. This 16-year-old boy was admitted with paraplegia and hyperspasticity of lower extremities and weakness of both upper extremities after a football injury. Spinal radiographs showed no evidence of a fracture or dislocation in entire spine. **A,** AP and, **B,** lateral cervical myelograms show congenital spinal stenosis and narrowing of subarachnoid space. There is mild widening of spinal cord at C4-6, probably caused by swelling. Note generalized narrowing of AP diameter of cervical spinal canal.

Technique

A number of different myelographic techniques in spinal cord injury have been described in the literature.[33,37,52] The choice of a standard technique or the modification of various techniques differs greatly in different institutions according to the facilities and personal preference of the neuroradiologists and neurosurgeons involved. These techniques vary as well according to the chronicity and site of injury and neurologic findings. The technique used in a patient with old trauma to the lumbar region differs from that used for the patient with thoracic injury or acute cervical injury associated with quadriplegia.

Patients with suspected spinal injury are brought to the radiology department on a Stryker frame while under traction using Crutchfield or Gardner-Wells tongs in cervical or thoracic cases. In many instances the patient can be moved carefully and safely to the x-ray table without the frame but with adequate traction maintained. Under the supervision of the neuroradiologist and an always-present neurosurgeon, a group of nurses and radiologic technologists will do the transferring. Most of the patients are transferred in the prone position. Lumbar route is preferred in all instances if possible. In cervical cord injuries where the lumbar route is chosen, the patient is transferred in the prone position while on the frame and a chin holder is added to the frame. The holder is used for head support and to eliminate neck movements. An 18-gauge spinal needle is used when Pantopaque is chosen as contrast material. For metrizamide (Amipaque) a 20-gauge spinal needle is preferred.

Lumbar region. With the patient in the prone position, spinal puncture is made two levels above or below the injured level. Pantopaque, 3 ml, is introduced into the subarachnoid space when complete blockage is suspected. Under fluoroscopy the contrast material is directed to the injured level by tilting the table cephalad or caudad or both. If no blockage or partial blockage is discovered, an additional 10 ml of Pantopaque is injected. The contrast medium is removed after completion of the study. If a complete blockage is present, the needle will be removed and frontal and cross-table lateral views in both the supine and prone positions will be obtained using a grid cassette and the overhead x-ray tube. When Amipaque is chosen as the contrast agent, 10 ml of 170 to 190 mg I/ml concentration is used.

Thoracic region. A lumbar route with the patient in the prone or lateral decubitus position is preferred. Either Pantopaque or Amipaque can be used. When Pantopaque is chosen, the possible blockage can be demonstrated by the introduction of 3 ml. If partial or no blockage is observed, up to a total amount of 36 ml of the contrast medium is injected and frontal and cross-table lateral views are obtained. In the event that the length of the obstruction is questioned, the upper level of the block is evaluated via the cervical route. For Amipaque myelography, 12 to 14 ml of 220 mg I/ml is injected via a lumbar puncture.[50] The flow of the contrast medium should be monitored constantly by fluoroscopy.

Cervical region. Since Kelly and Alexander's[33] first introduction of lateral cervical puncture for myelography, a number of authors have described the benefits of using this method in cervical spinal injuries.[37,50,52] The puncture is made at the C1-2 level with the patient in either the supine, prone, or decubitus position. Although the supine position requires less patient manipulation and is considered to be safer, the prone position is preferred in most cases for complete evaluation of the cervical subarachnoid space. This is especially true when Pantopaque is used because it layers down on the posterior margin of the spinal canal. Thus the anterior margin of the spinal cord may not be fully evaluated (Fig. 5-30).

When a complete block is suspected, 3 ml of Pantopaque or 10 ml of 250 mg I/ml of Amipaque is used with the patient in the supine position. Frontal and lateral views are obtained with the overhead x-ray tube. Pantopaque is preferred when the cerebrospinal fluid is not bloody, to avoid the possibility of severe reactions to Amipaque. These reactions include severe headache, vomiting, meningismus, and occasional seizure, any of which will add to the patient's problems.[44,50] If the cerebrospinal fluid is bloody as is occasionally the case with acute cord injuries, Amipaque is used to avoid possible development of arachnoiditis. The clinical and experimental studies show that arachnoiditis may develop by introduction of and especially by retention of Panatopaque within the subarachnoid space.[28,29] Although histologic reactions are present in all cases, most of them do not show clinical evidence of arachnoiditis. The most severe clinical symptoms with retained Pantopaque develop in cases that have blood in the cerebrospinal fluid.[28] To avoid such a reaction, it is advised that Pantopaque be totally removed from the subarachnoid space whenever possible. Adhesive arachnoiditis has been seen experimentally in animals given excessively large volumes and concentrations of Amipaque.[23] However, no radiologic changes of arachnoiditis have yet been reported in patients who underwent Amipaque myelography either with or without bloody cerebrospinal fluid.[37,49]

When a complete block is not suspected and myelography is done to rule out extradural defects such as herniated disc or hematoma, the puncture is made with the patient in the prone position. Pantopaque, 12 to 15

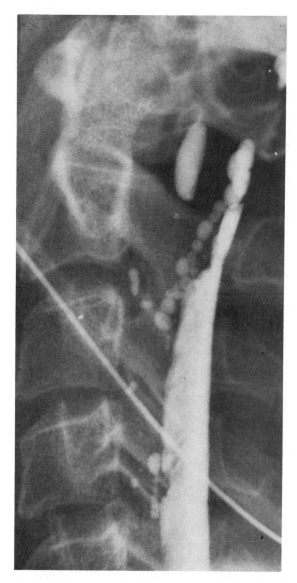

Fig. 5-30. Supine cervical myelogram. Cervical Pantopaque myelogram in supine position via lateral C1-2 puncture showing layering of contrast in posterior part of subarachnoid space. Anterior aspect of spinal cord cannot be evaluated.

ml, or Amipaque 12 ml of 250 mg I/ml, is injected into the subarachnoid space. Frontal and lateral views with the overhead x-ray tube are then obtained.

Gas myelography. Some investigators have stressed the benefits of gas myelography in spinal cord injuries.[40,42] Because of the difficulty and limitations of gas myelography, it is only used as a last resort in patients with a strong history of allergic reactions to iodinated contrast materials. We have not found any superiority of gas myelography over the use of Amipaque since it has become commercially available.

Gas myelography should be done on a tomographic table. The patient is placed in the lateral decubitus po-

sition with the head tilted down 10° to 15° from the horizontal plane. Via lumbar puncture, about 40 to 80 ml of air is injected slowly into the subarachnoid space in fractional doses after fractional removal of a total of 50 to 60 ml of cerebrospinal fluid. Lateral tomograms are made throughout the width of the canal in 2 to 3 mm intervals. At the end of the study, the excess gas is equilibrated with the atmosphere before the needle is removed.

Radiologic findings

The possible abnormal radiologic findings seen on myelography in spinal injury are as follows:
1. Complete blockage (Figs. 5-25, 5-26, and 5-32)
2. Partial blockage (Figs. 5-21 to 5-24)
3. Indentations on the contrast column without blockage (Figs. 5-11 to 5-15, 5-17, 5-18, 5-27 and 5-28)
4. Avulsion of nerve roots (Figs. 5-19 and 5-20)
5. Dural tear, leakage of cerebrospinal fluid and contrast into the soft tissues (Figs. 5-15, 5-24, 5-28, and 5-31)

Complete spinal block. Posttraumatic complete spinal block is usually caused by a combination of several factors, including a swollen spinal cord and other extramedullary compressive causes. A swollen spinal cord is shown on myelography as fusiform enlargement of the cord both on the frontal and lateral views, with a resultant narrowing of the subarachnoid space. The extramedullary causes for complete spinal block include extradural hematoma, bone fragments, vertebral dislocations, disc protrusions or herniations (Fig. 5-25), foreign bodies from penetrating wounds, and very rarely subdural hematoma. The blockage occurs because one or more of these factors are pressing and displacing the cord tightly against the opposite wall of the spinal canal (Fig. 5-26). The blockage can be opposite one disc space or one or more vertebral levels. It may be caused by a ventral, dorsal, or lateral compressing factor. Occasionally when the fracture-dislocation is unstable, the complete blockage shown when the spine is in one position may become incomplete in another position (Fig. 5-32). Thus whenever possible the patient should be studied in both supine and prone positions for complete evaluation of a blockage (Fig. 5-32). The gibbus deformity is exaggerated in the prone position to an extent that may cause a complete blockage and may lead to worsening of the patient's clinical status. Preexisting stenosis of the bony spinal canal from congenital or acquired causes is important since it increases the risk of block and damage of the spinal cord. A herniated disc can result in complete block in the lumbar region in cases of narrow spinal canal from degenerative changes and posterior bony spurs.

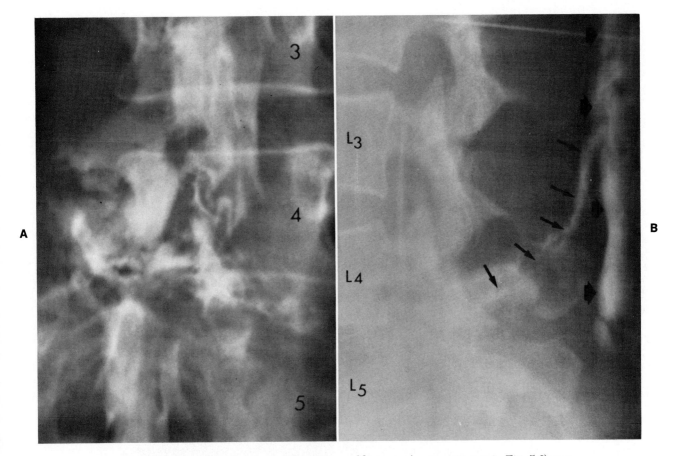

Fig. 5-31. Posttraumatic dural tear. This 38-year-old woman (same patient as in Fig. 5-6) was run over by a car. Plain film of lumbosacral spine shows fracture-dislocation at L4-5 level (see Fig. 5-6, A). **A,** AP and, **B,** lateral Amipaque lumbar myelograms show distortion of normal anatomy of lumbar subarachnoid space and extravasation of contrast material at L4-5 level resulting from dural tear. Long arrows indicate fistula tract, and short arrows indicate collection of contrast material in subcutaneous space of back.

Partial spinal block. Partial block occurs when the subarachnoid space is considerably narrowed by a swollen cord or is compressed by an extradural defect. The factors that cause partial block are similar to those for complete block (Figs. 5-21 to 5-24). Traumatic spinal swelling does not usually result in immediate complete block except when it is very severe. The primary pathoanatomic changes of swelling are edema and hemorrhage.[18] The severity is related to the magnitude of the force of injury. Hemorrhage usually starts in the central gray matter from tears in the walls of the venules. Hemorrhage, like edema, may be localized in the central portion of the cord and may extend peripherally to involve the white matter. Moreover, associated areas of hemorrhage rostrad and caudad to the site of impact may occur. These changes take place within several hours to several days after trauma. A partial block may progress to a complete block with deterioration of the neurologic status.

Extradural defects without block. Myelography may demonstrate extradural defects produced by bone dislocations or fragments, herniated intervertebral discs, epidural hematomas, or foreign bodies from penetrating wounds, with no evidence of spinal blockage (Fig. 5-28). These factors can produce varying degrees of myelopathy and radiculopathy, by compressing the cord or the nerve roots or both.

Bone fragments may or may not impinge on the nerve roots. Their defects shown on myelography may be at bone or disc space levels depending on the migration of the free fragment. Correlation with plain films and tomograms will help in reaching the diagnosis.

Intervertebral disc herniation may result from acute trauma with or without fracture of the vertebra (Figs. 5-13 to 5-15 and 5-18).[7,8,43] Disc herniation is more common in cases with preexisting disc degeneration.[8] Pain and other neurologic symptoms may be delayed as much as 24 to 48 hours. Plain films may show a nar-

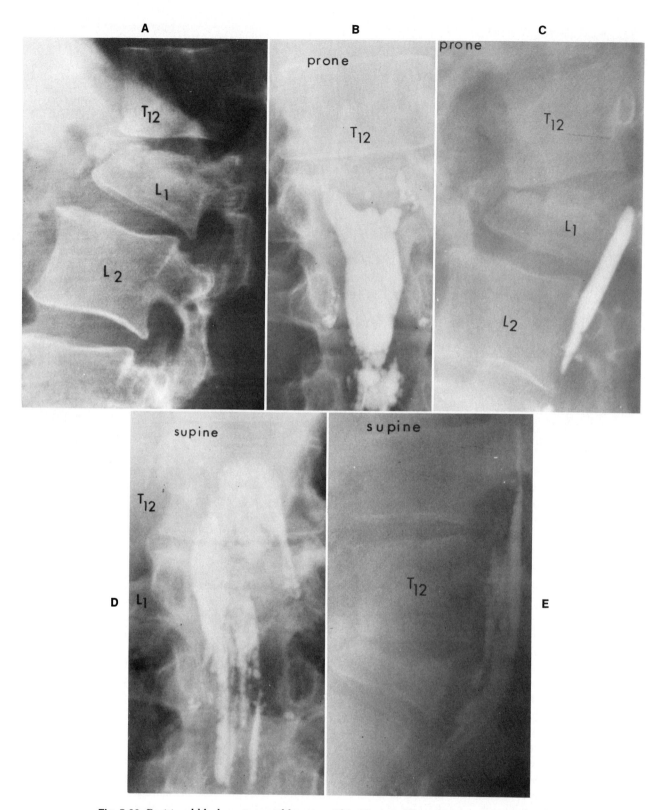

Fig. 5-32. Positional blockage in unstable spine. This 38-year-old man was seen 1 month after an automobile accident. **A,** Lateral view of thoracolumbar spine shows compression fracture of body of L1. **B,** AP and, **C,** lateral lumbar Pantopaque myelogram in prone position shows complete block at T12-L1 level as a result of a gibbus formation at this level. **D,** AP and, **E,** lateral views in supine position show free passage of contrast material.

rowed intervertebral disc space. Myelography usually reveals the defect to be at a disc level. Impingement on the cord or nerve roots by the herniated disc will cause myelopathy or radiculopathy. Herniated discs generally occur in one level but may be seen in different levels.

Epidural hematomas in the spine are usually venous in origin. They may develop after an apparently mild trauma (Figs. 5-11, 5-12, and 5-17).[41] Various bleeding diatheses, anticoagulant therapy, vascular tumors, or vascular malformations are predisposing factors. The site of the bleeding is usually not easily demonstrable.[41] On myelography, epidural hematomas may occur at any level and are demonstrated by the displacement of the dura mater away from the bones in a relatively long segment (Fig. 5-11). Diagnosis may be more difficult if the lesion is located ventrally and localized at a disc level. When the hematoma is associated with fracture or dislocation, the diagnosis may be possible by comparing the myelograms with the plain films and tomograms. This comparison helps to evaluate the proportion of displacement of the dura mater to the extent of impingement by the bony displacements. Progression of bleeding may result in complete block and progressive neurologic deterioration.

Avulsion of the nerve root plexus. Severe trauma to the shoulder with the arm in forced abduction will injure some of the lower cervical nerve roots.[62,65] The most common symptom seen in such an injury is Erb-Duchenne paralysis. In cases of injury to the first thoracic nerve root, Horner's syndrome may be seen because of involvement of the sympathetic fibers. A traumatic meningocele will develop as a result of avulsion of the nerve roots and can be shown on myelography (Fig. 5-19). If the study is done around the first 6 weeks after injury, the cerebrospinal fluid is usually xanthochromic in color, indicative of a subarachnoid hemorrhage. This probably results from avulsion of the nerve roots and their meningeal cuffs. After introduction of the contrast material into the subarachnoid space, flow of the contrast material is carefully observed while the patient is tilted with his head down. Contrast material will outline one or more irregular pockets that lie in a lateral and caudal direction from the subarachnoid space (Fig. 5-20). In some instances these pockets will fill better by having the patient cough or lie on the affected side. The radiolucent shadows of the nerve roots seen in normal contrast-filled nerve root sleeves will be absent. Multiplicity and irregularity of the lesions and their location in the lower cervical and upper thoracic regions are important factors in establishing the correct diagnosis. A single nerve root cyst (meningocele) can represent a normal anatomic variant.

Avulsion of the lumbosacral nerve roots is rare. This will occur in severe trauma to the pelvis that fractures the pelvic bone or separates the sacroiliac joint. The traction force on the lumbosacral plexus may result in the avulsion of the lumbosacral nerve roots.

Dural tear. A traumatic tear in the dura mater and arachnoid can occur in closed and penetrating wounds of the spine. In closed injury a bony fragment is the usual cause. However, overstretching of the membranes in an acute hyperflexion or hyperextension injury may result in a tear (Fig. 5-15). The subarachnoid space will be opened to the extradural space and surrounding tissues, leading to leakage of the cerebrospinal fluid. The contrast material will leak out of the subarachnoid space into blind pockets in the surrounding soft tissues or through a sinus tract into anatomic spaces, such as the pleura or the mediastinum.[60,64] Since these patients are more prone to infectious meningitis, early diagnosis of a dural tear is important. Myelography will demonstrate the leaking contrast material, the sinus tracts, and the level and extent of the tear (Figs. 5-24, 5-28, and 5-31). When a cerebrospinal fluid leakage is suspected, Amipaque is the contrast material of choice for myelography because it is easily absorbed from the soft tissues.

ANGIOGRAPHY IN SPINAL TRAUMA

Varying degrees of damage to the intraspinal as well as the extraspinal vessels can result from both penetrating and nonpenetrating trauma to the spine.* Although the intraspinal arterial injuries may occur anywhere along the spinal cord, the extraspinal arterial damage usually occurs in the cervical region and involves the carotid or the vertebral arteries or both. The vascular damage may result from a direct insulting physical factor, such as bone displacements or fragments or foreign bodies from penetrating wounds, or it may result from a blunt nonpenetrating trauma without fractures or dislocations.

The mechanism of vascular injury in a blunt trauma is believed to be a sudden forceful stretching of the artery over the hyperextended spine with contralateral flexion of the head. The vertebral arteries have been found to suffer damage to their walls even in minor traumatic neck movement such as yoga exercises or chiropractic manipulation.[21,38] It has been demonstrated experimentally that stretching of the arteries will result in tears in the intima and media while the adventitia remains intact. The extent of the traumatic tear and the degree of elevation of the intimal flap may cause partial or total occlusion of the artery affected or may result in a dissecting aneurysm.[51,63] In some cases intimal tears have been found as a nidus for thrombus. Trauma may dislodge a preexisting atheromatous plaque, or emboli

---

*References 1, 9, 20, 25, 35, 51, 63.

may separate from a posttraumatic arterial thrombosis, resulting in intracerebral vascular occlusion. The role of vascular spasm after trauma is not well defined and may be a factor in the progression to thrombosis.[20]

Since the symptoms of extraspinal vascular injury are usually those of intracranial vascular occlusive disease, the extracranial cause of the posttraumatic cerebral ischemia may be ignored. If cerebral ischemia developed after trauma to the spine, the posttraumatic stenosis of the cervical portion of the cranial vessels should be studied by angiography. Injury to segmental arteries contributing to the spinal cord circulation may bring up the risk of ischemic myelopathy depending on the number of the vessels involved. The midthoracic region has a relatively poor blood supply, and obstruction to the main contributing vessels in this area may result in spinal cord infarction.

Extraspinal arterial injuries by penetrating wounds are usually caused by gunshot or stab wounds. They result directly from the object initiating the wounds as well as from associated fractures and bone displacements. They may result in either partial or complete occlusion of one or more of the arteries with ischemia or hemorrhage or both affecting the central nervous system.

Normal angiographic anatomy

The spinal cord is supplied by three longitudinal arterial channels: the anterior and the posterolateral spinal arteries, as well as the perimedullary plexus that connects these arteries.[13,45,56,57] The anterior spinal artery is located in front of the anterior median fissure, and the posterolateral arteries lie in the dorsolateral sulci of the spinal cord. The anterior spinal artery is formed by the union of the two anterior spinal rami from the distal portions of the vertebral arteries. It is maintained as a single trunk along the entire length of the spinal cord. However, it may be quite small in the midthoracic region; sometimes actual discontinuity exists in this area. It is reinforced at different levels throughout the length of the spinal cord by the anterior radicular arteries. The posterior spinal arteries originate from vertebral arteries just proximal to the origin of the rami of the anterior spinal artery. They form two pos-

terolateral longitudinal arterial channels and are maintained throughout the lengths of the spinal cord by additional branches from the posterior radicular arteries. They are not usually seen in a normal angiogram.

The radiculospinal arteries in the neck arise from the cervical portion of the vertebral, the thyrocervical, and the costocervical arteries. In the thoracic region they arise from the intercostal and subcostal arteries, and in the lumbar region from the lumbar arteries. The largest of these radicular branches, the artery of Adamkiewicz (arteria radicularis magna) arises usually either from an inferior intercostal or a lumbar branch anywhere between T9 and L2 (85%) on the left side (75%). In 15% of cases it arises between T5 and T8. It is fairly large, giving off a cephalic and a caudal branch, the latter being the larger of the two. Because of this appearance it acquires a characteristic hairpin configuration.

The circumferential branches of the anterior and posterior spinal arteries form a perimedullary plexus of arterial networks. The nutrient vessels of the cord parenchyma are separated into a central and a peripheral arterial system. The central system is derived from the anterior spinal artery. The peripheral system is supplied mainly from the posterior spinal arteries and the perimedullary arterial plexus.[45,56,57]

The veins of the spinal cord follow essentially the same pattern as the arteries. The blood flows out of the spinal cord into the radicular veins to the vertebral venous plexus and the extraspinal network.

The circulation of the spinal cord can be divided into three major functional territories:

1. Cervical–upper thoracic territory, which corresponds to the cervical and the first two thoracic segments and is supplied by branches from the vertebral, thyrocervical, and costocervical arteries
2. Midthoracic territory, which covers down to the seventh thoracic spinal segment and represents a watershed with a marginal blood supply since it receives only a few thoracic radicular branches and some craniad flow from the lumbar area
3. Thoracolumbar territory, which extends from T8 to the filum terminale and is supplied mainly by the artery of Adamkiewicz

Technique

Selective catheterization of individual arteries is imperative for adequate visualization of the circulation of the spinal cord.[12,16] Midstream injections have been reported to occasionally produce paraplegia as a complication. This complication is probably caused by filling of all the arteries supplying the lower half or two thirds of the cord by contrast material simultaneously. The patient is lying on his back, and the contrast material, being heavier, will layer very quickly even in a rapidly moving stream. Selective catheterization angiography of the spinal cord vessels can be considered as a safe procedure and one that is rarely accompanied by significant complications. In the cervical region catheterization should be done to the vertebral artery and the costocervical and the thyrocervical trunks on both sides. In the thoracic and lumbar regions selective injections are done into the intercostal arteries, the subcostal ar-

tery, and the first two lumbar arteries on both sides to visualize the artery of Adamkiewicz. The midstream injection is necessary when young children are being examined because it is usually not possible to catheterize the individual vessels due to their small size. The same may be true in the elderly because of the presence of atheromatous narrowing of the origin of the vessels. In the presence of occlusion of the iliac arteries it is necessary to use the axillary route, although it is not nearly as convenient or satisfactory. While making the successive injections of the intercostal arteries, only 2 to 3 ml of iothalamate meglumine (Conray 60) is injected each time. When injecting the intercostal artery from which the artery of Adamkiewicz arises, the injection of contrast material should be followed immediately by a small amount of saline injection after which the catheter is withdrawn from the opening of the artery.

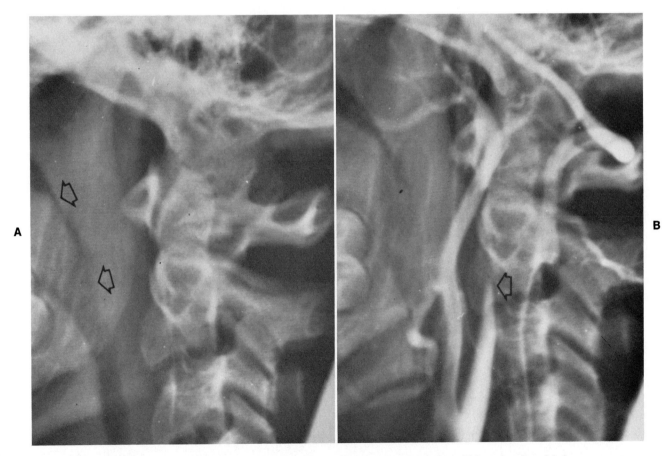

Fig. 5-33. Traumatic occlusion of internal carotid artery. This 17-year-old boy developed left hemiparesis and lethargy 8 hours after trauma to neck. **A,** Lateral plain film of cervical spine shows no evidence of a fracture or dislocation. Note anterior displacement of nasopharyngeal air shadow *(arrows)*. **B,** Right brachial arteriogram demonstrates complete occlusion *(arrow)* of internal carotid artery 3 cm above its origin. Anterior displacement of nasopharynx seen in plain film is probably caused by localized hematoma.

Indications

Since the first report of selective angiography of the spinal cord in postspinal trauma patients by Gargour and co-workers,[16] only 25 cases of spinal arteriography in patients with posttraumatic neurologic sequelae have appeared in the literature.[55] It is still too early to define precisely the application and indications of selective spinal cord angiography in spinal trauma. Almost all investigators agree that performing the procedure may help to evaluate the large vessels supplying the spinal cord but not the critically important intraspinal and intramedullary smaller vessels. It is generally felt that selective angiography in spinal cord injuries may give a clue to the prognosis and help in the choice of therapeutic management. When the other radiologic studies do not reveal extensive traumatic spinal damage in patients with neurologic deficits, the vascular component of the damage may be more important.[59]

Angiographic findings

Abnormal angiographic findings in spinal trauma include the following:
1. Extraspinal vessels (Figs. 5-33 to 5-37)
2. Intraspinal vessels
   a. Arterial disruption (Fig. 5-38)
   b. Arterial displacement (Figs. 5-39 and 5-40)
   c. Hyperemia
   d. Extravasation of contrast medium into the spinal meningeal spaces

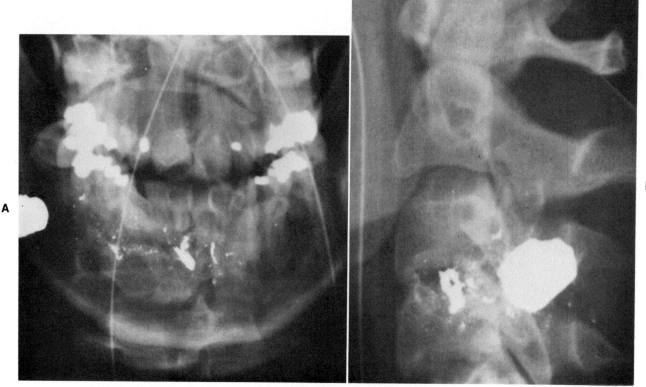

Fig. 5-34. Disruption of vertebral artery by penetrating wounds of spine. This 24-year-old man sustained a gunshot wound to cervical spine and became quadriplegic. **A,** AP and, **B,** lateral views of cervical spine demonstrate tract of bullet.

Extraspinal vessels. Posttraumatic vascular damage to the extraspinal vessels can occur in both penetrating and nonpenetrating (blunt) trauma (Figs. 5-33 to 5-37).* Multiple extracranial vessels can be involved.[25] The damage to the vessel or vessels ranges from varying degrees of stenosis to complete occlusion. The occlusive changes can result from intimal tear, thrombosis, dissecting aneurysm, or spasm. Cerebral ischemia can develop secondary to changes in extracranial vessels or from occlusion of the intracranial vessels as a result of embolism by an atheromatous plaque or thrombus frag-

ments propagated from the site of trauma. The internal carotid artery is usually occluded 1 to 3 cm above the bifurcation (Fig. 5-33).[51] The vertebral artery may be crushed by the vertebrae during neck injury, and all layers may be ruptured (Fig. 5-36). The ruptured intimal flap can result in direct, partial to complete occlusion, or it can progress to thrombotic occlusion of the artery. It is suggested that after a tear in the intimal and medial layers in which thrombosis does not occur, an aneurysm, either true or false, may develop (Figs. 5-35 and 5-36).[35,54] A traumatic false aneurysm occurs when the cavity is walled off and is connected to the true arterial lumen.

*References 20, 21, 25, 35, 38, 51, 54, 63.

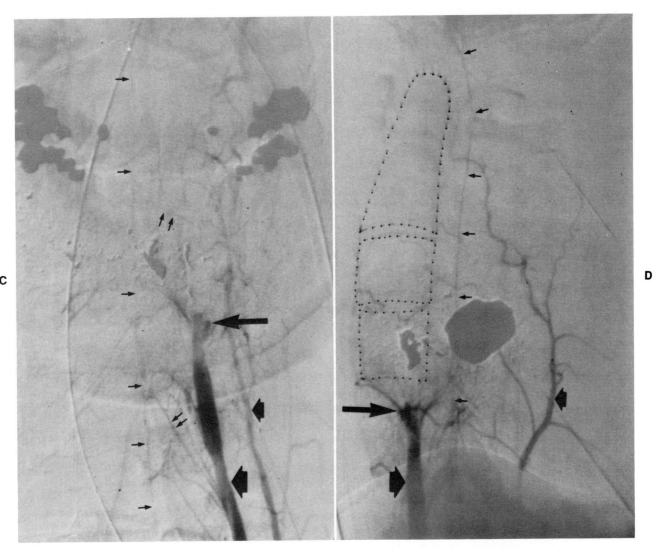

Fig. 5-34, cont'd. C, AP and, **D,** lateral views of neck during left vertebral arteriography *(lowest arrow)*. Note complete disruption of left vertebral artery at C4-5 level *(large arrow)*. Anterior spinal artery is visualized from C1 through C6 with no evidence of disruption or displacement *(small arrows)*. Deep cervical artery is visualized *(small thick arrow)*. Note visualization of radiculospinal arteries from left vertebral and deep cervical arteries *(double small arrows)*.

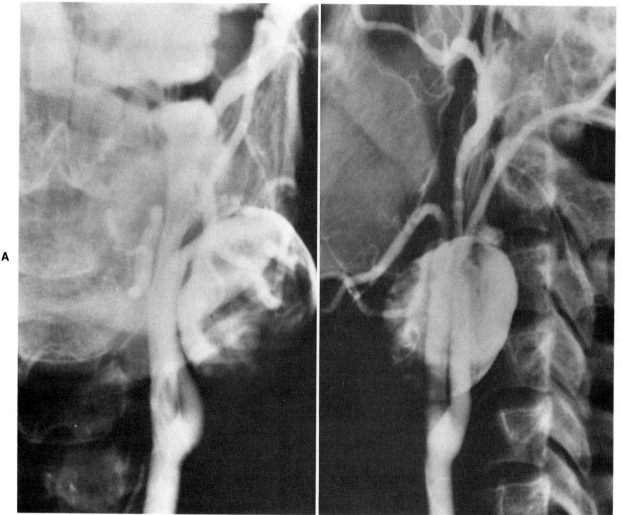

Fig. 5-35. Traumatic giant aneurysm of internal carotid artery. This 18-year-old man had a pulsatile mass on left side of neck. His history revealed a blunt trauma to left side of neck with no significant symptoms. **A,** AP and, **B,** lateral views of left common carotid arteriogram demonstrate giant aneurysm arising from posterior wall of right internal carotid artery about 4 cm above its origin.

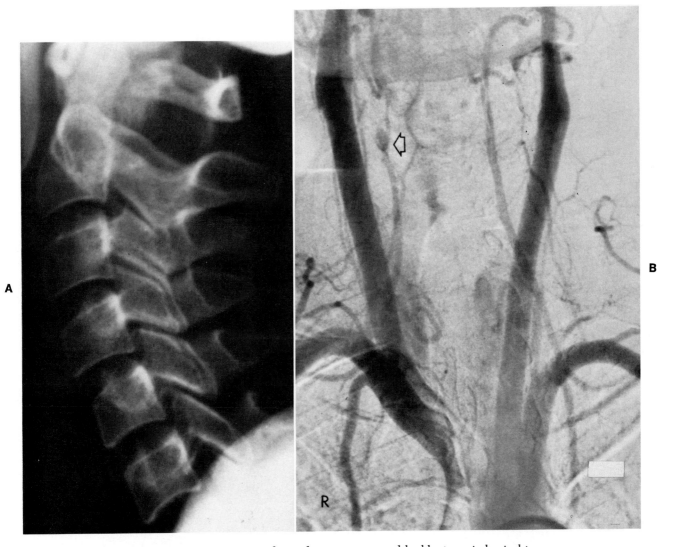

Fig. 5-36. Traumatic laceration and pseudoaneurysm caused by blunt cervical spinal trauma. This 23-year-old woman presented with bulbar signs and Wallenberg's syndrome after blunt trauma to the cervical spine. **A,** Plain film of cervical spine (lateral view) shows no evidence of fractures or dislocations. **B,** Initial aortic arch arteriogram suggests laceration of right vertebral artery at C4 level *(arrow).*

Continued.

The mechanism and the role of posttraumatic vascular spasm and segmental narrowing of the artery are not well known (Fig. 5-37). However, vascular spasm is a known sequela of trauma and can produce clinical symptoms. Whether the spasm may cause clinical symptoms depends on the degree of the spasm and the adequacy of the collateral blood supply if the affected artery is almost completely occluded during the spasm. Spasm can be temporary and may not result in lasting clinical symptoms. In other cases spasm may cause permanent damage because of infarction. The narrowing is usually localized, and there is a dilatation of the artery above the stenotic segment. It may last for several days to several weeks.

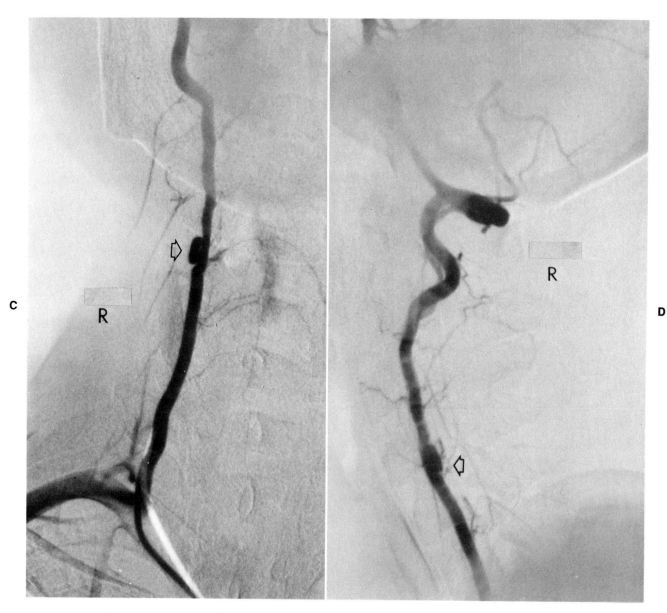

Fig. 5-36, cont'd. C and **D,** Selective right vertebral arteriogram 15 days after initial study demonstrates pseudoaneurysm *(arrows)* of right vertebral artery at C4 level at same site suggested by initial study.

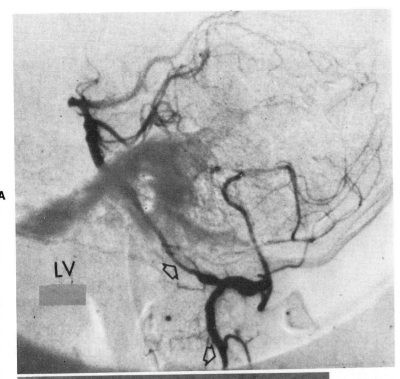

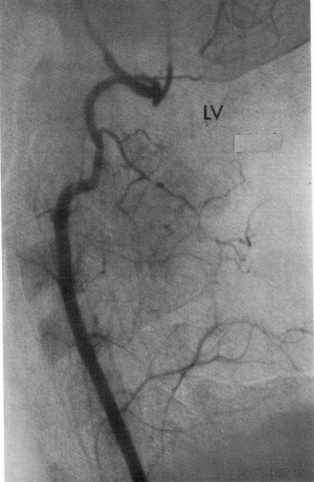

Fig. 5-37. Arterial spasm caused by blunt trauma to cervical spine (same patient as in Fig. 5-36). **A,** Lateral view of left vertebral arteriogram shows multiple segmental spasm in upper cervical portion of left vertebral artery (*arrows*). **B,** Repeat left vertebral arteriogram 15 days after initial study shows some improvement of previously seen segmental spasm of distal left vertebral artery.

Intraspinal vessels. Arterial disruption may occur in the anterior spinal artery or in a radiculospinal branch (Fig. 5-38). The interruption of the anterior spinal artery is very important, and if it occurs, it will cause severe, irreversible spinal cord damage with permanent loss of conduction of the long tracts. The interruption of the radiculospinal branches or even a vertebral artery has a better prognosis because of other collateral vessels supplying the anterior spinal artery. It should be kept in mind that failure of visualization of the anterior spinal artery does not necessarily indicate occlusion of that artery. Because of anatomic variations in the differ-

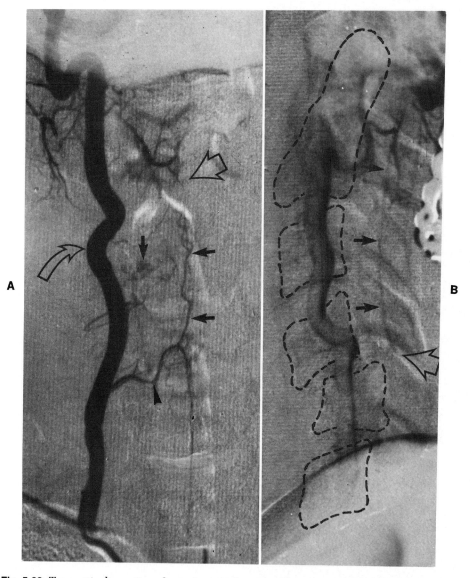

Fig. 5-38. Traumatic disruption of anterior spinal artery. This 18-year-old man sustained fracture-dislocation at C4-5 level. There was immediate motor and sensory quadriplegia. **A,** AP view of right vertebral arteriogram demonstrates deformity of vertebral artery *(open curved arrow)* at C4 and traumatic extravasation *(vertical arrow)*. Anterior spinal artery *(horizontal arrows)* appears tortuous and interrupted at posterior superior edge of C4 *(large open arrow)*, as localized on corresponding lateral view, **B;** its supply is provided by main radiculo-medullary artery *(arrowhead* in **A)** arising from right vertebral artery and passing through C6-7 right lateral foramen. **B,** Lateral view (late phase) shows opacification of anterior spinal vein *(arrows)*. There is interruption of vein at posterior superior edge of C4 *(large open arrow)* and deformity of vertebral artery caused by displacement (subluxation) of C5. (From Theron, J., et al.: Neuroradiology **15:**201, 1978.)

ent levels and collateral supplies to the artery, even in nontraumatic and normal cases it may not be demonstrated by arteriography. Gargour and co-workers[16] reported visualization of the anterior spinal artery by selective catheterization in 75% to 80% of cases. Di Chiro and Wener[12] were successful in demonstrating the anterior spinal artery in 80% of cases in the cervical region and 98% of cases in the thoracolumbar region by selective catheterization. Wener and co-workers[59] reported visualization of the anterior spinal artery in the cervical region in 90% of cases by selective injection of all the contributing vessels.

Arterial displacement is more frequent and may occur as a result of fracture-dislocation, displaced bony fragment, herniation of an intervertebral disc, hematoma, or a foreign body (Figs. 5-39 and 5-40). Displacement of the anterior spinal artery seems to have a better prognosis than arterial disruption. However, the inability of the current angiographic techniques to demonstrate the more important and more clinically critical intrinsic vasculature of the cord prevents one from making any definitive statement about the patient's prognosis. Severe neurologic syndromes can occur in spite of an angiographically uninterrupted anterior spinal artery. There is no correlation between the preservation of the anterior spinal artery and the neurologic prognostic improvement because neurologic functional damage can result from the direct effect of the frac-

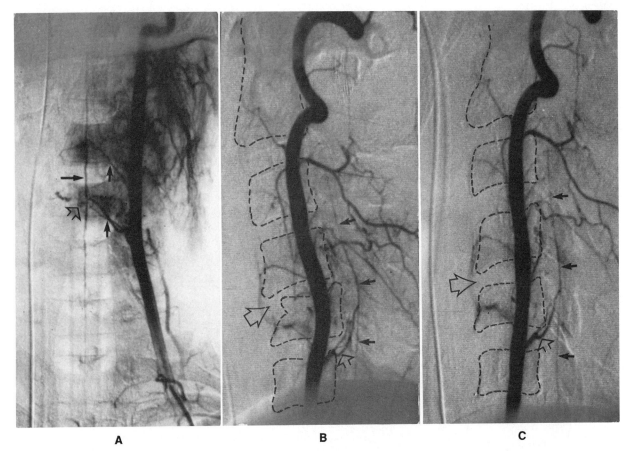

A   **B**   **C**

Fig. 5-39. Displacement of anterior spinal artery during fracture-dislocation. This 34-year-old man had a fracture-dislocation at C4-5 level and was found to be quadriplegic. Left vertebral arteriogram was performed 24 hours after trauma. **A,** AP view shows that two radiculospinal arteries are opacified (C4-5 and C5-6 left lateral foramina) *(vertical arrows)*. Anterior spinal artery *(horizontal arrow)* appears dilated but not interrupted. There is traumatic extravasation of contrast medium at C5 level *(open arrow)*. Lateral views before, **B,** and after, **C,** axial traction of cervical spine. Anterior spinal artery *(small arrows)* is displaced posteriorly by C5 vertebral body at C4-5 subluxation *(large open arrow)* before traction but returns to almost normal position after reduction of subluxation by traction. Anterior spinal artery *(small arrows)* is supplied mainly by C5-6 radiculomedullary artery *(small open arrow)*. (From Theron, J., et al.: Neuroradiology **15:**201, 1978.)

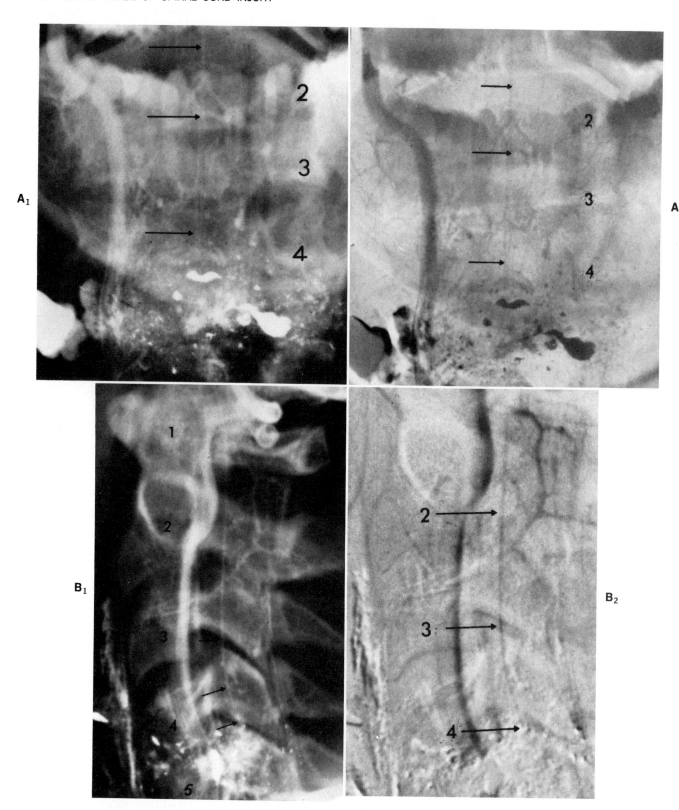

Fig. 5-40. Displacement of anterior spinal artery by penetrating wound (same patient as in Fig. 5-27). **A,** AP and, **B,** lateral views of cervical spine during left vertebral arteriography. Anterior spinal artery *(arrows)* is displaced posteriorly at C4 level. This corresponds to posterior displacement of spinal cord seen in myelography in Fig. 5-27. There is complete disruption of anterior spinal artery at level of C4-5 *(lowest arrow).*

tures-dislocations and may not be mediated through injury of the larger vessels.

Hyperemia and dilatation of the anterior spinal and radicular arteries are often observed after spinal trauma (Fig. 5-39). They appear early, can be extensive, and may persist for several months after injury. They have no prognostic significance. It is not possible to reach a definite conclusion concerning the local spinal blood flow from the morphologic modifications of dilated small spinal vessels alone.

Extravasation of contrast medium from meningeal arteries into the epidural or subdural spaces can be shown, indicating disruption of the meningeal vessels (Figs. 5-38 and 5-39). The clinical significance of this finding is not clear.

REFERENCES

1. Assenmacher, D. R., and Ducker, T. B.: Experimental traumatic paraplegia, J. Bone Joint Surg. [Am.] 53:671, 1971.
2. Babcock, J. L.: Cervical spine injuries, Arch. Surg. 111:646, 1976.
3. Barnes, R.: Paraplegia in cervical spine injuries, J. Bone Joint Surg. [Br.] 30:234, 1948.
4. Becker, D. H., Conley, F. K., and Anderson, M. E.: Quadriplegia associated with narrow cervical canal, ligamentous calcification and ankylosing hyperostosis, Surg. Neurol. 11:17, 1979.
5. Breig, A.: Biomechanics of the central nervous system: some basic normal and pathological phenomena, Stockholm, 1960, Almquist & Wiksell Förlag.
6. Breig, A., and El-Hadi, A. F.: Biomechanics of the cervical spinal cord, Acta. Radiol. 4:602, 1966.
7. Brooke, W. S.: Complete transverse cervical myelitis caused by traumatic herniation of an ossified nucleus pulposus, J.A.M.A. 125:117, 1944.
8. Brown, T., Hanson, R., and Yorra, A.: Some mechanical tests on the lumbo-sacral spine with particular reference to the intervertebral discs, J. Bone Joint Surg. [Am.] 39:1135, 1957.
9. Bussat, P., Rossier, A. B., Djindjian, R., et al.: Spinal cord angiography in dorsolumbar vertebral fractures with neurological involvement, Radiology 109:617, 1973.
10. Coin, C. G., Chan, Y. S., Keranen, V., and Pennink, M.: Computer assisted myelography in disk disease, J. Comput. Assist. Tomogr. 1:398, 1977.
11. Coin, C. G., Pennink, M., Ahmad, W. D., and Keranen, V. J.: Diving-type injury of the cervical spine: contribution of computed tomography to management, J. Comput. Assist. Tomogr. 3:362, 1979.
12. Di Chiro, G., and Wener, L.: Angiography of the spinal cord. A review of contemporary techniques and applications, J. Neurosurg. 39:1, 1973.
13. Djindjian, R.: Angiography of the spinal cord, Surg. Neurol. 2:179, 1974.
14. Epstein, J. A., Carras, R., Epstein, B. S., and Levine, L. S.: Myelopathy in cervical spondylosis with vertebral

15. Gargano, F. P., Meyer, J., Houdek, P. V., and Charyulu, K. K. N.: Transverse axial tomography of the cervical spine, Radiology 113:363, 1974.
16. Gargour, G. W., Wener, L., and Di Chiro, G.: Selective arteriography of the spinal cord in post-traumatic paraplegia, Neurology 22:131, 1972.
17. Geehr, R. B., Rothman, S. L. G., and Kier, E. L.: The role of computed tomography in the evaluation of upper cervical spine pathology, Comput. Tomogr. 2:79, 1978.
18. Gonsalves, C. G., Hudson, A. R., Horsey, W. J., and Tucher, W. S.: Computed tomography of the cervical spine and spinal cord, Comput. Tomogr. 2:279, 1978.
19. Goodman, J. H., Bingham, W. G., and Hunt, W. E.: Ultrastructural blood-brain barrier alterations and edema formation in acute spinal cord trauma, J. Neurosurg. 44:418, 1976.
20. Gurdjian, E. S., Audet, B., Sibayan, R. W., and Thomas, L. M.: Spasm of the extracranial internal carotid artery resulting from blunt trauma demonstrated by angiography, J. Neurosurg. 35:742, 1971.
21. Hanus, S. H., Homer, T. D., and Harter, D. H.: Vertebral artery occlusion complicating yoga exercises, Arch. Neurol. 34:574, 1977.
22. Hashimoto, I., and Tak, Y. K.: The true sagittal diameter of the cervical spinal canal and its diagnostic significance in cervical myelopathy, J. Neurosurg. 47:912, 1977.
23. Haughton, V. M., Ho, K. C., Larson, S. J., et al.: Experimental production of arachnoiditis with water-soluble myelographic media, Radiology 123:681, 1977.
24. Heiden, J. S., Weiss, M. H., Rosenberg, A. W., et al.: Penetrating gunshot wounds of the cervical spine in civilians, Neurosurgery 42:575, 1975.
25. Heilbrun, M. P., and Ratcheson, R. A.: Multiple extracranial vessel injuries following closed head and neck trauma, Neurosurgery 37:219, 1972.
26. Hinck, V. C., and Sachdev, N. S.: Developmental stenosis of the cervical spinal canal, Brain 89:27, 1966.
27. Hinkel C. L., and Nichols, R. L.: Opaque myelography in penetrating wounds of the spinal canal, Am. J. Roentgenol. 55:689, 1946.
28. Howland, W. J., and Curry, J. L.: Experimental studies of pantopaque arachnoiditis, Radiology 87:253, 1966.
29. Howland, W. J., and Curry, J. L.: Pantopaque arachnoiditis, Acta Radiol. 5:1032, 1966.
30. Jacobson, R. E., Gargano, F. P., and Rosomoff, H. L.: Transverse axial tomography of the spine. I. Axial anatomy of the normal lumbar spine, J. Neurosurg. 42:406, 1975.
31. Jacobson, R. E., Gargano, F. P., and Rosomoff, H. L.: Transverse axial tomography of the spine. II. The stenotic spinal canal, J. Neurosurg. 42:412, 1975.
32. Kaplan, C. J.: Cervical hyperextension injuries with paraplegia, J. Bone Joint Surg. [Br.] 35:97, 1953.
33. Kelly, D. L., and Alexander, E.: Lateral cervical puncture for myelography, J. Neurosurg. 29:106, 1968.
34. Laasonen, E. M., and Riska, E. B.: Preoperative radiological assessment of fractures of the thoracolumbar spine

causing traumatic paraplegia, Skeletal Radiol. 1:231, 1976.

35. Lai, M. D., Hoffman, H. B., and Adamkiewicz, J. J.: Dissecting aneurysm of internal carotid artery after nonpenetrating neck injury, Acta Radiol. 5:290, 1966.

36. Lee, B. C. P., Kazam, E., and Newman, A. D.: Computed tomography of the spine and spinal cord, Radiology 128:95, 1978.

37. Leo, J. S., Bergeron, R. T., Kricheff, I. I., and Benjamin, M. V.: Metrizamide myelography for cervical spinal cord injuries, Radiology 129:707, 1978.

38. Mehalic, T., and Farhat, S. M.: Vertebral artery injury from chiropractic manipulation, Surg. Neurol. 2:125, 1974.

39. Nagashima, C.: Cervical myelopathy due to developmental stenosis of the cervical spinal canal. 1. The sagittal diameter of the spinal canal, Neurol. Surg. (Japan) 1:163, 1973.

40. Pay, N. T., George, A. E., Benjamin, M. V., et al.: Positive and negative contrast myelography in spinal trauma, Radiology 123:103, 1977.

41. Pear, B. L.: Spinal epidural hematoma, Am. J. Roentgenol. 115:155, 1972.

42. Rossier, A. B., Berney, J., Rosenbaum, A. E., and Hachen, J.: Value of gas myelography in early management of acute cervical spinal cord injuries, J. Neurosurg. 42:330, 1975.

43. Rothman, R. H., and Marvel, J. P.: The acute cervical disk, Clin. Orthop. 109:59, 1975.

44. Sackett, J. F., Strother, C. M., Quaglieri, C. E., et al.: Metrizamide—CSF contrast medium, Radiology 123:779, 1977.

45. Schechter, M. M., and Zingesser, L. H.: The anterior spinal artery, Acta Radiol. 3:489, 1965.

46. Schneider, R. C., and Kahn, E. A.: Chronic neurological sequelae of acute trauma to the spine and spinal cord. IV. Problems pertaining to the treatment of retained foreign bodies, J. Bone Joint Surg. [Am.] 41:457, 1959.

47. Schneider, R. C., and Knighton, R.: Chronic neurological sequelae of acute trauma to the spine and spinal cord. III. The syndrome of chronic injury to the cervical spinal cord in the region of the central canal, J. Bone Joint Surg. [Am.] 41:905, 1959.

48. Scotti, L. N., Marasco, J. A., Pittman, T. A., et al.: Computed tomography of the spinal canal and cord, Comput. Tomogr. 1:229, 1977.

49. Skalpe, I. O.: Adhesive arachnoiditis following lumbar radiculography with water-soluble contrast agents, Radiology 121:647, 1976.

50. Skalpe, I. O., and Amundsen, P.: Thoracic and cervical myelography with metrizamide, Radiology 116:101, 1975.

51. Sullivan, H. G., Vines, F. S., and Becker, D. P.: Sequelae of indirect internal carotid injury, Radiology 10:91, 1973.

52. Sypert, G. W., and Mozingo, J. R.: A technique for early pantopaque myelography in cervical spinal cord injuries, Surg. Neurol. 6:221, 1976.

53. Takahashi, S.: Atlas of axial transverse tomography and its clinical application, New York, 1969, Springer-Verlag.

54. Teal, J. S., Bergeron, R. T., Rumbaugh, C. L., and Segall, H. D.: Aneurysms of the cervical portion of the internal carotid artery associated with nonpenetrating neck trauma, Radiology 105:353, 1972.

55. Theron, J., Derlon, J. M., and de Preux, J.: Angiography of the spinal cord after vertebral trauma, Neuroradiology 15:201, 1978.

56. Tveten, L.: Spinal cord vascularity. I. Extraspinal sources of spinal cord arteries in man, Acta Radiol. 17:1, 1976.

57. Tveten, L.: Spinal cord vascularity. III. The spinal cord arteries in man, Acta Radiol. 17:257, 1976.

58. Vallebona, A.: Nouvelle methode roentgenstratigraphique, Radiol. Clin. (Basel) 16:279, 1947.

59. Wener, L., Di Chiro, G., and Gargour, G. W.: Angiography of cervical cord injuries, Radiology 112:597, 1974.

60. Wilson, C., and Jumer, M.: Traumatic spinal-pleural fistula, J.A.M.A. 179:813, 1962.

61. Yashon, D., Jane, J. A., and White, R. J.: Prognosis and management of spinal cord and cauda equina bullet injuries in sixty-five civilians, J. Neurosurg. 32:163, 1970.

62. Yeoman, P. M.: Cervical myelography in traction injuries of the brachial plexus, J. Bone Joint Surg. [Br.] 50:253, 1968.

63. Zilkha, A.: Traumatic occlusion of the internal carotid artery, Radiology 97:543, 1970.

64. Zilkha, A., Reiss, J., Shulman, K., and Schechter, M. M.: Traumatic subarachnoid-mediastinal fistula, J. Neurosurg. 32:473, 1970.

65. Zorub, D. S., Nashold, B. S., and Cook, W. A.: Avulsion of the brachial plexus. I. A review with implications on the therapy of intractable pain, Surg. Neurol. 2:347, 1974.

CHAPTER 6

Closed reduction of spinal fractures and dislocations

PAUL R. MEYER, Jr., M.D.

Methods of regaining spinal column realignment are recorded as early as 400 BC (Hippocrates)[8] and the first century AD (Celsus)[10] but are best described and illustrated by Vidus Vidius in 1544.[15] Hippocrates and Celsus described the use of a winch table, or "extension bench," capable of producing spinal distraction by simultaneous traction in opposite directions at the foot and axilla.

Postural reduction of fracture-dislocations of the thoracic and lumbar spine began in the 1920s and 1930s. The prone patient was hyperextended by means of slings, frames, or hammocks.[9,25] Hanging the patient by the upper or lower extremities, utilizing the body weight as countertraction, was described by Bohler in 1935.[2] Watson-Jones[27] described spinal reduction by the prone placement of the patient between two tables, manipulation of the spine, and application of an extension plaster body cast or "plaster bed." The use of the plaster bed is no longer advocated for use in the patient with absent sensation because of the threat of skin breakdown. Frankel and co-workers[13] and Guttmann[14,15] advised "postural reduction" of thoracic and lumbar fractures by prolonged bed rest in a position of hyperextension for up to 11 to 13 weeks or until bone healing occurred.

The performance of manipulative reduction of fracture-dislocations of the thoracic and lumbar spine in the neurologically injured patient has been questioned by several authors.[15,16,23] The consensus is one of concern, although no reports of neurologic deterioration are attributed to manipulation. Other authors deny any increase in the level of neurologic deficit after spine manipulation and reduction.[10,21,22] Stanger[26] reports a high recurrent dislocation rate where such spines have been managed conservatively.

Early operative intervention in acute spinal injuries with vertebral column malalignment and associated neurologic dysfunction has been advocated by some authors[11,28] as an emergency or day-of-injury procedure. Other authors advise surgical stabilization between the day of injury and 2 weeks after injury.* There is uniform agreement that laminectomy alone adds significantly to further spinal instability and has little if any beneficial effect on the enhancement of neurologic return. In our series extension of neurologic injury secondary to manipulation and stabilization of the spine did not result, although such complications can occur and frequently go unrecognized or unreported. Recent consultations and case reviews have revealed three postoperative neurologic deteriorations: two incomplete and one complete; each occurred after spinal instrumentation at 4 days, 9 days, and 2 weeks after injury. The most plausible cause is either direct or indirect vascular alteration to the cord. For example, a vertebral injury at T11 that results in a T6 neurologic deficit is

---

*References 4, 12, 16, 17, 19-22.

181

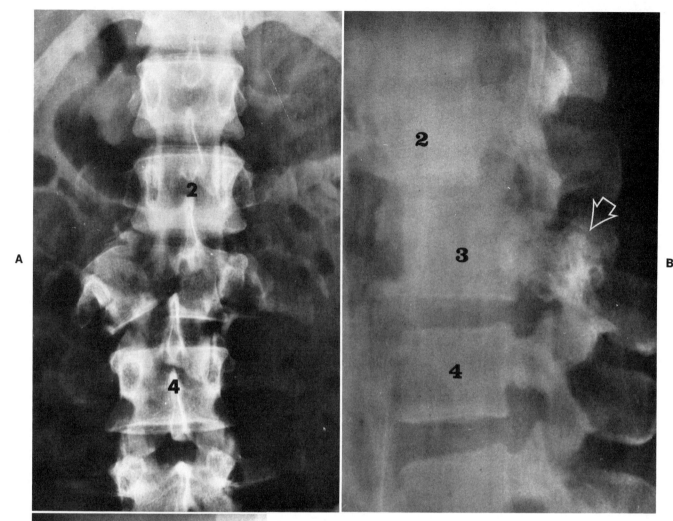

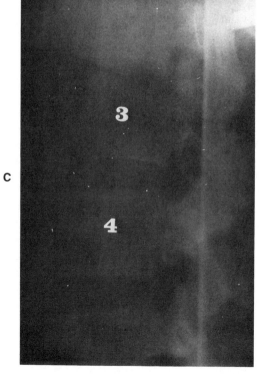

Fig. 6-1. Bursting fracture of L3 with dislocation of L2 on L3 and incomplete cauda equina injury. **A** and **B,** Prereduction and, **C,** postmanipulation cross-table lateral radiographs. Note fractures of multiple transverse processes, **A,** and posterior elements (*arrow* in **B**).

more likely to be caused by spinal cord ischemia secondary to vascular embarrassment (the vessel of Adamkiewicz).[1,18] For this reason the immediate objective of spinal injury care is reduction of spinal malalignment and either reduction of or prevention of neurologic embarrassment secondary to compression. Whether early surgical realignment and decompression of the spine are required is a matter of personal opinion, philosophy, or patient assessment. Most authors agree that appropriate, timely surgery will reduce spinal instability and length of required recumbency and enhance rehabilitation.[7,11,12,16,20]

NEUROLOGIC ASSESSMENT

Injuries to the thoracic cord, between vertebral bodies T1 and T10, which result in an immediate complete

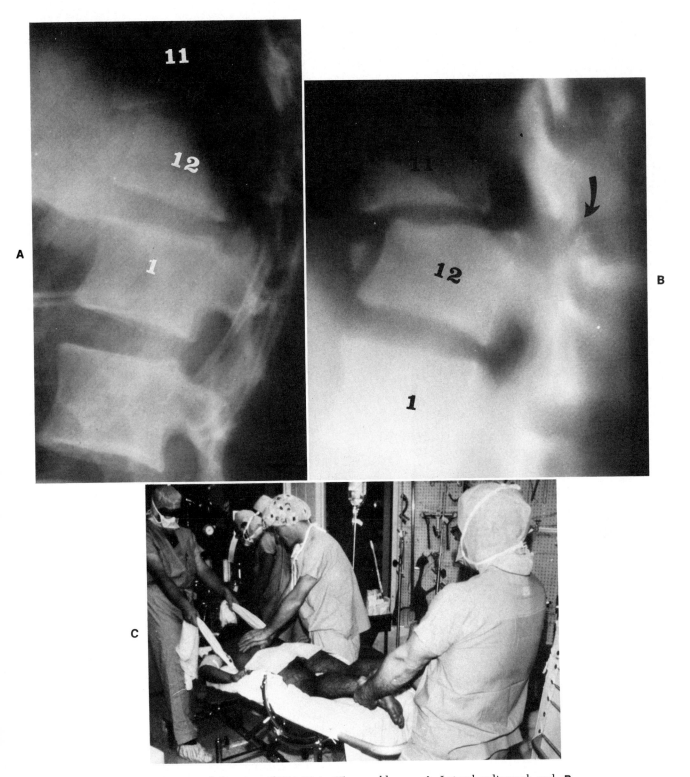

Fig. 6-2. Fracture-dislocation of T11-12 in 27-year-old man. **A,** Lateral radiograph and, **B,** polytomogram show compression of T11, wedge fracture of T12, dislocation, and locked facets (*arrow* in **B**). **C,** Closed manipulation under general anesthesia.

Continued.

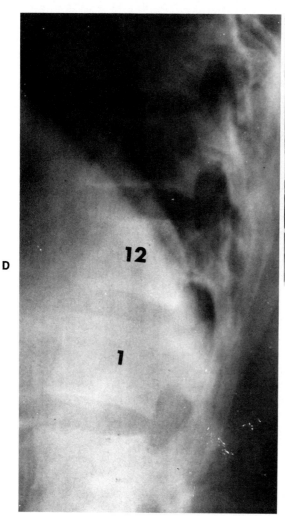

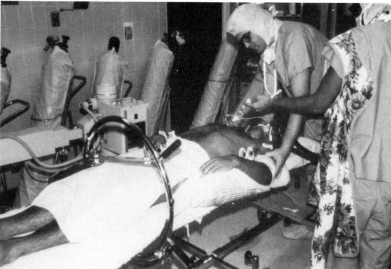

Fig. 6-2, cont'd. D, Postreduction lateral radiograph. **E,** Maintenance of thoracolumbar hyperextension with patient turned in supine position. Note pillow opposite injury site.

or ascending neurologic injury, appear to be irreversible regardless of the treatment rendered. This includes drug therapy (steroids, mannitol), fluid therapy, or immediate surgery. It can also be stated emphatically that if there is neurologic improvement, spontaneous surgery without due cause is ill advised. Circumstantial evidence does seem to indicate that in the absence of some obvious cause surgical manipulation alone may, in the acutely traumatized spinal cord, be all that is required to bring about neurologic extension. Fortunately many of these changes, when insidious in onset, are noted to be temporary but unable to be changed. Because the finding of a complete obstruction on myelogram, above the level of the conus medullaris and cauda equina, has not been found to result in neurologic improvement when "decompressed,"[5,6,11] both the surgery and the myelogram serve little purpose. This particularly applies to the *complete* neurologic injury.

Trauma to the vertebral column at the level of the conus medullaris (T12-L1), like trauma to the spinal

cord, is quite predictable. The extent of the injury normally dictates whether the injury to the lumbar and sacral segments of the cord will be complete or incomplete. On the other hand, injury to the cauda equina is quite unpredictable. Injuries occurring below the level of the initial root exit (T10) down to the level of the conus medullaris (L1) require careful neurologic assessment. However, when neurologic findings are incomplete and inconsistent, stabilization should be delayed. This is not to say that improvement in spinal realignment should not be attempted early by either closed manipulation or postural reduction.[13-15] Certainly, significant fracture-subluxation-dislocation of the vertebral column should not be allowed to exist for more than 2 weeks. Longer than this, even open attempts at realignment often fail because there is extensive fibrosis about the fracture-trauma site. In those instances where secondary complications of trauma occur, such as deep venous thrombosis requiring heparin, hemopneumothorax, pulmonary embolism, or sepsis, every effort should be made to gain an early, adequate reduction by either postural reduction or spinal manipulation. The alternative is acceptance of the spinal malalignment as it exists. In the absence of contraindications, postural reduction or closed manipulation substantiates the rationale for achieving early spinal realignment. Thus alternate management techniques depend on the need for (1) immediate surgery in the presence of an increasing neurologic deficit in the neurologically incomplete

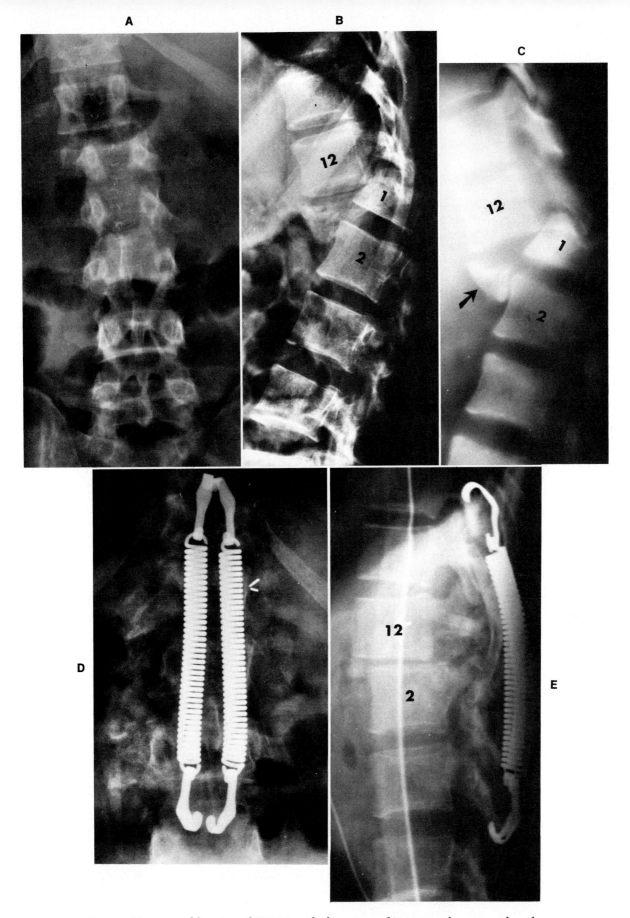

Fig. 6-3. Fracture-subluxation of T12-L1 with disruption of posterior elements and wedge compression fracture of L1 in a 21-year-old man (initial radiographs not shown). **A** to **C,** Four months after injury and laminectomy. Progressive loss of position has resulted in fragmentation of L1 *(arrow)* and total dislocation. Spine realignment was obtained by total resection of L1 through combined anteroposterior approach. **D** and **E,** Weiss compression springs were utilized for internal fixation. Note absence of hyperextension deformity. (See text.)

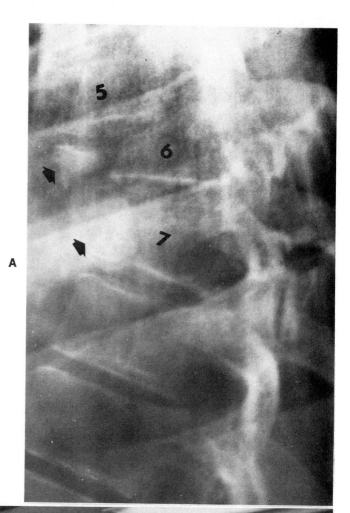

Fig. 6-4. Fracture-dislocation of T5-6 with comminuted wedge fracture of T6 and T7 (*arrows* in **A**). **B,** Closed manipulation technique. Note traction both proximally and distally while vertical pressure is applied over prominent proximal spinous process of distal segment.

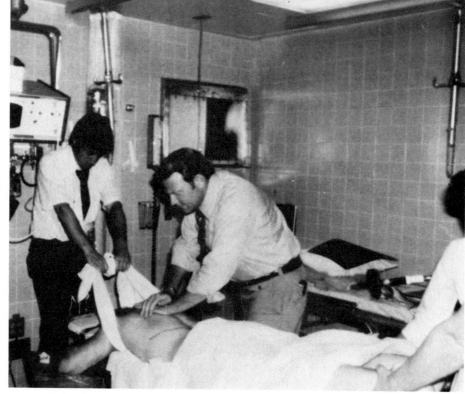

patient, (2) postural reduction in the complete neurologically injured patient with fracture and dislocation, or (3) closed manipulation in the neurologically complete thoracic injury or incomplete lumbar injury, followed by surgical stabilization with internal fixation and bone graft, at 2 to 3 weeks. The third alternative may be the plan of choice, although it is contraindicated by the presence of associated injuries, that is, rib fractures with intra-abdominal or intra-thoracic injuries. Such injuries preempt immediate spinal reduction, although spinal reduction by closed manipulation was done in two of 22 patients in the series herein reported 48 hours after injury, and reduction was successfully done on one patient 2 weeks after injury. One patient's closed reduction was done 36 hours after splenectomy (Fig. 6-1), and one required a general anesthetic for reduction of his dislocation (Fig. 6-2). One patient died from pulmonary embolism, a complication related to his multiple-system trauma, 2 weeks after surgery and 5 weeks after the initial trauma.

TREATMENT

Heretofore, the identification of an acute thoracic or lumbar vertebral fracture with associated gross vertebral column malalignment was tantamount to an immediate posterior surgical "decompression." The result of such a laminectomy was often further vertebral column instability with a gradual worsening of the malalignment (Fig. 6-3).[4,20] Seldom was the extent of the neurologic injury considered, and less often was the decompressive procedure accompanied by a simultaneously performed spine-stabilizing procedure. A supplementary alternative to the above management scheme is correction of vertebral column malalignment by manipulation and closed reduction of the acute thoracic or lumbar fracture-dislocation (Figs. 6-2, 6-4, and 6-5). The objective is immediate restitution of spinal alignment hopefully resulting in spinal canal and neurologic tissue decompression. Attainment of spinal alignment without a deteriorating neurologic picture circumvents the need for immediate surgical intervention, although surgical stabilization is uniformly performed at a later date. The decision for conservative care is based on a carefully performed neurologic evaluation on admission. When gross malalignment of the vertebral column with bony comminution about and within the neural canal is present and is accompanied by a well-delineated neurologic level consistent with the vertebral injury, early surgical intervention may be indicated.

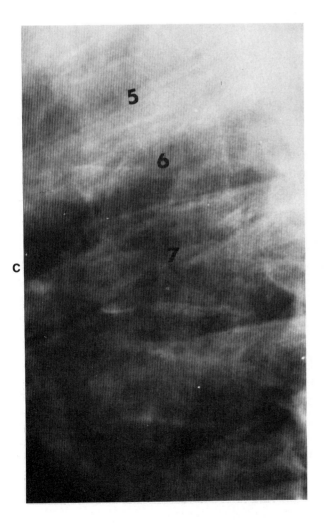

Fig. 6-4, cont'd. C, Postreduction lateral radiograph.

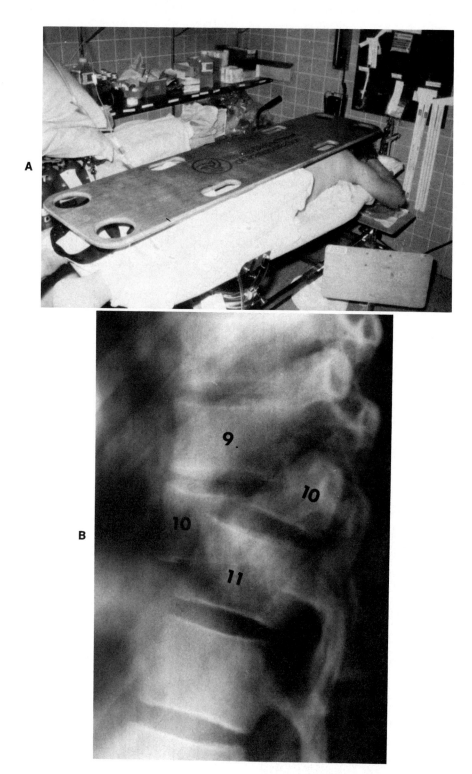

Fig. 6-5. A, Twenty-one-year-old complete paraplegia trauma victim turned to prone position on Stryker frame. Spine board was used for transportation in supine position. **B,** Lateral radiograph demonstrates fracture-dislocation of T9-10.

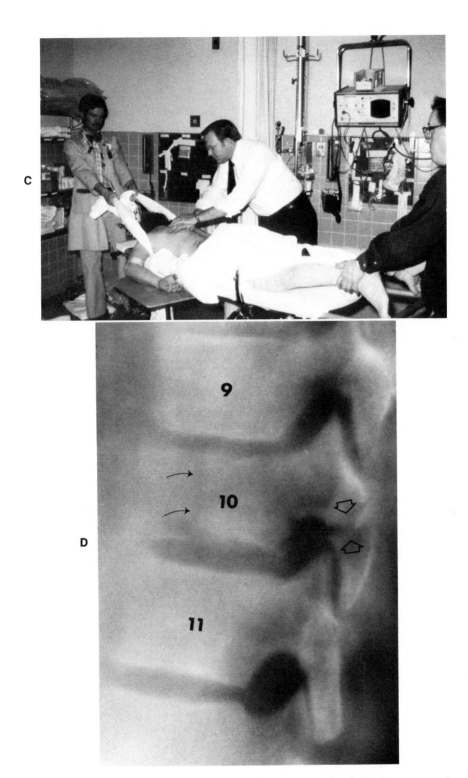

Fig. 6-5, cont'd. C, Method of closed reduction using proximal and distal traction and pressure at fracture site. **D,** Postreduction polytomogram shows reduction of T9-10 dislocation and close approximation of two fragments of T10 *(small arrows)*. Note fracture of lamina *(open arrows)*.

ANATOMIC CONSIDERATIONS

Numerous factors must be taken into account when deciding on the most appropriate method of managing a fracture-dislocation of the thoracic or lumbar spine. Philosophy, experience, or teaching does influence the choice of management technique. Personal observations following complete excision of an entire vertebral body (anterior and posterior elements) in order to regain vertebral column realignment (Fig. 6-3) demonstrate less of a concern for the presence or absence of the anterior longitudinal ligament than heretofore expressed. It has always been considered that this structure was necessary in (1) spinal column stability, (2) maintenance of spinal reduction, and (3) the prevention of overdistraction or hyperextension when using either distraction or compression fixation devices. Without question, the structure must be considered. Hyperextension has resulted in this structure's absence on one occasion, requiring removal of the compression device and insertion of a distraction device. The prime consideration remains the presence or absence of neurologic integrity.

FRACTURE CLASSIFICATION

Flesch and co-workers[12] and Rogers and co-workers[24] describe three types of thoracic and lumbar vertebral column injuries with associated ligamentous fracture-dislocations and subluxation components similar to those identified in our series.

1. Flexion-rotation, comminuted vertebral body fractures with fracture and disruption of the posterior bone and ligamentous structures (usually forward subluxation of the superior vertebral body on the inferior vertebral body [Fig. 6-5])
2. Wedge-compression fracture of the vertebral body with associated fracture of the posterior elements and subluxation of the superior vertebral body on the inferior body (Figs. 6-6 and 6-7)
3. Vertebral body bursting fracture (Fig. 6-1)

In our series we identified an additional type 4 injury: posterior element (facet) dislocation associated with disruption of the posterior ligamentous structures (Figs. 6-2, 6-8, and 6-9).

Of 22 fracture-dislocations of the thoracic and lumbar spine described later in this chapter and managed by initial manipulation and closed reduction, 3 (14%) were type 1, 15 (68%) were type 2, 1 (4%) was type 3, and 3 (14%) were type 4 (Table 6-1).

Text continued on p. 196.

Table 6-1. Fracture classifications in 22 patients treated by closed reduction

Type	Description	No.	%
1	Fracture-disruption of posterior elements; comminuted vertebral fracture of inferior vertebra and forward subluxation-dislocation of superior vertebra on inferior vertebra	3	14
2	Fracture of posterior elements; wedge-compression or no fracture of inferior vertebra, forward subluxation of superior vertebra on inferior vertebra	15	68
3	Bursting vertebral fracture with vertebral body dislocation	1	4
4	Posterior element (facet) dislocation with forward subluxation of superior vertebra on inferior vertebra	3	14

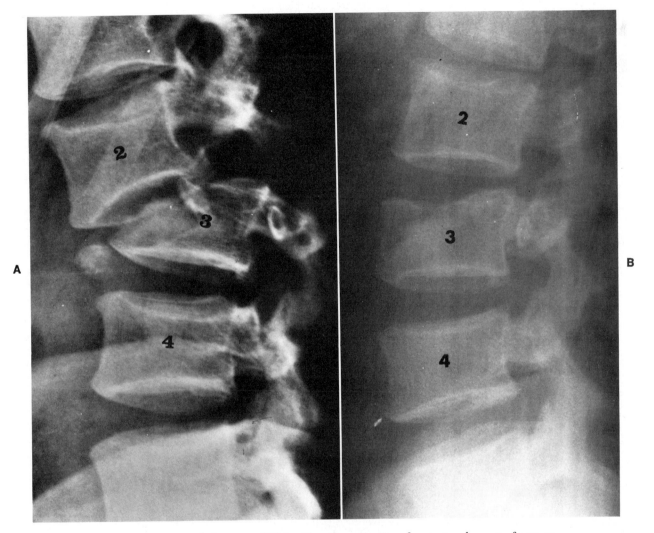

Fig. 6-6. A, Fracture-dislocation of L2-3 with wide separation of posterior elements, fractures of facets, and comminuted wedge fracture of body of L3. **B,** Cross-table lateral view after closed reduction shows excellent alignment of L2-3.

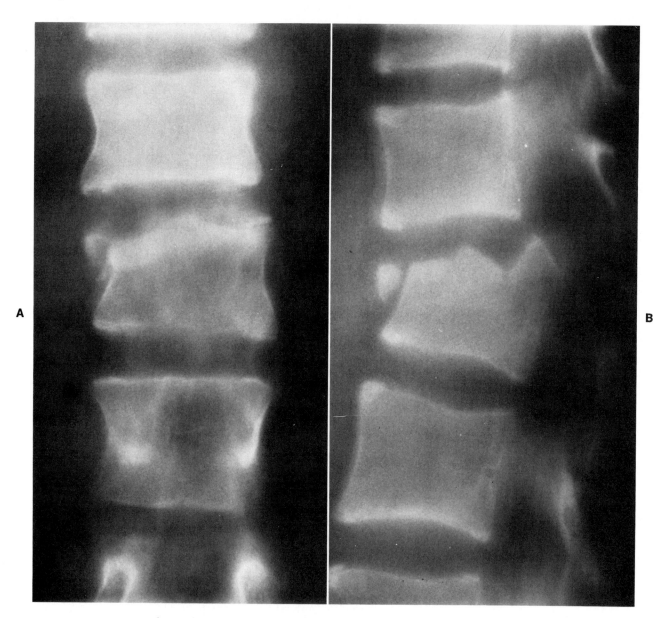

Fig. 6-7. Chance fracture of L2. **A** and **B,** Polytomograms show fracture through posterior and anterior elements and associated forward displacement of L1 on L2. Patient had additional fractures of cervical spine and femurs, requiring general anesthesia.

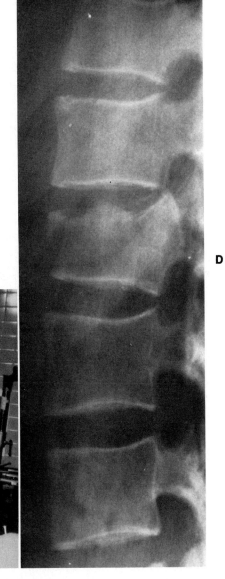

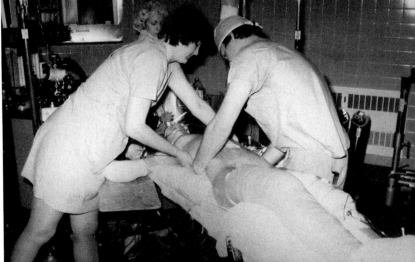

Fig. 6-7, cont'd. C, Lumbar spine manipulation was done in supine position. **D,** Postreduction cross-table lateral radiograph.

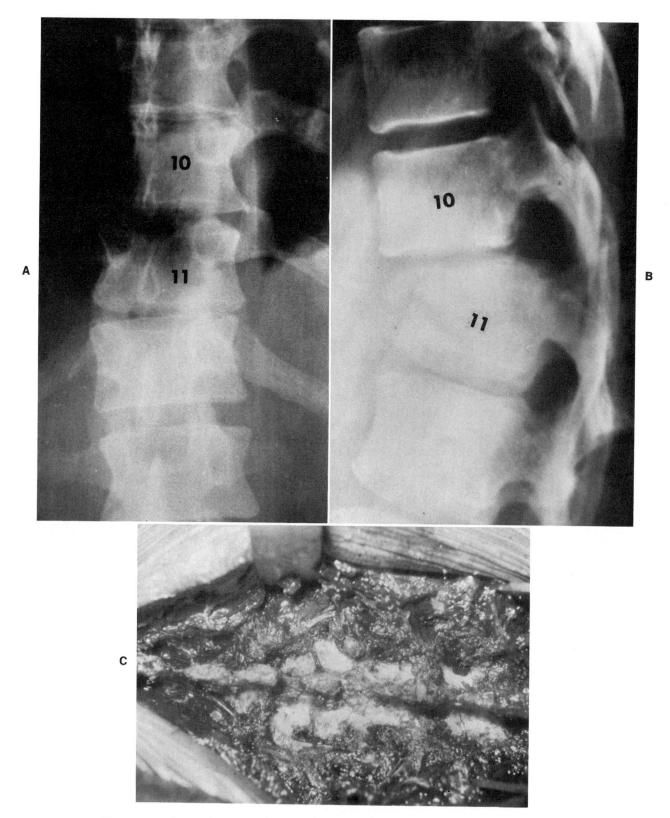

Fig. 6-8. **A** and **B,** Dislocation and locked facets of T10-11 with incomplete neurologic injury. Closed reduction failed. **C,** Open reduction reveals bilateral dislocated and locked facets.

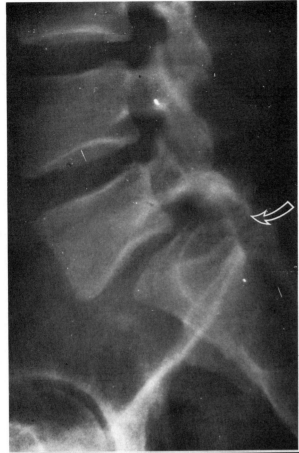

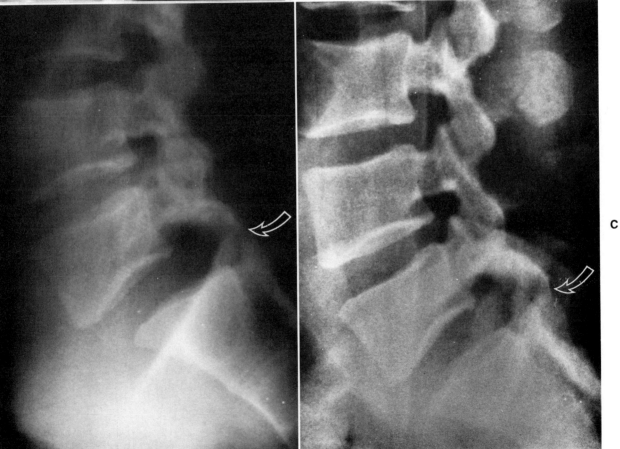

Fig. 6-9. Fracture-dislocation of L5-S1 with fracture of superior facets *(arrows)*. **A,** Prereduction radiograph. Closed manipulation resulted first in partial, **B,** and then in complete, **C,** reduction of dislocation.

CLOSED MANIPULATION-REDUCTION TECHNIQUE

The decision for closed spine fracture manipulation is made after careful patient physical and neurologic assessment and determination of the presence or absence of associated injuries. There being no overriding contraindications, an intravenous line is maintained and the patient is kept NPO (nothing by mouth). Intravenous diazepam (Valium), 10 mg, in conjunction with an appropriate analgesic such as morphine sulfate or meperidine (Demerol), is very effective in producing sufficient relaxation to perform the closed reduction maneuver. If head injury is suspected, narcotics are contraindicated.

The patient, placed on a Stryker wedge frame, is in the prone position. Within 10 to 15 minutes of administering both the muscle relaxant and the analgesic, one assistant is placed at each ankle to provide longitudinal (caudal) traction, while a third assistant provides cephalad traction by means of a transverse sheet placed beneath the upper chest and brought dorsally over the posterior shoulders via both axillae (Figs. 6-2, C; 6-4, B; and 6-5, C). During traction, the arms are maintained at the patient's side. The fourth and most experienced assistant, after careful evaluation and localization of the spinal defect level, applies perpendicularly directed pressure over the most prominent spinous process (Figs. 6-2, C; 6-4, B; and 6-5, C). This prominence coincides with the gibbus produced by the most

proximal vertebral spinous process of the distal spinal segment (Figs. 6-2, A and B). Direct pressure is applied for one or two brief periods. Occasionally one may palpate the reduction as it occurs. To determine the effect of the attempted reduction, a cross-table lateral (horizontal beam) radiograph is obtained while the patient is in the prone position (Figs. 6-1, C; 6-2, D; 6-4, C; 6-5, D; 6-6, B; and 6-7, C). If the reduction has failed the procedure is repeated as described. The patient is told what neurologic sensations he might experience and asked to report if any of these sensations occur during the procedure. If a repeat reduction attempt fails, no further attempt should be made.

After manipulation the patient is maintained in hyperextension (Fig. 6-2, E) while turning him from prone to supine and supine to prone every 2 hours. This is done to relieve the weight on the skin overlying bony prominences and to prevent skin breakdown. It is achieved by placing two pillows opposite the level of dislocation while the patient is supine and two pillows opposite the chest and lower pelvis when he is prone. Whether spinal alignment has or has not been improved with manipulation, the patient should be maintained in hyperextension until surgery. If the closed reduction or postural reduction has failed and gross spinal malalignment persists, surgery is indicated. Where gross spinal deformity exists in the presence of neurologic function, it is prudent to delay surgery until the patient's neurologic condition stabilizes.

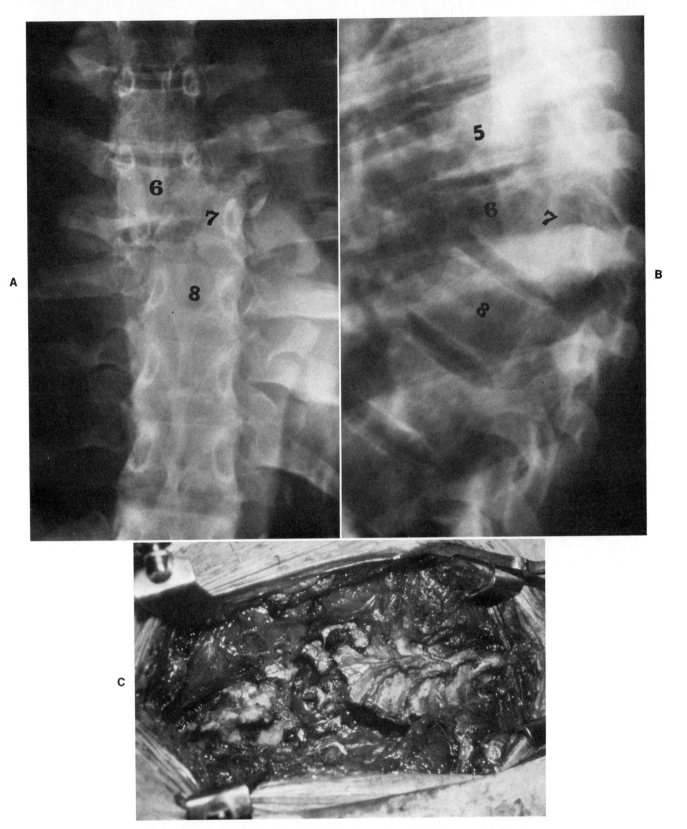

Fig. 6-10. A and **B,** Fracture-dislocation of T6-7 after acute flexion injury in 21-year-old automobile accident victim. Note fracture of left transverse processes. This type of vertebral injury is unreducible by closed manipulation. **C,** Surgical photograph shows total separation of T6-7 posterior elements, laceration of dura mater and spinal cord, and fractures of posterior elements of T7-10. Head is to left.

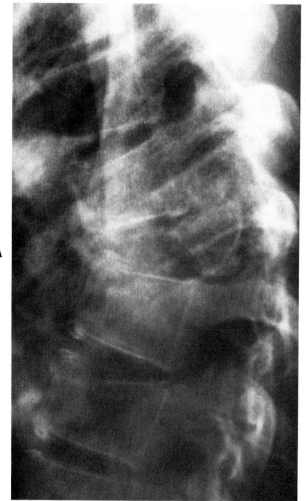

A

Table 6-2. Outcome of 22 closed reductions*

Outcome	No.	%
Successful closed reductions	19	86
Failure reductions (locked facets-fragments)	3	14
Recurrent facet dislocation: preoperative/ postmanipulation	3	14
Number stabilized and fused	22	100
Death secondary to multiple trauma	1	4.5

*Closed reductions were as follows: 9 (41%) thoracic, 7 (32%) thoracolumbar, and 6 (27%) lumbar.

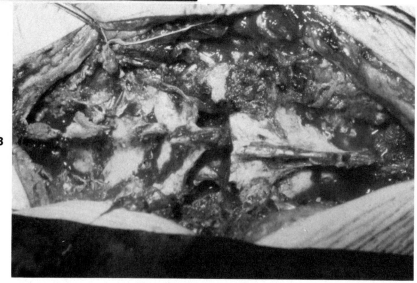

B

Fig. 6-11. A, Flexion injury to midthoracic spine with disruption of posterior elements and impingement of pedicle of T7. This type of vertebral injury is unreducible by closed manipulation. **B,** Surgical photograph shows separation of posterior elements, fracture of pedicle of T7 and upper facets of T8, and exposure of dura mater.

CONCERNS OVER CLOSED MANIPULATION TECHNIQUE

The potential for extension of neurologic injury does exist, although it is remote, whether an acute spinal cord injured patient is managed conservatively, with manipulation, or surgically. Careful analysis of the fracture and its neurologic injury, if present, is required. Experience with the closed reduction-manipulation technique reveals that in the presence of bilateral facet dislocation (locked facets) without fracture, closed reduction will not likely be achieved without the use of general anesthesia (Table 6-2; Figs. 6-8, 6-10, and 6-11). Anesthesia is not necessary for fracture-dislocation reduction where fractures of the facets have occurred. A delay of up to several days between injury and attempted reduction, whether with or without facet fractures, generally dictates a need for anesthesia. Should failure of reduction under general anesthesia occur, a decision is then required as to whether postural positioning or immediate open reduction is required. We have found that immediate operative intervention is required only when there is evidence of significant bone or disc encroachment on neurologic tissue in the presence of an *incomplete* neurologic injury[20]; others feel more comfortable with immediate open reduction.[11,12,16,17]

An associated complication of closed manipulation and reduction of a thoracic or lumbar fracture-dislocation is the loss of that reduction (Table 6-2). Holdsworth and Hardy[16] described spine instability as existing with (1) fractured facets, (2) rupture of interlaminar and interspinous ligaments, and (3) rupture of the anterior longitudinal ligament. Dickson and co-workers[11] and Davis[9] question this latter structure's rupturing with flexion injuries to the spine (Fig. 6-12), although a case may be made in some instances (Figs. 6-1 and 6-10). For such injuries Guttmann[14] advocated conservative management with bed rest and "postural reduction" in hyperextension for periods up to 3 months. In our series using this method of postreduction "maintenance of reduction," three cases underwent recurrent facet dislocation between 2 and 3 weeks (Table 6-2). This occurred in patients in whom there were neither facet fractures nor apparent disruption of the anterior longitudinal ligament. Those patients in whom facet fractures did exist and were reduced also underwent moderate but noncompromising vertebral body–posterior element displacement (Fig. 6-6). These findings substantiate the need for careful postural positioning or spine stabilization during the early posttrauma period.

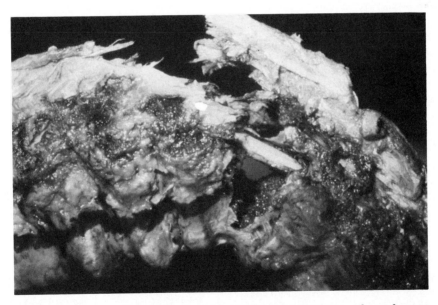

Fig. 6-12. Fresh cadaver spine under vertical load. Flexion deformity results in disruption of posterior ligamentous and bony posterior elements, followed by rupture of ligamentum flavum and posterior longitudinal ligament and distraction-slice fracture through vertebral body. Note remaining integrity of anterior longitudinal ligament.

CASE MATERIAL

Between 1972 and 1978 the Midwest Regional Spinal Cord Injury Care System cared for 349 acute thoracic, thoracolumbar, or lumbar spine fractures within 72 hours of injury. The Illinois Emergency Medical System[3] has served as an integral part of the system, particularly in early retrieval of victims, with an average admission time of 8.6 hours. One half had complete neurologic injuries (48%), and the remainder were incomplete (52%).[22] Of the 349 patients, 109 (31%) underwent spine stabilization during their initial hospitalization.

Of the 349 acute thoracic and lumbar injuries 22 (6%) had a fracture-dislocation that was amenable to manipulation and closed reduction (Tables 6-1 to 6-3; Figs. 6-13 and 6-14) followed by spine stabilization and fusion.

Of the 22 thoracic and lumbar fracture-dislocation manipulations, 8 (36%) sustained a complete neurologic injury and 11 (50%) an incomplete neurologic injury. Of those with incomplete injury, six (55%) improved, and five (45%) were unchanged; no patient showed deterioration after manipulation. Three patients (14%) had normal neurologic findings on admission and remained normal after manipulation (Table 6-3).

In the patient population undergoing closed reduction, nine (41%) were thoracic fracture-dislocations, seven (32%) were thoracolumbar fracture-dislocations, and six (27%) were lumbar fracture-dislocations (Table 6-2). Nineteen (86%) were successfully treated by reduction (Figs. 6-1, 6-2, 6-4 to 6-7, and 6-9), and three (14%) could not be reduced either because of locked facets (Fig. 6-8), bone impingement (Fig. 6-11), or extensive dislocation and fracture posteriorly, not amenable to closed manipulation, or did not have any residual stability (Fig. 6-10).

Radiologic analysis of the 22 fracture-dislocations revealed four major injury types: (1) flexion-rotation vertebral body fractures: three (14%); (2) wedge-compression vertebral body fractures: 15 (68%); (3) vertebral body bursting fracture: one (4%); and (4) pure ligamentous disruption with facet dislocation: three (14%) (Table 6-1).

Of 349 fractures of the thoracic, thoracolumbar, and lumbar spines, 109 (31%) required spinal stabilization. Within this group were 22 (6%) fracture-dislocations of the thoracic and lumbar vertebral column, which underwent closed manipulation and reduction of spinal injuries resulting from severe flexion–rotation–axial load or translatory horizontal shear injuries to the vertebral column. Of this group, 8 sustained complete neurologic injuries at the time of the injury (7 thoracic and 1 thoracolumbar), 11 had incomplete injuries (seven mixed conus medullaris–cauda equina lesions and four cauda equina lesions), and three had a normal neurologic sta-

Table 6-3. Clinical conditions of 22 patients treated by closed reduction

Before reduction	No.	%
Normal neurologic status	3	14
Neurologically complete	8	36
Neurologically incomplete*	11	50

*After reduction, six (55%) improved, five (45%) were unchanged, and none deteriorated.

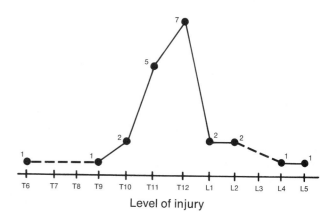

Fig. 6-13. Graphic presentation of level of fracture-dislocations in 22 patients treated by closed reductions.

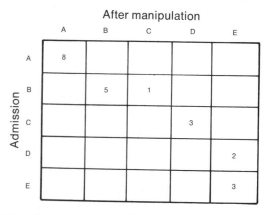

Fig. 6-14. Neurologic status of 22 patients before and after closed reduction. *A,* Complete absence of motor and sensory function; *B,* sensory function intact with absent motor function; *C,* sensory function intact with no useful motor function; *D,* sensory function intact with useful motor function; *E,* normal neurologic function. Neurologic classification according to Frankel and co-workers.[13]

tus resulting from injuries at the L1-2 and L2-3 vertebral levels.

Twenty-two fracture-dislocations of the thoracic and lumbar vertebral column were analyzed. The integrity of the anterior longitudinal ligament (Figs. 6-1, 6-5, 6-10) was not thought to play a vital role in bringing about a successful reduction, although its contribution cannot be disputed. Where facet fractures accompanied posterior element fractures and ligamentous disruption, with vertebral column malalignment, closed reduction was found to be relatively simple, quick, and successful. The opposite was noted when facets were found to be intact and dislocated. Closed manipulation was uniformly unsuccessful on these, as was the case of significant vertebral column displacement at the T6-7 level, accompanied by significant posterior element fracture and displacement (Fig. 6-10). Three spines initially thought to be adequately reduced were redisplaced within 3 weeks of reduction. Following manipulation and reduction all 22 fracture-dislocation spines underwent a posterior spinal instrumentation, fusion procedure at 2 or 3 weeks. One patient died from a pulmonary embolus while in physical therapy 2 weeks postoperatively and 5 weeks after multiple injury.

REFERENCES

1. Adamkiewicz, A.: Die Blutgefässe des Menschlichen Rückenmarkes Tiel, Die Gafässe der Ruckenmarkoberflache, S. B. Heidelberg, Akad. Wiss. **85**:101, 1882.
2. Bohler, L.: The treatment of fractures, Bristol, England, 1935, John Wright and Sons.
3. Boyd, D. R., and Flashner, B. A.: The critically injured patient concept and the Illinois statewide plan for trauma centers, Springfield, Ill., 1971, Department of Public Health Printers.
4. Bradford, D. S., Akbarnia, B. A., Winter, R. B., and Seljeskog, E. L.: Surgical stabilization of fractures and fracture dislocations of the thoracic spine, Spine **2**:185, 1977.
5. Comarr, A. E.: Laminectomy in patients with injuries to the spinal cord, J. Int. Coll. Surg. **31**:437-442, 1959.
6. Comarr, A. E., and Kaufman, A. A.: A survey of the neurological results of 858 cord injuries. A comparison of patients treated with or without laminectomy, J. Neurosurg. **13**:95-106, 1956.
7. Convery, F. R., Minteer, M. A., Smith, R. W., and Emerson, S. M.: Fracture dislocation of the dorsal-lumbar spine—acute operative stabilization by Harrington instrumentation, Spine **3**:160, 1978.
8. Covall, D. A., Clipper, I. S., Hoem, T. I., and Rusk, H. S.: Early management of patients with spinal cord injury, J.A.M.A. **151**:89, 1953.
9. Davis, A. G.: Tensile strength of the anterior longitudinal ligament in relation to treatment of 132 crush fractures of the spine, J. Bone Joint Surg. **20**:429, 1938.
10. Dick, T. B. S.: Traumatic paraplegia pre-Guttman, Paraplegia **7**:173-177, 1969.
11. Dickson, J. H., Harrington, P. R., and Erwin, W. D.: Results of reduction and stabilization of the severely fractured thoracic and lumbar spine, J. Bone Joint Surg. [Am.] **60**(6):799, 1978.
12. Flesch, J. R., Leider, L. L., Erickson, D. L., et al.: Harrington instrumentation and spine fusion for unstable fractures and fracture-dislocation of the thoracic and lumbar spine, J. Bone and Joint Surg. [Am.] **59**:143, 1977.
13. Frankel, H. L., Hancock, D. O., Hyslop, G., et al.: The value of postural reduction in the initial management of closed injuries of the spine with paraplegia and tetraplegia, Paraplegia **7**:179, 1969.
14. Guttman, L. J.: The management of the paraplegic patient, Practitioner **176**:157, 1956.
15. Guttmann, L. J.: Spinal deformities in traumatic paraplegics and tetraplegics following surgical procedures, Paraplegia **7**:38, 1969.
16. Holdsworth, F. W., and Hardy, A. G.: Early treatment of paraplegia from fracture of the thoracolumbar spine, J. Bone Joint Surg. [Br.] **35**:540, 1953.
17. Kaufer, H., and Hayes, J. T.: Lumbar fracture-dislocation. A study of twenty-one cases, J. Bone Joint Surg. [Am.] **48**:712, 1966.
18. Lazorthes, G., Gouaze, A., Zadek, J. D., et al.: Arterial vascularization of the spinal cord, J. Neurosurg. **35**:253, 1971.
19. Leidholt, J. D., Young, J. J., Hahn, H. R. E., et al.: Evaluation of late spinal deformities with fracture-dislocations of the dorsal and lumbar spine in paraplegics, Paraplegia **7**:16, 1969.
20. Meyer, P. R.: Complications of treatment of fractures and dislocations of the dorsolumbar spine. In Epps, C. H., Jr., editor: Complications in orthopaedic surgery, vol. 2, Philadelphia, 1978, J. B. Lippincott Co., pp. 643-715.
21. Meyer, P. R., and Dobozi, W.: Fracture-dislocation of the dorsolumbar spine. Hampartzoum Kelikian Symposium, Northwestern University, Chicago, Dec. 1975.
22. Meyer, P. R., Rosen, J. S., and Hamilton, B. B.: Midwest Regional Spinal Cord Injury Care System. RSA-OHD-HEW grant no. 13P-55864/5-03. Progress Reports II, III, IV, Chicago, 1973, 1974, 1975, Northwestern University.
23. Munro, D.: Thoracic and lumbosacral cord injuries, J.A.M.A. **122**:1055, 1943.
24. Rogers, L. F., Thayer, C., Weinberg, P. E., and Kim, K. S.: Acute injuries of the upper thoracic spine associated with paraplegia, Am. J. Roentgenol. **134**:67, 1980.
25. Rogers, W. A.: Cord injury during reduction of thoracic and lumbar vertebral body fracture and dislocation, J. Bone Joint Surg. **20**:689, 1938.
26. Stanger, J. K.: Fracture-dislocation of the thoracic lumbar spine with special reference to reduction by open and closed operation, J. Bone Joint Surg. **29**:107, 1947.
27. Watson-Jones, R.: The treatment of fractures and fracture-dislocations of the spine, J. Bone Joint Surg. **16**:30, 1934.
28. Whitesides, T. E., and Alishah, S. G.: On the management of unstable fractures of the thoracolumbar spine: rationale for use of anterior decompression and fusion and posterior stabilization, Spine **1**:99, 1976.

CHAPTER 7

Surgical stabilization of spinal cord injury

SECTION A. Cervical spine

LEONARD J. CERULLO, M.D.

SECTION B. Thoracic and lumbar spine

PAUL R. MEYER, Jr., M.D.

SECTION A. Cervical spine

INDICATIONS FOR FUSION

Nonphysiologic motion, the result of injury to cervical vertebrae and their associated ligaments, subjects the local nerve roots and the cervical spinal cord segments to the risk of further deterioration by physical trauma and vascular compromise. The risks are a function of both range of abnormal motion and the degree of stress required to produce abnormal movement. The very stable and very unstable injuries present no judgmental problem. The "middle ground" stability injuries are surrounded by controversy concerning the desirability, or lack thereof, of surgical fusion to pave the way for a more rapid and certain attainment of the same fusion as nature will achieve gradually.[4] Early fusion allows early mobilization and rehabilitation, hopefully preventing the physical and psychologic morbidity associated with prolonged immobilization in skeletal traction.[8] On the other hand, the medical risks of general anesthesia and the neurologic risks of intubation, manipulation, surgical trauma, and hypotension must be weighed against these potential benefits. Occasionally a seemingly stable injury will reveal its true nature when an external appliance is applied (Figs. 7-1 and 7-

2) or when a radiograph is taken prior to rehabilitation (Fig. 7-3). Early posterior or anterior decompressive surgery, advocated in certain centers, may transform an otherwise stable injury into a precarious one.

Following the decision to surgically stabilize the cervical spine, the choice of approach must be considered. The options include anterior, posterior, and combination approaches.[2] The indications and relative advantages of each approach will be considered.

Regardless of the route of operation, preoperative radiologic evaluation includes multidirectional tomography of the entire segment of spine to be dealt with and plain radiography of the entire spine to rule out unsuspected noncontiguous fractures. Myelography is indicated when the neurologic damage outweighs the bony disruption, when the neurologic condition is deteriorating, and prior to surgery on all incomplete spinal cord lesions (Fig. 7-4).

The operation is performed in a position of maximal stability, that is, in skeletal traction on a stable operating table (in our institution, with the Stryker frame). Intraoperative monitoring of fluid and electrolytes requires an indwelling urinary bladder catheter, continuous measurement of arterial blood pressure, and in certain instances, the ability to monitor spinal cord function by somatosensory evoked response. Adequate respiratory control is ensured by endotracheal intubation or tracheostomy. The intubation of the cervical spine injured patient is performed with the patient awake, although sedated, in order to assure minimal mobilization of the injured spine and to detect any change of neurologic function that may result from the procedure. Pharmacologic protection against further cord injury by physical manipulation is unproven, although steroids and barbiturates may be effective in this regard. Hypotension, deliberate or untoward, is to be avoided. The choices of bone graft, donor site, and surgical approach are determined by the mechanism of injury, the area of instability, associated injuries, concomitant complications of spinal cord injury (e.g., deep venous thrombosis, pressure sores), and preference of the surgeon.

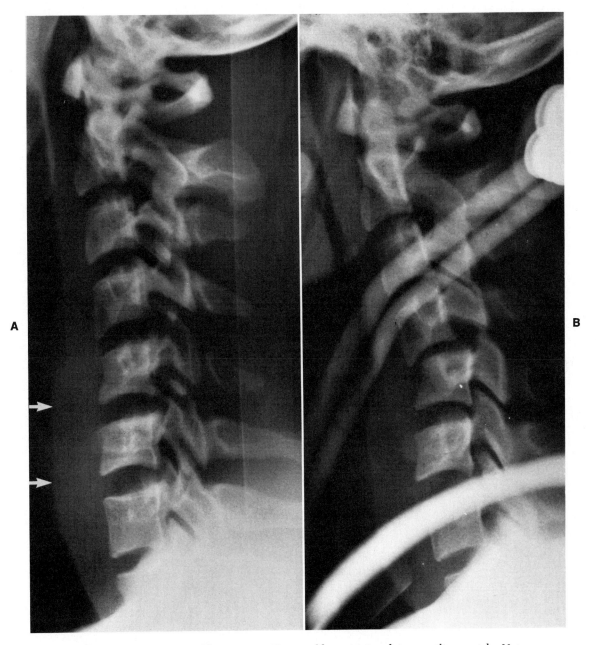

Fig. 7-1. A, Seemingly stable spine in 20-year-old man injured in wrestling match. Note, however, prevertebral soft tissue swelling *(arrows)*. **B,** Instability at level of C4-5 is revealed when patient was mobilized in SOMI orthosis.

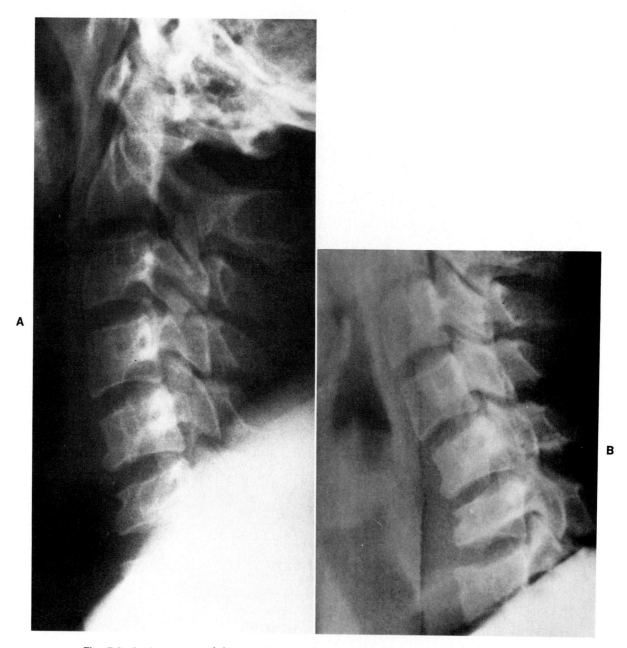

Fig. 7-2. A, Apparent stability in 23-year-old man injured in automobile accident with compression fractures of C5 and C6. **B,** Instability became manifest when patient was elevated in supportive collar.

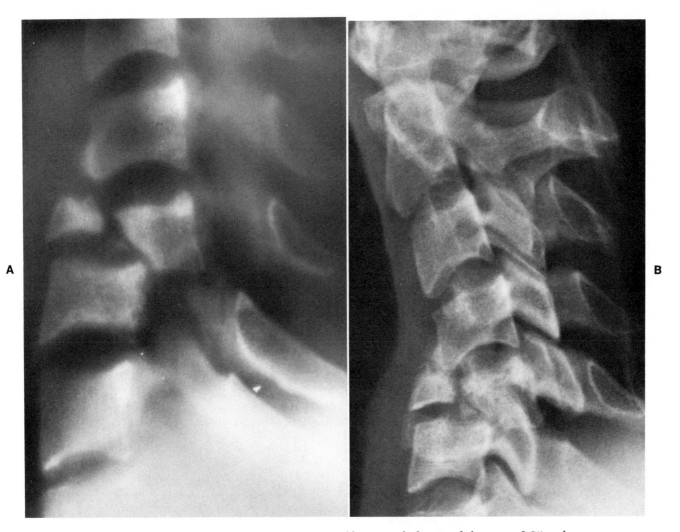

Fig. 7-3. A, Lateral polytomogram of 24-year-old man with fracture-dislocation of C5 and 50% reduction of spinal canal. **B,** Radiograph after 6 weeks of treatment with halo device and 6 weeks of supportive collar shows cervical spine fixed in kyphosis.

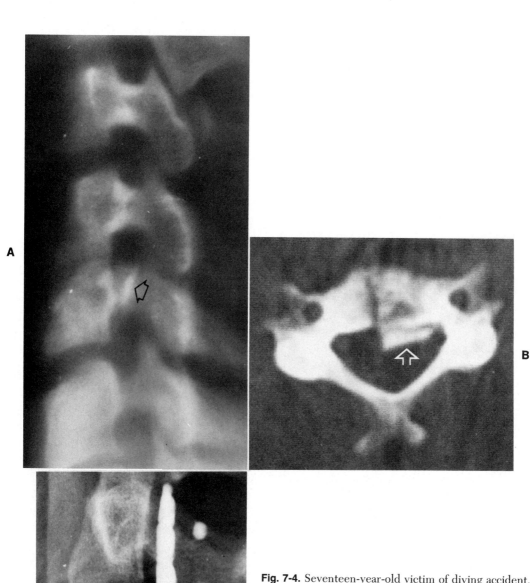

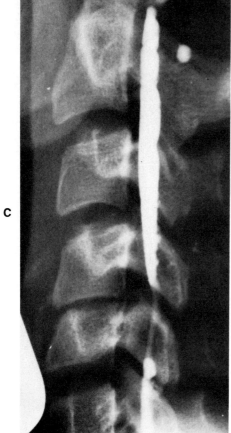

Fig. 7-4. Seventeen-year-old victim of diving accident. **A,** Lateral polytomogram and, **B,** CT scan show bony fragment in spinal canal at level of C5 *(arrows)* and narrowing of C4-5. **C,** In addition, myelogram shows posterior displacement of cord by fragment, extruded disc, and hematoma. These findings dictate anterior cervical approach.

CERVICAL FUSION: ANTERIOR APPROACH

The anterior route to cervical spine exposure offers the surgeon a direct and rapid access to the vertebral body and intervertebral disc with minimal need for muscle and soft tissue dissection and negligible postoperative patient discomfort. The presence of nearby infection, such as that threatened by tracheostomy, is a relative contraindication to the approach. Surgical complications include damage to the great vessels, perforation of the esophagus, vocal cord paralysis from damage to the recurrent laryngeal nerve, and postoperative respiratory embarrassment secondary to a wound hematoma with tracheal compression. The choice of the type of anterior fusion depends on the pathology. Simple removal of the intervertebral disc and maintenance of the intervertebral space by an iliac graft are the essence of the *Smith-Robinson procedure* (Fig. 7-5).[6,10] The *Cloward procedure*[3] offers the opportunity to decompress both the intervertebral disc and large portions of vertebral body with replacement of both by a bone dowel,

either autogenous or heterogenous (Fig. 7-6). The strut graft, obtained from cortical iliac bone or tibia, allows replacement of the entire vertebral body with fusion to the bodies above and below (Fig. 7-7).

The anterior approach is seldom necessary for lesions of the upper cervical spine where the attraction of ease of exposure is lost by the need for a transoral or transmandibular approach. Occasionally a severely dislocated odontoid process compressing the upper cervical cord or lower medulla must be removed by this route, but actual stabilization procedures are rare. Intraoperative radiologic control is necessary to verify the anatomic level since the more limited view and/or similar anatomy makes the anterior approach less obvious than the posterior from a localization point of view. Discography and discoresistance can be determined at the same time. Postoperatively, radiologic control is used to verify proper neck position in an orthosis and to confirm the proper depth of bone plug localization (Fig. 7-8). When using less radiopaque dowel materal (Kiel

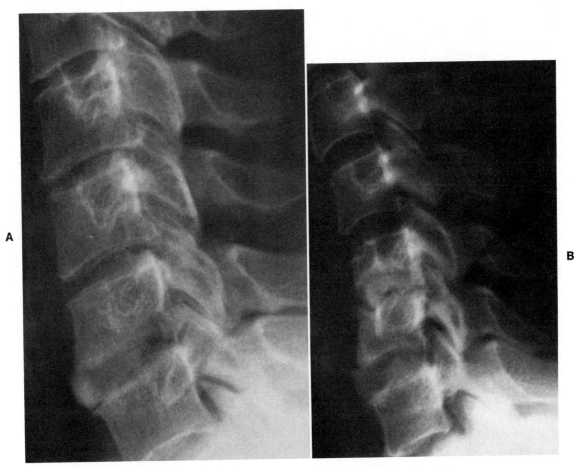

A

B

Fig. 7-5. Intervertebral disc space is maintained after removal of disc and insertion of slice of iliac crest: *Smith-Robinson procedure*. **A,** One disc space. **B,** Two disc spaces in another patient.

bone graft*), an adherent radiopaque marker, such as tantalum in bone wax on the "leading edge" of the dowel, is useful (Figs. 7-6 and 7-9). This is seldom necessary when cortical bone is utilized. After an appropriate period of time, ranging from 8 to 12 weeks, tomography of the cervical spine is repeated to demonstrate bone fusion. It may be helpful at this time to also obtain flexion-extension radiographs to confirm stability.

---

*Kiel Surgibone is the registered trade name for a specially cleaned cancellous bovine bone.

The use of anterior cervical fusion by any of the previously described techniques or modifications of them[11] presumes posterior stability. If the latter is lacking or has not been previously verified, and the patient is mobilized, slippage of the bone plug with resultant kyphosis and potential aggravation of cord injury can result (Fig. 7-10). When the indications for anterior fusion or decompression are obvious, as in posterior subluxation of the vertebral body or fragments thereof, instability does not contraindicate the procedure but must be dealt with. In order to ensure the permanence of bone graft placement, a posterior spinous wiring can be performed (Figs. 7-11 and 7-12).

Text continued on p. 214.

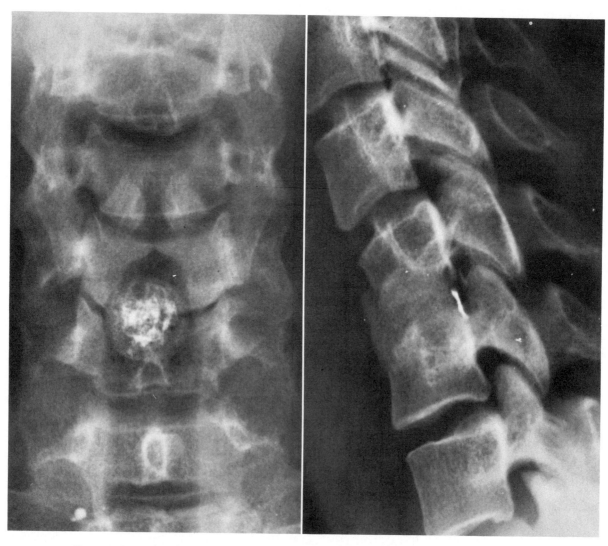

Fig. 7-6. Bone dowel at C5-6 after *Cloward procedure* in 46-year-old woman injured in automobile accident. Note opaque tantalum powder marking Kiel bone.

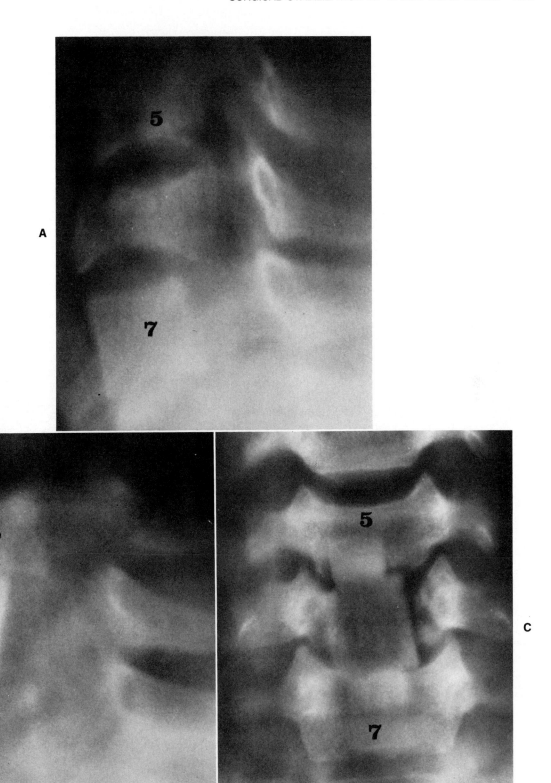

Fig. 7-7. A, Twenty-year-old man injured in diving accident with fracture of C6 and 20% narrowing of spinal canal. **B** and **C,** Sixth vertebra was removed and replaced by tibial strut, which is notched into C5 and C7.

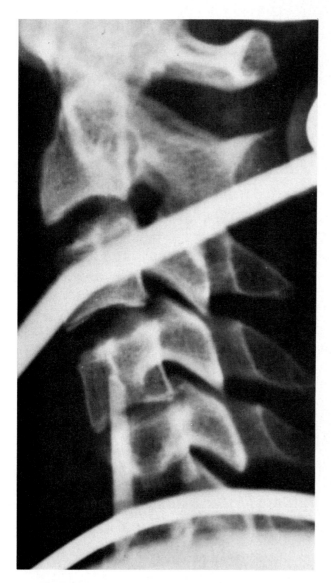

Fig. 7-8. Kyphosis of cervical spine after anterior fusion in 15-year-old diving accident victim with fracture-dislocation of C5 and 20% narrowing of spinal canal. Kyphosis resulted from posterior instability.

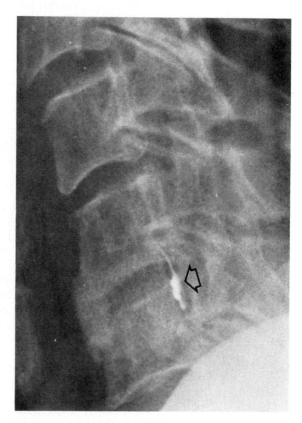

Fig. 7-9. Opaque tantalum powder (*arrow*) defines posterior limit of Kiel bone graft after *Cloward procedure*.

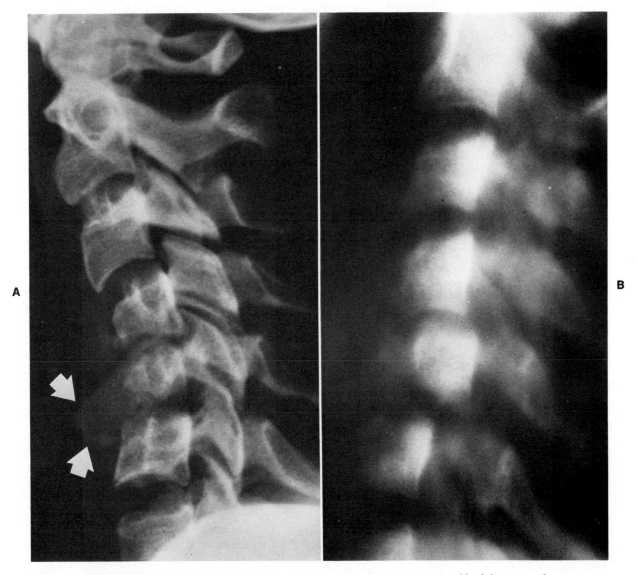

Fig. 7-10. A, Slipped bone plug *(arrows)* from anterior fusion in 17-year-old adolescent with fracture of C5. **B,** Posterior instability became obvious during follow-up polytomography when neck was extended.

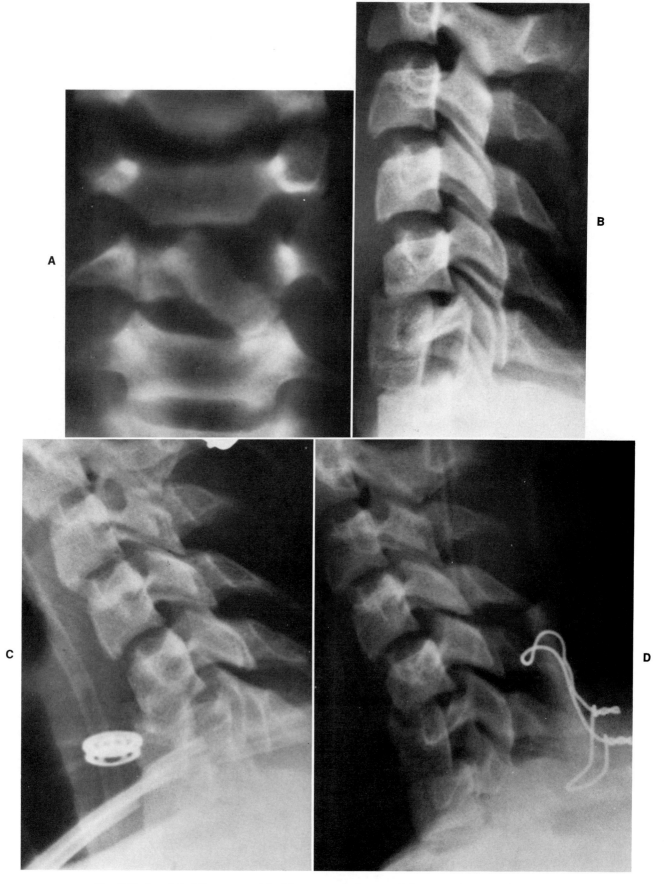

Fig. 7-11. A and **B,** Fifteen-year-old adolescent with fracture-dislocation of C5-6 and anterior fusion. **C,** Posterior instability allowed progressive kyphosis. **D,** Posterior fusion and wiring reduced deformity and prevented further angulation.

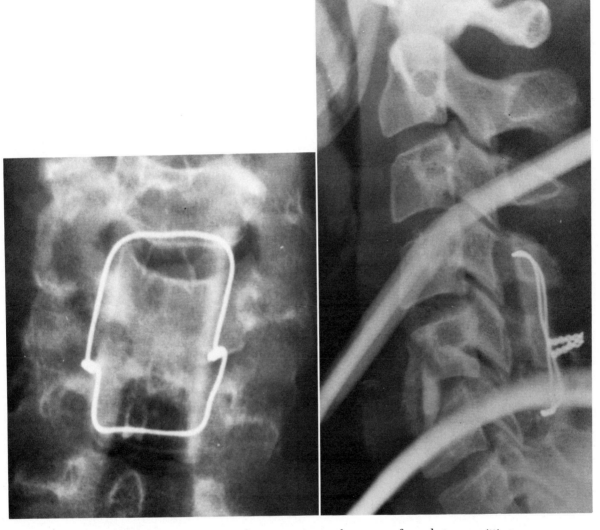

Fig. 7-12. Ideally both anterior and posterior approaches are performed at same sitting, as seen in this 32-year-old man with extension-rotation injury at C5-6.

CERVICAL FUSION: POSTERIOR APPROACH

Fractures of the upper cervical spine are generally best treated with external fixation devices (Minerva cast, halo jacket), reserving surgery for those cases in which fusion fails to occur (Fig. 7-13). Surgical stabilization using the posterior route is also indicated for congenital nonfusion of the odontoid process (os odontoideum) (Fig. 7-14) and for C1-2 instability secondary to rheumatoid arthritis.[9] Both conditions frequently become manifest after head and neck injury. *McLaurin technique*[5] consists of wire fixation of the arch of C1 to the spinous process of C2 with lateral onlay bone taken from either iliac crest or tibia (Fig. 7-15). If the free-lying odontoid process produces symptoms of medullary compression, it can be removed through a transoral (anterior) surgical approach. It is imperative to determine preoperatively the dynamic interaction between atlas and the base of the skull on the one hand and atlas and axis on the other hand prior to deciding in favor of surgical intervention. This is best accomplished through fluoroscopy or cinefluoroscopy rather than flexion-extension radiographs, which really demonstrate only the end positions and not the contortions arrived at to achieve the final resting place. Postoperative radiologic examinations are necessary to verify solid fusion without motion (Fig. 7-16). When the posterior arch of C1 has failed to fuse or is hypoplastic, surgical fusion must be carried to the posterior rim of the foramen magnum or occipital squama.

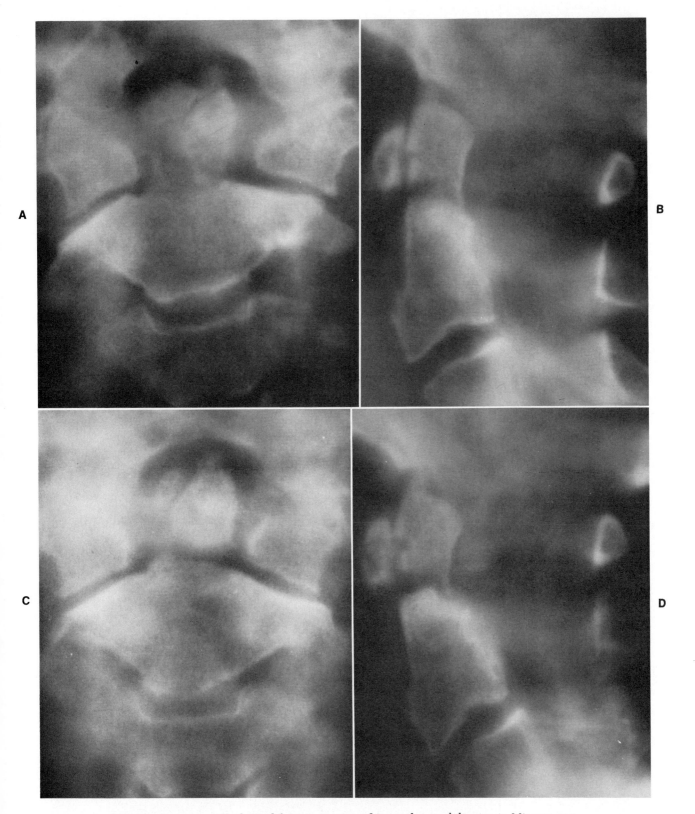

Fig. 7-13. Nonunion of odontoid fracture in spite of 3-month immobilization in Minerva cast in 56-year-old man who fell onto Chicago "L" train tracks. **A** and **B,** October 1977. **C** and **D,** August 1978.

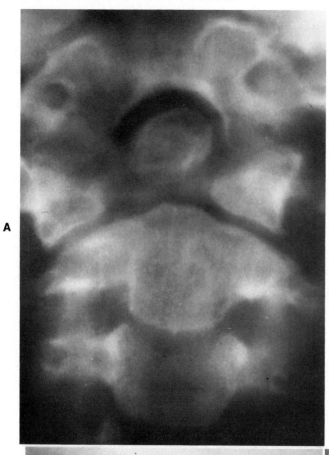

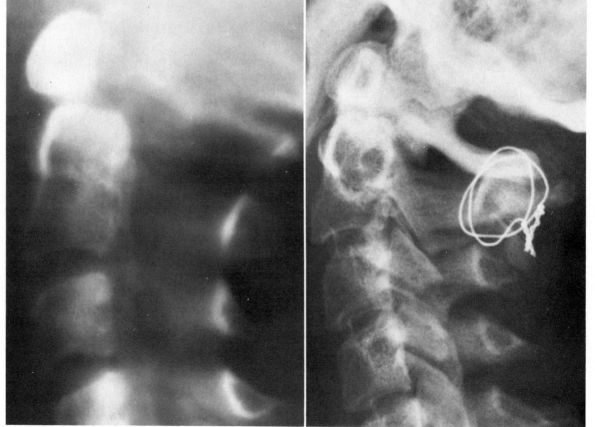

Fig. 7-14. A and **B,** Os odontoideum in 27-year-old woman with multiple skeletal fractures from automobile accident. **C,** Asymptomatic os odontoideum became symptomatic after accident and required posterior fusion.

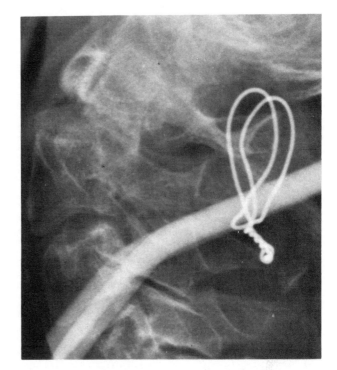

Fig. 7-15. *McLaurin procedure* in 51-year-old man injured in automobile accident.

Fig. 7-16. Flexion-extension lateral radiographs after posterior fusion of C1-2 in 46-year-old man with old odontoid fracture show persistent instability. **A,** Flexion view shows good position of odontoid process but separation of spinous processes *(arrow)* despite wiring. **B,** Extension view shows approximation of spinous processes and posterior displacement of odontoid process.

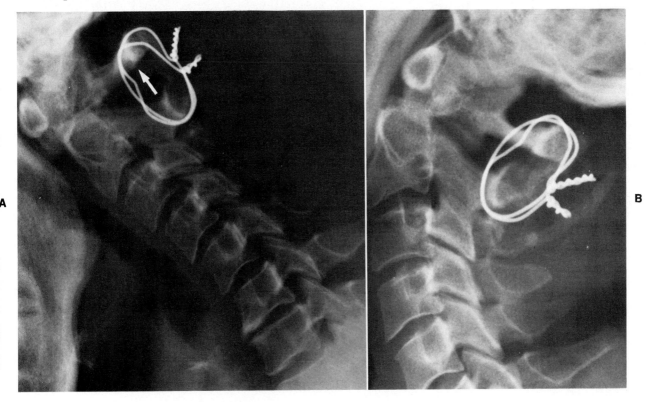

Fracture-dislocations involving the cervical spine below C3 are generally amenable to reduction by skeletal traction with gradually increasing force. Extreme caution should be taken, however, to avoid overdistraction at the site of injury (Fig. 7-17). In the early hours following the injury, while reduction is being attempted, frequent cervical spine radiographs must be obtained and compared. Should unilateral or bilateral facet reduction be impossible by noninvasive means, surgical reduction can be accomplished at the time of elective fusion (Fig. 7-18). If the degree of malalignment is se-

vere enough to constrict the spinal canal sufficiently to produce further neurologic deterioration, anatomic realignment becomes a surgical emergency (Fig. 7-19). When surgery is performed early, the reduction is generally a simple one and the reduced elements are maintained in position by wire and bone fusion. A later operation because of fibrous and neo-osseous buildup occasionally requires the surgical removal of the tip of the superior facet in order to enable the remaining joint components to be snapped into place. Here, too, reduction is maintained by wire and bone fusion.

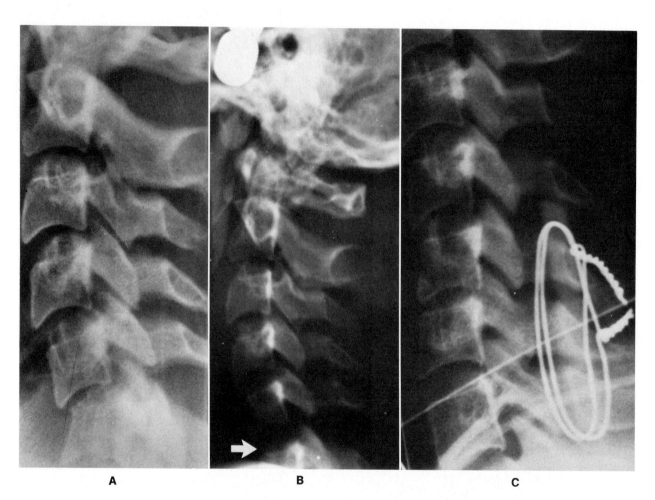

Fig. 7-17. A, Nineteen-year-old woman with fracture-dislocation of C5-6. **B,** Overdistraction *(arrow)* is seen when patient is placed in tongs, which dictated early fusion to avoid damage to vertebral arteries, **C.**

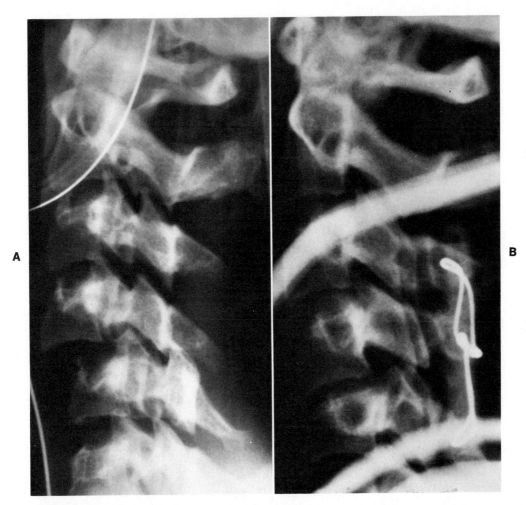

Fig. 7-18. Bilateral locked facets of C4-5 and significant canal narrowing, **A,** required emergency surgical reduction and stabilization, **B.**

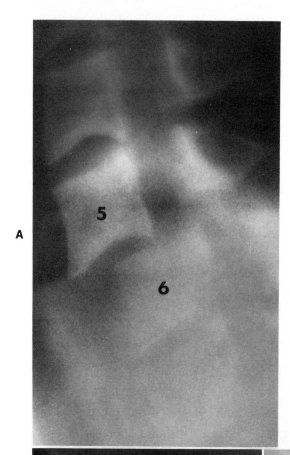

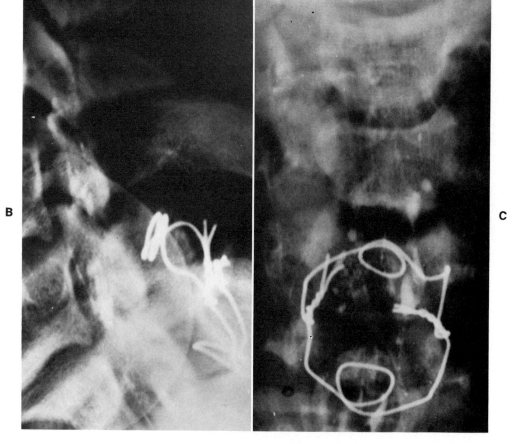

Fig. 7-19. A, Fracture-dislocation of C5-6 in 22-year-old man with locking facets and compromised spinal canal. **B** and **C,** Immediate surgical stabilization resulted in satisfactory alignment.

The techniques for posterior cervical fusion are numerous, but all basically depend on stabilization between intact laminae. Disrupted laminar arches are sandwiched between intact processes, and a bridge is fashioned over the fractured elements. *Sublaminar fusion*, a term that refers to the location of the stabilizing metallic elements rather than the actual bony bridge, requires passage of stainless steel wire either under a single lamina, *Alexander technique*,[1] or under a series of adjacent laminae, *Meyer technique* (Fig. 7-20). The supporting structure thus created holds into place and stabilizes the bone "bridge" of tibia or iliac crest. The *Rogers' fusion*[7] (Fig. 7-21) avoids entering the epidural space by fixing the wires at the base of the spinous processes above and below, then bridging the gap with bone graft taken from tibia or iliac crest (Fig. 7-22). The "*Yale*" *fusion* joins the facets at each level and is useful when previous laminectomy has eliminated the possibility for laminar or spinous process fixation. The radiologic picture of the various types of fusion should be straightforward. Certainly the sublaminar fusion is the most stable. However, overapproximation may result in a loss of a "level" by foraminal encroachment on the nerve root, and the bowing of the sublaminar wires may narrow the spinal canal to the degree that myelopathy results.

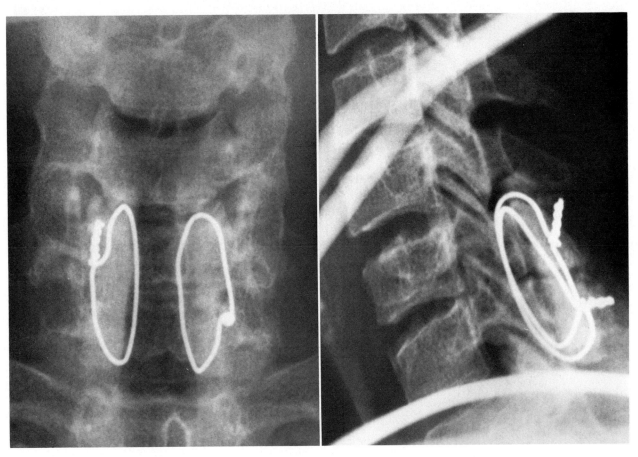

Fig. 7-20. *Sublaminar fusion* in 31-year-old man with fracture-dislocation of C6-7 and unilateral locked facets.

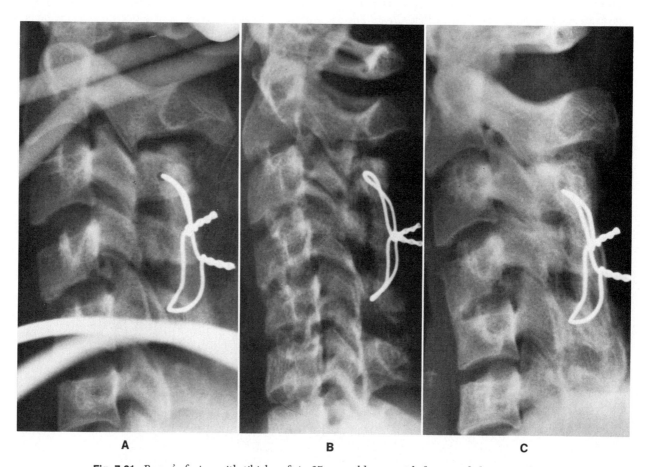

A   B   C

Fig. 7-21. *Roger's fusion* with tibial graft in 25-year-old man with fracture-dislocation of C4-5. Serial radiographs show progressive incorporation of graft. **A,** August 1978. **B,** October 1978. **C,** June 1979.

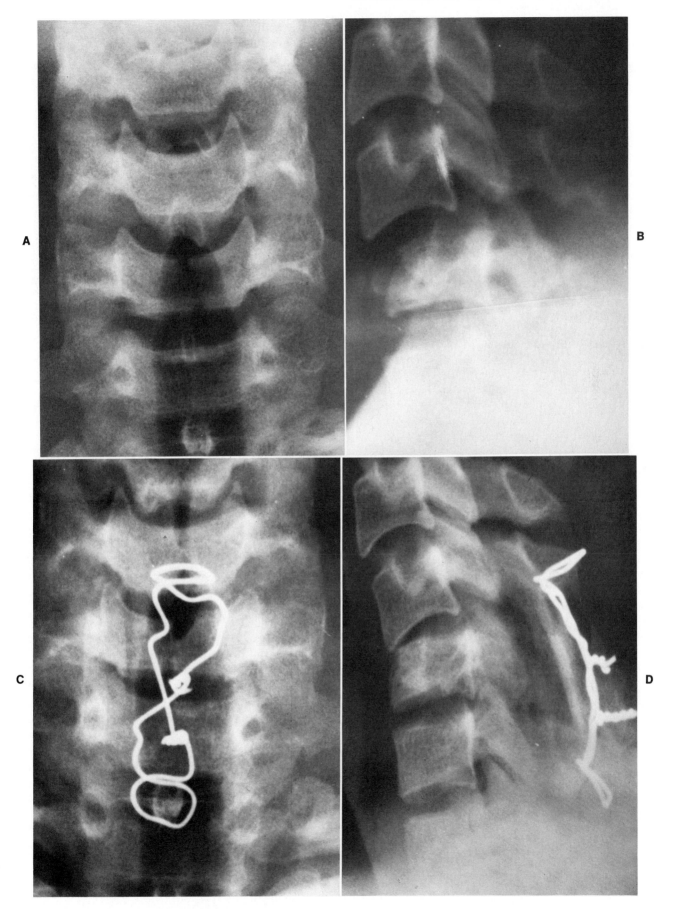

Fig. 7-22. A and **B,** Twenty-year-old man with fracture-dislocation of C5-6. **C** and **D,** Roger's fusion was achieved 3 months later.

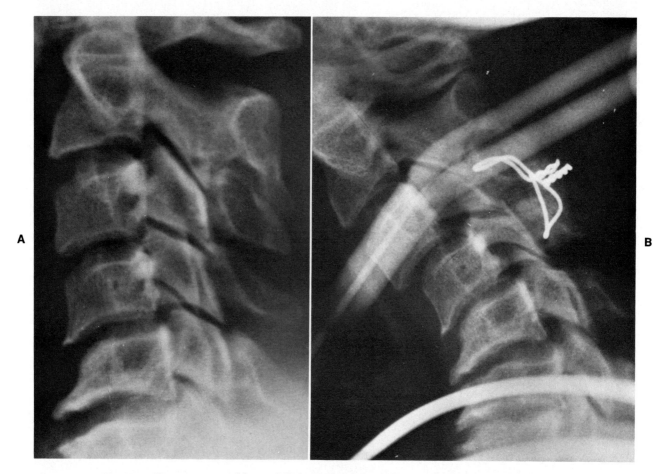

Fig. 7-23. Forty-two-year-old man fell down the stairs and showed fracture of right facet of C3 on tomography (not shown) but apparent stability on plain radiograph, **A. B,** Despite posterior fusion, there is continuous instability 3 months after surgery.

After surgical stabilization the patient is maintained in a device to reduce head and neck motion and thereby diminish the chance for pseudoarthrosis. Various appliances including the Minerva cast, halo jacket, SOMI brace, and a variety of cervical collars can be used. At a suitable period postoperatively tomography should demonstrate fusion, and following removal of the orthosis flexion-extension radiographs are obtained to verify stability (Fig. 7-23).

In order to prevent excessive immobility of the spine, long grafting procedures are to be avoided. Should the posterior elements of several contiguous spinal segments be involved, thus mitigating against a short (two to three segments) fusion, it is frequently desirable to wait for bony healing, anticipating that ligamentous disruption might not be overwhelming (Fig. 7-24). When, because of failure of ligamentous repair or overwhelming vertebral body collapse, the resultant

angulation is unacceptable, stabilization through surgery after bony healing can be attempted. If the medical condition of the patient precludes surgery for significant period of time, it is usually desirable to wait the remaining few weeks in order to ascertain the possibility of nonsurgical fusion prior to the more invasive route.

The objectives of open reduction and spinal fusion are to ensure physiologic alignment of the spine, to eliminate excessive motion and instability, and to avoid late development of kyphosis. These objectives may be achieved through closed or open techniques, the choice being dictated by the pathophysiology in the individual situation. Preoperative, intraoperative, and postoperative radiologic analysis of the static and dynamic situation is the sine qua non for rational choice of treatment.

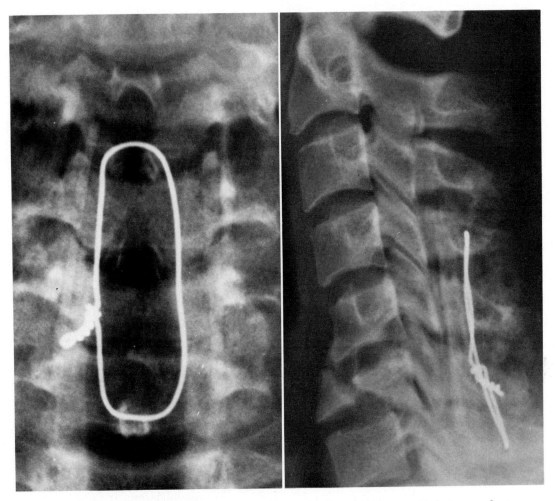

Fig. 7-24. Unusually long posterior fusion was required in this 25-year-old diving accident victim with fracture of C6 because of persistent instability after bony healing.

REFERENCES

1. Alexander, E., Davis, C. H., and Forsyth, H. F.: Reduction and fusion of fracture dislocation of the cervical spine, J. Neurosurg. 27:588-591, 1967.
2. Bick, E. M.: An essay on the history of spine fusion operations, Clin. Orthop. 35:9-15, 1964.
3. Cloward, R. B.: The anterior approach for removal of ruptured cervical disks, J. Neurosurg. 15:602, 1958.
4. De Quervain, F., and Hoessley, H.: Operative immobilization of the spine, Surg. Gynecol. Obstet. 24:428, 1917.
5. McLaurin, R. L., Veind, R., and Salmon, J. H.: Treatment of fractures of the atlas and axis by wiring without fusion, J. Neurosurg. 36:773-780, 1972.
6. Robinson, R. A., and Smith, G. W.: Anterolateral cervical disc removal and interbody fusion for cervical disc syndrome, Johns Hopkins Med. J. 96:233, 1955.
7. Rogers, W. A.: Fractures and dislocations of the cervical spine. An end result study, J. Bone Joint Surg. [Am.] 39:341-376, 1957.
8. Schurmann, K.: The importance for rehabilitation of the interbody fusion and stabilization operation in fracture/dislocation of the cervical spine, Scand. J. Rehab. Med. 4:114-122, 1972.
9. Sherk, H. H., and Snyder, B.: Posterior fusions of the upper cervical spine: indications, techniques, and prognosis, Orthop. Clin. North Am. 9:1091-1099, 1978.
10. Smith, G. W., and Robinson, R. A.: The treatment of certain cervical spine disorders by anterior removal of the intervertebral disc and interbody fusion, J. Bone Joint Surg. 40:607-623, 1958.
11. Stouffer, E. S., and Rhoades, M. E.: Surgical stabilization of the cervical spine after trauma, Arch. Surg. 111:652-657, 1976.

SECTION B. **Thoracic and lumbar spine**

Fractures of the thoracic and lumbar spine vary widely in type and site of injury. If one considers that there are 12 thoracic vertebrae and five lumbar vertebrae, it is of interest to note that a preponderance of fractures result at the thoracolumbar junction T12 (15.6%) (Fig. 7-25) and L1 (13.8%), with a second area of frequency at T10 (10.1%).[5] The reason for this relatively high occurrence at the thoracolumbar area is the presence of the greatest range of available spine motion (in flexion and extension) at the junction between levels of relative spine rigidity (thoracic chest cage and spine) and spine flexibility (lumbar spine). A second level of frequent injury to the thoracic spine occurs at T8 (7.3%) (Fig. 7-26). This higher thoracic spine injury site probably is in some way related to the normal anatomic presence of upper thoracic spine kyphosis. This, coupled with the forced application of an excessive axial load, results in a variety of upper thoracic vertebral fractures. The type of fracture will vary with the direction and magnitude of the force vectors applied. As an example, the application of acute flexion and axial load forces to the spine, with a rotational component (as is likely to occur with a victim upside down, with the head and neck flexed, and with an associated rotational component to the upper thoracic cage and shoulders) can result in an oblique, laterally displaced compression fracture of either or both vertebrae at the T4 or T5 level (Fig. 7-27). A second common variety is that of a pure dislocation between two vertebrae, in the presence of a sudden high velocity lateral translatory force (Fig. 7-26). The third most common site of injury to the thoracic or lumbar spine is L3. The more plausible rationale for injury to this area is the presence of either an erect or a normal lordotic lumbar spine, to which a sudden high axial load is applied, as in jumps or falls from great heights. The type of fracture of the vertebra that usually results is a blow-out or bursting fracture (see Fig. 6-1).

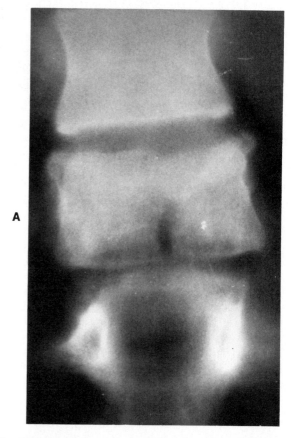

A

Fig. 7-25. **A,** Severe comminuted fracture-dislocation of vertebral body of T12 with fracture of pedicle and posterior extrusion into neurocanal *(arrow* in **B**). This resulted in partial obstruction to flow of contrast medium on myelogram, **C.** Neurologic injury: incomplete.

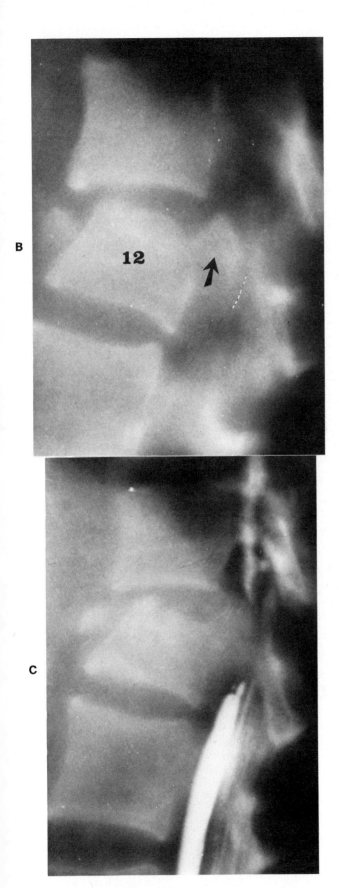

Fig. 7-25, cont'd. For legend see opposite page.

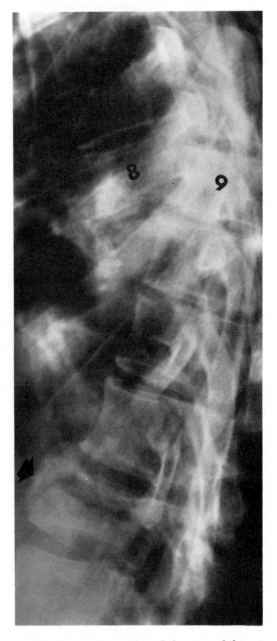

Fig. 7-26. Fracture and complete dislocation of thoracic vertebra T8 on T9 with disruption of posterior elements of T8 in 48-year-old man. Injury was secondary to fall and landing on object. Note secondary-level fracture of L1 *(arrow)*. Neurologic injury: complete. (See also Fig. 7-30.)

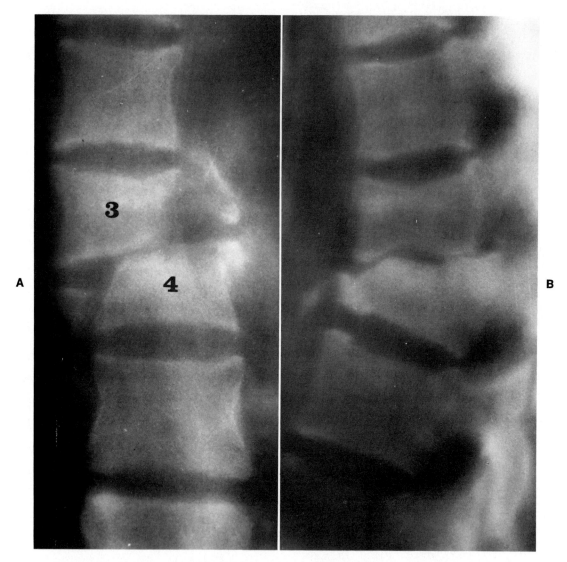

Fig. 7-27. Anteroposterior and lateral polytomograms of axial load, flexion, and rotation injury to upper thoracic spine (T3 and T4) in 27-year-old paraplegic injured in motorcycle accident. Note oblique fracture of T3 with associated lateral displacement, **A,** forward displacement, **B,** and invagination of T3 into T4. Neurologic injury: complete.

FORCE VECTORS AND FRACTURE CLASSIFICATION

Injuries to the thoracic and lumbar spine are the result of five basic directional loads:

1. Axial
2. Flexion
3. Extension
4. Rotation
5. Translatory

The resultant direction or composite effect, therefore, cannot be predicted with regularity, although certain types of vertebral injury occur more often than others. Thus the type of vertebral fracture will often indicate the direction of the inflicting force and to some extent its magnitude.

Review of 349 injuries to the thoracic and lumbar spine revealed the presence of six basic fracture- and dislocation-type injuries (Table 7-1).[6] Each is the result of one or more of the five above directional forces. The fracture types are:

1. Wedge-compression fracture
2. Vertebral bursting fracture
3. Posterior-anterior (Chance) shear fracture
4. Bilateral posterior element vertebral body fracture
5. Unilateral posterior element vertebral body fracture
6. Bilateral facet dislocation with or without minor vertebral body fracture

The three primary fracture-dislocation-subluxation types of the thoracic and lumbar spine[3,7] described in Chapter 6 basically become a combination of one or more of the six above individual fracture-dislocation types.

It should be stressed that injuries to the thoracic and lumbar spine, particularly in the presence of translatory or lateral shear of one vertebra on another, with or without

Table 7-1. Directional forces and vertebral column injuries

Force (load)	Vertebral fracture
Axial	Bursting fracture
Axial/flexion	Wedge-compression fracture
Flexion	Posterior distraction, anterior wedge-compression fracture
Axial/flexion/rotation	Compression/oblique/lateral displacement fracture
Extension	Posterior element fracture, anterior distraction
Translatory	Posterior-anterior shear (Chance) fracture or facet, vertebral body dislocation

fracture of either the anterior or posterior bone elements, ligamentous disruption of the interspinous, interlaminar (ligamenta flava) or posterior and anterior longitudinal ligaments, can and often do result (Fig. 7-26). When this occurs, instability is to be anticipated. Of 349 fractures of the thoracic and lumbar spine identified, 109 underwent spine stabilization. Of those undergoing stabilization, 22 were dislocated at the time of initial evaluation and could be reduced by closed manipulation (Chapter 6). In the presence of vertebral element dislocation, where neither anterior nor posterior bone fracture occurs, instability should be anticipated and is likely to result in abnormal vertebral column motion. In our experience, as well as that of others, these injuries frequently require spine stabilization.[1,2]

SURGICAL RATIONALE

Operative intervention and stabilization as an emergency or immediate management alternative are rarely required except when there is evidence of bone encroachment on neurologic tissue, in the presence of an incomplete neurologic injury. Whether operative intervention is early or late, the concern for appropriate neurologic decompression is always considered. As a rule, where the incompletely injured spinal cord or conus medullaris is compromised by bone or intervertebral disc material, the most appropriate approach for decompression is anteriorly. When dealing with encroachment of the cauda equina by bone or disc, however, most often the more appropriate approach will be posterior. This is not a hard and fast rule, although it should be recognized that the reason for "decompression" of viable spinal cord tissue is to reduce the vascular compromise on this very sensitive neurologic tissue. Because the major vascular supply to the spinal cord[4] lies along its anterior surface, only anterior decompression is likely to result in successful relief of this compromise. The greater abundance and lesser importance of the vascular supply to the cauda equina make up one explanation for the rationale that this peripheral nerve tissue is more resistant to trauma than the spinal cord. Certainly the type of nervous tissue (axon with neural sheath) contributes to this increased viability and resistance. Thus the posterior approach is the more appropriate. In addition, it has been frequently recognized that in the presence of fracture of the posterior elements, particularly when associated with displacement of one vertebral element on another, dural lacerations can be anticipated (Fig. 7-28). These are best repaired via the posterior approach. It should be appreciated that either a staged or combined anterior-posterior approach may be simultaneously required for the management of certain fracture-dislocations of the spine (Fig. 7-29).

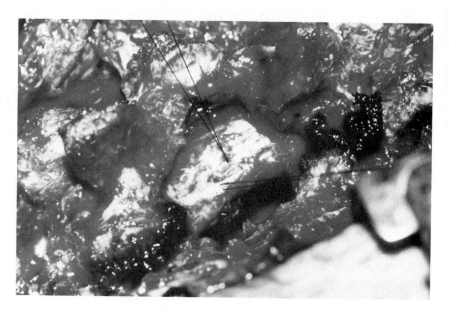

Fig. 7-28. Laceration of dura mater at thoracolumbar junction secondary to fracture of T12-L1 facets with vertebral dislocation. Anterior lateral approach with space anterior to dural area of vertebral body resection; inferior to laminectomy is transverse process, with lamina passing superiorly. Harrington distraction apparatus at bottom of illustration.

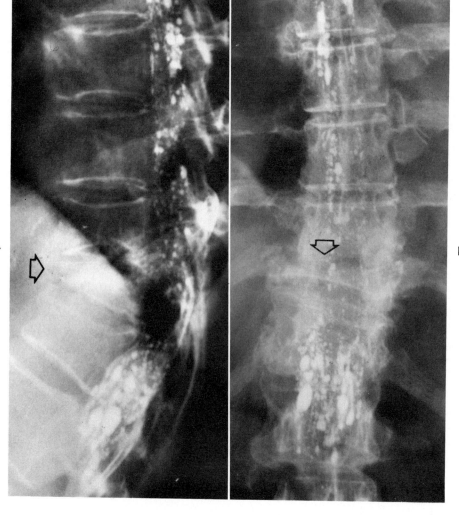

A

B

Fig. 7-29. For legend see opposite page.

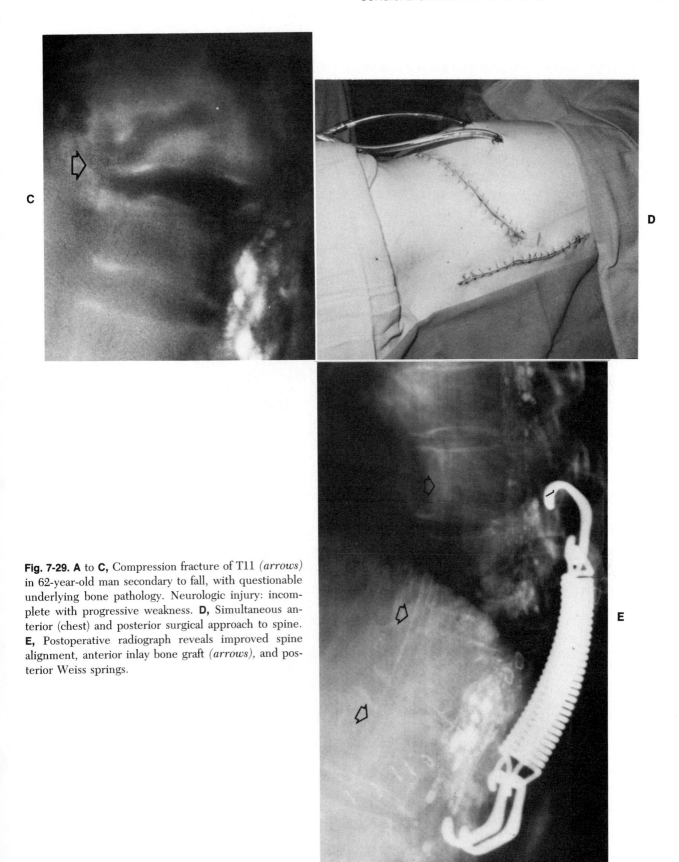

Fig. 7-29. A to **C,** Compression fracture of T11 *(arrows)* in 62-year-old man secondary to fall, with questionable underlying bone pathology. Neurologic injury: incomplete with progressive weakness. **D,** Simultaneous anterior (chest) and posterior surgical approach to spine. **E,** Postoperative radiograph reveals improved spine alignment, anterior inlay bone graft *(arrows),* and posterior Weiss springs.

COMBINED ANTERIOR-POSTERIOR SPINE APPROACH

On occasion, trauma to the vertebral column may be of such severity that total dislocation between two vertebral elements will occur (see Fig. 6-3). Usually this kind of injury results in gross spinal instability and malalignment, as well as a complete neurologic injury.

Early restoration of vertebral column realignment is required, either by manipulation (Chapter 6), postural positioning, or surgical reduction. Because of the rapid onset of scar formation, reduction must be accom-

plished within the first 2 weeks; otherwise, even with surgery, realignment of the vertebral column becomes difficult. Because of the difficulty of vertebral realignment, a very effective means of approaching such a fracture has been the use of the combined anterior (chest or retroperitoneal approach)–posterior (spinal) approach (Fig. 7-30). The selection of the most appropriate internal fixation device for this type of spinal injury varies among the Harrington compression rods, Harrington distraction rods, and the Weiss springs. The preferred selection has a great deal to do with the re-

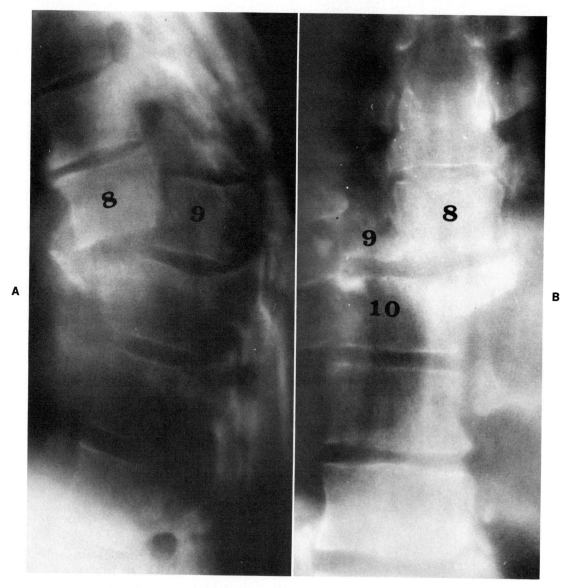

Fig. 7-30. Complete fracture-dislocation of T8-9 (same patient as in Fig. 7-26). **A** and **B,** Polytomograms show severity of injury.

maining inherent stability (rib cage) of the spine, as well as personal preference. Our experience using Weiss springs in such fractures has to date been successful in maintaining compression across the fracture reduction site, maintaining postoperative alignment, and allowing for early spinal healing ($2\frac{1}{2}$ to 3 months). Always during the postoperative period, a Knight-Taylor orthosis (Fig. 7-31) or body cast (Fig. 7-32) is utilized for external immobilization. The device is worn until the spine is deemed healed (minimum of 3 months).

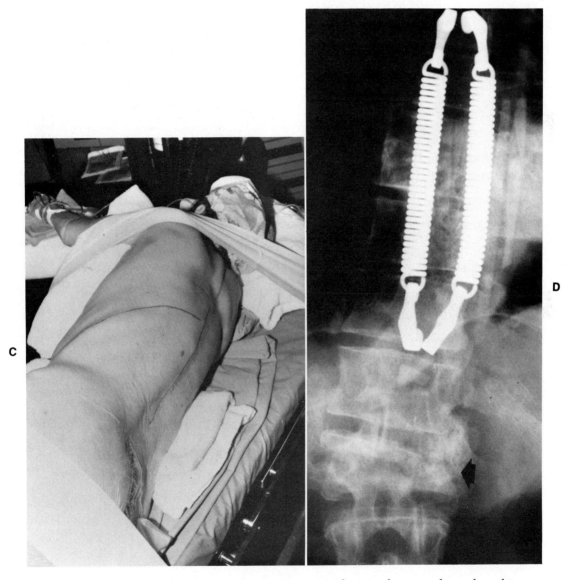

Fig. 7-30, cont'd. C, Simultaneous anteroposterior surgical approach was used to reduce this 3-week-old dislocation. **D,** Postreduction radiograph reveals improved spine alignment. Note second-level fracture at L1 *(arrow)*.

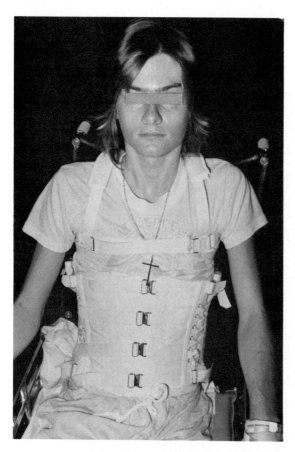

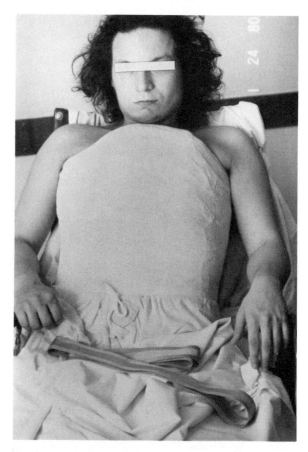

Fig. 7-31. *Knight-Taylor orthosis.* This type of orthosis is primarily indicated for external stabilization of fractures between T7 and L5. It is particularly helpful in providing abdominal and lumbar support in presence of high paraplegia.

Fig. 7-32. *Plaster of Paris body jacket.* This type of external immobilization is utilized when rigid stabilization of thoracolumbar junction is required. Care must be taken to pad iliac crest well if protective sensation is absent. This orthosis can be interchanged with laminated plastic thoracolumbar jacket, which is removable.

Table 7-2. Type of vertebral injury and stabilization procedures utilized

Injury	Stabilization procedures
Wedge-compression	Harrington distraction rods
	Harrington compression rods*
	Weiss springs*
Vertebral bursting fracture	Harrington distraction rods
Posterior-anterior translatory shear fracture	Harrington distraction rods
	Weiss springs
Bilateral facet/pedicle/vertebral body fracture	Harrington distraction rods
	Weiss springs*
Bilateral dislocated facets	Harrington distraction rods
	Combination Harrington distraction rod and Weiss spring
Unilateral facet/pedicle/ vertebral body fracture	Weiss spring
	Harrington compression rods

*Complete neurologic injury.

SELECTION OF INTERNAL FIXATION

Generally, recognition of (1) the type of mechanical force responsible for the spinal injury; (2) the type of fracture-dislocation-subluxation that has resulted; and (3) the status of the neurologic injury will indicate the most appropriate method of accomplishing operative spinal stability (Table 7-2). Depending on these requirements, the three most commonly utilized methods of obtaining spinal realignment, internal fixation, and stability are the following:

1. Harrington distraction rods (Fig. 7-33)
2. Harrington compression rods (Fig. 7-34)
3. Weiss compression springs (Fig. 7-35)

Occasionally, in the presence of unusual fractures or dislocations, the combined use of distraction using the Harrington rod and the Weiss compression devices may be indicated (Fig. 7-36). The Murig-Williams plate (Fig. 7-37) is no longer recommended for use as an internal fixation device because of the frequency of failure with this method due to the pulling away of the posterior spinous processes from the metal transfixing bolts and plate, with a resulting increase in spine deformity.

Text continued on p. 242.

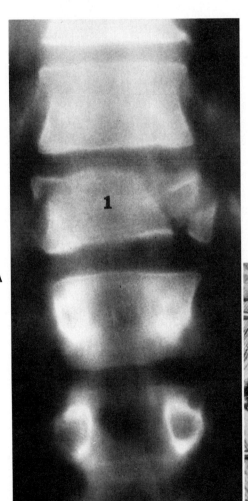

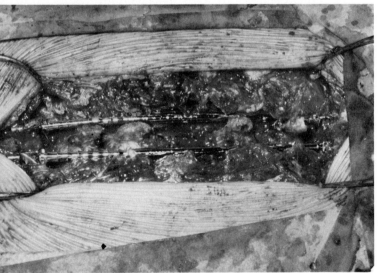

Fig. 7-33. *Harrington distraction rods.* Utilized to support vertebral column in fracture of L1 vertebral body and left pedicle, **A**. Open reduction and insertion of Harrington rods, **B**. Note hooks at proximal and distal ends attached to laminae. Spinous processes lie between Harrington rods.

Continued.

C 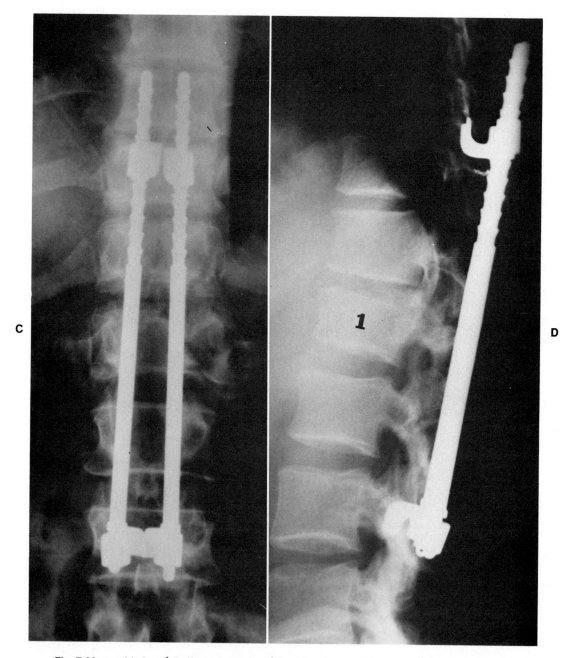 D

Fig. 7-33, cont'd. C and **D,** Postoperative radiographs show satisfactory stabilization of spine.

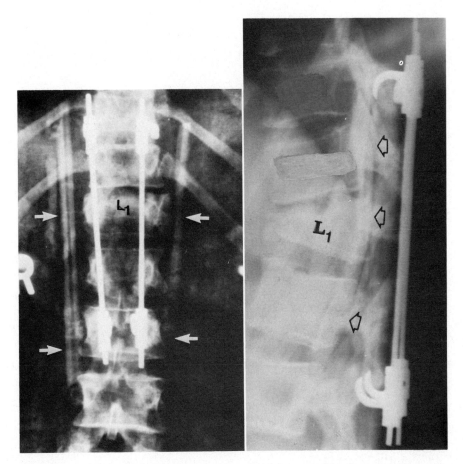

Fig. 7-34. *Harrington compression rods.* Comminuted fracture of L1 6 months after operative laminectomy, requiring insertion of Harrington compression rods. Because of posterior instability, kyphosis has occurred. Note posterolateral fibular bone grafts *(arrows)*.

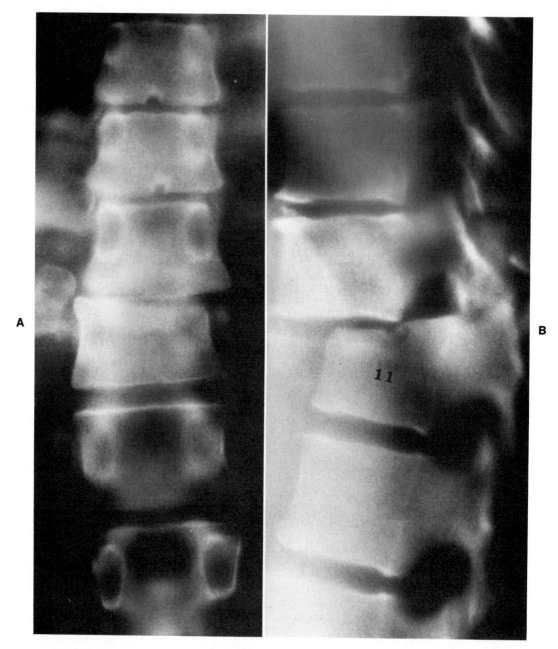

Fig. 7-35. *Weiss springs.* **A** and **B,** Fracture-dislocation of vertebral bodies at T10-11 with fracture of posterior elements and dislocation of facets (same patient as in Fig. 3-5). **C,** Open reduction, Weiss springs internal fixation is used to maintain compression across previously dislocated facets. **D** and **E,** Postoperative radiographs reveal reduction of spine and internal fixation.

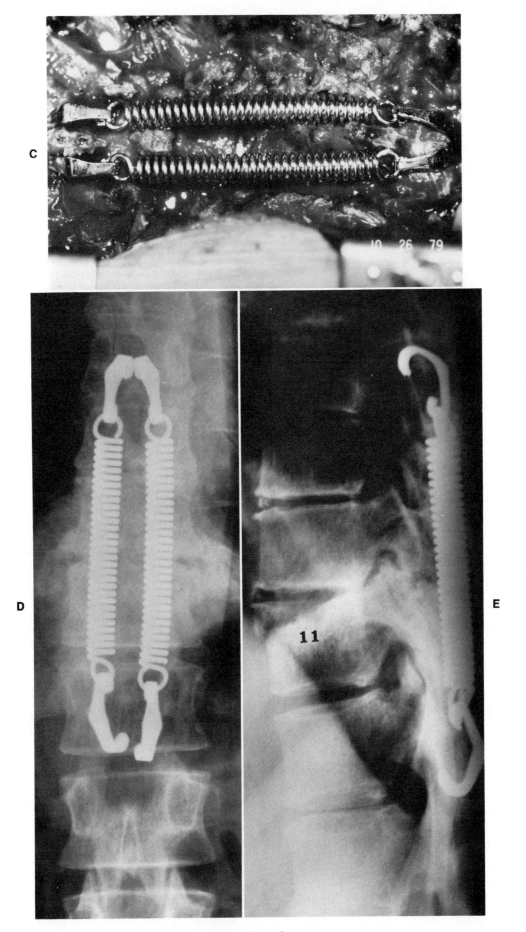

Fig. 7-35, cont'd. For legend see opposite page.

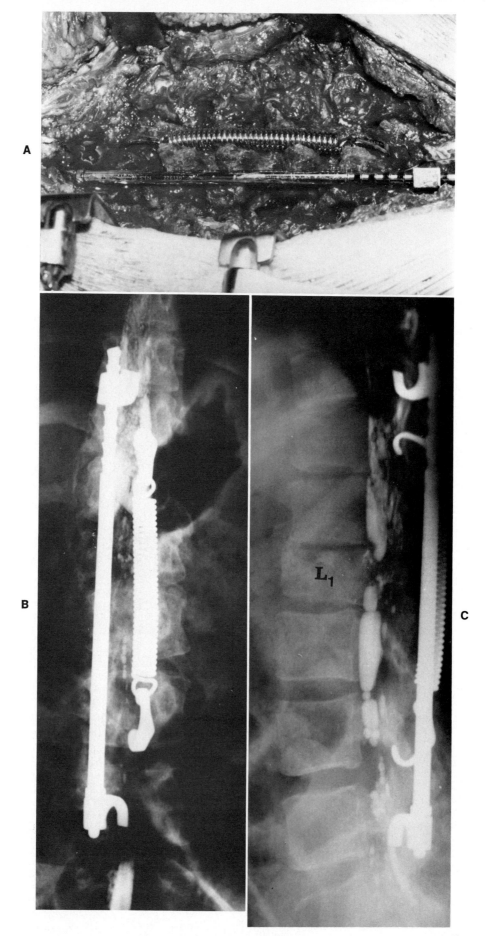

Fig. 7-36. *Combination Weiss spring and Harrington distraction rod.* **A,** Operative photograph of Weiss compression spring and Harrington distraction rod. Both are attached to lamina by means of hooks. **B** and **C,** Postoperative radiographs reveal good spinal alignment. This type of internal fixation is utilized in unbalanced spinal fractures.

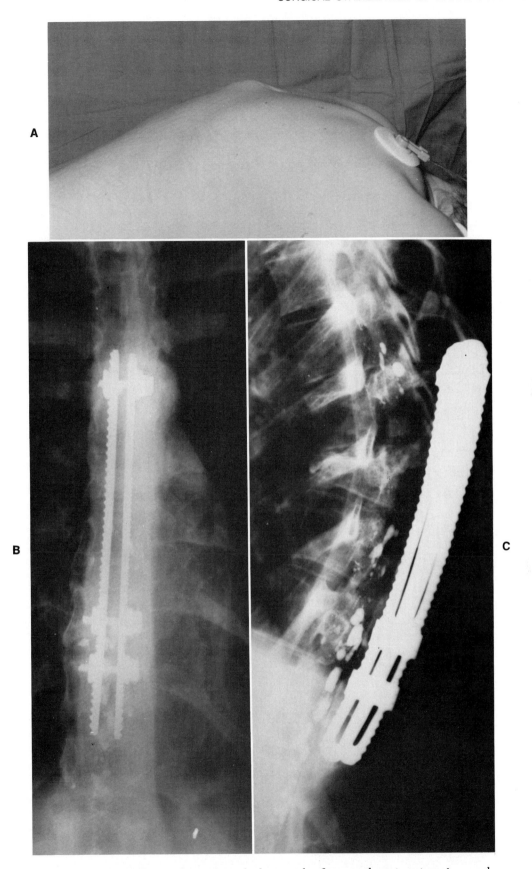

Fig. 7-37. *Murig Williams plates.* Lateral photograph of upper thoracic spine, **A,** reveals significant thoracic kyphosis. Note prominence of skin where end of plate is lying in subcutaneous tissue. **B** and **C,** Radiographs reveal upper thoracic spine subluxated forward at level of upper end of plates. Result is loss of fixation because of fracture of spinous processes, through which bolts connecting plate to bone pass.

COMPLICATIONS OF INTERNAL FIXATION

Technical factors that may contribute to the failure of internal fixation devices are the following:

1. If the transition of the smooth and notched portion of the Harrington distraction apparatus is placed to coincide with the level of injury, fatigue fracture of the rod may occur (Fig. 7-38). Effort should be made to ensure that this potentially weakened area of the internal fixation device does not lie opposite the fracture site.

2. A potential cause for delay in spine fracture–internal fixation–fusion healing is overdistraction of vertebral body fracture fragments, usually within the area of the upper lumbar spine with overvigorous use of the Harrington distraction rod. This is likely to occur while attempting to gain improved spinal alignment (Fig. 7-39, C). Although it has not been revealed in the literature that overdistraction is a problem to be contended with, it is our opinion that such may prevent amalgamation of comminuted vertebral body fragments into the final, stable, healed vertebral body callus. For this same reason the potential exists for settling across the comminuted vertebral body, while posterior element distraction is maintained by the Harrington rods. The result is the development of a flexion deformity at the fracture site in spite of stable rod-hook fixation (Fig. 7-39, D).

3. There may be a hyperextension deformity of the vertebral column at the level of injury, resulting from the application of a compression force across the posterior elements (Harrington compression rods or Weiss springs) (Fig. 7-40), caused by the loss of continuity of the anterior vertebral column ligamentous structures, specifically the anterior longitudinal ligament.

4. Iatrogenic production of lateral angulation scoliosis at the level of injury is likely to result from the insertion of bilateral compression devices (Weiss springs or Harrington compression rods) in the presence of a vertebral fracture with (a) a unilateral fracture of one half of the vertebral body and (b) a unilateral fracture of one pedicle and facet on the same side. The result is a convex scoliosis to the side of the unilateral fracture. This complication can be prevented by either the use of two Harrington rods (Table 7-2; Fig. 7-33) or one rod (on the side of the body-pedicle fracture) and a compression device on the opposite side (Fig. 7-36).

Text continued on p. 248.

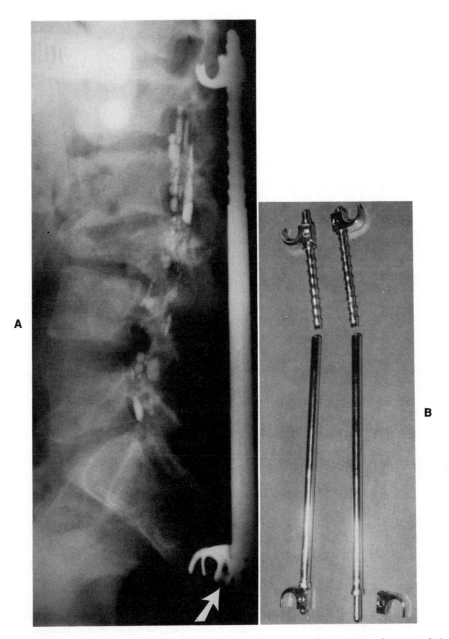

Fig. 7-38. A, Bursting fracture of L3 stabilized with Harrington distraction rods. Note dislocated lower hook *(arrow)*. Eleven months later a fatigue fracture of Harrington rods at level of fracture occurred. **B,** Fractured Harrington rods were removed. Fracture resulted at transition between smooth and notched segments of rod. Note dislocated lower hook.

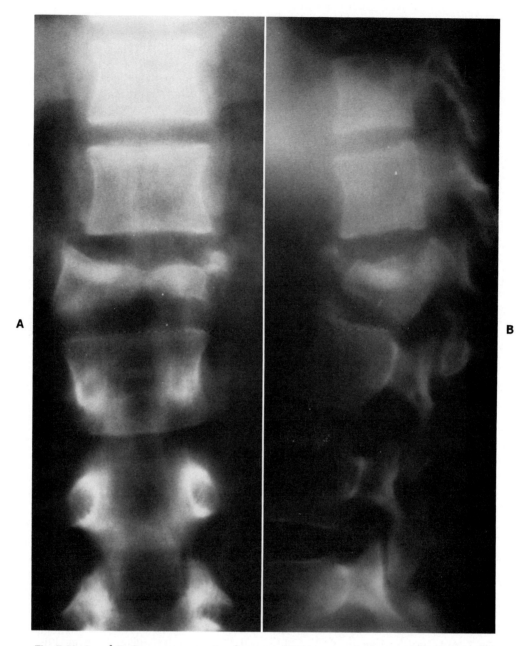

Fig. 7-39. A and **B,** Severe compression fracture of L1 (same patient as in Fig. 4-17) treated with Harrington distraction rods.

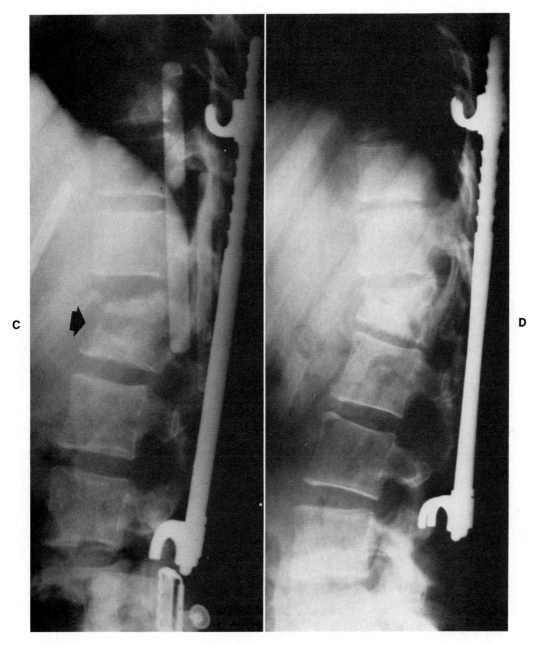

Fig. 7-39, cont'd. This initially resulted in overdistraction of comminuted fragments of L1 (*arrow* in **C**). In such instances loss of spinal alignment, delay in healing, and occasional "breaking away" of hooks from lamina may occur with recurring kyphosis, **D.** While L1 is collapsed, distraction is maintained across posterior elements.

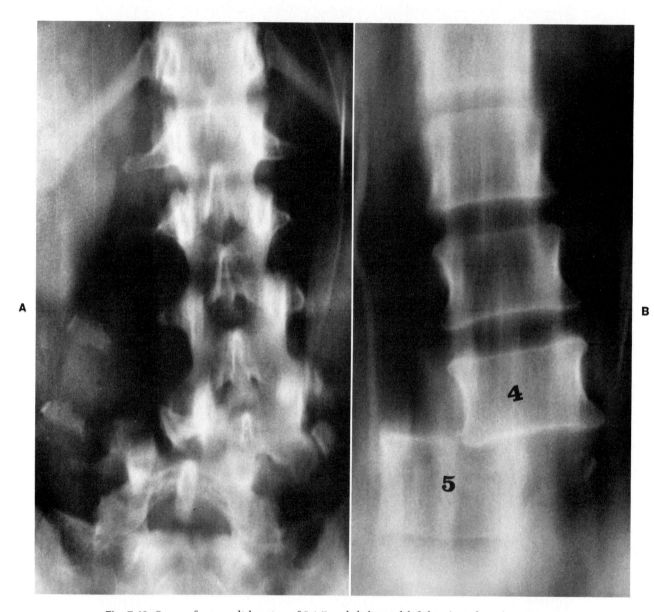

Fig. 7-40. Severe fracture-dislocation of L4-5 and dislocated left hip (not shown) in 38-year-old woman run over by a car (same patient as in Figs. 5-6 and 5-31). **A** and **B,** Polytomograms show extent of injury.

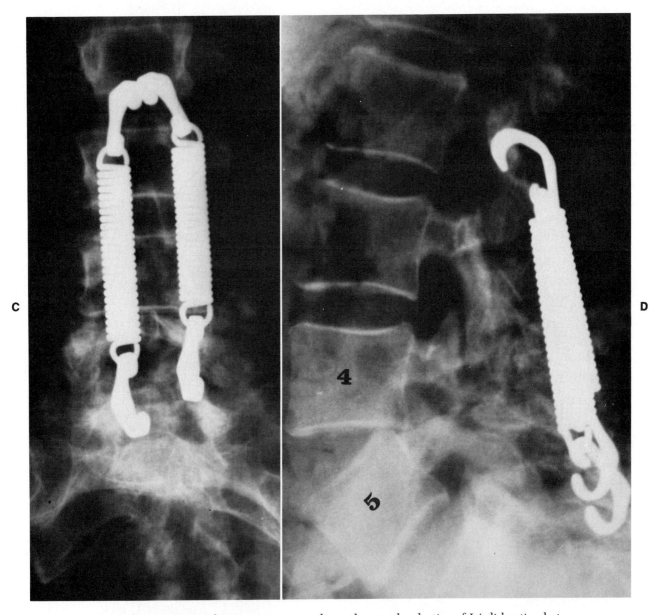

C

D

Fig. 7-40, cont'd. C and **D,** Postoperative radiographs reveal reduction of L4 dislocation but widening of L4-5 interspace anteriorly because of loss of anterior longitudinal ligament and extension moment across lumbosacral spine. Patient was managed in flexion body cast for 3 to 5 months. Injury healed without complication.

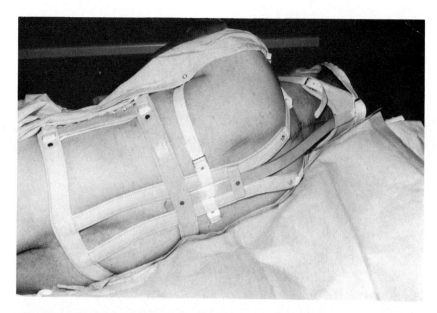

Fig. 7-41. *Knight-Taylor orthosis with cervical extension*. This orthosis is utilized for fractures of thoracic spine above T7. Cervical extension maintains alignment of head and neck with thoracic spine and prevents flexion moment across fracture site.

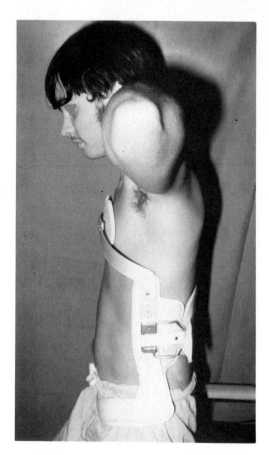

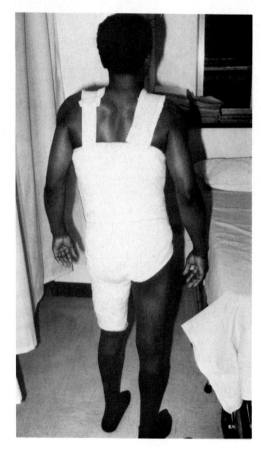

Fig. 7-42. *Three-point hyperextension (Jewett) brace*. This orthosis is used for external immobilization of spine fractures between T7 and L5. It is most effective for protection of either stable or surgically stabilized fractures, where neurologic system is intact.

Fig. 7-43. *Body cast with thigh extension*. Fractures about lumbosacral joint are difficult to immobilize because of pelvic motion. Standard lumbosacral orthoses are not successful in preventing pelvic rotation. The author has successfully used a combination of a body cast and a one thigh spica in such instances. Uniform fracture healing has resulted.

EXTERNAL (ORTHOTIC) SPINAL IMMOBILIZATION

Regardless of the use of the conservative or surgical approach to spinal reduction and fracture healing, each patient will require the wearing of some type of external stabilizing orthosis until the fracture has healed.

Fractures above the level of T6 require the addition of a head-neck support along with the thoracolumbar orthosis (Fig. 7-41). For fractures of the thoracic and lumbar spine from T6 to L5, either the Knight-Taylor (Fig. 7-31) or a Jewett hyperextension orthosis (Fig. 7-42) may be utilized. If the spinal internal fixation stability is questioned or the patient is difficult and unreliable, a body cast is preferred (Fig. 7-32). When the injury involves the lumbosacral joint, immobilization is best attained by means of the combined body cast and one-leg spica to the knee (Fig. 7-43). Each orthosis is worn for a minimum of 3 months.

Management of vertebral column fractures varies with the presence of unilateral or bilateral vertebral element fractures, the presence of vertebral body comminution, the presence of vertebral body facet dislocation, and the presence or absence of neurologic injury (Table 7-2). The number of the above variables will be the primary determinant of the stabilization technique to be used. Each fracture must be individualized and managed either conservatively by bed care and orthotic management or surgically with both internal fixation and bone grafting, followed also by external orthotic immobilization until stable.

REFERENCES

1. Bradford, D. W., Akbarnra, B. A., Winter, R. B., and Seljeskog, E. L.: Surgical stabilization of fractures and fracture dislocations of the thoracic spine, Spine **2**:185, 1977.
2. Dickson, J. H., Harrington, P. R., and Erwin, W. D.: Results of reduction and stabilization of the severely fractured thoracic and lumbar spine, J. Bone Joint Surg. [Am.] **60**:799, 1978.
3. Flesch, S. R., Leider, L. L., Erickson, D. L., et al.: Harrington instrumentation and spine fusion for unstable fractures and fracture-dislocation of the thoracic and lumbar spine, J. Bone Joint Surg. [Am.] **59**:143, 1977.
4. Lazorthes, G., et al.: Arterial vascularization of the spinal cord, J. Neurosurg. **35**:253, 1971.
5. Midwest Regional Spinal Cord Injury Care System: Annual Progress Report VII. Grant no. 13P-55864, Washington, D.C., 1978, Rehabilitation Services Administration, Department of Health and Human Services.
6. Meyer, P. R.: Complications of fractures and dislocations of the dorsolumbar spine. In Epps, C. H., Jr., editor: Complications in orthopaedic surgery, vol. 2, Philadelphia, 1978, J.B. Lippincott Co., pp. 643-709.
7. Rogers, L. F., Thayer, C., Weinberg, P. E., and Kim, K. S.: Acute injuries of the upper thoracic spine associated with paraplegia, Am. J. Roentgenol. **134**:67, 1980.

CHAPTER 8

Pulmonary and other chest complications

RICHARD A. MINTZER, M.D., and RICHARD M. GORE, M.D.

The thorax is rarely spared from complications in patients with spinal cord injury. Indeed, most of the complications observed during the acute stage of injury are related to disturbances in respiratory function and these problems are frequently life threatening. Four major categories of patients are at particular risk: (1) quadriplegics deprived of their major respiratory muscles; (2) patients with thoracic or lumbar spine injuries associated with rib or sternal fractures resulting in a hemothorax or hemopneumothorax; (3) patients with concomitant closed heart, lung, vascular, or esophageal trauma; and (4) patients with preexisting chronic respiratory disease. These complications will be placed in the perspective of their temporal sequence.

During the period immediately after spinal cord injury, pulmonary edema, paralysis of respiratory muscles, flail chest, aspiration of gastric contents, atelectasis, hemothorax and pneumothorax, pulmonary embolism and infarction, and the adult respiratory distress syndrome are the major contributors to patient morbidity and mortality. Although pulmonary complications become less important during the later stages of the patient's disability, recurrent pneumonia and bronchiectasis do contribute to patient morbidity. Injuries to the esophagus, tracheobronchial tree, heart, aorta, great vessels, and pulmonary ligament are not commonly seen in patients admitted with spinal cord injury, since trauma significant enough to damage the vital organs usually results in death.

PATHOPHYSIOLOGIC ASPECTS OF RESPIRATORY DISTURBANCES

Normal respiratory function is a complicated process involving both voluntary and involuntary muscles. There is general agreement that the intercostal and abdominal muscles are the major accessory muscles of respiration.[10] During the period of spinal shock that follows injury to the cervical and upper thoracic spinal cord, the innervation to these muscles is lost, so that the trapezius and the sternocleidomastoid muscles become the main accessory muscles of respiration.[23] After the acute injury subsides, there is restoration of the intercostal muscles. This is apparently related to a spinal reflex in which the passive stretching of the intercostal muscles caused by motion of the diaphragm acts as an afferent stimulus to intercostal contraction.[11]

As a consequence of loss of the normal accessory muscles of respiration, spinal cord injured patients demonstrate a decrease of vital capacity, reduced maximum ventilatory volume, and an increase in the residual space of the lungs. These three changes are related to the supine position of the injured patient, a flaccid abdomen from loss of the abdominal muscles, and a depressed diaphragm.[12]

Further respiratory problems arise as the adynamic status of the gastrointestinal tract leads to gastric dilatation, which in turn causes some elevation of the diaphragm. The gastric dilatation, together with the supine position, renders the spinal cord injured patient susceptible to aspiration of gastric contents into the lungs. Aspiration may lead to pulmonary edema from chemical irritation or from the introduction of unusual organisms into the lungs, resulting in a pneumonia that is refractory to normal antibiotic therapy. In addition to the ventilatory changes, the pneumonias, and chemical irritation of aspiration, a loss of normal vasoconstrictors in the lung parenchyma can result in pulmonary edema. This pulmonary edema is frequently made worse by the large volume of fluid often given to spinal cord injured patients to treat the peripheral hypotension that results from the loss of vasoconstrictor tone. However, it has been shown that patients with spinal cord injury without excessive fluid therapy still may develop pulmonary edema as a result of hypoxemia.

The recumbent position combined with the loss of cough reflex and the inability to clear secretions results in atelectasis. This also leads to elevation of the diaphragm with decreased excursion and a progressive loss of pulmonary function. Respiratory function may further be compromised by metabolic alkalosis secondary to losses of gastric juices through the nasogastric tube.

TECHNICAL CONSIDERATIONS

Good portable chest radiographs are vital if patients with spinal cord injury and associated pulmonary complications are to be appropriately diagnosed and treated (Figs. 8-1 and 8-2). Since these patients are frequently immobilized by various traction devices, movement of them by the radiologic technologist is limited. Complete cooperation of trained nursing personnel, physicians, and the radiologic technologist is required to obtain optimal radiographs.

In addition to the problems associated with patient positioning, the presence of multiple tubes and appliances complicates taking radiographs of the patient with spinal cord injury. All tubes and appliances not in use should be removed from the overlying anterior or from the posterior chest wall. Since spinal cord injured patients may have associated injuries of the chest caused by their trauma or by complications of therapy, it is important not to confuse artifacts such as skin folds with pathologic processes such as pneumothorax. Skin-fold artifacts can be eliminated by placing a pillowcase over the x-ray cassette before positioning.

Many patients require frequent radiographs to monitor their rapidly changing pulmonary status. Proper evaluation requires consistency of technique. This in turn requires a reliable portable x-ray unit with sufficient power to penetrate patients in body casts. Fast film-screen combinations are essential to ensure proper penetration, prevent motion unsharpness, and reduce patient exposure. Use of "fast" conventional calcium tungstate screens degrades image quality, producing films with a great deal of mottle. Furthermore, since there are a wide variation of densities in the chest that must be evaluated, a "long scale" film is the obvious choice. We are currently using a GE AmX portable x-ray unit, Kodak Lanex–Ortho G screen-film combination, and approximately 80 kV with a 10:1 grid for our portable chest radiographs. The GE AmX unit provides adequate power for consistent exposures. The Lanex screens are of the rare-earth type and are more efficient "trappers" of the available radiation without degrading the image by mottle. The Ortho G film with its wide latitude is excellent for the range of densities in chest radiography. After the initial exposure the film is evaluated by a radiologist and determination of the optimal milliampere-seconds (mAs) is made. The technique is then recorded on a chart kept near the patient's bed. This ensures consistency in exposure, and subtle changes in the chest that may have been ascribed to "technical differences" are thus properly assessed.

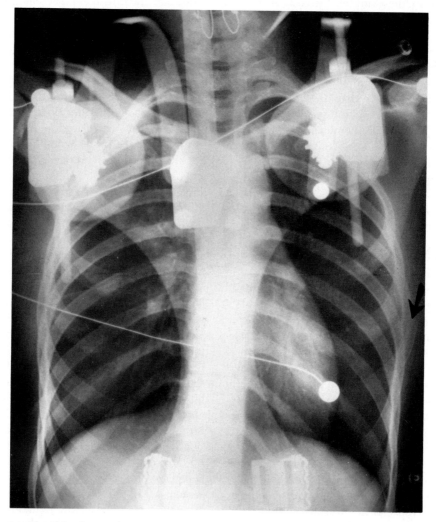

Fig. 8-1. Portable chest radiograph of 19-year-old woman who became C5 quadriplegic as a result of a motor vehicle accident. Film was taken after cervical fusion. There is good penetration of mediastinum. Lung parenchyma and pulmonary vascularity are well seen even with brace in position. Note fracture of fifth left rib (arrow).

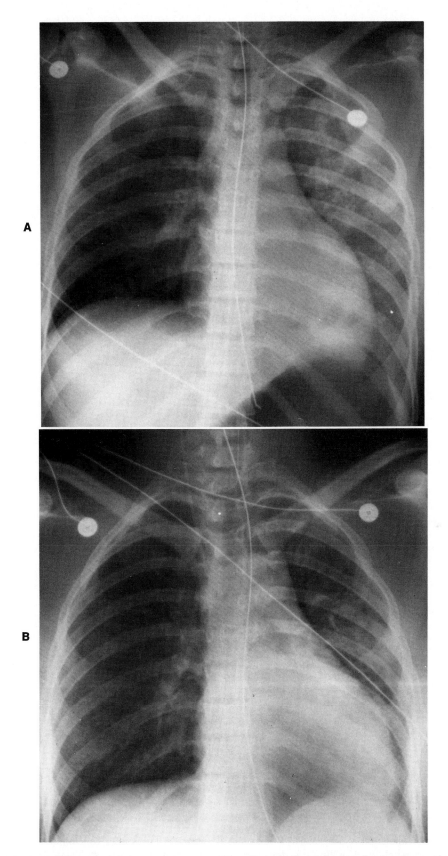

Fig. 8-2. Same patient as in Fig. 8-1. **A,** Radiograph was taken 6 hours after accident. Alveolar infiltrate is present in left upper lobe. Pulmonary contusion is most likely cause. **B,** Four days later there is nearly complete clearing of contused left lung.

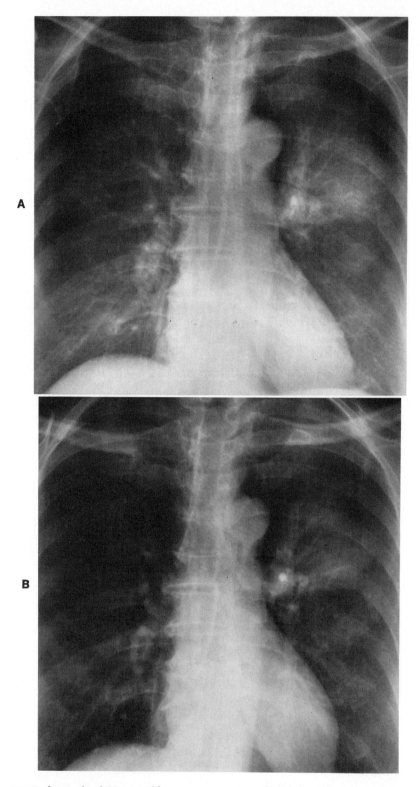

Fig. 8-3. Radiograph of 74-year-old woman approximately 6 hours after concomitant trauma to left lateral chest. **A,** Infiltrate is demonstrated in left perihilar region. **B,** Three days later infiltrate is still present and there is no evidence of clearing.

CONCOMITANT INJURIES TO THE THORACIC ORGANS

Traumatic lung injuries including contusion, hematoma, and laceration frequently accompany spinal cord injury, and any spinal cord injured patient should be carefully assessed to rule out any of these lesions, which may pass unnoticed.

Pulmonary contusion

Contusion is probably the most common radiologic finding in nonpenetrating chest trauma and actually occurs more frequently than rib fractures.[21] Contusion is produced by rupture of alveoli and blood vessels with resultant interalveolar and interstitial hemorrhage and edema. Although not present initially, radiologic changes usually develop within 6 hours of injury. The area of contusion appears as an ill-defined infiltrate that directly underlies the portion of the chest wall that has sustained injury (Fig. 8-2). Contrecoup injury is less frequently seen. In uncomplicated contusion, clearing begins approximately in 48 hours. If significant clearing has not taken place by 72 hours, another cause of the infiltrate, such as lung bleeding, atelectasis, or pneumonia, must be considered.

Pulmonary hematoma

Pulmonary hematoma is the next most frequently encountered chest injury in patients who have sustained blunt chest trauma. In addition to the finding of contusion, there is a macroscopic collection of blood within the lungs.[24] This collection usually occurs because of the presence of a small pulmonary laceration. The appearance of pulmonary hematoma is initially quite similar to that of lung contusion in that there is usually an ill-defined infiltrate that develops approximately 6 hours after injury (Fig. 8-3). Unlike pulmonary contusions, the lung infiltrate persists 5 to 6 weeks. These hematomas may resolve in a manner reminiscent of pulmonary embolism, with a "shrinking nodule" that diminishes in size for several months and ultimately leaves a small fibrotic scar.

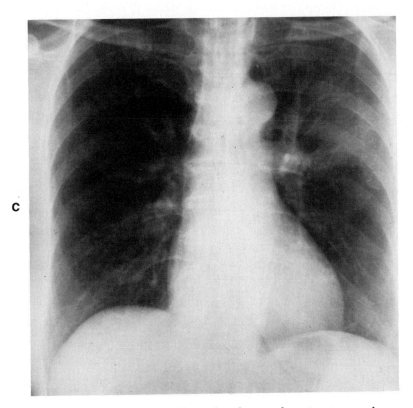

Fig. 8-3, cont'd. C, Two weeks later infiltrate has decreased in size, is more homogeneous, and typifies appearance of a *pulmonary hematoma* in that it appears to be "melting" rather than clearing from within.

Pulmonary laceration

Pulmonary lacerations, less common than either hematomas or contusions, can also occur in patients with chest trauma and spinal cord injury. Motor vehicle accidents or falls from significant heights are usually the cause. A pulmonary laceration, unlike a contusion or a hematoma, demonstrates an area of infiltrate on the initial chest radiograph. Shearing forces tear the lung, producing the laceration. Sudden compression of an area of lung results in explosive pressure buildup when there is occlusion in a segment in the peripheral bronchial tree. This explosive force ruptures alveolar walls, tearing blood vessels and liberating air into the interstitium of the lung. Air-fluid levels may occur with blood filling ruptured alveoli.[24]

Although hematoma and contusion are generally seen as ill-defined areas of infiltrate that are relatively homogenous centrally, pulmonary lacerations demonstrate both areas of infiltrate and central, cystic, air-containing structures. Ultimately the hemorrhage walls off the hematocele formed by the laceration. Lacerations resolve slowly over the course of several weeks.

Pneumothorax and hemothorax

Pneumothorax (Fig. 8-4), hemothorax (Fig. 8-5), and hemopneumothorax are frequently seen in association with penetrating wounds of the thorax in patients with spinal cord injury but also may be seen in closed injuries of the chest. Patients with fractures of the thoracic and upper lumbar spine often have concomitant injury to the pleural space. The rupture of small alveoli thought to be responsible for pulmonary laceration can cause hemopneumothorax in the absence of any obvious injury to the chest wall. Furthermore, patients may develop a pneumothorax as a result of too vigorous ventilatory therapy (Fig. 8-6).

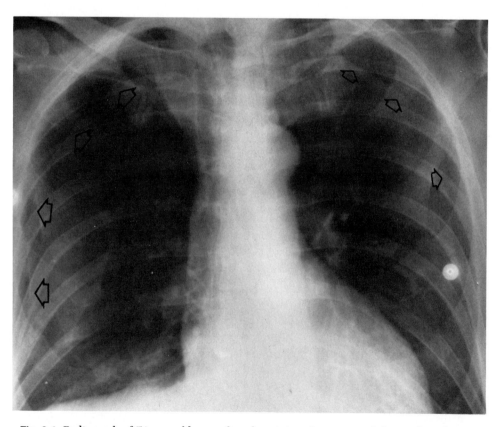

Fig. 8-4. Radiograph of 74-year-old man after chest injury from automobile accident demonstrates right-sided *pneumothorax (large arrows)* and skin fold simulating pneumothorax of left hemithorax *(small arrows)*.

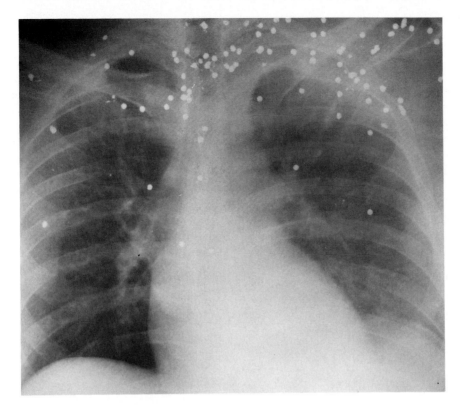

Fig. 8-5. Portable chest radiograph of 34-year-old man after gunshot wound to cervical spine and chest. Relative opacification of entire left side of chest is caused by *free-flowing hemo-thorax*, layering posteriorly on this supine film.

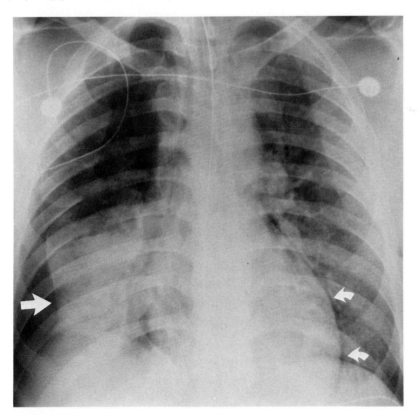

Fig. 8-6. Pneumothorax *(large arrow)* and pneumomediastinum *(small arrows)* developed in C5 quadriplegic as a result of vigorous ventilatory therapy. In addition, there is pneumonia of partially collapsed right lower lobe.

Trauma affecting the pulmonary ligament

Traumatic pneumatoceles of the pulmonary ligament have been reported to occur after laceration of the lung.[7] Although we have seen only one posttraumatic pulmonary ligament pneumatocele, we have seen numerous examples of triangular densities simulating left lower lung collapse, which have proven to be pleural hematomas trapped between the posterior aspect of the heart and the anterior surface of the pulmonary ligament in patients with a thoracic vertebral fracture (Fig. 8-7).[15] The fluid nature of this triangular density beneath the left hilum can be differentiated from collapse by turning the patient into the left lateral decubitus position. Fluid that creates the triangular density between the heart and the ligament when the patient is supine will flow to the left lateral pleural space in the left lateral decubitus position.

Pneumomediastinum

Few patients were seen at our spinal cord injury unit with a radiologic finding of pneumomediastinum. Nevertheless, mediastinal or deep cervical emphysema following blunt trauma to the thorax is among the most important signs of tracheobronchial laceration.[15] The presence of either finding in a patient who has not had positive pressure ventilation is strongly suggestive of tracheobronchial fracture, and bronchoscopy is required.[14] Because the tracheobronchial tree is a rigid structure it is far more likely to rupture than the mobile and elastic esophagus. In the absence of demonstrable laceration to the tracheobronchial tree by bronchoscopy, an esophageal rupture should be sought as the next most likely cause of deep cervical or mediastinal emphysema (Fig. 8-13).

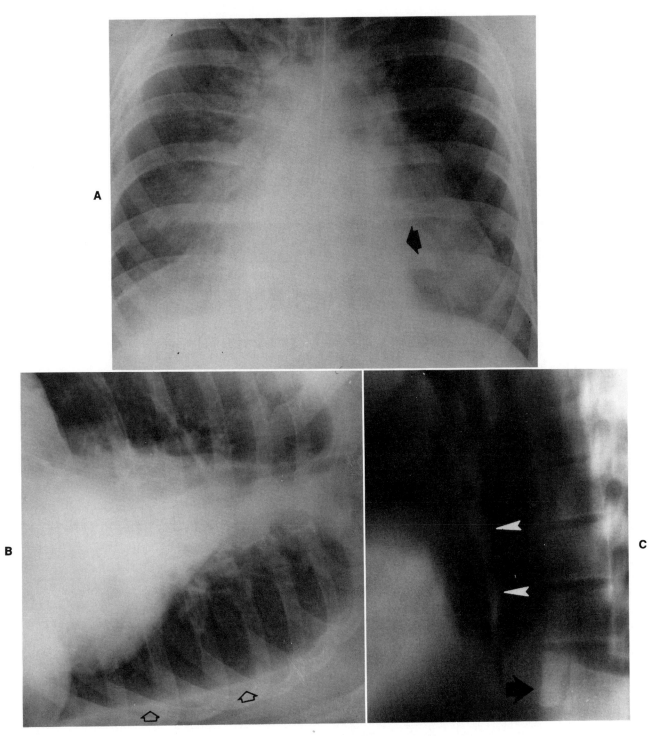

Fig. 8-7. Six hours after motor vehicle accident, portable chest radiograph in supine projection, **A,** shows triangular density medial to left ventricular border *(arrow)*. **B,** Decubitus film with left side dependent indicates triangular density behind heart is no longer present and there is free-flowing pleural effusion now present along left lateral chest wall *(arrows)*. **C,** Tomogram of lower chest demonstrates presence of fracture of tenth thoracic centrum *(black arrow)* and *fluid trapped by pulmonary ligament (white arrowheads)*. This fluid simulated left lower lobe collapse with patient supine. (From Mintzer, R. A., et al.: Chest **76:**401-405, 1979.)

Injury to the tracheobronchial tree

Tracheobronchial lacerations usually affect the main bronchi, typically within 2.5 cm of the carina.[17] Two different presentations may be seen with a tracheobronchial lesion: total disruption or partial tear (incomplete). With total disruption of the bronchus and free communication with the pleural space, a large pneumothorax will result (Fig. 8-8). The lung will not reexpand despite appropriate suctioning, chest tubes, or thoracostomy. With total rupture of a main bronchus, the collapsed airless lung, rather than retracting about the hilus, occupies a dependent position within the thorax when the patient is in the upright position. The collapsed lung is situated inferiorly and medially with maintenance of vascular connection to the hilus. Pneumothorax is absent or small and undetectable radiographically when disruption of the bronchus is incomplete.[5] In either the total or incomplete situation, gas may escape through the bronchial wall and peribronchial connective tissues directly into the mediastinum. The peribronchial tissues remain sufficiently intact in incomplete disruption to permit at least partial ventilation of the affected lung. Mediastinal gas may be virtually impossible to detect radiographically so that the fracture of the bronchus may remain occult until either atelectasis or pulmonary infection develops distal to the obstruction at the site of laceration. The obstruction in this case develops from the accumulation of granulation tissue at the fracture site and may occur as early as 1 week after injury.[14] Tomography may be required to demonstrate the linear collections of air that insinuate between the peribronchial connective tissue sheet in the outer surface of the bronchial tube.[24] Delay in diagnosis of a rupture of the bronchus generally leads to stenosis or complete occlusion of the bronchus. Ultimately bronchiectasis or atelectasis or both will occur.[24]

In the absence of injury to the airway and the neck, gas in the deep cervical fascial plane should be considered an extension of the mediastinal emphysema even without radiologic evidence of a mediastinal component after closed chest injury.[6,14] Mediastinal or subcutaneous emphysema occurs in more than 60% of cases of tracheobronchial laceration.[18] Although pulmonary lacerations permit gas to enter the pulmonary interstitium and then the mediastinum, it is extremely unusual for large amounts of gas to be forced into the mediastinum unless the patient has been subjected to positive pressure ventilation.

Tension pneumothorax and subcutaneous emphysema may develop after rib fractures have lacerated the visceral and parietal pleura; pneumomediastinum of this origin has never been documented.[14]

Additional radiologic findings in patients with ruptures of the trachea are also associated with injuries to the aorta and great vessels and include fractures of the first three ribs, an apical pleural cap, and a widened mediastinum.

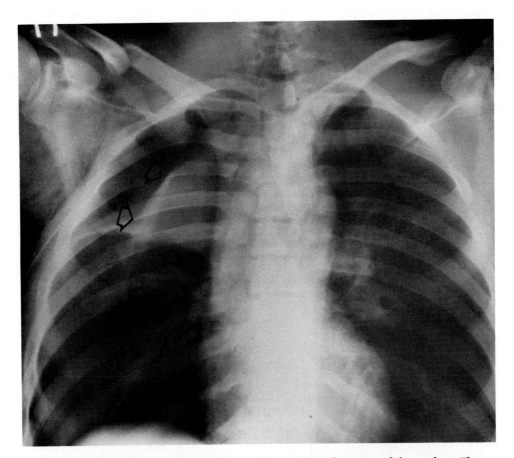

Fig. 8-8. Portable chest radiograph of 27-year-old man injured in automobile accident. There is a massive pneumothorax on the right with right lung collapsed and seen as perihilar mass *(arrows)*. Subcutaneous emphysema and fracture of right clavicle are also noted. Despite placement of chest tube and suctioning, right lung failed to reexpand. Bronchoscopy revealed rent in right upper lobe bronchus, which communicated with pleural space.

Cardiovascular injuries

Although at the Midwest Regional Spinal Cord Injury Care System we have seen few cardiovascular lesions in patients with spinal cord injury, inclusion of these complications is necessary since motor vehicle accidents responsible for most spinal cord injuries are also the most common cause of cardiovascular injury. Numerous cardiovascular lesions can result from nonpenetrating chest trauma. They include pericardial rupture or hemorrhage with or without tamponade,[16] transmural myocardial infarction,[13] rupture or injury to portions of the valvular apparatus, injury to the conduction system with acute or chronic arrhythmias, rupture or laceration of coronary arteries, thrombosis of the coronary artery saphenous vein graft, traumatic coronary artery fistulas,[8] ventricular aneurysm formation, and postpericardiotomy syndrome. Ruptures of the aorta occur at the isthmus at the site of the ligamentum arteriosum in 95% of traumatic ruptures. The radiologic signs related to ruptures in this location include widening of the mediastinum causing shift of the trachea to the right, blurring of the normal sharp aortic contour, and opacification of the aorticopulmonary window, as well as depression of the carinal angle. As stated earlier, an apical pleural cap accompanied by fractures of the first three ribs is seen in association with tracheobronchial fractures but may also be seen in traumatic rupture of the aorta and great vessels (Figs. 8-9 and 8-10).

Rupture of smaller vessels about the mediastinum also results in mediastinal hematoma (Figs. 8-11 and 8-12). Small vessel rupture is a much more frequent cause of mediastinal widening than is aortic rupture. Nonetheless, because of the overlap in signs between traumatic rupture of the aorta and great vessels and mediastinal widening from rupture of small vessels, when mediastinal widening is demonstrated on plain films of the chest, aortography should be obtained.

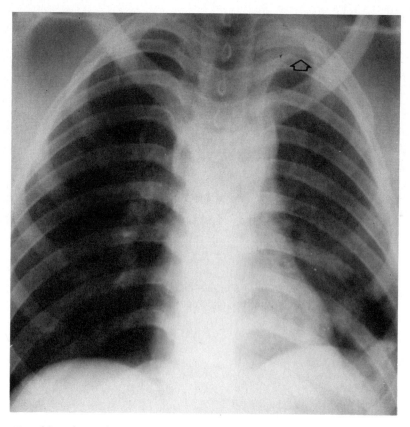

Fig. 8-9. Portable radiograph in 16-year-old boy after multiple gunshot wounds demonstrates widened mediastinum, left apical pleural cap *(arrow)*, and fracture of left second and eighth ribs. All of these findings suggested presence of laceration of aorta or great vessel. Aortography failed to demonstrate such a process.

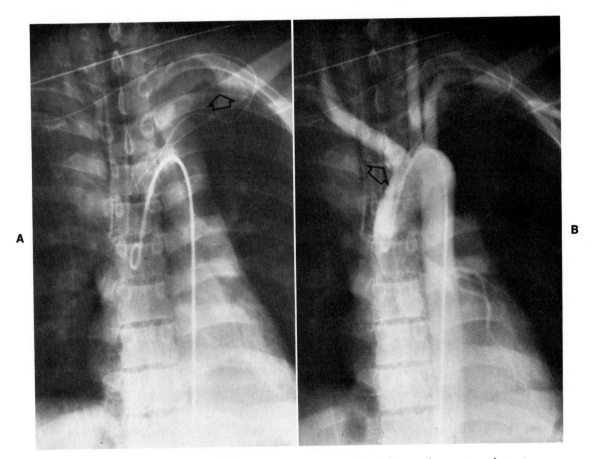

Fig. 8-10. A, Preliminary film before aortography in 23-year-old man after motorcycle accident demonstrates apical pleural cap *(arrow)*, mediastinal widening, and loss of normal aortic contour. These findings were also present on initial chest radiograph. **B,** Aortography demonstrates *pseudoaneurysm* with intimal flap at origin of innominate artery *(arrow)*.

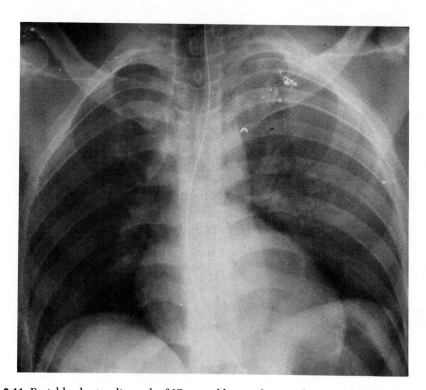

Fig. 8-11. Portable chest radiograph of 27-year-old man after gunshot wound to upper cervical spine. Metallic fragments are seen overlying right shoulder, left upper chest, and abdomen. Widening of superior mediastinum proved to be secondary to *laceration of small mediastinal vessels*.

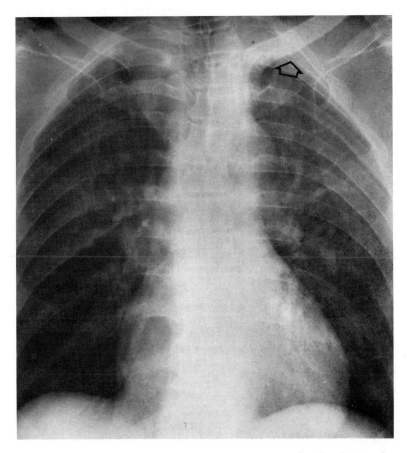

Fig. 8-12. Portable chest radiograph of 64-year-old patient immediately after accident. Widening of superior mediastinum, fractures of the left first and second ribs, and apical pleural cap *(arrow)* are demonstrated. Aortic contour is sharp, and no aortic or great vessel lacerations were demonstrated. Widened superior mediastinum and apical pleural cap are presumably related to *laceration of small mediastinal vessels.*

Injury to the esophagus

In our experience at the Midwest Regional Spinal Cord Injury Care System, rupture of the esophagus has occurred in spinal cord injured patients only when there was penetrating injury to the cervical or upper thoracic region (Fig. 8-13). We have not seen esophageal ruptures secondary to blunt trauma. As stated earlier, it would be unusual for a mobile and elastic structure such as the esophagus to rupture from blunt trauma.

Rupture of the esophagus secondary to chest or cervical trauma is associated with an exceedingly high mortality. The most common injury to the esophagus is the result of iatrogenic instrumentation.[24] Complete esophageal rupture, a life-threatening situation, is indicated by pain, prostration, dyspnea, and shock, and it inevitably results in mediastinitis, requiring prompt surgical drainage.[1] Infrequently the infection becomes localized and forms an abscess near the site of rupture. More commonly, however, vomiting, mediastinitis, and empyema develop rapidly.[24]

The location of esophageal disruption is related to the site of trauma. The distal esophagus can be ruptured with sharp blows to the lower chest or upper abdomen. The upper esophagus can be ruptured by trauma to the upper thorax. Iatrogenic injures to the esophagus usually occur in the proximal region but can occur at the site of a hiatal hernia or other areas of abnormality. Radiographic findings in esophageal rupture (Fig. 8-12) include (1) mediastinal or deep cervical emphysema, (2) widened mediastinum, and (3) an air-fluid level in the mediastinum. Although the mediastinum is minimally widened initially, its width increases rapidly because of the fulminating mediastinitis or abscess.[24] With extension of the process into the adjacent pleural space, hydropneumothorax and then empyema develop. Iodinated contrast agents (Gastrografin) rather than barium sulfate should be used for the definitive diagnosis of esophageal rupture to minimize the risk of granuloma formation in the event of an esophagomediastinal communication.

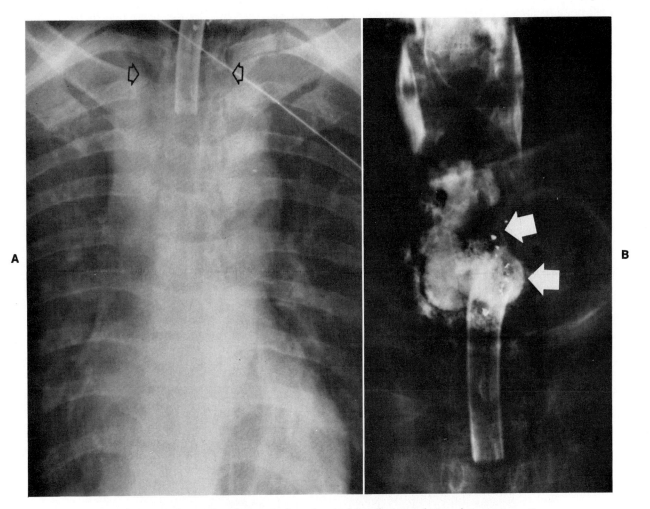

Fig. 8-13. A, Mediastinal widening and mediastinal emphysema *(arrows)* are apparent on portable radiograph obtained after gunshot wound to cervical spine and neck. **B,** After ingestion of contrast material, *esophageal laceration (arrows)* at site of gunshot wound is apparent, as is mediastinal and deep cervical emphysema.

Injury to the diaphragm

Although the incidence of diaphragmatic rupture in patients with multiple injuries after blunt trauma is estimated to be about 4% to 5%, the presence of diaphragmatic injury is virtually nonexistent in patients with concomitant spinal cord injury. In our review of more than 500 patients admitted to the spinal cord injury unit at Northwestern Memorial Hospital, we have detected a single case of diaphragmatic rupture.

The left hemidiaphragm is ruptured in approximately 90% of diaphragmatic ruptures, and 10% involve either both diaphragms or the right hemidiaphragm. This rel-ative sparing of the right hemidiaphragm is due to the presence of the liver in the right upper abdomen. Radiologic findings include hemothorax, herniation of a hollow viscus into the left chest, unusual contour of the hemidiaphragm, and contralateral shift of the mediastinum. All of these findings can be demonstrated on supine radiographs of the chest (Fig. 8-14).[22]

Because of the tremendous force required to rupture the diaphragm, there are nearly always other serious injuries, causing the diaphragmatic injury to be overlooked. Long delays in diagnosing this process are frequent.

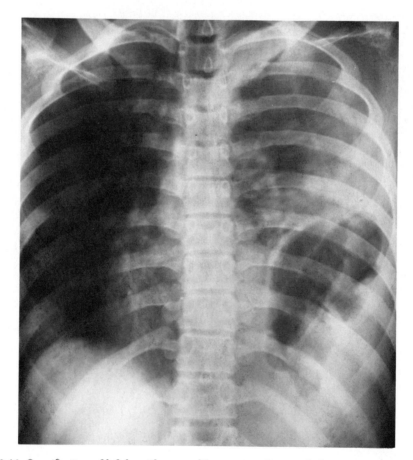

Fig. 8-14. Opacification of left hemithorax and herniation of stomach, bowel, and spleen with mediastinal shift are apparent in this 19-year-old man with concomitant blunt abdominal trauma.

Phrenic nerve stimulation

Although direct diaphragmatic injuries and herniations are rare, significant respiratory compromise from diaphragmatic paralysis or paresis is fairly common in patients with high cervical cord lesions. The diaphragm innervated by the phrenic nerve accounts for over 60% of effective ventilation at rest; the remainder is supplied by the intercostal muscles, with a small contribution from the accessory muscles of respiration: the sternocleidomastoid and trapezius.[2] Either component can maintain adequate ventilation at rest. In most cases of cervical spine trauma, the intercostal muscles are lost during the period of spinal shock. Diaphragmatic innervation and function are maintained so that until intercostal reflexes are reestablished, patients with lesions at or below the level of C4 can live without appreciable symptoms or signs of respiratory insufficiency.[9] Transection of the cord above the origin of the phrenic nerve (third through fifth cervical segments), however, results in abolition or diminution of diaphragmatic action and the patient will require artificial ventilation.

In patients with lesions above C4, with a paralyzed or a paretic diaphragm, the return of intercostal function may be insufficient to provide adequate ventilation. The respiratory status of these patients can frequently be improved by phrenic nerve stimulation. Since approximately 100 times the energy needed from cardiac pacing is required for even unilateral phrenic nerve stimulation, the power source must be external.[3] Radio frequency electronic stimulators with implanted electrodes and receivers (Fig. 8-15) and external transmitters, antennas, and power source are used with modest success in spinal cord injured patients.

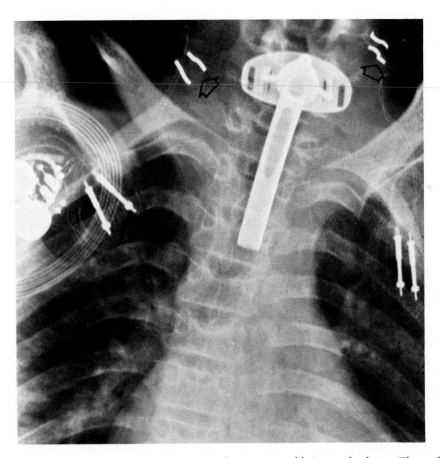

Fig. 8-15. *Phrenic nerve stimulators* implanted in 14-year-old C4 quadriplegic. Electrode-stimulating leads are held to phrenic nerves by vascular clips *(arrows)*. Note transmitting antenna and radiofrequency receiver over each shoulder.

ACUTE COMPLICATIONS

In the acute phase of spinal cord injury, patients are prone to develop pulmonary edema, pulmonary embolism, acute adult respiratory distress syndrome, aspiration pneumonia, or migratory atelectasis. The last two complications also occur in the chronic stages and will be discussed later.

Pulmonary edema

During the immediate postinjury period, many patients become hypoxic secondary to the various respiratory insults. The clinical findings of hypoxemia are manifested prior to the appearance of radiologic findings. The hypoxemia present is often much greater than the radiologic abnormalities would suggest. This suggests that shunting occurs, leading to hypoxia, which is the result of interalveolar edema undetectable on the chest radiograph.[24]

Pulmonary edema in spinal cord injured patients has been attributed to the overzealous administration of large volumes of fluids frequently given to treat the peripheral hypotension that results from generalized loss of vasoconstrictor tone. This explanation, however, does not account for the immediate pulmonary edema found in battle casualities who die instantaneously of head wounds. Pulmonary edema is a frequent autopsy finding in patients with acute injuries of the cervical spinal cord.[1] In all likelihood, patients with upper spinal cord injury may have a sudden increased intercranial pressure with a subsequent massive sympathetic outpouring or a hormonal response leading to pulmonary edema. In general, a classic "bat wing" pulmonary edema pattern develops within 12 to 30 hours after injury (Fig. 8-16). The pulmonary edema seen with spinal cord injured patients responds rapidly to correction of hypoxia by intubation, oxygen, positive pressure

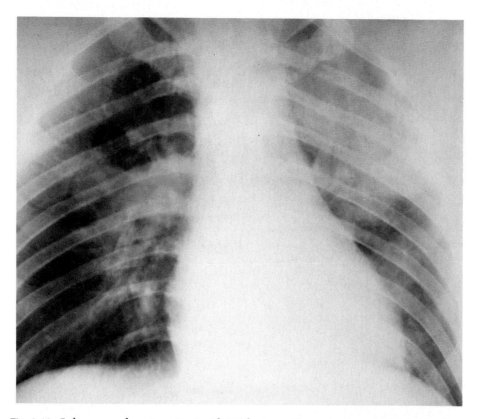

Fig. 8-16. *Pulmonary edema* in patient with C5 fracture. Heart size is normal. No significant amounts of fluid had been given to patient, who had an emergency myelogram that demonstrated impingement on spinal cord. In light of relatively normal heart size this represents pulmonary edema from spinal cord injury.

ventilation, bronchodilators, and diuretics. The heart may or may not be enlarged in the pulmonary edema seen in high spinal cord injuries.

Pulmonary edema in the spinal cord injured patient may not always be bilateral and diffuse. Unilateral pulmonary edema (Fig. 8-17), often confused with other unilateral alveolar or interstitial infiltrates, may result from increased hydrostatic pressure in the dependent lung when the patient is maintained in the lateral decubitus position for extended periods, often done to promote bronchial drainage or to prevent aspiration of gastric juice.[4] Unilateral pulmonary edema can also occur secondary to the pulmonary hypertension that results in the contralateral lung when there is a massive embolism of one pulmonary artery.[4]

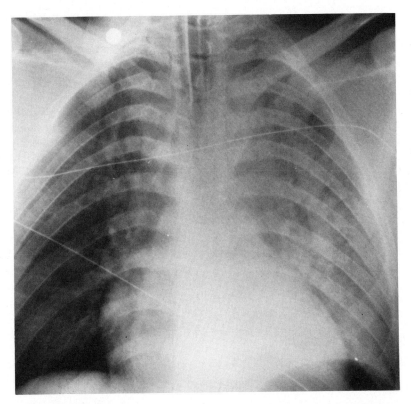

Fig. 8-17. Unilateral pulmonary edema on left in C5 quadriplegic man: possible cause for unilaterality—pulmonary embolism on right, resulting in poorly perfused right lung.

Pulmonary embolism

Patient immobility and the hypercoagulable state that frequently follows trauma predispose the spinal cord injured patient to deep venous thrombosis.[24] The incidence of fatal pulmonary thromboembolism has been placed between 0.6% and 4.7% during the acute stage of injury. Nonfatal embolism occurs in approximately 15% of patients. Prophylactic anticoagulation has been found useful in reducing this incidence when administered early in the course of the disease. Thromboembolism is rare during the chronic stage of disease.[19]

Plain chest film diagnosis of pulmonary embolism is difficult in the general population and virtually impossible in the spinal cord injured patient. In most cases the chest film is unremarkable. The subtle ancillary signs of embolism, such as loss of lung volume, elevation of the diaphragm, platelike atelectasis, effusion, and patchy infiltration, which are suggestive in other patients, are nonspecific findings in the spinal cord injured patient in whom these findings are quite common even in the absence of pulmonary embolism. A high index of suspicion must be maintained and radionuclide ventilation-perfusion scans and angiography should be employed as indicated.

Acute adult respiratory distress syndrome

With improved respiratory care in patients after spinal cord injury, the grim prognosis of the acute adult respiratory distress syndrome (AARDS; pulmonary surfactant disease) noted several years ago has improved. Nonetheless, this syndrome still is seen all too frequently and remains an important life-threatening process. Clinically there is an initial phase of well-being. This is followed by a loss in pulmonary function that rapidly accelerates, leading to progressively more difficult ventilation, which leads to hypoxia and dyspnea.

The radiologic findings during this phase include a pulmonary edema pattern with interstitial infiltration initially and then diffuse bilateral pulmonary densities in a perihilar distribution (Fig. 8-18).

The causes of the clinical and radiologic findings are quite variable. AARDS can be found in patients (1) who have been in cardiogenic shock or septic shock, (2) who have fat emboli from major trauma to the pelvis, or (3) who took an overdose of drugs or who aspirated gastric contents. The clinical and radiologic findings are similar in all three conditions, because the lung reacts in a nonspecific and limited way to injury. Pulmonary capillary dysfunction is the common etiology.

In the subacute phase there may be some initial improvement after intubation, but hypoxia may again appear and be profound enough to require mechanical ventilatory assistance including positive end expiratory pressure ventilation (PEEP), high oxygen concentration, and therapy related to the underlying cause of the AARDS. At this point, there appear to be two main pathophysiologic problems: increased pulmonary vascular permeability and abnormal gas distribution in the lungs. These two pathophysiologic processes result in a reduction of the functional residual capacity, a decreased pulmonary compliance, and a ventilation-perfusion mismatch.

The radiologic findings at this point include those seen in the immediate postinjury period with radiologic evidence of a ventilation-perfusion mismatch manifested as large areas of lung being hyperventilated and other areas quite opaque with no evidence of significant ventilation.

Up to this point, all of these changes are reversible. In the subacute phase, which begins approximately 5 days after the initial symptoms, hilar membranes are formed and the patient remains profoundly hypoxic in spite of intubation, PEEP, and high oxygen concentration. This stage is irreversible, and it is of interest that at least superficially, the radiologic findings appear to improve. More areas of ventilated lung are present, and there is less evidence of consolidation. On close inspection of the radiographs (Fig. 8-18, B) this improved pattern (with worsening clinical findings) demonstrates that the usual air bronchogram seen in the early and mid phases has been replaced by a bubbly pattern with interstitial air rather than alveolar air predominating.[20]

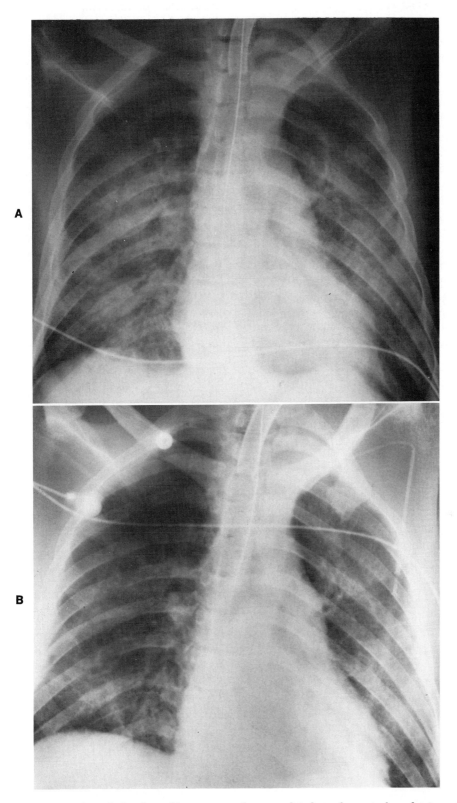

Fig. 8-18. A, Bilateral alveolar infiltrates were discovered 3 days after spinal cord injury. **B,** Seventy-two hours later, areas of consolidation have been replaced by bubbly appearance due to interstitial air. Patient's condition continued to worsen. He now has acute *adult respiratory distress syndrome*.

CHRONIC COMPLICATIONS

Pulmonary complications that appear chronically in spinal cord patients are related to poor clearing of secretions, atelectasis resulting from an absent cough reflex, increased mucous secretions, and aspiration of gastric contents.

Migratory atelectasis

Increased mucous secretions appear to be related to the presence of endotracheal or tracheostomy tubes. When migratory atelectasis is seen in spinal cord injured patients, it is nearly always in patients with these tubes (Fig. 8-19). It is our opinion that these tubes are responsible for the production of thick, tenacious mucus, which ultimately leads to the migratory atelectasis so frequently demonstrated in spinal cord injured patients. The atelectasis is refractory to normal measures and frequently requires bronchoscopy (Fig. 8-20). Vigorous therapy, including bronchodilators, broad-spectrum antibiotics, and respiratory therapy to induce cough, is imperative when infection or atelectasis develops in order to prevent any destruction of the bronchial tree.

Aspiration pneumonia

Aspiration pneumonia in the ambulatory population usually involves the lower lobes. The dependent portion of the lung becomes the site of aspiration in quadriplegic patients who are on Stryker frames. It is not unusual for a quadriplegic to demonstrate a lingular or right middle lobe aspiration pneumonia or even upper lobe aspirations in the anterior or posterior segments. Aspiration of gastric contents is a consequence of the patient's supine position and the pathophysiologic alterations found in the gastrointestinal tract, including the precipitous development of hiatus hernia and reflux. Aspiration pneumonia should be treated promptly with steroid therapy and other supportive measures, as well as broad-spectrum antibiotic coverage. Bronchiectasis can be avoided with prompt attention to all respiratory complications.

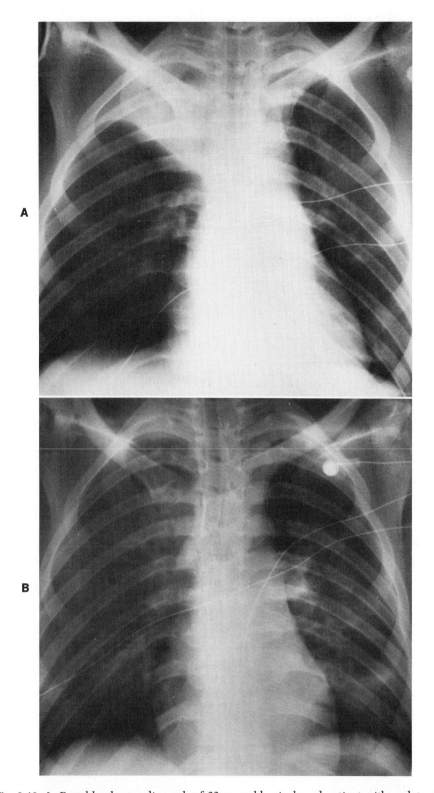

Fig. 8-19. A, Portable chest radiograph of 22-year-old spinal cord patient with endotracheal tube in proper position. There is *atelectasis* of right upper lobe. Bronchoscopy revealed thick, tenacious mucus occluding RUL bronchus. **B,** Seventy-two hours later, there has been complete reexpansion of right upper lobe atelectasis, but atelectasis and infiltrate are now present in left lower lobe. After second bronchoscopy, endotracheal tube was removed and no further atelectatic changes occurred.

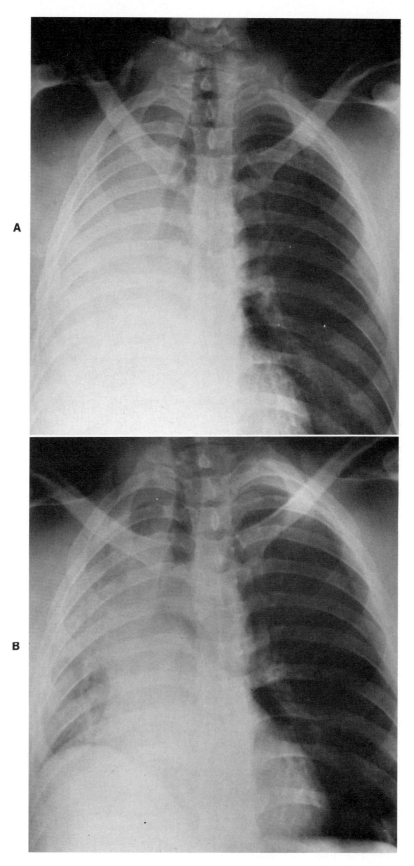

Fig. 8-20. A, Right-sided atelectasis in 34-year-old C7-T1 dislocation quadriplegic man injured in automobile accident. **B,** Twenty-four hours later, following bronchoscopy and removal of a mucous plug, there is partial aeration of atelectatic lung but still shift of mediastinum and elevation of right hemidiaphragm.

REFERENCES

1. Brisman, R., and Clemmer, T.: Pulmonary hemodynamics and intracranial hypertension, Proc. Am. Assoc. Neurol. Surg., no. 57, 1973.
2. Burke, D. C., and Murray, D. D.: Handbook of spinal cord medicine, New York, 1975, Raven Press, pp. 32-33.
3. Calenoff, L., and Kruglik, G. D.: Implanted radio-frequency electonic stimulators, Am. J. Roentgenol. **124:**1-6, 1975.
4. Calenoff, L., Kruglik, G. D., and Woodruff, A.: Unilateral pulmonary edema, Radiology **126:**19-24, 1978.
5. Davies, D., and Hopkins, J. A.: Patterns in traumatic rupture of the bronchus, Injury **4:**261-264, 1973.
6. Eijgelaar, A., and van der Heide, J. H. N.: A reliable early symptom of bronchial or tracheal rupture, Thorax **25:**120-125, 1970.
7. Fagan, C. J., and Swischuk, L. E.: Traumatic lung and paramediastinal pneumatoceles, Radiology **120:**11-18, 1976.
8. Forker, A. D., and Morgan, J. R.: Acquired coronary artery fistula from non-penetrating chest injury, J.A.M.A. **215:**289-291, 1971.
9. Fugel-Meyer, A. R.: The respiratory system. In Handbook of neurology, New York, 1976, American Publishing Co., pp. 335-337.
10. Guttman, L.: Respiratory disturbances. In Spinal cord injuries, Oxford, England, 1973, Blackwell Scientific Publications, pp. 182-193.
11. Guttman, L., and Bell: Suspension therapy. In Hollis, M., and Roper, M., editors: Suspension therapy in rehabilitation, London, 1958, Ballière, Tindale Publishers, pp. 107-108.
12. Hemmingway, A., Bors, E., and Hobby, R. P.: An investigation of the pulmonary function of paraplegics, J. Clin. Invest. **37:**773-782, 1958.
13. Lehmus, H. F., Sundquist, A. B., and Giddings, L. W.: Coronary thrombosis with myocardial infarction secondary to nonpenetrating injury to the chest wall, Am. Heart. J. **47:**470-473, 1954.
14. Lotz, P. R., Martel, W., Rohwedder, J. J., and Green, R. A.: Significance of pneumomediastinum in blunt trauma to the thorax, A.J.R. **132:**817-819, 1979.
15. Mintzer, R. A., Hendrix, R. W., Johnson, C. J., and Neiman, H. L.: The radiologic significance of the left pulmonary ligament: experience with 26 patients, Chest **76:**401-405, 1979.
16. Parmley, L. F., Manion, W. C., and Mattingly, T. W.: Nonpenetrating traumatic injury of the heart, Circulation **18:**371-396, 1958.
17. Payne, W. S., and DeRemee, R. A.: Injuries of the trachea and major bronchi, Postgrad. Med. **49:**152-158, 1971.
18. Silbiger, M. L., and Kushner, L. N.: Tracheobronchial perforation: its diagnosis and treatment, Radiology **85:**242-246, 1965.
19. Silver, J. R.: Prophylactic anticoagulant therapy in the prevention of pulmonary emboli in patients with acute spinal injuries. Presentation at the Annual Clinical Spinal Cord Injuries Conference, 1971, pp. 154-186.
20. Teplitz, C.: The core pathology and integrated medical science of adult respiratory insufficiency, Surg. Clin. North Am. **56:**1091, 1976.
21. Wilson, R. F., Murray, C., and Antonerko, D. R.: Nonpenetrating thoracic injury, Surg. Clin. North Am. **5:**16, 1977.
22. Wisc, L., Connorl, J., Hwang, Y. N., et al.: Traumatic injuries to the diaphragm, J. Trauma **13:**946, 1973.
23. Yashon, D.: Spinal injury, New York, 1978, Appleton-Century-Crofts, pp. 277-281.
24. Zylak, C. J.: Radiologic aspects of thoracic trauma syllabus. Radiology of the chest. Presentation at the Sixty-fourth Scientific Meeting of the R.S.N.A., 1978.

CHAPTER 9

Gastrointestinal complications

RICHARD M. GORE, M.D., and RICHARD A. MINTZER, M.D.

Gastrointestinal complications occur with distressing frequency in patients with spinal cord injuries. The diagnosis and treatment of these abnormalities pose a challenge because the profound neurologic deficit diminishes visceral sensitivity and alters the physiologic parameters (i.e., pulse, blood pressure) on which one relies for diagnosis. As overall mortality has declined with improvements in the immediate postinjury care and respiratory and genitourinary management, previously unrecognized alimentary tract pathology is becoming apparent and now accounts for up to 10% of fatalities among spinal cord injured patients.[7,22]

Every segment of the gastrointestinal tract can be a site of complication. Serious complications, including ileus, peptic ulcer disease with hemorrhage and perforation, gastric dilatation, and pancreatitis, generally occur during the immediate postinjury period. Fecal impaction, the superior mesenteric artery syndrome, amyloidosis, and the precocious appearance of hiatus hernia, gastroesophageal reflux, and diverticulosis may be seen as chronic complications of spinal cord injury.

Early detection of these abnormalities is essential but is frequently hampered by the nonspecificity of the signs and symptoms of abdominal pathology in the spinal cord injured patient. This justifies a vigorous diagnostic approach that may include plain films, various contrast examinations, ultrasonography, computed tomography, angiography, or whatever modality seems appropriate in a given clinical setting.[13] We will review the experience of others collected from the literature and will present an overview of our own experience with the gastrointestinal complications that have been encountered in the spinal cord injured patients at the Midwest Regional Spinal Cord Injury Care System and the Rehabilitation Institute of Chicago.

VISCERAL INNERVATION

A basic understanding of the innervation of the gastrointestinal tract is vital to an appreciation of the spectrum of visceral complications of spinal cord injury. Although the alimentary tract has an inherent automaticity that is mediated by various hormones, peptides, and the intrinsic plexuses of Meissner and Auerbach, profound and often pathologic changes result when external nervous input is withdrawn.[2,14] The first and last portions of the gastrointestinal tract are controlled by voluntary muscles and reflexes, that is, the voluntary muscles for mastication and deglutition and the external anal sphincter. The intervening gut receives sympathetic and parasympathetic innervation from the autonomic nervous system (Fig. 9-1). Imbalances between the two components of the autonomic system and release of the external anal sphincter from central control are responsible for the majority of gastrointestinal complications in the spinal cord injured patient.

Parasympathetic innervation of the stomach, small bowel, and proximal one half to two thirds of the colon is supplied by the vagus nerve. The descending colon, sigmoid, and rectum are subserved by the pelvic nerves originating in the sacral segments S2-4 (Fig. 9-1).[2,14]

Since the vagus and pelvic nerves usually survive injury, parasympathetic activity is preserved in spinal cord injured patients, although the pelvic nerves are released from central control.[14] Sympathetic input, however, is usually disrupted since the preganglionic fibers are located in the thoracolumbar intermediomedial and intermediolateral cell column of the spinal cord from T4 to L2.[2,14] The degree of separation of the gastrointestinal tract from central sympathetic control is determined by the level of spinal cord injury up to the level of T4-6, above which separation is complete.

Spinal cord injury therefore results in unchallenged parasympathetic activity up to the region of the transverse colon distal to which the pelvic parasympathetic nerves act independently. Since parasympathetic stimulation enhances intestinal tone, relaxes junctional sphincters (i.e., cardia, pylorus, ileocecal valve), and stimulates glandular secretion,[2] it is not surprising that peptic ulcer disease, gastroesophageal reflux, and pancreatitis complicate spinal cord injury. The fact that the stimulatory effect of the vagus nerve terminates at the transverse colon also explains the occurrence of high fecal impactions peculiar to spinal cord injured patients. The more distal colon, subserved by the pelvic nerves, does not receive the stimulus to peristalsis from the vagus nerve and thus tends to have more sluggish motility.[2]

Since the impulses that subserve visceral reflexes and carry painful sensations (ischemia, excessive stretch, violent contraction) are transmitted by sympathetic fibers, these warning, homeostatic signals are lost after injury.[22] This makes patient awareness and clinical diagnosis of abdominal abnormalities most difficult. The problem is compounded by the fact that reflexes, abdominal muscle tone, heart rate, and temperature, important clinical parameters on which one relies for diagnosis, are often altered in these situations even in the absence of alimentary tract pathology.[7] For this reason, radiology assumes a critical role in the early diagnosis of gastrointestinal disorders in the spinal cord injured patient.

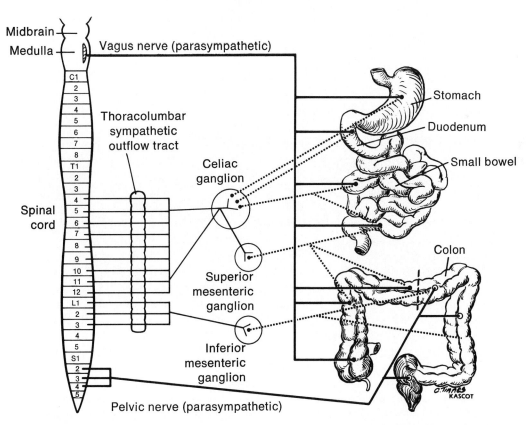

Fig. 9-1. Diagram of visceral innervation. Thick solid lines are parasympathetic fibers; dotted and thin solid lines represent sympathetic fibers. Preganglionic neurons are shown as solid lines and postganglionic neurons as dotted lines.

RADIOLOGIC STUDIES

A chest radiograph and plain film of the abdomen should routinely be obtained on all patients with suspected abdominal pathology. The chest film will not only identify certain lung abnormalities such as pulmonary embolism or pneumonia, which may symptomatically simulate an intra-abdominal process, but also will demonstrate the presence of a pneumoperitoneum if the chest film is done in the upright position. The abdominal film may demonstrate the presence of ileus, obstruction, nephrolithiasis, cholelithiasis, pancreatitis, fecal impaction, or perforation.

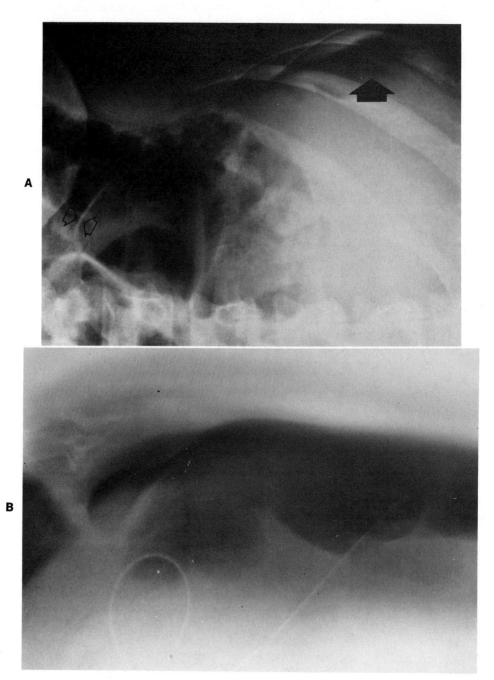

Fig. 9-2. A, Extraluminal gas *(large arrow)* collected between liver and abdominal wall in left lateral decubitus film. Pneumoperitoneum was unexpected finding in this 21-year-old C5 quadriplegic patient with vague abdominal pain in whom a perforated ulcer was subsequently found at laparotomy. Note air outlining of both walls of intestine *(small arrows).* **B,** Pneumoperitoneum evident on portable cross-table lateral film. Patient was a 77-year-old man with hangman's fracture and perforated duodenal ulcer.

Perforation of a viscus with subsequent peritonitis is the most common gastrointestinal cause of death in the spinal cord injured patient; thus every effort should be made to establish the presence of free intraperitoneal air.[7,17] The upright chest film is the most sensitive radiologic examination for the demonstration of pneumoperitoneum, but this view is frequently unobtainable in the patient with acute injuries. In these instances, small volumes of free intraperitoneal air can be detected with a left lateral decubitus view of the abdomen. The patient should remain in the left side dependent position for 5 minutes before the radiograph is taken. This allows time for free air to accumulate between the lateral margin of the liver and the abdominal wall (Fig. 9-2, A). Decubitus films will also demonstrate air-fluid levels, important considerations when ileus or obstruction is suspected (Fig. 9-2, B).

When only a supine film is available pneumoperitoneum can occasionally be recognized if the air outlines both the inner and outer walls of the intestines, outlines the falciform ligament to suggest the seams of a football, or outlines the lateral umbilical ligaments in the pelvic region appearing as an inverted V (Fig. 9-3). Menuck and Siemers[20] have noted that more commonly, intraperitoneal air is visible as a linear or triangular lucency in the right upper quadrant. This lucency at the posterior inferior liver margin or projected over the superior margin of the kidney represents free air in the right anterior subhepatic space or its posterior extension (Morison's pouch).

Appropriate additional radiologic procedures (i.e., contrast examinations, ultrasonography, computed tomography, radionuclide scans) should be obtained following thorough evaluation of the plain films. Ultrasonograms, iodine-containing contrast examinations, and radionuclide scans should precede barium sulfate studies, since residual barium will reduce the diagnostic yield of these examinations.

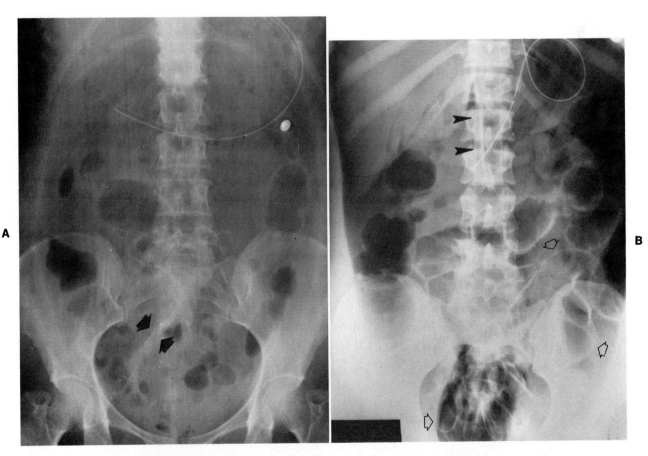

Fig. 9-3. *Pneumoperitoneum.* **A,** Intraperitoneal air outlines right umbilical ligament *(arrows)* and gives "football" appearance to abdomen on supine film of this T4 paraplegic patient with abdominal pain caused by perforated gastric ulcer. **B,** Unsuspected massive pneumoperitoneum demonstrated on plain abdominal film. Note excellent visualization of both walls of intestines *(arrows)* and outlining of falciform ligament *(arrowheads)*. Perforated gastric ulcer was found at laparotomy.

Methods for performing contrast studies on spinal cord injured patients

Despite the obvious difficulties in performing any diagnostic procedure in the spinal cord injured patient, very satisfactory studies can be obtained. The success of the examination depends more on the adequacy of preparation than on patient mobility. Retained gastric secretions and fecal material are the nemesis of diagnostic contrast studies in these patients. A clear liquid diet for at least 2 to 3 days accompanied by mild laxatives and the liberal use of cleansing enemas should be used as preparation for the lower gastrointestinal series. In preparing for the upper gastrointestinal examination or ultrasonography, the length of restriction of oral intake must take into account the diminished gastric motility frequently seen in these patients, and intravenous hydration should be considered in some instances.

Upper gastrointestinal examinations should begin in the right lateral decubitus position, since this position permits filling of the duodenum and minimizes the risk of aspiration. Once the patient has completed ingestion of the barium preparation, spot films of the duodenum may be obtained in the decubitus position and the remainder of the examination may proceed normally.

When performing oral cholecystography, the administration of contrast pills must take into account the sluggish motility and delayed gastric emptying frequently encountered in the spinal cord injured patient. The patient should be placed in the right lateral decubitus position for several hours after contrast ingestion to encourage gastric emptying and avoid the pooling of contrast material in the gastric fundus (Fig. 9-4).

The barium enema examination only requires very slight alterations when studying the spinal cord injured patient. A digital rectal examination will establish the presence of feces and give some indication as to the competency and size of the anal sphincter. A Bardex balloon-type enema tip should be used routinely especially in patients who have had trauma to the sacral plexuses because the rectum is usually patulous. The barium should be administered from a closed plastic bag rather than from a barium can because the former facilitates barium evacuation for the postevacuation film. The examination may otherwise proceed in a normal fashion, and large spot films (i.e., 10 × 12 in, 14 × 14 in) should be used to salvage as much information as possible in patients who often are unable to retain the enema for any great length of time. Evacua-

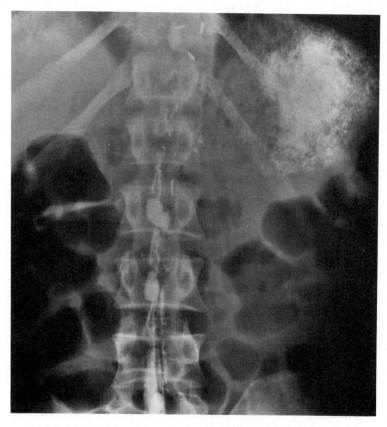

Fig. 9-4. Nonvisualization of gallbladder in 32-year-old C7 quadriplegic. Note pooling of contrast medium in gastric fundus. Patient was not placed in right lateral decubitus position after contrast ingestion.

tion is performed by placing the barium bag below the level of the fluoroscopic table. The patient's clinical status should be carefully monitored during the barium enema examination, particularly when there is a history of autonomic dysreflexia as described in Chapter 20.

ACUTE GASTROINTESTINAL COMPLICATIONS
Ileus

Reflex ileus is the most common gastrointestinal complication of the acute stage of spinal cord injury. It is related to the period of spinal shock in which there is a generalized diminution of reflex activity producing a disruption in the intrinsic rhythmicity of the intestines. This transient depression in segments distal to the cord lesion is caused by the sudden withdrawal of the predominantly facilitative or excitatory influences of supraspinal centers from the spinal cord.[14] Ileus accom-

panied by fecal retention is especially common when cord transection occurs at or above the level of segmental innervation of the abdominal viscera, generally considered to be T5 to L2.[14]

The duration, extent, and time of onset of ileus depend on the level and completeness of injury. Ileus is generally present immediately after thoracolumbar cord injury, but its onset may be delayed 24 hours in midthoracic lesions and up to 48 hours in cervical injuries.[5,11] Ileus usually lasts 3 to 4 days but persists up to 7 days in patients with cervical lesions.[11] The severity and duration of ileus are usually greater in patients with cervical lesions and are usually more severe in complete as opposed to incomplete cord transection.[5,11]

In the absence of peritoneal inflammation, paralytic ileus radiographically manifests as generalized gas and fluid distention of the entire gastrointestinal tract (Fig.

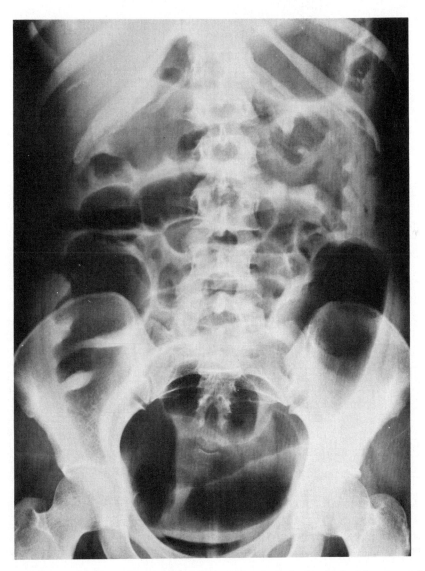

Fig. 9-5. Adynamic ileus in 22-year-old woman with spinal shock who had fractures of C5, T12, and L2. Note dilated small bowel loops and colon.

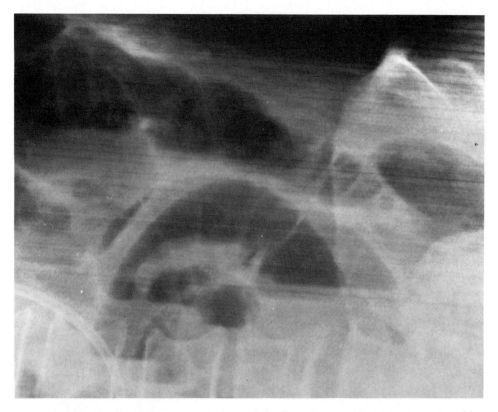

Fig. 9-6. Adynamic ileus of acute stage of spinal shock in 59-year-old quadriplegic. Portable decubitus film reveals air-fluid levels in multiple loops.

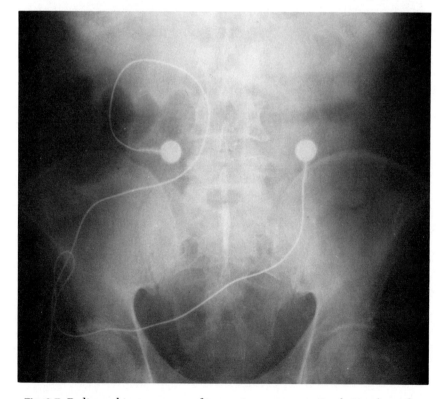

Fig. 9-7. Radiographic appearance of transcutaneous neurostimulation electrodes.

9-5). Differentiation from mechanical obstruction may be difficult especially in patients who have undergone abdominal surgery for associated injuries. The colon often shows a relatively greater degree of distention than the small bowel in ileus, and postural films show air-fluid levels that tend to be on the same level in each loop (Fig. 9-6). This is in contrast to mechanical obstruction in which the air-fluid levels are more prominent and are at different levels in the same loop. There is also greater distention of the small intestine in obstruction. Sequential films will show little change in patients with paralytic ileus but may show marked changes when obstruction is present. In the absence of surgery, however, bowel obstruction is uncommon in the immediate postinjury period since insufficient time has elapsed for the formation of fecal impaction.

In patients with an upper thoracic or cervical cord lesion, ileus represents a potentially fatal complication. A distended viscus interferes with diaphragmatic excursion, greatly increasing the respiratory distress in patients already compromised by paralysis of the intercostal and abdominal muscles. Indeed, aspiration of vomitus from an unrecognized ileus is probably the most common cause of sudden death in the quadriplegic patient in the first 48 hours after injury.[3] The patient is unable to cough adequately, and sudden death may result from respiratory failure. Another serious complication of ileus is deposition of large volumes of fluid and electrolytes in the gut, so-called "third spacing," which

may lead to electrolyte imbalance and dehydration. Nasogastric suction and vigorous intravenous replacement are imperative to reduce gut distention and the risk of vomiting.

The incidence of paralytic ileus is so high and its attendant risks so large that transcutaneous electrical neurostimulation is now routinely used as prophylaxis during the period of spinal shock at the Midwest Regional Spinal Cord Injury Care Center. In this protocol, intermittent currents are transmitted through small electrodes attached to the abdominal wall (Fig. 9-7). By enhancing spinal reflex activity, neurostimulation has demonstrated gratifying results in the reduction of gastrointestinal complications during the period of spinal shock, for example, avoidance of the nasogastric tube entirely or its early discontinuance, prevention of ileus and gastric dilatation, and prevention of stasis of fluid in the alimentary tract.[31] The incidence of paralytic ileus has declined at this center from 15% to 1% or 2% of spinal cord injuries at all levels since the addition of transcutaneous neurostimulation to the immediate care protocol.[31]

Acute gastric dilatation

Following upper thoracic and cervical cord injury, acute dilatation of the stomach often occurs with or without a generalized ileus. Two factors are believed to be responsible for this complication: one anatomic and the other neurologic. In the immediate postinjury pe-

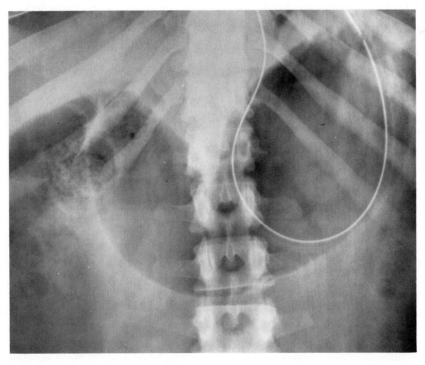

Fig. 9-8. Gastric dilatation with very little gas present distally in 36-year-old man several hours after T3 cord injury resulting in paraplegia.

riod, patients with spinal cord injury may be placed in a body cast or be kept in a hyperextended position for stabilization of a vertebral fracture. This may cause compression of the midtransverse duodenum against the aorta by the superior mesenteric artery, the so-called body cast syndrome.[1,10] This phenomenon will be discussed in greater detail in the section on the superior mesenteric artery syndrome. This anatomic feature, when combined with the reflex inhibition of peripheral gastric motor activity mediated by the vagus nerve, results in acute gastric dilatation.[1] As in the case of ileus, massive gastric dilatation may cause respiratory distress by compromise of diaphragmatic excursion or by aspiration of vomitus.

Radiologic recognition and prompt decompression are urgent in this complication. The abdominal film demonstrates a huge gastric shadow containing air, fluid, and retained food. Frequently, air can be seen in the duodenal bulb as well (Fig. 9-8). When the patient is supine, the fluid-filled stomach may appear as a large upper abdominal mass displacing the intestines caudad. When large amounts of fluid are present, the entire stomach may be outlined.

Peptic ulcer disease, hemorrhage, and perforation

Although the association of peptic ulcer and central nervous system disease was first made by Rokitansky in 1841, it was not until 1933 that gastric ulceration was first acknowledged as a complication of spinal cord injury.[25] Since that time there have been sporadic reports attesting to the increased incidence of peptic ulcer disease in spinal cord injuries, figures ranging between 3% and 51%.[5,21,25,27,30] The discrepancy in statistics relates to the severity and level of cord damage, the presence of associated injuries, the history of surgery, and the presence of renal abnormalities. Peptic ulcer disease is observed in both the acute and chronic stages of spinal cord injury.

Acute peptic ulceration occurs in 3% to 7% of acute spinal cord injuries and is indicated by acute gastrointestinal hemorrhage.[5] Although pale or hyperemic mucosal changes can be observed endoscopically within 24 hours of severe trauma, most patients seen are 6 to 19 days after injury with multiple superficial erosions along the greater curvature of the stomach, so-called stress ulcers.[11,25] These ulcers may not only cover the entire gastric mucosa but involve the esophagus and duodenum as well. Fiberoptic endoscopy appears to be the diagnostic procedure of choice in the detection of these stress ulcers since they are beneath the resolution of standard barium studies. Double-contrast techniques are impractical in these patients, many of whom are on Stryker frames. Early recognition is vital since the mor-

tality from this complication can be as high as 15% to 20% and even higher in children.[5]

Perforation of a peptic ulcer is often related to injudicious nasogastric tube placement and represents a disastrous complication in the spinal cord injured patient. Since 25% of perforated ulcers do not demonstrate pneumoperitoneum, contrast studies may be needed to document the presence and site of perforation. Water-soluble iodinated contrast material rather than barium sulfate should be administered through a nasogastric tube, since the latter has a tendency to form peritoneal granulomas and adhesions in the event of perforation. No more than 60 to 100 cc of contrast material should be used so as to facilitate removal and to minimize the risk of dehydration from the osmotic sequestering of intravascular fluid in the gut by the very hyperosmolar tri-iodinated contrast agents employed.

The etiology of stress ulcers is unclear. They may be in part caused by endogenous steroids released after trauma or therapeutically administered steroids given to reduce spinal cord edema. Parasympathetic-sympathetic imbalance has also been implicated, since after complete cord transection all inhibitory sympathetic influences are lost, which leaves the vagal action unopposed.[3,20,25,33] This leads to increased gastrin secretion and hydrochloric acid production, as well as mucosal vasodilation, excellent substrates for ulcer disease.[3,20,25] Indeed, Pollack and Finkelman[28] observed a significant elevation of gastric acidity in 19.8% of a group of paraplegics. This finding was only seen in patients with lesions at or above the lower level of gastric sympathetic input, T5, which may explain the higher incidence of peptic ulcer disease observed in patients with cervical injuries, placed as high as 22% in one series, as compared to those patients with lesions below T5 (3% to 6%).[5,20,27]

To decrease the incidence of peptic ulcer disease during the acute stage of spinal injury, intravenous cimetidine, 300 mg four times daily, and the periodic administration of antacids through the nasogastric tube have been added to the acute spinal cord injury protocol at the Midwest Regional Spinal Cord Injury Care Center.

Pancreatitis

Pancreatic dysfunction is occasionally seen in patients with spinal cord injury.[6] This condition is frequently overlooked because the neurologic deficit often precludes patient appreciation of epigastric pain and because of the nonspecificity of the clinical and radiologic signs. Ileus, abdominal distention, fever, protracted nausea, and vomiting, although signs of pancreatitis, are more commonly the direct result of spinal cord injury.

Ultrasonography and computed tomography are helpful in the radiologic evaluation of these patients and are frequently diagnostic. Unfortunately there is often an abundance of gastric and intestinal gas even in the healthy, compensated spinal cord injured patient so that ultrasound visualization of the pancreas is difficult. The presence of significant quantities of gas in the stomach, small bowel, and colon must be viewed with suspicion (i.e., ileus, obstruction), but it should be kept in mind that these patients often normally have gassy abdomens (Fig. 9-9).

On ultrasound examination, acute pancreatitis is most commonly seen as a generalized enlargement of the gland. With influx of inflammatory edema, the pan-creas, which is normally more echogenic than the liver, becomes less echogenic than the liver. The edema also increases through transmission and produces strong back wall shadows (Fig. 9-10). Ultrasonography is ideal for identification of pancreatic pseudocysts.

In those patients in whom ultrasonography is nondiagnostic, computed tomography is necessary. Acute pancreatitis is characterized by a generalized enlargement of the pancreas and influx of fluid producing a decrease in the attenuation number (Fig. 9-11). Inflammatory edema or thickening of the peripancreatic fascial planes is often seen. Chronic and severe pancreatitis may produce obliteration of fat planes around the major vascular structures.

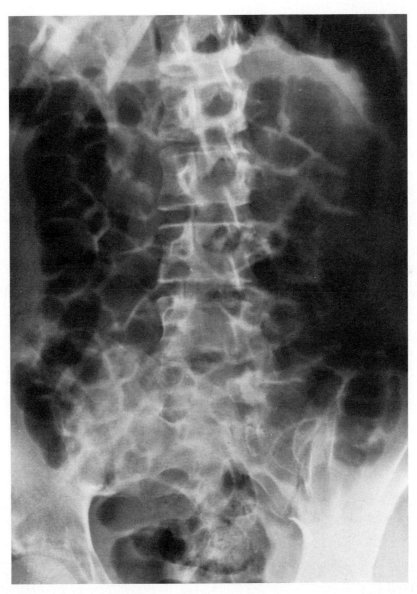

Fig. 9-9. Typical, nonobstructive "gassy abdomen" frequently observed in stabilized, healthy spinal cord injury patients. Patient is a well-compensated 16-year-old C6 quadriplegic girl.

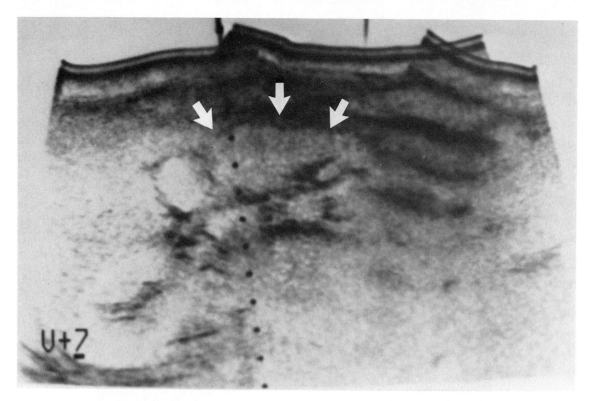

Fig. 9-10. Classic ultrasound characteristics of acute pancreatitis with enlargement of entire pancreas *(arrows)* and fewer than normal internal echoes.

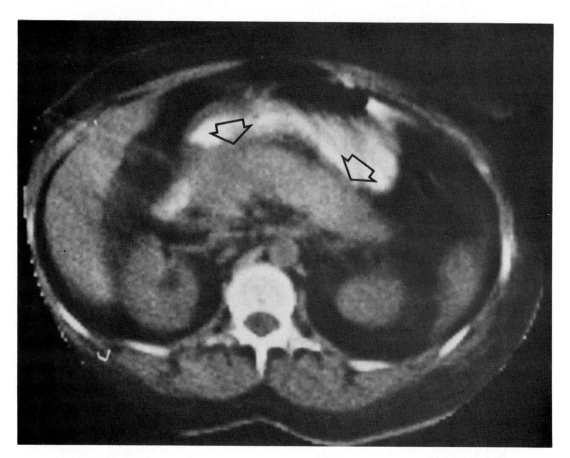

Fig. 9-11. Acute pancreatitis. CT scan showing markedly enlarged pancreas *(arrows)* and decreased attenuation of head.

The proposed mechanism of pancreatitis in spinal cord injury is related to sympathetic-parasympathetic imbalance, which results in overstimulation in the sphincter of Oddi and the production of viscid but enzymatically potent pancreatic juices. This leads to stasis and ultimately pancreatitis.[26]

Acute abdomen

The profound motor and sensory impairment in the spinal cord injured patient makes recognition and evaluation of the acute abdomen difficult. The early pain of abdominal distress in the spinal cord injured patient is dull, oppressive, and poorly localized and may be indicated only by a vague complaint of something wrong in the abdomen.[15,22] This is usually preceded by a subtle loss of appetite and nausea. The pain may be (1) abdominal or referred to a distant site sharing the same embryonic or neurologic segment as the viscera; (2) from the stomach, duodenum, and gallbladder to the interscapular area; (3) from the diaphragm, liver, or spleen to the neck or shoulder mantle; or (4) from the appendix to the periumbilical region.[23] A neurogenic origin of the pain can usually be excluded because in this condition the pain is sharp, knifelike, and often bilateral.[12,15,22]

The differential diagnosis of abdominal distress in the spinal cord injured patient includes acute pyelonephritis, fecal impaction, obstruction, appendicitis, abdominal abscess, rupture of the urinary bladder, peptic ulcer disease, pancreatitis, gallbaldder disease, and perforation.[16,26] If the plain chest and abdominal films do not suggest a diagnosis, an intravenous urogram should then be performed to exclude genitourinary tract pathology. Calculi and obstruction will be readily apparent on the intravenous urogram. One fourth of patients with acute pyelonephritis demonstrate radiologic abnormalities including renal enlargement, diminished pyelogram, inhomogeneous nephrogram, or striations of the ureter and pelvis.

Peptic ulcer disease and pancreatitis are investigated as described earlier. Acute cholecystitis can be readily identified using either ultrasonography or the nuclear medicine study ^{99m}Tc-HIDA scan. Gallstones are indicated by a strong echo producing masses within the dependent portion of the gallbladder on ultrasound examination (Fig. 9-12). In the majority of cases a characteristic acoustic shadow is produced posterior to the stone, the result of almost complete absorption of the incident beam. Gallstones characteristically migrate to the dependent portion of the gallbladder.

Recently ^{99m}Tc-HIDA (technetium 99m dimethyl acetanilide iminodiacetic acid) cholescintigraphy has been

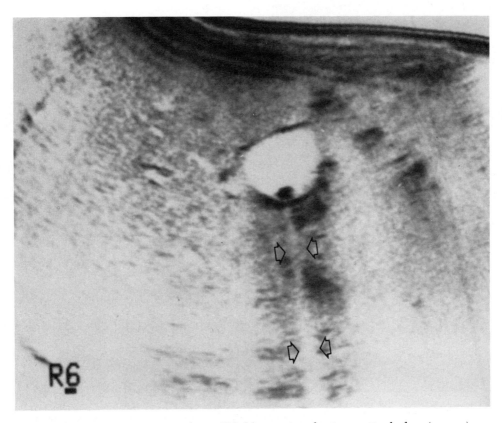

Fig. 9-12. Gallstone present within gallbladder causing classic acoustic shadow (arrows).

added to the diagnostic armamentarium. This radionuclide technique is discussed in Chapter 19.

CHRONIC GASTROINTESTINAL COMPLICATIONS
Neurogenic colon

After the period of spinal shock, the return of peristalsis and bowel sounds is accompanied by the appearance of the defecation reflex, a reflex spinal arc in which skin stimulation about the perineum will cause automatic rectal emptying.[14] This occurs in patients with lesions above the sacral segments. Normal control and sensitivity, of course, will be lost and the external anal sphincter will become hypertrophic and spastic as in any upper motor neuron lesion.[14] In a lower motor neuron lesion caused by a lumbosacral injury, the sacral segments of the defecation reflex are lost and the external anal sphincter becomes patulous.[14]

At the beginning of bowel training, a complete contrast radiologic examination of the alimentary tract is indicated. This will reveal previously unsuspected congenital or acquired abnormalities, such as diverticulosis, enteroptosis, megacolon, or chronic gastric or duodenal ulcer, all of which may adversely affect the reconditioning of the gastrointestinal tract.[14] The techniques for these examinations have been previously described.

Fecal impaction is the most frequent gastrointestinal tract complication of chronic spinal cord injury. Patients with lesions in the cervical, thoracic, and upper lumbar region tend to have proximal obstruction particularly at the level of the transverse colon (Fig. 9-13, *B*), whereas lumbosacral lesions are frequently associated with rectal impaction (Fig. 9-13, *A*).[11] The proximal impaction is explained by the fact that the transverse colon is the boundary between vagal and pelvic nerve control; vagal stimulation promotes peristalsis, but this impetus is lost in the more distal colon, which is subserved by the pelvic nerves (Fig. 9-1). Lesions of the sacral segments are associated with fecal retention because the defecation reflex is lost. In cauda equina lesions, rectal stagnation results from paralysis of the pelvic musculature.

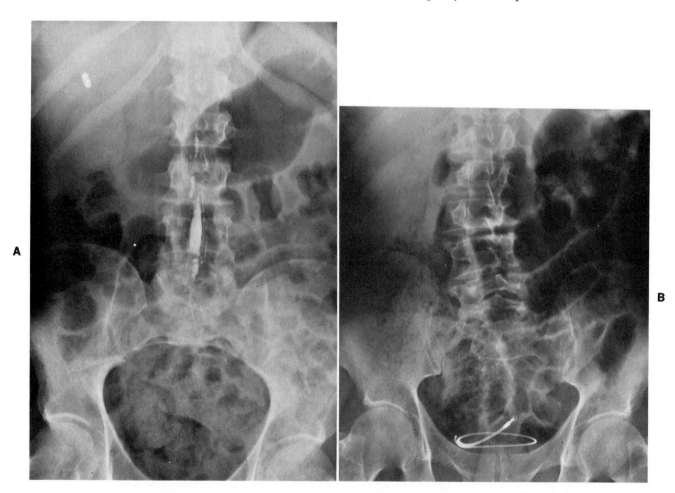

Fig. 9-13. Fecal impaction. **A,** Rectal impaction in 44-year-old man with cauda equina syndrome. **B,** "High" proximal fecal impaction with small bowel dilatation in 64-year-old man with paraplegia.

Radiographically, fecal impaction may be recognized by the bubbly appearance of feces in the region of the transverse colon or rectum with proximal dilatation. Impaction not infrequently will cause obstruction to the retrograde flow of barium on the lower gastrointestinal series (Fig. 9-14).

Peptic ulcer disease

An increased incidence of peptic ulcer disease is found among spinal cord injured patients during the chronic stage of their disability. In a recent prospective study, gastroduodenal endoscopic abnormalities, including mucosal congestion, submucosal hemorrhages, erosions, ulcerations of gastric mucosa, as well as duodenal ulcers, were observed in 51.4% of patients.[30]

In contrast to the predominantly gastric location of the ulcers occurring during the immediate stage of injury, most ulcers seen over the long term are located in the duodenum.[4] Declining renal function secondary to recurrent infections and vesicoureteral reflux, unopposed vagal-parasympathetic activity producing hypersecretion of gastric juice, bile reflux, ingestion of an-

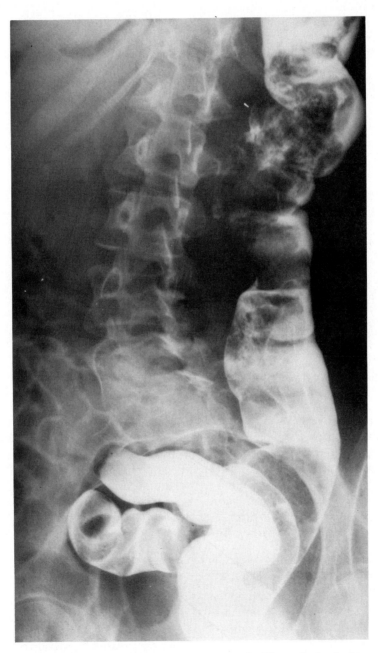

Fig. 9-14. Fecal impaction causing obstruction to retrograde filling of colon by barium enema at splenic flexure in 20-year-old T7 paraplegic woman.

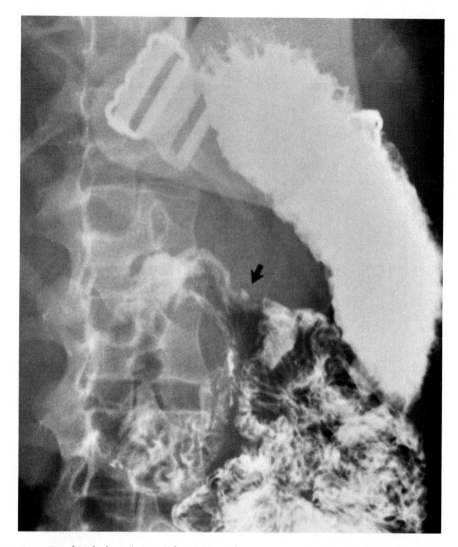

Fig. 9-15. Duodenal ulcer *(arrow)* demonstrated on upper gastrointestinal series in 17-year-old C6 quadriplegic girl with nausea and vomiting.

ti-inflammatory drugs for muscle aches, and calcium metabolism abnormalities have been implicated in the etiology of peptic ulcer disease in these patients.[4,5,8,14]

The duodenal ulcers of the spinal cord injured patient are radiographically identical to those found in the general population, with an ulcer crater surrounded by thickened folds often in a radiating pattern. When seen in profile, the ulcer appears as a niche of barium projecting beyond the bulb (Fig. 9-15).

Superior mesenteric artery syndrome

Recurrent occlusion of the third portion of the duodenum by vascular compression of the superior mesenteric artery, the superior mesenteric artery syndrome or arteriomesenteric occlusion of the duodenum, may occur in both the acute and chronic stages of spinal cord injury. The etiology of this syndrome remains partially obscure but is related to a small vascular angle as the superior mesenteric artery takes origin from the abdominal aorta at the level of the first lumbar vertebra.[10,29] In its downward course the superior mesenteric artery crosses the duodenum and may cause compression of the midtransverse portion against the aorta.

This vascular angle may be reduced congenitally, but certain acquired predisposing factors have been identified: loss of retroperitoneal fat, exaggerated lumbar lordosis, laxity of the muscle tone of the abdominal wall, and excessive traction on the mesentery by the small bowel.[10,29,32]

Acutely the superior mesenteric artery syndrome is usually related to a body cast or hyperlordosis of the lumbar spine (Fig. 9-16).[1] This situation was previously described in the section on the body cast syndrome.

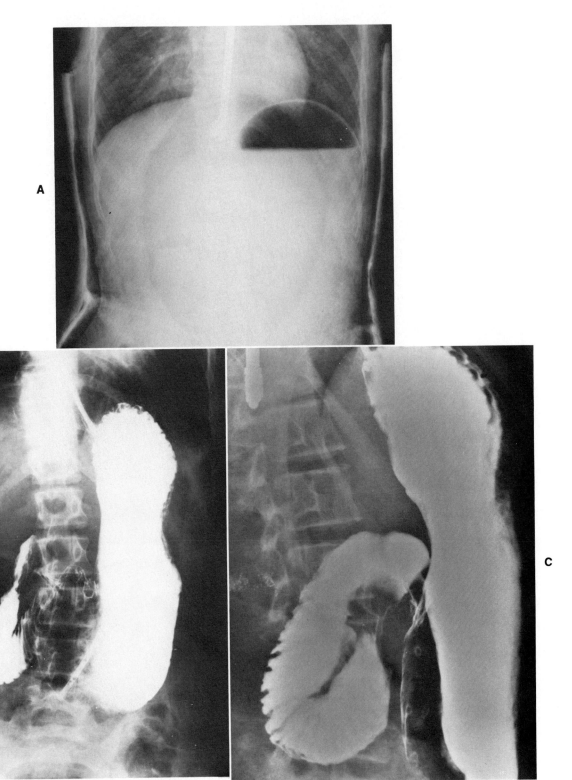

Fig. 9-16. Body cast syndrome in 12-year-old girl with abrupt onset of vomiting 1 day after application of body cast. **A,** Upright plain film shows air-fluid levels in stomach and duodenum. Lucent area represents window in cast. **B** and **C,** Upper gastrointestinal studies demonstrate obstruction with verticle linear extrinsic pressure defect of third portion of duodenum.

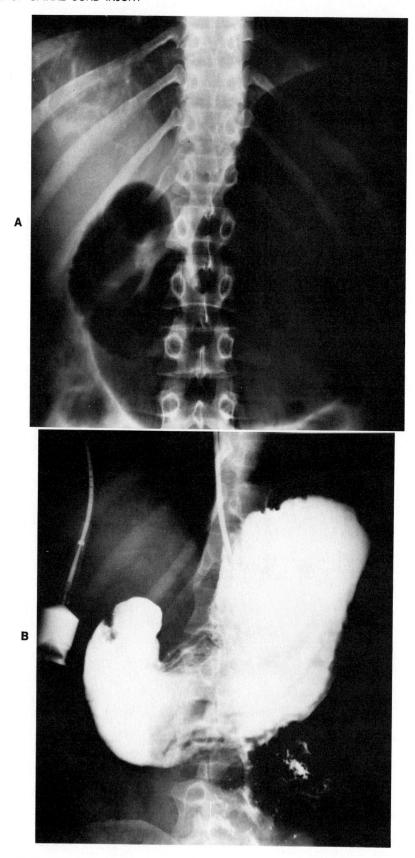

Fig. 9-17. Superior mesenteric artery syndrome in 27-year-old C5 quadriplegic woman who lost 30% of her body weight after injury. **A,** Plain supine abdominal film shows massive gastric dilatation. **B,** Upper gastrointestinal examination shows retention of barium in stomach.

Arteriomesenteric occlusion of the duodenum may occur more chronically and insidiously, especially in the chronically debilitated patient, for example, severe burn victims and patients with spinal cord injury (Fig. 9-17).[11,29,32] It is postulated that the severe wasting and weight loss so prevalent in these conditions reduce the retroperitoneal areolar tissue around the duodenum, decreasing the vascular angle.[29,32] When this diminutive vascular angle is accompanied by prolonged periods in the supine position, recurrent duodenal occlusion may occur.

Clinically the superior mesenteric artery syndrome is heralded by pernicious vomiting, which is usually sudden and copious.[10] Chronically these patients have nausea, vomiting, and distention 1 to 2 hours postprandially. Food increases the weight of the small intestine, which places traction on the mesentery, further decreasing the vascular angle.[10,29]

Radiographically the diagnosis can frequently be made on the plain film by demonstrating a markedly dilated stomach containing food and fluid (Figs. 9-16, A, and 9-17, A). Barium contrast studies reveal dilatation of the first and second portions of the duodenum associated with a vertical linear extrinsic pressure defect of the third portion (Figs. 9-16, B, and 9-17, B). The lumen is narrowed and compressed, but the mucosal folds remain intact. Retention of the barium is noted in the stomach and duodenum, and there frequently is a to-and-fro motion of the barium as it is refluxed into the stomach. A categorical diagnosis can be made by placing the patient in the left lateral decubitus position, prone position, or knee-chest position, thus reducing the drag of the mesentery on the duodenum. In these positions the duodenal contents should drain promptly. A resumption of the supine position should reproduce the radiologic abnormalities.

Prompt recognition of this entity is essential because sudden relaxation of the cardia may result in vomiting with aspiration and cardiac arrest.[10,29]

The treatment of superior mesenteric artery syndrome is conservative, with avoidance of the supine position after meals and upward manual displacement of the abdominal muscles with adequate support of the abdominal wall.[10,29] In the acute situation, gastric decompression is necessary. If conservative measures fail, a surgical bypass procedure may be needed.

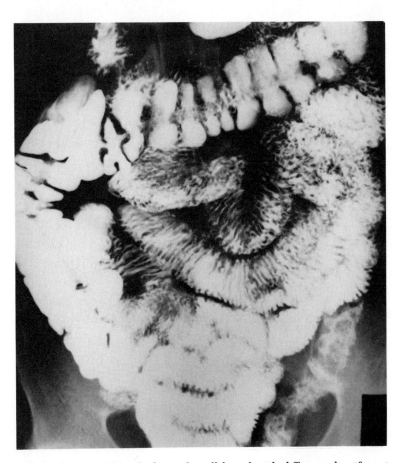

Fig. 9-18. Classic features of amyloidosis of small bowel with diffuse and uniform increased thickening of valvulae conniventes. Note "jejunalization" of ileum.

Amyloidosis

Amyloidosis is often present in patients dying from the complications of spinal cord injury.[9] Amyloidosis is a systemic disease characterized by the deposition of the abnormal mucopolysaccaride protein complex amyloid in certain body tissues.[9,18] It may occur in a primary form representing a plasma cell dyscrasia. More commonly, amyloidosis is seen as a secondary form caused by chronic reticuloendothelial stimulation by chronic debilitating disease or long-standing inflammation such as in rheumatoid arthritis, ulcerative colitis, syphilis, or tuberculosis.[9,18] The spinal cord injured patient usually develops the secondary form between 5 and 15 years after injury. There appears to be no relationship between the level of spinal cord injury and the incidence of amyloidosis, but the duration of complications, such as chronic recurring pressure sores, osteomyelitis, or chronic pyelonephritis, does influence its onset.[9,18,24]

Gastrointestinal involvement is common in secondary amyloidosis, and infiltration occurs at all levels of the alimentary tract.[18,19] The diagnosis is made with a biopsy by demonstrating staining of the amyloid with Congo red.[18] The tongue and rectum are the primary sites for biopsy. During the early stages of the disease visceral infiltration by amyloid may only occur in and about the blood vessels of the submucosa. Later, amyloid is found in the wall, especially in the muscularis mucosa.[19]

The primary radiologic finding in amyloidosis is the thickening of the valvulae conniventes. The enlargement tends to be symmetric, uniform, and diffuse, extending into the ileum and producing a "jejunal" appearance to the ileum (Fig. 9-18).[19]

Miscellaneous gastrointestinal complications

Chronic spinal cord injury appears to accelerate the aging process of the alimentary tract in that hiatus hernia, gastroesophageal reflux, and diverticulosis, generally associated with middle and old age, appear prematurely in these patients during the third and fourth decades (Fig. 9-19).[3,11] This tendency to reflux must al-

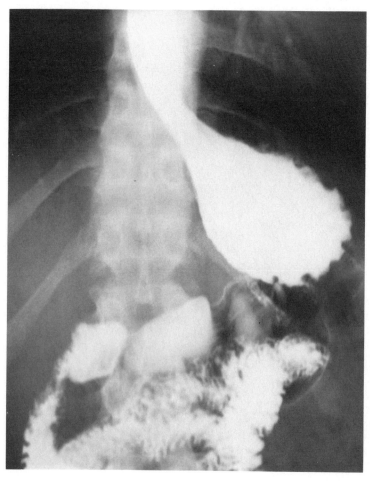

Fig. 9-19. Gastroesophageal reflux demonstrated in 25-year-old C5 quadriplegic man during gastroduodenal examination.

ways be kept in mind when performing gastroduodenal studies to minimize the risk of aspiration. Limitation of motion of the diaphragm, atrophy of the muscles and dehiscence of some of the fibrous tissue at the esophagogastric junction chronically raised intra-abdominal pressure, and the sphincterolytic effect of unapposed vagal action may all have a role in the production of hiatus hernia and reflux. Chronic fecal sludging and raised intraluminal pressure proximally are suggested etiologies for the precocious appearance of diverticula.

REFERENCES

1. Berk, R. N., and Coulson, D. B.: The body cast syndrome, Radiology **94:**303-305, 1970.
2. Bhagat, B. D., Young, P. A., and Biggerstoff, D. E.: Fundamentals of visceral innervation, Springfield, Ill., 1977, Charles C Thomas, Publisher, pp. 51-56, 152-153.
3. Bowen, J. C., Fleming, W. H., and Thompson, J. C.: Increased gastrin following penetrating central nervous system injury, Surgery **75:**720-724, 1974.
4. Brock, J. A.: X-ray survey: upper gastrointestinal disease—284 spinal cord injury patients, Proc. Annu. Clin. Spinal Cord Injury Conference **11:**1-6, 1967.
5. Burke, D. C., and Murray, D. D.: Handbook of spinal cord medicine, New York, 1976, Raven Press, pp. 29-32, 53-56.
6. Carey, M. E., Nance, F. C., and Dirgis, M. D.: Pancreatitis following spinal cord injury, J. Neurosurg. **47:**917-922, 1977.
7. Charney, K. J., Juler, G. L., and Comarr, A. E.: General surgery problems in patients with spinal cord injuries, Arch. Surg. **110:**1983-1988, 1975.
8. Claus-Walker, J., Carter, R. E., Campos, R. J., and Spencer, W. A.: Hypercalcemia in early traumatic quadriplegia, J Chronic Dis. **28:**81-90, 1975.
9. Comarr, A. E.: Secondary amyloidosis in injuries to the spinal cord, Am. J. Surg. **95:**843-844, 1958.
10. Eaton, S. B., and Ferrucci, J. T.: Radiology of the pancreas and duodenum, Philadelphia, 1973, W.B. Saunders Co., pp. 318-325.
11. Gore, R. M., Mintzer, R. A., and Calenoff, L.: The radiology of gastrointestinal complications of spinal cord injury. Presentation at the Sixty-fifth Scientific Assembly and Annual Meeting of the Radiological Society of North America, Atlanta, Nov. 27, 1979.
12. Greenfield, J.: Abdominal operations on patients with chronic paraplegia: report of cases, Arch. Surg. **59:**1077-1087, 1949.
13. Griffiths, H. H.: The radiology of spinal cord injury: a review article, Proc. Annu. Clin. Spinal Cord Injury Conference **21:**43-52, 1971.
14. Guttman, L.: Spinal cord injuries, Oxford, England, 1973, Blackwell Scientific Publications, pp. 430-455.
15. Hoen, T. I., and Copper, I. S.: Acute abdominal emergencies in paraplegics, Am. J. Surg. **75:**19-24, 1948.
16. Holden, E. M.: Intestinal obstruction in spinal cord injury patients, Proc. Annu. Clin. Spinal Cord Injury Conference **15:**110-112, 1966.
17. Inberg, H. O., and Prust, F. W.: The diagnosis of abdominal emergencies in patients with spinal cord lesions, Arch. Phys. Med. Rehabil. **49:**343-345, 1968.
18. Malement, M., Friedman, M., and Pschibul, F.: Amyloidosis of paraplegia, Proc. Annu. Clin. Spinal Cord Injury Conference **12:**33-41, 1963.
19. Marshak, R. H., and Linder, A. E.: Radiology of the small intestine, Philadelphia, 1976, W. B. Saunders Co., pp. 63-68.
20. Menuck, L., and Siemers, P. T.: Pneumoperitoneum: importance of right upper quadrant features, Am. J. Roentgenol. **127:**753-756, 1976.
21. Mihaldzic, N., and Frederick, W.: Peptic ulcer in paraplegia, Proc. Annu. Clin. Spinal Cord Injury Conference **13:**68-71, 1964.
22. Miller, L. S., Staas, W. E., and Herbison, G. J.: Abdominal problems in patients with spinal cord lesion, Arch. Phys. Med. Rehabil. **56:**405-408, 1975.
23. Moeller, B. A.: Perforated duodenal ulcer in quadriplegia, Proc. Annu. Clin. Spinal Cord Injury Conference **7:**1-3, 1958.
24. Moses, D. S.: Secondary amyloid disease in paraplegia, Proc. Annu. Clin. Spinal Cord Injury Conference **3:**14-17, 1954.
25. Nuseibeh, I. M.: Stress ulcerations in spinal injuries. In Vinken, P. J., and Bruyn, G. W., editors: Handbook of clinical neurology, vol. 26. Injuries of the spine and spinal cord, part II, Amsterdam, 1976, North-Holland Publishing Co.
26. O'Hare, J. M.: The acute abdomen in spinal cord injury patients, Proc. Annu. Clin. Spinal Cord Injury Conference **15:**113-117, 1966.
27. Perret, G., and Solomon, A.: Gastrointestinal hemorrhage and cervical cord injuries, Proc. Annu. Clin. Spinal Cord Injury Conference **11:**1-6-110, 1967.
28. Pollack, L. J., and Finkelman, I.: The digestive apparatus in injuries to the spinal cord, Surg. Clin. North Am. **34:**259-268, 1954.
29. Ramos, M.: Recurrent superior mesenteric artery syndrome in a quadriplegic patient, Arch. Phys. Med. Rehabil. **56:**86-88, 1975.
30. Ranaka, M., Vchiyami, M., and Kitano, M.: Gastroduodenal disease in chronic spinal cord injuries, Arch. Surg. **114:**185-187, 1979.
31. Richardson, R. R., Meyer, P. R., and Raimondi, A. J.: Transabdominal neurostimulation in acute spinal cord injuries, Spine **4:**47-51, 1979.
32. Wallace, R. G., and Howard, W. B.: Acute superior mesenteric artery syndrome in the severely burned patient, Radiology **94:**307-310, 1970.
33. Yashon, D.: Spinal injury, New York, 1975, Appleton-Century-Crofts, pp. 247-276.

CHAPTER 10

Venography in acute spinal cord injury

HARVEY L. NEIMAN, M.D.

Lower extremity deep venous thrombosis and pulmonary embolism are well-described complications of acute spinal cord injury. The incidence of thrombosis of the deep veins of the lower extremities in the spinal cord injured is approximately 15% as determined clinically and as high as 90% with the use of iodine 125 fibrinogen scanning.[2,13,14,18] This high incidence of venous disease in the patient with acute spinal cord injury can be anticipated because of the multiple risk factors that are present. Several investigators have shown a decrease in venous flow in the lower limbs of bedridden and paralyzed patients.[15,20] Prolonged pressure on the veins of immobile limbs can also cause intimal injury, which further enhances the thrombosis potential.[17] Finally, the relationship of deep venous thrombosis and surgical procedures has been well described.[19]

The risk of fatal pulmonary embolism in this same group of patients within a 3-month period of spinal cord injury is also very high, having been reported to be 2% to 16%.[10,16,18] The importance of early diagnosis is therefore readily apparent. At the same time, the problem is compounded in many patients by the need for immediate operative intervention for fracture reduction and stabilization of the spine, making anticoagulant therapy relatively contraindicated. The need for accurate diagnosis of deep venous thrombosis therefore becomes critical.

Contrast venography has been the traditional imaging technique for identification of venous thrombosis.[8] More recently, however, the use of transcutaneous

Doppler ultrasonography, impedance plethysmography, and ^{125}I fibrinogen radionuclide studies (Chapter 19) has changed the spectrum of indications for lower extremity contrast examinations. The noninvasive procedures can be utilized as screening studies. Venography, however, remains the standard for judging the other procedures; it also has several clear-cut indications,[5] including (1) equivocal noninvasive flow studies, (2) noninvasive flow studies in variance with the clinical situation, (3) the period prior to vena caval interruption, (4) documented pulmonary emboli without a source, and (5) chronic venous insufficiency. In patients with acute spinal cord injury any of the first four indications frequently warrants contrast venography.

TECHNICAL CONSIDERATIONS

In a routine examination on a nonparalyzed patient, a modification of the Rabinov and Paulin[8] technique is utilized. This involves the use of a radiographic tilt table with spot film capabilities and an overhead tube. The patient is examined in a semiupright 60° position with the leg that is not being examined bearing the weight of the individual. In addition, a rolled towel is placed behind the Achilles tendon of the examined extremity. The procedure is carried out without a tourniquet in this completely non-weight-bearing position. Contrast material is injected into a vein on the dorsum of the foot with subsequent contrast filling of both the superficial and deep systems (Fig. 10-1). Radiographs are obtained beginning at the ankle and extending

298

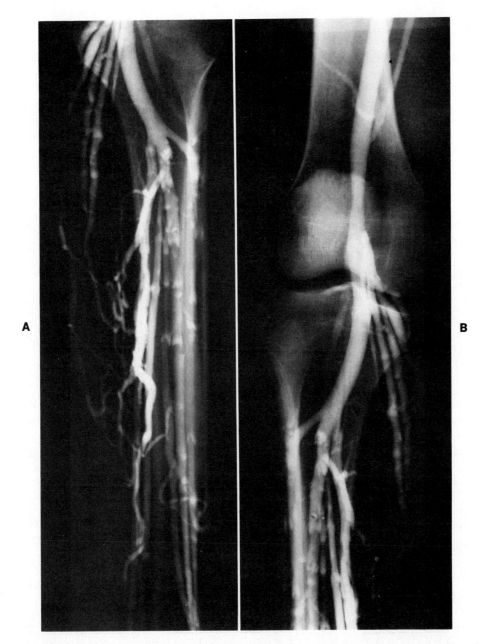

Fig. 10-1. Normal venous anatomy of leg, **A,** and distal thigh, **B.** Note that veins are free of intraluminal filling defects and have a normal course and caliber and normal valve architecture.

through the iliac veins. Approximately 100 ml of contrast material is injected for each lower extremity.

In the patient with acute spinal cord injury, however, there are unique conditions that negate this upright, non-weight-bearing, nontourniquet technique. For obvious reasons the patient cannot be examined in an upright position and frequently, in fact, must be examined while positioned in a Stryker frame. This obligatory recumbent position means that contrast material cannot flow in a normal physiologic manner in the deep venous system. This complicates the diagnostic technique since it has been clearly shown that flow artifacts and incomplete filling of the deep venous system occur when contrast material is injected with the patient in the supine position.[3,4] Physiologic changes in flow that appear to be unique to the spinal cord injured patient also occur. These limitations not only create difficulty in diagnosis by contrast venography but also make the radionuclide venogram with technetium 99m albumin microspheres or macroaggregated albumin similarly limited.

As a result, the tourniquet as described by Rogoff and DeWeese[9] was initially utilized in order to force contrast material into the deep venous system.

At Northwestern University, however, we found that this too created difficulties in that there were frequently flow defects attributable to the tourniquets. More importantly, however, there remained inconsistent and incomplete filling of the deep venous system, suggesting the presence of a thrombus in an uninvolved site. Therefore in the last 2 years we have utilized an inflatable plastic boot that was initially designed for

lower extremity immobilization after trauma. When this boot is inflated, the effect is to create an increase in pressure within the superficial venous system of the lower extremity that is equal throughout. This in turn forces contrast material into the deep venous system (Fig. 10-2). In the nonparalyzed individual lower extremity venous flow is preferentially via the deep system and to a lesser extent via the superficial venous system. However, as previously noted, there is always some degree of shunting of the contrast material from the deep venous system to the superficial system with

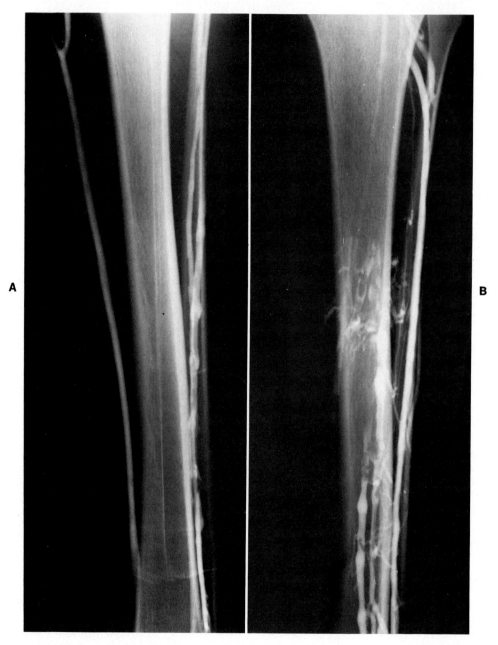

Fig. 10-2. A, Superficial venous filling with patient in supine position. **B,** Inflated boot forces contrast material into deep venous system, demonstrating significant calf vein thrombosis.

the recumbent position. In the spinal cord injured individual, however, there appears to be almost total shunting of contrast material and therefore presumably blood away from the normal patterns that are expected. It is postulated that with flaccid paralysis the tone of the superficial veins is decreased, creating a system of diminished peripheral resistance as compared to the deep venous system, and therefore preferential flow is via the superficial veins. With spastic paraplegia it is postulated that there may be an increase in muscular tone about the deep venous system. This again would

allow the superficial venous system to have a relative decrease in resistance and would permit preferential flow via the latter route.

The basis for the above postulates is the clinical setting. To date we have not tested these concepts in a research environment. Contrast material injected into the dorsum of the foot in a spinal cord injured individual flows with marked preference via the superficial venous system unless its route is altered by external factors. This has been noted to be true in both the spastic and the flaccid forms of paralysis. We have noted,

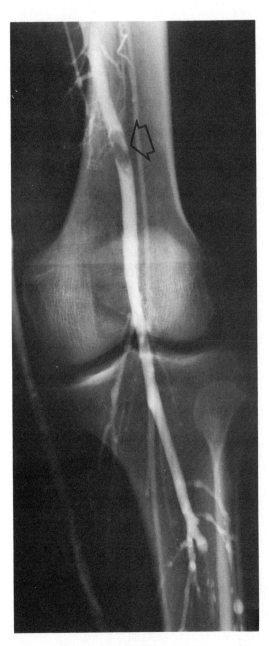

Fig. 10-3. Well-circumscribed filling defect *(arrow)* in popliteal vein is characteristic of thrombosis.

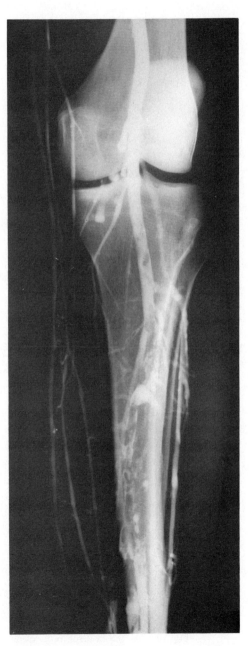

Fig. 10-4. Extensive thrombosis involving entire deep venous system of leg.

therefore, a great deal of difficulty in producing a diagnostic quality contrast venogram in the spinal cord injured patient. The technique as described, however, has markedly improved the quality of the examination and, in fact, now allows us to examine the patient on the Stryker frame. This means that unstable spinal fractures are not manipulated, and there is no chance of exacerbating the injury. It allows for an easy examination for both patient and physician and means that contrast venography is an easily performed procedure.

A radiographic cassette is placed under the examined limb and a mobile overhead x-ray tube is used for filming. The inflatable boot is commercially available (Jobst) and is operated by a foot pump. We additionally place tourniquets at the ankle and the thigh and inject from 75 to 125 ml of 60% iodinated contrast material. Radiographs are obtained from the ankle to the pelvis, demonstrating excellent visualization of the venous anatomy.

After the procedure much effort is expended to flush

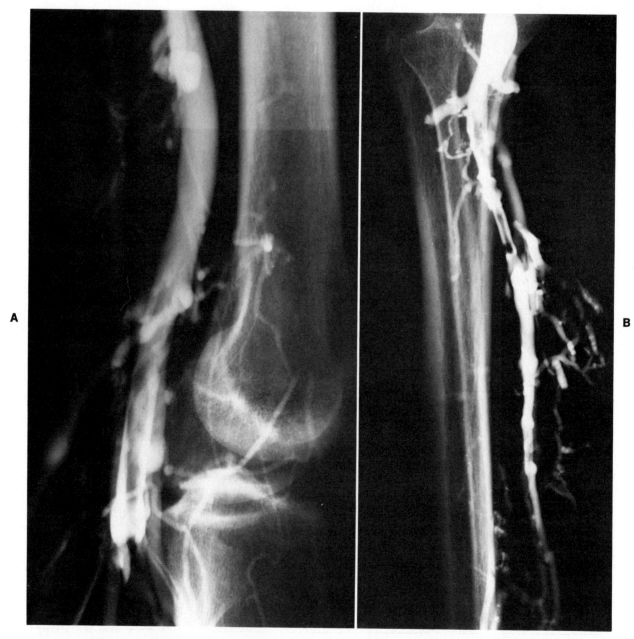

Fig. 10-5. A, Tail of thrombus extending into popliteal vein demonstrating railroad track sign. **B,** Thrombus in calf vein with intraluminal filling defect centrally located and contrast material along margins.

the contrast material from the veins of the lower extremity with the use of heparinized saline.

RADIOLOGIC MANIFESTATIONS

The normal anatomy of the deep venous system of the lower extremity has been well described and is available in standard anatomy textbooks. The venographic diagnosis of thrombosis is based on the demonstration of an intraluminal filling defect within an opacified vein (Figs. 10-3 and 10-4). Acute thrombus appears as a radiolucent defect within the vein with a surrounding white rim of contrast material. This frequently takes the appearance of a railroad track (Fig. 10-5). As a thrombus ages, the contrast rim is lost along one margin, indicating adherence to the adjacent wall. Subsequently the thrombus retracts, allowing the opposite rim of contrast material to become thicker. A partially recanalized vein demonstrates stranding within the lumen, giving transverse or vertical webs. A more completely recanalized vein may have irregular mar-

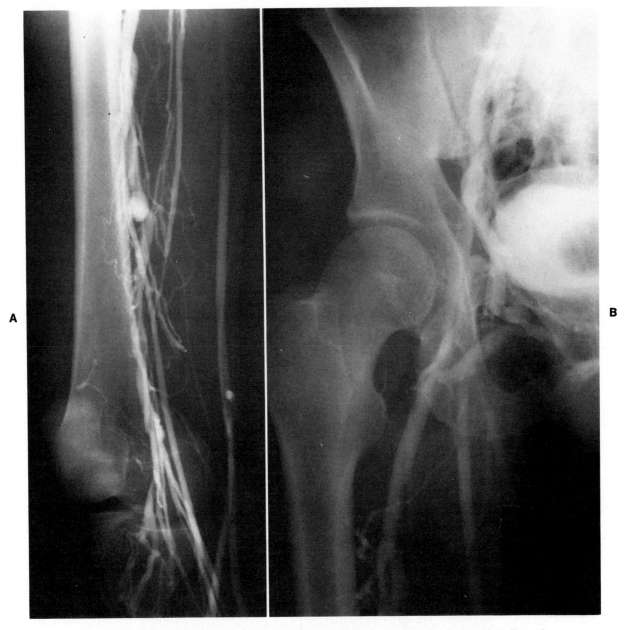

Fig. 10-6. A, Note tortuous, valveless recanalized femoral vein with multiple tiny collateral veins also present. **B,** Recanalized iliac veins are present in this patient with well-developed collateral channels. These findings are indicative of chronic disease.

gination with loss of normal valvular architecture (Fig. 10-6).

Abrupt cutoff of a normally filled venous channel is also a sign of acute thrombosis. The vessel, however, must be filled proximally and distally, separated by a nonopacified segment.

Division of flow from a segment or the entire deep venous system is further evidence of thrombosis in a nonparalyzed individual. Since division of flow is frequently seen in the patient with acute spinal cord injury, as noted previously, this sign is of less importance.

Delineation of the entire extent of the disease is important because thrombosis with a nonadherent tail, particularly in the iliofemoral region, is more likely to cause pulmonary embolism (Fig. 10-7). This ability of contrast venography to "stage" the disease process is clearly an advantage over all the noninvasive tests. Rational therapy can then be based on demonstration of both the proximal and distal extents of the disease process and the likelihood of central embolization.

Contrast venography is the most accurate method for evaluation of the venous system of the lower extremity because it directly visualizes veins. It is extremely un-

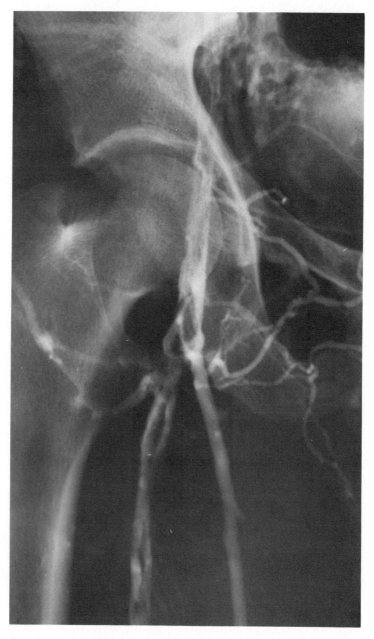

Fig. 10-7. Thrombus is present filling common femoral and iliac veins, demonstrating acute disease.

likely that a thrombus in the iliofemoral region or in the area of the main veins of the calf would be missed. Although it is almost impossible to create an adequate model by which to judge contrast venography, since it is usually considered the "gold standard," subjective evaluation with clinical follow-up or operative findings confirms its accuracy.[6,7,8,11,12] The practical advantage of venography is that it demonstrates the thrombus and its extent, as well as the age of the disease process.

COMPLICATIONS

Although complications of contrast venography are rare, the study is not entirely without risks. Inadvertent extravasation of contrast material at the injection site in a patient with sensation is associated with pain and burning. However, if there is also a compromised arterial supply to the lower extremity, there may be local tissue damage and ulceration of the skin.[6]

Pain, tenderness, and localized swelling after the venogram have been noted occasionally. Thrombosis secondary to the contrast material is another reported complication. Albrechtson and Olsson have noted a high incidence of thrombosis after venography, as documented by ^{125}I fibrinogen uptake studies.[1] In their recent work, however, the contrast material was not flushed from the vein vigorously with heparinized saline. Presumably this high rate of thrombosis would be markedly diminished given the latter situation. Massive pulmonary embolism after phlebography has not been a concern.

REFERENCES

1. Albrechtson, U., and Olsson, C. G.: Thrombotic side effects of lower limb phlebography, Lancet 1:723-724, 1976.
2. Brach, B. B., Moser, K. M., Cedar, L., et al.: Venous thrombosis in acute spinal cord paralysis, J. Trauma 17:289-292, 1977.
3. Greitz, T.: The technique of ascending phlebography of the lower extremity, Acta Radiol. [Diagn.] (Stockh.) 42:421-427, 1954.
4. Limdblum, K.: Phlebographische Untersuchung des untereschenkels bei Konstastinjektion in eine subkutane Vene, Acta Radiol. [Diagn.] (Stockh.) 22:288-292, 1941.
5. Neiman, H. L.: Phlebography in the diagnosis of venous thrombosis. In Bergan, J. J., and Yao, J. S. T., editors: Venous problems, Chicago, 1978, Year Book Medical Publishers, pp. 111-122.
6. Nicholides, A. N.: Diagnosis of venous thrombosis by phlebography. In Bergan, J. J., and Yao, J. S. T., editors: Venous problems, Chicago, 1978, Year Book Medical Publishers, pp. 123-140.
7. Nicholides, A. N., Kakkar, V. V., Field, E. S., and Renny, J. T. G.: The origin of deep vein thrombosis: a venographic study, Br. J. Radiol. 44:653-659, 1971.
8. Rabinov, K., and Paulin, S.: Roentgen diagnosis of venous thrombosis in the leg, Arch. Surg. 104:134-141, 1972.
9. Rogoff, F. M., and DeWeese, J. A.: Phlebography of the lower extremity, J.A.M.A. 172:1599-1603, 1960.
10. Silver, J. R.: The prophylactic use of anticoagulant therapy in the prevention of pulmonary emboli in 100 consecutive spinal injury patients, Paraplegia 12:188-193, 1974.
11. Thomas, J. L., McAllister, V., and Tonge, K.: The radiological appearance of deep venous thrombosis, Clin. Radiol. 45:199-205, 1971.
12. Thomas, M. K., Fletcher, G. W. L., Cockett, F. B., and Negus, D.: Venous collaterals in the external and common iliac vein obstruction, Clin. Radiol. 18:403-407, 1967.
13. Todd, J. E., Frisbie, J. H., Rossier, A. B., et al.: Blood flow laboratory, Paraplegia 14:50-57, 1976.
14. Tribe, C. R.: Causes of death in the early and late stages of paraplegia, Paraplegia 1:19-47, 1963.
15. Wakim, K. G., Terrier, J. C., Elkins, E. C., et al.: Effect of percutaneous stimulation of the circulation in normal and paralyzed lower extremities, Am. J. Physiol. 153:183-186, 1948.
16. Walsh, J. J., and Tribe, C.: Phlebothrombosis and pulmonary embolism in paraplegia, Paraplegia 3:209-212, 1965.
17. Warlow, C., Ogston, D., and Douglas, A. S.: Venous thrombosis following stroke, Lancet 2:1305-1306, 1972.
18. Watson, N.: Venous thrombosis and pulmonary embolism in spinal cord injury, Paraplegia 6:133-139, 1968.
19. Wessler, S.: Small dose of heparin in a new concept of hypercoagulability, Thromb. Haemost. 33:81-84, 1974.
20. Wright, H. P., Osborn, S. D., and Hysen, M.: Venous velocity in bedridden medical patients, Lancet 1:669-671, 1952.

PART III

Rehabilitation of spinal cord injury

CHAPTER 11

Rehabilitation process

JOEL S. ROSEN, M.D.

Radiologic evaluation of spinal cord injured patients is best achieved when correlated with the clinical conditions at the time of the radiologic examination. This is equally valid for the early hours after the injury as during the following weeks, months, and years of medical and surgical rehabilitation care. The clinical conditions of spinal cord injured patients are best understood when the rehabilitation process, with all its facets, is known to physicians involved in direct or indirect care of spinal cord injury.

The rehabilitation process starts with the extrication of a spinal cord injured patient from the scene of an accident and concerns itself with the following areas: physical management, level of function, cardiovascular reflexes, the neurogenic bladder, the neurogenic bowel, spasticity, osteoporosis and pathologic fracture, psychology, sex, and pregnancy and labor.

PHYSICAL MANAGEMENT

During the early period of spinal cord injury and immobilization, the rehabilitation process is focused on prevention rather than treatment. The importance of prevention of pressure sores applies both in the intensive care unit and on the rehabilitation floor. Use of assistive devices such as sheepskin, skin oil, turning frames, and electric beds is helpful, but these *cannot* substitute for good nursing care. Avoidance of localized prolonged pressure over a bony prominence is the only effective means of pressure sore prevention. Frequent skin checks, regardless of the turning method, are es-

sential. It takes only a few hours of neglect to start what may become an irreversible process. Complete range of motion of the joints in all affected extremities is essential at least twice daily to prevent contractures. Where partial paralysis exists, the patient should move the joint as much as possible with the therapist completing the range of motion. Bed clothes must be loose and undersheets tight to avoid creases over anesthetic skin areas. Therapeutic muscle-strengthening exercises must begin as soon as the patient is conscious. In those extremities immobilized by arm-boards or casts, isometric exercises are effective.

Attaining the upright position is essential for either ambulation with braces or wheelchair activities. Whether one uses a tilt table or full reclining wheelchair to train the patient is immaterial as long as it is realized that accommodation may be a slow, gradual progress. If the recumbency phase was prolonged by treatment of a complication, such as a pressure sore, it will likewise take longer to adjust to the upright position. Assumption of the upright position requires stability of the bony spine lesion. Initial treatment of the acute cervical spine injury will have been by skeletal traction in definitely or until surgical stabilization has been accomplished. The length of time of use of external support varies with the kind and site of injury. The type and effectiveness of surgical stabilization should be verified radiographically when patients are transferred from an acute treatment facility to a rehabilitation center (Fig. 11-1).

The decision to remove external support is made when

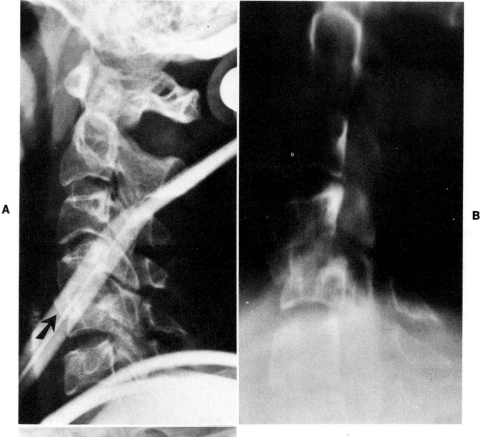

Fig. 11-1. Radiographic verification of spinal fusion in 23-year-old quadriplegic man with fracture-dislocation of C5-6. **A,** Lateral view taken before removal of external support shows short anterior bone graft *(arrow)*. **B,** Tomogram demonstrates inadequate anterior fusion failing to establish stability. **C,** Posterior spinal fusion extending from C4-6 was then performed.

callus formation is visible on the radiographs. In many circumstances, however, no callus will be visible radiographically and the decision must be based on other factors. In the cervical spine, with the history of a fracture-dislocation, supports are used for approximately 3 months from the time of trauma. At that time, flexion-extension films can be obtained to ensure stability (Fig. 11-2). If no motion is present at the injured area, the orthosis can be removed. Use of isometric exercises while the patient is still wearing the orthosis will significantly decrease the morbidity when it is removed. In the presence of a dislocation, early attempts at motion films yield little benefit, since the spine must be stabilized anyway to allow for adequate stability to occur. Stability of the bony lesion occurs long before actual bone fusion. Before assuming a sitting or upright position, all patients should have total spine radiographs to exclude a secondary unrecognized spinal fracture.[28]

Temporary assistive devices, such as built-up utensils,

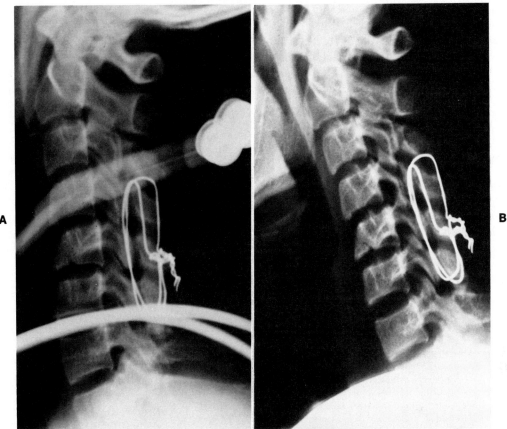

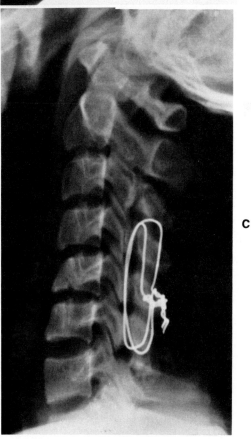

Fig. 11-2. Ensuring stability of spinal fusion prior to removal of orthosis in 21-year-old quadriplegic. **A,** Lateral view with SOMI brace on shows good position of posterior spinal fusion. **B,** Flexion and, **C,** extension lateral views with patient's head carefully flexed and extended show stability of fusion.

tenodesis splints, and sling suspension for weak upper extremity proximal muscles, all help to allay the feelings of helplessness and allow the patient to participate actively in his own program. Application of devices to assist activities of daily living and training should start while the patient is still in the intensive care unit. Prescription of definitive orthotic devices for long-term use may wait until the patient has attained an upright position.[24]

Strengthening residual functioning muscles, teaching regular or motorized wheelchair techniques, and teaching activities of daily living, prevention of complications, and good bowel, bladder, and skin care are the basic principles of physical treatment.

For the patient to attain these goals required are the interest, dedication, and close cooperation of a team of allied health specialists: physical therapist, occupational therapist, nurse, psychologist, social worker, and recreational therapist.

Drivers' education and vocational exploration are interrelated in this patient population and must be made available as early as realistically feasible. No hard and fast rules are available as to (1) the specific vocations available to the spinal cord injured individual and (2) the correct time to introduce intensive exploration. Critical to realistic exploration in this area is the matter of home accessibility, available transportation, and availability of necessary equipment and possible attendant care.[10,21,26]

LEVELS OF FUNCTION

Initially the treatment must be focused on life-saving techniques and preventing complications (pressure sores, pyelonephritis, contractures, etc.). These are critical, since the ultimate level of independence of the patient with spinal cord injury will frequently depend on how many of these problems have been avoided. Extensive pressure sores or contractures can easily con-

Table 11-1. Activities of daily living related to functional level

Functional level	Activities of daily living
C3 and above	Respirator dependent; requires total assistance for transfers and self-care; independent in mobility in motorized wheelchair and communication
C4	Independent from respiratory assistance; can assist with simple activities of daily living only with the assistance of externally powered assistive devices
C5	Can perform upper extremity activities of daily living with assistive devices and some physical assistance; can propel wheelchair short distances functionally
C6	May be able to independently transfer or to do so with minimal or moderate assistance; independent upper extremity activities, but usually receives assistance for lower extremity activities and bowel and bladder care; uses standard wheelchair without difficulty
C7	Independent self-care, transfers, wheelchair function, and bowel and bladder care because of the presence of triceps and finger flexors and extensors
C8	Completely independent in all activities; some residual weakness in intrinsic hand muscles
T1-7	Normal upper extremities; trunk balance is poor and patient may require the assistance of his upper extremities for stability
T8-10	Normal respiratory control with good trunk balance; ambulation not usually a realistic functional goal
T10-L1	May ambulate with bilateral long-leg braces and crutches; ambulation may be functional for short distances because of the presence of pelvic control; patient still requires a wheelchair for most activities
L2-S1	Independent in ambulation with below-the-knee braces only, and two canes or forearm crutches
S2	May ambulate without lower extremity orthosis
S3	Complete voluntary bowel and bladder function

vert an individual with the potential for independent living to one who needs extensive attendant care.

The actual level of functional independence with activities of daily living depends on the level of spinal cord injury but varies greatly with the individual and attendant circumstances, that is, spasticity, ectopic bone, age, other medical complications, weight, pain, motivation, architectural barriers, and so on[6]; for example, a short individual but one who is very agile with better than normal strength in his upper extremities may be able to ambulate with braces even though he may have a higher spinal cord lesion than a comparable individual who is unable to ambulate.

General levels of function with regard to activities of daily living to be expected by a young healthy individual without the above problem are given in Table 11-1.

CARDIOVASCULAR REFLEXES

Most high spinal cord injured patients will be seen immediately after injury with profound shock and bradycardia secondary to the traumatic sympathectomy with subsequent loss of supraspinal influence over the sympathetic nervous system and its peripheral vasoconstrictor activity.[14] In the early stages it may be necessary to use a parasympatholytic (atropine) to treat the profound bradycardia and to use vasopressor drugs to raise the blood pressure. The condition does resolve with time as the autonomic nervous system regains its stability.

As the patient becomes mobilized, the question of profound postural hypotension is encountered in all patients with lesions above the midthoracic level.[29] Peripheral venous and splanchnic bed pooling occurs as a result of lack of muscle tone and poor skin turgor. Reduced venous return to the heart, orthostatic hypotension, and decreased cerebral blood flow also occur. If the condition is acute and is not treated as an emergency, cerebrovascular accidents have been known to occur.

Gradual progressive elevation of the lower extremities to higher degrees and for longer periods of time gradually allows the cardiovascular system to adapt. Compressive stockings, abdominal binders, and low doses of ephedrine have been effective in relieving symptoms.

Lower extremity edema, particularly during the flaccid stage, is a constant problem secondary to the previously mentioned factors, as well as decreased lymphatic return. The edema is usually symmetric below the knees, soft and pitting in character, and responds to treatment by periodic elevation during the day and night. Use of elastic stockings is frequently required, and occasionally low doses of diuretics are employed. Other complicating factors, such as hypoproteinemia, anemia, and previous deep venous thrombosis, must be ruled out.

NEUROGENIC BLADDER

Immediately after the injury, during the stage of spinal shock, the urinary bladder is described as being areflexic and flaccid, even though there is certain amount of tone preserved through the effects of the autonomic nervous system. This tone can be destroyed by periodic overdistention of the bladder. Continuous drainage of the bladder is usually required within the first few days of injury or until life-threatening conditions have been stabilized.

Thereafter, an intermittent catheterization program can be instituted in which the bladder is emptied at 4-hour intervals with a rigidly controlled fluid intake, the primary goal being to avoid overdistention and infection.[15]

As the bladder regains its tone and the patient starts to void, the frequency of intermittent catheterization can be decreased. If within a reasonable period of time the patient does not adequately empty his bladder (postvoiding residuals less than 70 ml), surgical intervention in the form of a sphincterotomy or bladder neck procedure or both to reduce outflow obstruction may be considered.[18] In addition to sufficiently low residuals, it must be ensured that the individual does not have a marked elevation in intravesical pressure, which may ultimately lead to reflux, hydroureter, and hydronephrosis. Frequently because of spasticity of the external sphincter or increased urethral resistance the patient may not be able to void spontaneously. Antispasticity drugs or those that decrease urethral resistance may be tried. Lifelong intermittent catheterization is another alternative for the individual who is continent and does not wish to consider using external urine-collecting devices. Because of the absence of an effective external collecting device for females, catheterization may be the only effective alternative to continuous drainage.[22] Recurrent leakage of urine, autonomic dysreflexia, difficulty with attendant care, pressure sores from use of an external collecting device, or ease of socialization may prompt some patients to elect to use continous drainage. With use of continuous drainage, the catheter should be taped to the upper thigh or lower abdominal wall to decrease traction and decrease the penile-scrotal angle to lessen the chance of periurethral abscess.[16] In the presence of a Foley catheter in the bladder, maintenance of an adequate fluid intake is necessary to prevent frequent plugging of the catheter. Maintenance of a sterile urine in the presence of a catheter balloon is virtually impossible. Routine use of antibiotics in a patient with an indwelling catheter is not indicated. The old practice of giving antibiotics to patients who have an asymptomatic bacteriuria is subject to question. Semiannual or annual lifetime urologic follow-up is required to prevent such problems as reflux, hydroureteronephrosis, fistulas, and diverticula. During these evaluations, intravenous urography and voiding cystourethrography are required to outline both upper and lower urinary tracts. Urodynamic studies will also be required to ensure against high-pressure voiding.

NEUROGENIC BOWEL

Immediately after injury the patient will usually have an ileus and oral intake will be contraindicated. Even before spinal shock wears off, some degree of peristalsis occurs. This stage is further delayed with destruction of the sacral cord or cauda equina.[9] Initial attempts at bowel control are focused on keeping the patient clean and avoiding skin irritation and impaction. The majority of patients will experience some degree of diarrhea during the acute phase.

After the initial acute state in which ileus and acute abdominal trauma must be dealt with and when the nasogastric tubes are discontinued, a formal therapy program may be instituted. Even when the individual is lying in bed, use may be made of the gastrocolic and rectocolic reflexes to help establish a pattern of evacuation.

The principal goals in bowel training are twofold: (1) to avoid impaction and (2) to avoid incontinence. An initial program utilizing stool softeners, mild laxatives, medicated suppositories, and digital stimulation on a daily basis is frequently effective. As the individual is mobilized and is able to participate more in physical activity and control his own diet, many of the medications may be eliminated. With assumption of the erect position in bed or a commode chair, use of gravity will greatly facilitate the program. As the individual comes out of spinal shock, gentle dilatation of the anal sphincter will stimulate peristalsis of the colon and rectum to evacuate (mediated by S2, S3, and S4). Eventually this may be the only means necessary for bowel evacuation. Digital stimulation may also assist by tending to reflexly cause increased intra-abdominal pressure and straining. The ability to voluntarily increase intra-abdominal pressure to facilitate defecation will have been lost because of spinal cord paralysis.[8] Most patients ultimately decide on an every-other-day program either very early in the morning or evening as the preferred method of long-term management. The correct program for the individual patient is the one that prevents impaction, incontinence, and excessive trauma to the tissues and is realistic from a psychosocial point of view.

In preparation for any radiologic or direct visualization of the gastrointestinal tract, attention must be given to the altered tone of the tissues and proper preparation must take place, usually over a 3-day period.

SPASTICITY

Immediately after onset of the spinal cord lesion, the patient goes into a stage of spinal shock in which all reflexes below the level of the injury are depressed. As this stage starts to resolve (3 to 6 weeks), most patients will experience the annoying occurrence of "spasms" in skeletal muscles below the lesion.[6] This gradually increases to a point of increase in muscle tone, hyperreflexia, and clonus. The skeletal muscles below the lesion have been released from the supraspinal inhibitory impulses from the brain. Patients frequently interpret the onset of spasticity as the return of voluntary function. There is no relationship between the onset of spasticity and voluntary motor control.

Spasticity may ultimately provide a useful function in that many patients may voluntarily or by eliciting specific reflexes produce spasticity that may lead to stability of the lower extremities that can assist in transfers or ambulation. More frequently, however, the spasticity is uncomfortable, leads to difficulty in positioning, and may even lead to pressure sores by the repeated rubbing of skin on the bed or wheelchair. Severe lower extremity and abdominal spasms have been known to throw patients out of bed and out of wheelchairs. Upper extremity spasticity in quadriplegics may significantly interfere with activities of daily living.[19]

Medical treatment of spasticity by diazepam (Valium), baclofen (Lioresal), and dantrolene sodium (Dantrium), or a combination of these drugs is at best marginal and is very rarely useful in the severely spastic patient. Patients do tend to develop a tolerance to drug management over a period of time.

Destructive procedures, such as phenol, peripheral nerve, and motor point blocks, intrathecal phenol, radiofrequency rhizotomy, and myelotomy, are frequently needed as lifesaving procedures, that is, to relieve spasticity and allow for surgical closure of pressure sores. They may also be used to eliminate spasticity that is dangerous to the patient and significantly interferes with activities of daily living. Because of the possibility of producing pain with these procedures, as well as the fact that they are destructive of neural tissue, their use must be individualized with each patient. Because of the alteration in bladder and sexual function with intrathecal procedures, patients will rarely accept this treatment soon after onset of the injury.

PAIN

In the acutely spinal cord injured patient, the pain that is perceived is that of the basic injury, namely, torn ligaments, broken bones, and local muscle spasm. It is best managed by immobilization in traction and

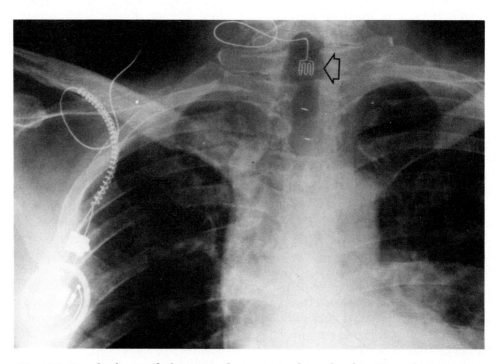

Fig. 11-3. Dorsal column radiofrequency electronic simulator placed in C4 quadriplegic man with intractable pain. Modified bilateral laminectomy of T1-3 was performed to insert electrode head *(arrow)* into dural pocket. Receiver is implanted subcutaneously on right chest wall.

analgesics. In the long-term spinal cord injured patient, with the exception of the severely depressed or cauda equina patient, severe pain is not usually a major factor in the rehabilitation process. There are many bizarre sensations, frequently perceived as pain, below the level of the lesion that some believe are caused by scar formation at the distal end of the proximal stump of the spinal cord. This pain is frequently described as diffuse and burning in nature and usually does not follow a dermatome distribution. It is very resistant to treatment. Occurrence of discomfort with spasticity is very common and often described as painful. When the spasticity is not very severe, this discomfort will frequently respond to the antispasticity drugs, positioning, and range of motion; when the spasticity is very severe, there is little available for treatment other than the radical procedures described previously.

Local or nerve root pain is always possible at the site of injury secondary to instability, scar tissue, or improper reduction. The pain is treated the same as any other neuritic pain once the diagnosis is made.

When pain is accompanied by anxiety and depression in the individual unable to cope with life in a wheelchair, the patient may respond to small doses of mild tranquilizers plus tricyclic antidepressants. Indiscriminate use of drugs must be avoided, since the individual who is incapacitated by the pain is very likely to be the one to become drug dependent. Use of therapy is beneficial to prevent painful contractures and reduce spasticity by range of motion.

Intermittent nerve blocks with a local anesthetic are useful for diagnostic purposes and possibly as a means of conservative treatment of an acute problem. Alcohol or phenol nerve blocks are occasionally used but must be approached with care since they may cause neuropathy themselves. Local injections of an anesthetic and steroids followed by manipulation may be useful in relieving discomfort in the paraspinal areas.

Use of surgical procedures, such as neurectomy or root section, has a small but definite place. Posterior rhizotomy may be useful for spasticity or cauda equina pain while sparing the sacral segments. Occasionally a spinal-thalamic tractotomy may be done to relieve pain below the level of the lesion. In order for this to be effective, it must be done several segments above the lesion, and it does carry the risk of raising the level of paralysis. Use of dorsal column stimulators (Fig. 11-3) and transcutaneous nerve stimulators is new, and their true role in chronic pain management in the spinal cord injured individual has yet to be established.[5]

OSTEOPOROSIS AND PATHOLOGIC FRACTURES

Immediately after injury, there is a profound mobilization and loss of calcium and protein from the skeleton, most prominent in the area below the level of paralysis. Loss of protein and minerals is most severe during the first few weeks of injury, and thereafter the process continues, but at a slower rate, for several months. Eventually a new state of bone turnover is reached and maintained.[7,30]

The massive mobilization of calcium and minerals plus the usual presence of urinary infection lead to the formation of urinary tract stones. Patients with lower motor neuron lesions have a much more profound degree of osteoporosis than those with upper motor neuron lesions, since the spasticity provides muscle tone leading to more preservation of bone substance. Quadriplegics will frequently have lesser degrees of osteoporosis of the upper extremities.[1]

Pathologic fractures secondary to "soft bones" are very common, especially in the femur (Fig. 11-4, A) and usually are caused by a relatively mild degree of trauma, that is, bumping a leg during a transfer, a sudden twisting motion with ambulation, and so on.[3]

Agressive therapeutic efforts at maintaining range of motion in a joint restricted by contractures or ectopic bone are also a relatively common cause of pathologic fractures. When the patient reports a "pop," sudden increase in range of motion, or sudden swelling, radiologic evaluation is indicated. Conservative treatment is usually indicated unless it would cause an unreasonable period of immobility, in which case surgical fixation and resumption of the rehabilitation program are the treatments of choice. When open reduction and internal fixation are indicated, care must be exercised to ensure that the surgical wound is not placed over a weight-bearing surface, for example, the posterior aspect of the greater trochanter (Fig. 11-4, B).

PSYCHOLOGY

Although it is generally agreed that there is no such thing as a spinal cord personality, the general characteristics of spinal cord patients warrant mention. They are typically young (average age, 27), male (male-to-female ratio, approximately 5:1), with some evidence of major psychosocial disruption in their lives recently, such as an arrest, divorce, loss of employment, or school problems.

Subsequent to the onset of injury, there are a series of stages that the patient passes through:

1. Anxiety and fear: these emotions are seen early as the patient wonders about life and death, hospital environment, impending surgery, and so on.

2. Denial: depression is absent as the patient goes through a stage where he cannot accept the permanence of what has happened; he cannot accept his physician's statement that he will not recover. This may be useful early, because the patient will frequently work

very hard at his rehabilitation program during this period.

3. Anger: this frequently follows the period of denial when the truth can no longer be ignored. The patient becomes angry at the world, at those causing his injury, the staff, God, or anything or anyone available.

4. Bargaining: a bargain is struck with himself, his surroundings, or God. "If only my fingers will function, I will be satisfied," or "If only I could walk I would not

ask for more." As each stage is reached, a new bargain is made for the next stage.

5. Grief and mourning: all patients with a permanent degree of disability go through a stage where they mourn the loss of body functions. This frequently occurs after several months when the patient no longer sees evidence of neurologic return.

6. Adjustment: while there is no actual stage of "acceptance" of the disability, ultimately many patients re-

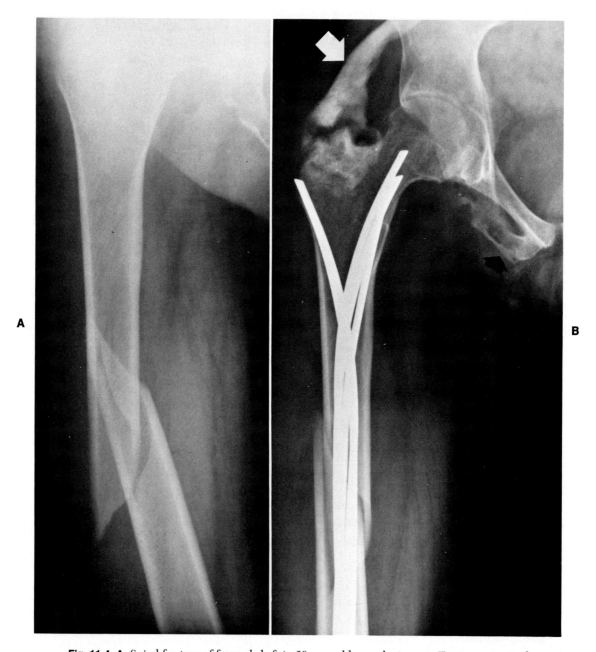

Fig. 11-4. A, Spiral fracture of femoral shaft in 20-year-old paraplegic man. Fracture occurred during range of motion exercises. **B,** Surgical stabilization was achieved by insertion of Ender rods. Insertion is in lower femur away from sensible areas: ectopic bone at hip *(white arrow)* and pressure sore and previously resected and regenerated ischial tuberosity *(black arrow).*

alize the permanence of their lesion and adjust to the fact that they have to make the best of what they have. Once this realization comes, the patient frequently becomes a good vocational candidate and actively takes a permanent and true interest in taking care of himself and in community reintegration. This process may take as long as several years.[6]

Psychologic adjustment to a permanent disability is always a real or potential problem. To attempt to minimize these problems, an early, realistically optimistic prognosis must be given by the physician. It is necessary to be as explicit as possible. Communication among the staff is equally crucial, since it is important that all staff members know what has been said to minimize the chance of the patient's playing one staff person off against the other. Group conferences among patients or families or both are frequently useful when they are run by an appropriately trained staff person. For a short period of time, small doses of amitryptyline have been reported to be useful for treating depression.

Suicide attempt during rehabilitation or immediately after discharge are rare. Those individuals who have a spinal cord injury as a result of a self-inflicted wound require close psychiatric attention and follow-up.[2,26]

SEX

Voluntary control of the sex act depends on an intact neural axis, as well as an adequate balance of the hormone level and the proper psychologic makeup. As many as 50% of men with spinal cord injury may have testicular atrophy, presumably secondary to loss of autonomic temperature control in the scrotum and frequent urinary tract infections.

There are several centers in the spinal cord having to do with the sexual functions of erection, emission, and ejaculation. The two centers for erection are the peripheral or reflexly activated center (parasympathetic S2 through S4 via the pelvic nerves), and the central or psychogenically activated center (sympathetic T11 through L2 via the hypogastric nerves). The S2 through S4 area is responsible for ejaculation via the somatic pudendal nerve.[27]

A comprehensive discussion of altered neurophysiology of the sexual act in spinal cord injury is beyond this discussion, but as many as 75% of spinal cord injured men can achieve an erection, 35% successful coitus, and 10% ejaculation. The patients with the higher level spinal cord lesions have a better chance of achieving an erection, but those with a lower level lesion have a better chance of achieving ejaculation and orgasm. The degree of success with regard to sexual intercourse will vary greatly with the degree of completeness of the lesion; the more incomplete the lesion, the greater the chance of success.

The issue of sexuality and sexual function in the spinal cord injured is certainly one that must be dealt with in a thorough manner and that cannot wait until the patient raises the issue. On the other hand, it must not be explored at an inappropriate time during the rehabilitation program, or more harm than good may result. Although sex is one of the many functions altered in spinal cord injury, attitudes about it vary so greatly among individuals that it assumes different degrees of importance in each patient. The whole issue of sexual satisfaction for the patient and partner must be considered in the context of what is satisfactory to both individuals and does not violate the social or moral codes of either.[13,17]

PREGNANCY AND LABOR

Frequently after the onset of a major spinal cord injury, a woman may miss her menstrual period for as long as several months. In the absence of anemia or complicating medical problems, normal menses will usually restart and continue uneventfully. An occasional patient will have difficulty with autonomic dysreflexia at the time of menses. In the absence of complicating medical factors, a spinal cord injured woman with normal menses may be assumed to have also resumed normal ovulation cycles and should not have an impairment in fertility.

The course of pregnancy may be uneventful except for the increased difficulty in performing normal activities of daily living. Further along in the pregnancy if the patient has bacteriuria, the chance of symptomatic genitourinary infection increases as does the chance of upper tract involvement caused by the enlarging uterus. The actual course of labor may be painless if the lesion is above the somatic innervation to the abdomen. In patients with upper motor neuron lesions, labor tends to be very precipitate. In those patients with lesions above T5, the onset of labor also carries with it the chance of the onset of autonomic crisis (autonomic dysreflexia). For these two reasons most physicians will hospitalize a pregnant woman with spinal cord injury at 32 weeks' gestation. Indications for cesarean delivery are the same as in an individual without a spinal cord injury.[20,23]

LONGEVITY AND MORTALITY

Survival in the spinal cord injured person has improved dramatically since the establishment of the first spinal cord injury center at Stokes-Mandeville Hospital in the 1940s. Following World War I only 10% of soldiers with spinal cord injuries survived more than 1 year. Recent studies indicate that the overwhelming number of spinal cord patients that die do so within the first 2 months of injury as a result of respiratory causes. Once the patient is past the initial few months, the chances of long-term survival increase dramatically.

The major causes of death in long-term spinal cord injured patients are renal failure, cardiovascular disease, and respiratory problems, respectively.[11] It is likely that with the advent of increased interest in spinal cord injury and the use of antibiotics, intermittent catheterization, and the more widespread availability of spinal cord centers the incidence of death from these causes may decrease with time.[12]

REFERENCES

1. Abramson, A. S., and Delagi, E. F.: Influence of weight-bearing and muscle contraction in disuse osteoporosis, Arch. Phys. Med. Rehabil. **42**:147-151, 1961.
2. Athelstan, G. T., Mitchell, C. J., Dickerson, A., and Sell, G. H.: Psycho-social and vocational programs, Proc. Annu. Clin. Spinal Cord Injury Conference, pp. 119-139, 1978.
3. Benassy, J.: Associated fractures of the limbs in traumatic paraplegia and tetraplegia, Paraplegia **5**:209, 1968.
4. Buchwald, E.: Physical rehabilitation for daily living, New York, 1952, McGraw-Hill Book Co.
5. Burke, D. C.: Pain in paraplegia, Paraplegia **10**:297, 1973.
6. Burke, D. C., and Murray, D. D.: Handbook of spinal cord medicine, London, 1975, Macmillan International, pp. 67-70.
7. Claus-Walker, J., Spencer, W. A., Carter, R. E., et al.: Bone metabolism in quadriplegia: dissociation between calciuria and hydroxyprolinuria, Arch. Phys. Med. Rehabil. **56**:327-332, 1975.
8. Comarr, A. E.: Bowel regulation for patients with spinal cord injury, J.A.M.A. **167**:18-21, 1958.
9. Connell, A. M., Frankel, H., and Guttmann, L.: Motility of pelvic colon following complete lesions of spinal cord, Paraplegia **1**:98-115, 1963-1964.
10. Ford, J. R., and Duckworth, B.: Physical management for quadriplegic patient, Philadelphia, 1974, F. A. Davis Co.
11. Freed, N. M., Bakst, H. J., and Barrie, D. L.: Life expectancy, survival rates, and causes of death in civilian patients with spinal cord trauma, Arch. Phys. Med. Rehabil. **47**:457-463, 1966.
12. Geisler, W. O., Jousse, A. T., and Wynne-Jones, M.: Survival in traumatic transverse myelitis, Paraplegia **14**:262-275, 1977.
13. Griffith, E. R., and Trieschmann, R. B.: Sexual function-ing in women with spinal cord injury, Arch. Phys. Med. Rehabil. **56**:18-21, 1975.
14. Guttmann, L.: Spinal cord injuries. Comprehensive management and research, Oxford, England, 1973, Blackwell Scientific Publications.
15. Guttmann, L., and Frankel, H.: Value of intermittent catheterization in early management of traumatic paraplegia and tetraplegia, Paraplegia **4**:63-84, 1966-1967.
16. Hardy, A. G.: Complications of the indwelling urethral catheter, Paraplegia **6**:6, 1968.
17. Hohmann, G. W.: Considerations and management of psycho-sexual readjustment in cord-injured male, Rehabil. Psychol. **19**:50-58, 1972.
18. Lee, I. Y., Ragnarsson, K. I., Sell, G. H., et al.: Trans-urethral bladder neck surgery in spinal cord injured patients, Arch. Phys. Med. Rehabil. **59**:80-83, 1978.
19. Pedersen, E.: Clinical assessment and pharmocologic therapy of spasticity, Arch. Phys. Med. Rehabil. **55**:344-354, 1974.
20. Robertson, D. N. S., and Guttmann, L.: Paraplegic patient in pregnancy and labour, Proc. R. Soc. Med. **56**:381-387, 1963.
21. Rossier, A. B.: Rehabilitation of the spinal cord patient, Documenta Geigy Acta Clinica, Basel, 1973.
22. Rossier, A. B.: Neurogenic bladder in spinal cord injury. Management of patients in Geneva, Urol. Clin. North Am. **1**:125, 1974.
23. Rossier, A. B., Ruffieux, M., and Ziegler, W. H.: Pregnancy and labour in high traumatic spinal cord lesions, Paraplegia **7**:210-216, 1969.
24. Ruge, D.: Spinal cord injury, Springfield, Ill., 1969, Charles C Thomas, Publisher.
25. Rusk, H. A.: Rehabilitation medicine, ed. 4, St. Louis, 1977, The C. V. Mosby Co.
26. Smith, C. R.: Home planning for severely disabled, Med. Clin. North Am. **53**:703-711, 1969.
27. Tarabulcy, E.: Sexual function in the normal and in paraplegia, Paraplegia **10**:201-208, 1972.
28. Toerge, J. E., Rosen, J. S., and Calenoff, L.: Secondary spinal lesions in spinal cord injury patients, Arch. Phys. Med. Rehabil. **59**:343, 1978.
29. Valbona, C., Spencer, W. A., Cardus, D., and Dales, J. W.: Control of orthostatic hypotension of quadriplegic patients with pressure sores, Arch. Phys. Med. Rehabil. **44**:7-18, 1963.
30. Viau, A. P., Naftchi, N. E., St. Paul, H. M., et al.: Mineral metabolism in spinal cord injury, Fed. Proc. **37**:926, 1978.

CHAPTER 12

Clinical evaluation of the neurogenic bladder

PAUL E. KAPLAN, M.D.

In order to evaluate the neurogenic bladder, it is necessary to understand the applied physiology of the normal bladder. Quantitative as well as qualitative information about the bladder's function is vital. This information must be obtained serially so that any alteration of bladder function can be monitored. The evolution of bladder function is a constant finding in patients with neurogenic bladders. Accordingly, a brief summary of the applied physiology will first be necessary.

APPLIED PHYSIOLOGY

The bladder's innervation is through the parasympathetic portion of the autonomic nervous system.[10] It is cranial as well as sacral. Smooth muscle of the bladder's internal sphincter and bladder neck is not under any voluntary control but is normally in a state of contraction. It has a resting tone. The parasympathetic nervous system and the sympathetic nervous system are not necessarily competitive in all aspects. The interaction between the parasympathetic and sympathetic nervous systems is not one of simple facilitation or inhibition. It is sometimes an additive relationship and subject to cranial modification. Brain stem and cerebral lesions can augment or inhibit bladder contraction. The external urethral and anal sphincters are skeletal muscle and are responsive to voluntary control.[7] They are normally in a contracted state until relaxed. The micturition reflex is initiated by sphincteric relaxation, which is preceded by subjective sensations.[24] Cranial control therefore indirectly influences the tone of the bladder and

internal sphincter through the autonomic nervous system and may directly influence the relaxation of the external anal and urethral sphincters.[26] It is the cranial control that is reduced in the neurogenic bladder.

HISTORY AND PHYSICAL EXAMINATION

The first step in any evaluation of a patient with a neurogenic bladder is a complete history and physical examination. During the history taking any neurologic impairment that might affect the bladder, such as neuropathies, spinal cord injury, multiple sclerosis, and strokes, should be carefully documented. In addition, the history of the patient's bowel and bladder habits prior to the onset of the spinal cord injury should be investigated. It is vital to learn the state of the patient's present sensation in his bladder. Can he distinguish when his bladder is full or not? Can he tell when he is voiding? Is it painful when he tries to urinate? Must the patient help the urination along by pressing in on his abdomen? Has the patient ever had to use a catheter or any other appliance?

The history of any urinary dysfunction should be combined with the history of bowel habit dysfunction and the history of sexual dysfunction. On physical examination, a complete neurologic examination is essential, as is an examination of the genitals and a thorough anal examination. Sensation of the perineal area should be evaluated. Intact light touch and pinprick sensations are often associated with the ability to know when to void.

During the anal examination the presence or absence of the bulbocavernosus (BC) reflex and/or anocutaneous (AC) reflex should be determined. Since the innervation of the bladder is through the pelvic nerve, the presence of the BC reflex is very important in determining whether innervation is intact. In females the AC reflex is evaluated. These reflexes are not identical. However, the BC reflex has a very similar pathway to the AC reflex.[21] In the BC reflex, stimulation of the foreskin results in a contraction of the external urethral sphincter. For the AC reflex the skin around the anus is pinched and the external sphincter of the anus contracts. The BC and AC reflexes are similar enough that they are often used for determining (1) the intactness of the reflex arc involving the sensory return from the anal skin or foreskin to the S3 and S4 segments of the spinal cord and (2) the somatic innervation through the pudendal nerve to the anal or urethral sphincters.

RESIDUAL CAPACITY

Central to the evaluation of the neurogenic bladder is determination of the residual capacity of the bladder. The patient should be catheterized immediately after voiding. The urine volume must be measured. The urine obtained by catheterization should be sent for analysis and culture and sensitivity determinations. It has been suggested that a balanced bladder is one in which the ratio of total volume (residual and void) to residual volume is not more than 5:1 (maximal 60 ml) for "upper motor neuron" type neurogenic bladders and 10:1 (maximal 40 ml) for "lower motor neuron" type neurogenic bladders.[2,4] Serial residual volume determinations are usually obtained as a central part of intermittent catheterization management techniques.

CYSTOMETRY

Cystometry can be performed using a variety of equipment. The most reproducible method uses a mercury strain gauge and transducer attached to a polygraph. The direct cystometrogram is performed using suprapubic catheterization. The bladder could be catheterized through the urethra, drained, and its pressure measured in the indirect method. A sterile 5% glucose solution made of known volume might be used to fill the bladder and the pressure monitored in either method. The pulse and blood pressure should also be monitored, especially when evaluating tetraplegic patients. Several phases of micturition may be identified. These include precontraction, isometric contraction, isotonic contraction, decreased contraction, and the final phase.[20] The first desire to urinate will be at 175 ml with the fullness at 450 ml, and the capacity at approximately 450 ml. Accordingly, during intermittent catheterization, the total volume of the bladder is kept to 300 to 500 ml. The catheterizations or residual determinations are timed so that this objective is met.

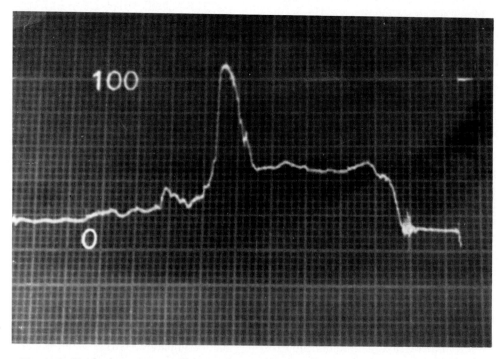

Fig. 12-1. Urethral pressure profile in patient with vesicosphincteric dysfunction. Bladder is empty and at rest. Catheter is slowly pulled out of bladder through urethra. External urethral sphincter pressure is in excess of 100 mm Hg.

Excretory cystometry might also be used to evaluate the neurogenic bladder. It is, however, more cumbersome than retrograde cystometry and does not notify the investigator as to the bladder volume at any one point in time. Pressure of the external urethral sphincter could be determined at any time before or after the evaluation (Fig. 12-1).

CLASSIFICATION

Using the BC/AC reflexes and cystometrogram results, it is possible to classify the neurogenic bladder. Four categories are suggested:

1. AC/BC positive (+) hypertonic neurogenic bladders (upper motor neuron)
2. AC/BC negative (−) hypotonic neurogenic bladders (lower motor neuron)
3. AC/BC positive (+) hypotonic neurogenic bladders (transitional state)
4. Normal bladder

To date, AC/BC (−) hypertonic neurogenic bladders are not at all common and are probably transitional or represent incomplete lesions. AC/BC (+) hypertonic neurogenic bladders have the highest probabilities of responding to intermittent catheterization programs and of becoming catheter free. AC/BC (−) hypotonic bladders have the lowest probabilities of becoming catheter free. Credé's maneuvers or abdominal pressure or both will be necessary.[3]

CYSTOURETHROGRAPHY

Voiding cystourethrography is extremely important in the evaluation of the neurogenic bladder.[9] Techniques are described in Chapter 13. Intravenous urogram allows evaluation of kidney function and the detection of hydronephrosis. Cystourethrography, using iced solutions of contrast medium, similar to the ice water test has been used to determine whether sensation from the bladder is intact. The ice water diagnostic test is, however, useless to evaluate bladder function.[22]

ELECTROMYOGRAPHY

The end organ of the micturition reflex, the bladder, is smooth muscle in a syncytium. Therefore it represents a compromise between the syncytial skeletal muscle that is in the heart and the smooth muscle that is in the gastrointestinal tract. It is laced with postganglionic parasympathetic neurons.[10] As early as 1936,[6] it was noted that electric activity could be recorded from the detrusor muscle. At first, it was recorded with bromide paper. Later, bladder electromyography was performed on animal and human subjects.[16] Modern techniques include the following. A fine kinesiologic wire may be threaded through a French urethral catheter, looped over a 25- or 22-gauge needle, and implanted in the bladder wall. The electric potentials are recorded using an electromyograph. A very sensitive recording appa-

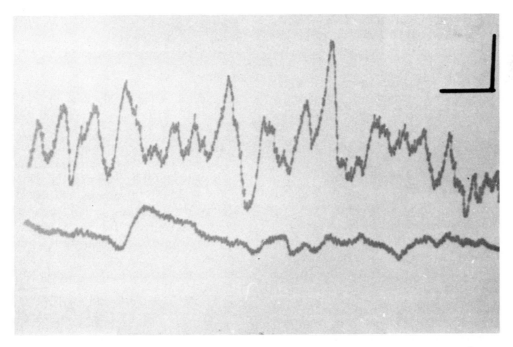

Fig. 12-2. Comparison of bladder and external urethral sphincter electromyogram. Top line is bladder (smooth muscle) electric activity potentials at 20 μV/vertical marker. Bottom line is external urethral sphincter electric potentials at 200 μV/vertical marker. Horizontal marker is 10 msec for each line. While bladder is active, external urethral sphincter is not. This recording was taken just at voiding.

ratus is necessary because the electric potentials are very small (8 to 60 μV) and brief (2 to 5 msec).[13,16]

Bladder electromyographic response from normal human bladders reveals that at rest the bladder still has electric activity.[18] This electric activity is comparable to the resting tone of the bladder wall. As a result, abnormally increased potential amplitude and frequency are noted in the AC/BC (+) hypertonic bladder, whereas the spastic muscle is silent with an electromyogram (EMG) examination.[13] AC/BC (+) or AC/BC (−) hypotonic neurogenic bladders have EMG responses of decreased amplitude and frequency.[14] Skeletal EMG activity and smooth muscle EMG activity are not parallel. Patients with active external urethral sphincters may have hypotonic bladders. Electromyography of the external urethral or anal sphincter or of the abdominal wall has been performed simultaneously with bladder electromyography.[17] External urethral or anal sphincter activity or abdominal wall EMG activity is not simultaneous with detrusor electric activity but is often inversely related to it. On the one hand, bladder EMG activity has been observed with the patient under general anesthesia[15] and with all skeletal muscles at rest. On the other hand, simultaneous contraction of the detrusor and external urethral sphincter is often observed. The pressure and electric activity of the external urethral sphincter are often greatly elevated throughout the examination of these cases (Fig. 12-2).[5,8]

The bladder EMG is not a standard evaluation for every patient. Cystourethrography, cystometry, and sphincter electromyography may be done. Bladder EMG is not performed on patients with infection who are not under treatment with an antibiotic. A small amount of microscopic hematuria may be seen after bladder EMG for the next 1 or 2 days but clears up spontaneously. Generally the indications for bladder EMG are those of a patient with a neurogenic bladder who has been evaluated with cystourethrography and intravenous urography and who is not undergoing successful decatheterization (Fig. 12-3).

Bladder EMG has been used to characterize the different types of neurogenic bladders on the basis of EMG activity. AC/BC (+) hypotonic and hypoactive bladders are found in patients from the first half year to the full year after their spinal cord injury. They usually evolve to normal or to AC/BC (+) hypertonic and hyperactive bladders. In the normal bladder group a frequency of 71 Hz, or cycles per second, a mean amplitude in the electric activity of 15 μV, and a duration of 4.6 msec of those motor unit potentials were recorded from smooth muscle. The wave is similar to fibrillation potential in skeletal muscle in duration and amplitude and has a regular periodicity.

In AC/BC (−) hypotonic and hypoactive bladders,

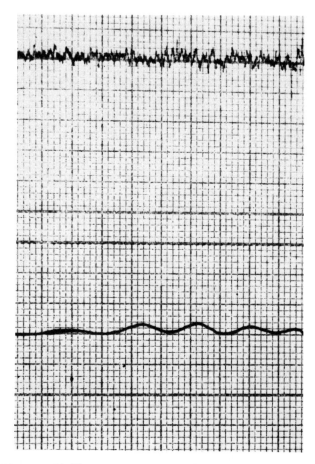

Fig. 12-3. Bladder cystometrogram and external urethral electromyogram are compared with patient starting to void. Top line is external urethral sphincter electromyogram. Sphincter is relatively silent during voiding. However, bladder pressure *(bottom line)* has greatly increased.

the electric activity of the smooth muscle is greatly diminished. The frequency, amplitude, and the duration are decreased. Because the duration is decreased in all of the other types of neurogenic bladders, the duration of the potentials recorded in smooth muscle (detrusor muscle) is probably related to the mass of the contracting muscle. The frequency and the amplitude of the electric potentials are greater in the AC/BC (+) and hypoactive bladders than in the AC/BC (−) hypotonic and hypoactive bladders; this is related to an increased contractile ability in the AC/BC (+) hypotonic bladders and foreshadows their better prognosis.

CYSTOMETRY AND ELECTROMYOGRAPHY

When the bladder is filled, its electric activity may be observed while it is at rest, half full, full, and voiding. With the stimulation of the increased pressure and volume, increased electric activity has been noted. In the normal bladder during EMG, the amplitude and

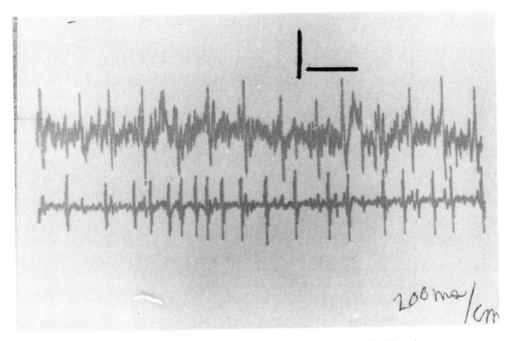

Fig. 12-4. External urethral sphincter electromyogram *(top line)* and bladder electromyogram *(bottom line)* are compared in patient with vesicosphincteric dysfunction. Two muscles are contracting simultaneously.

frequency of the bladder's electric potentials are increased, whereas the duration of each potential is decreased and a silent period of electric activity in the external urethral sphincter is noted during voiding. Quantitative correlations have been determined between the increase of bladder pressure, the bladder volume increase, and the electric activity of the bladder and external urethral sphincter in neurogenic and normal bladders.[14] As the pressure of the bladder increases, the electric activity of the bladder increases in amplitude and frequency but decreases in duration. As the volume goes up, the amplitude increases, the frequency increases, and the duration decreases. All of these correlations are statistically significant at a 1% level. In the AC/BC (−) hypotonic bladder, the bladder's electric activity is greatly reduced. As a result these correlations are less significant in AC/BC (−) hypotonic bladders than in the other types of neurogenic bladders.

AC/BC (+) hypotonic bladders eventually increase in tone. The decreased electrophysiologic tone noted initially is probably caused by the paralysis of the internuncial neurons of the spinal cord.[5,14] Indeed, after a spinal cord injury, bladder electrophysiologic tone may be decreased after appendicular skeletal muscular tone has returned. If flaccid paraplegia is present, the bladder will probably be hypotonic. The hypotonic bladder often exists along with an active external urethral sphincter in AC/BC (+) hypotonic neurogenic blad-

ders.[5] In addition, the comparative embryology of the external urethral sphincter is such that it is a flexor muscle of the tail.[25] Therefore it is kinesiologically similar to other flexor mass appendicular muscles, such as the medial hamstrings. As a result if a patient has very spastic medial hamstrings, he will usually have a spastic urethral sphincter.

Vesicosphincteric dysfunction occurs as a result of the obstruction to urine flow by the sphincters at the bladder neck.[27] This situation is most often found in AC/BC (+) hypertonic bladders. In spinal cord injured patients, the higher the level, the greater the possibility of developing vesicosphincteric dysfunction.[8,23] The silent period of the external sphincter during micturition is greatly shortened or eliminated. Hyperactivity of the urethral sphincter has also been noted in the AC/BC reflex. In effect, the bladder and sphincter are contracting together. The bladder evaluation of bladder EMG, external sphincter EMG, and cystometry will clearly indicate when this dysfunction exists (Fig. 12-4).[13]

BETHANECHOL TESTS

The bethanechol test is, at times, used to evaluate the neurogenic bladder.[24] In doing a cystometrogram in a normal person, if an injection of bethanechol is given, the patient will not be particularly sensitive to it. Uninhibited contractions will be absent, voiding midstream will not be interrupted, and residual urine will be less than 40 ml. A very great response to bethanechol is present in some AC/BC (+) hypertonic neurogenic bladders. The bethanechol in them will stimulate vesicosphincteric dysfunction with uninhibited bladder and sphincter contractions and interrupted urine flow. In AC/BC (−) hypotonic neurogenic bladders the bethanechol increases bladder contraction. The explanation for the positive test results is that the extreme decentralization of the bladder makes it very sensitive to bethanechol.

AUTONOMIC NERVOUS SYSTEM IMBALANCE

Bladder EMG and cystogram have been used to evaluate hyperactive neurogenic bladders seen in patients with stroke or multiple sclerosis. Electric potential amplitudes and frequencies of these two groups are increased over those of normal bladders but are not as great as in the AC/BC (+) hypertonic bladder in the patient with spinal cord injury; this is probably because this partial increase in electrophysiologic tone represents a partial interruption of the nerve supply in stroke and multiple sclerosis.[11] The greatly increased total electric activity in spinal cord injured hypertonic bladders represents a complete injury. Therefore in AC/BC (+) hypertonic bladders the increased electrophysiologic tone recorded by bladder EMG parallels the spasticity of the bladder. In these neurogenic bladders, the increased electrophysiologic tone probably mirrors an imbalance in the neuronal innervation so that spasticity represents an augmented stimulatory neuronal excitation.

BIOASSAY PROCEDURES

Bethanechol can increase amplitudes and frequencies of electric potentials of AC/BC (+) or AC/BC (−) hypotonic bladders.[15] Similarly, bladder EMG and cystometrograms have recorded the decrease of electrophysiologic tone in AC/BC (+) hypertonic neurogenic bladders after atropinization. Mecamylamine and phenoxybenzamine have been used in patients with spinal cord injury, neurogenic bladders, and autonomic hyperreflexia.[12] With the use of mecamylamine, there was a reduction in electric potential amplitude and frequency and of the pressure at capacity of the detrusor muscle. Although autonomic hyperreflexia was decreased, so was the contractile ability of the detrusor muscle. The same result was noted with the use of phenoxybenzamine. Phenoxybenzamine has been used for the treatment of autonomic hyperreflexia and also vesicosphincteric dysfunction. However, the administration of phenoxybenzamine also resulted in a reduced contractile ability of the detrusor muscle. Although the pressure of the external urethral sphincter was decreased, so was the maximal pressure produced by the bladder at capacity. The response to phenoxybenzamine reflects a reduction in the overabundant facilitory excitation of the bladder.

BLADDER KINESIOLOGY

Bladder EMG has been performed with placement of electrodes under direct visualization on some of our patients who had either the bladder removed because of tumors or are having transurethral resections and cystoscopies because of prostatic hypertrophy.[14] Since the bladder is a syncytium, bladder EMG may be performed with one wire implanted in the bladder wall. If two electrodes are implanted, the distance between them does not make a significant difference. Additionally, the largest electric potentials were generated on the serosal surface of the bladder. Since the concentration of ganglia and postganglionic neurons is greater on the serosal surface, this result suggests that the electric activity in the detrusor muscle may be produced by postganglionic neurons.[6,14] Another factor increasing electric activity was the tension directly applied to the bladder wall. This factor would correlate well with the increased amplitude and frequency of the electric potentials recorded from the bladder noted with increasing bladder volume and pressure.

OTHER METHODS OF INVESTIGATION

Cystometry with or without bladder electromyography may be supplemented by a number of different procedures either with or without the use of radioisotopes.[2,29] One of them is measurement of the urine flow. The various methods of determining the urine flow depend on attempted urination with and without a catheter. In both instances the amount of urine passed per unit of time may be plotted on a graph and the urine flow rate determined. The urine flow curve may be plotted on the same paper with the cystometrogram, pulse, and blood pressure.

Cystometry may be combined with external sphincter electromyography. In many urodynamic studies, cystometry is combined with electromyography of the external urethral sphincter and urine flow rate determinations. This last combination is particularly valuable for determining the presence of vesicosphincteric dysfunction. In this instance, simultaneous bladder contractions and muscular activity of the external urethral sphincter will be seen. The silent period of the external urethral sphincter during voiding will be absent.[3,30] The urine flow curve without a catheter will be flat as contrasted to the normal curve with a catheter. Often, without a catheter, the flow rate will be interrupted.

An electromyographic evaluation of the lumbosacral extensor spinae muscles, the gluteus maximus bilaterally, the gluteus medius bilaterally, and the anal sphincter is frequently extremely helpful.[1,28] On the one hand, the presence of denervation and a neuropathic interference pattern might help identify a lower motor neuron–type disease process.[19] On the other hand, decreased voluntary control over the skeletal muscles of the L5-S3 myotomes could accurately reflect the ability of the patient to regain full bowel and bladder control.

Abnormalities in the intravenous urogram may lead to a more detailed investigation of kidney function. In any case urinalysis, urine culture, and BUN, serum creatinine, and serum electrolyte determinations are indicated. However, in addition to these tests, the radioisotope scintiscan and renogram may be extremely helpful if kidney dysfunction is suspected. The creatinine clearance and the amount of protein in the urine over a 24-hour period are valuable in the determination of kidney function. If there is a significant amount of protein in the urine, it will then be important to determine the protein electrophoresis of that urinary protein. The presence of globulin in the urine denotes a much more serious urinary dysfunction than if albumin is present. The 24-hour clearance of sodium potassium will also, on occasion, be indicated.

Every patient should be approached on an individual basis. When the diagnosis is in doubt, the test should be repeated during the first several months after a spinal cord injury. In this period, shock may be diminishing and tone returning to the bladder and external sphincters. The management of the neurogenic bladder will only be effective if it is known what type of neurogenic bladder is being treated. In addition, treatment of the neurogenic bladder must be adapted to each patient's needs. A thorough, thoughtful evaluation will clarify the status of the neurogenic bladder. An appropriate regimen can then be instituted to manage that specific neurogenic bladder.

REFERENCES

1. Bailey, J. A., Powers, J. J., and Waylonis, G. W.: A clinical evaluation of electromyography of the anal sphincter, Arch. Phys. Med. Rehabil. 51:403, 1970.
2. Boss, E.: Neurogenic bladder, Urol. Surv. 7:177, 1957.
3. Boss, E.: Intermittent catheterization in paraplegic patients, Urol. Int. 22:236, 1967.
4. Comarr, A. E.: The practical urological management of the patient with spinal cord injury, Br. J. Urol. 31:1, 1959.
5. Diokno, A. C., Koff, S. A., and Bender, L. F.: Periurethral striated muscle activity in neurogenic bladder dysfunction, J. Urol. 112:743, 1974.
6. Evans, J.: Observations on the nervous supply to the bladder and urethra of the cat, with a study of the action potentials, J. Physiol. (Lond.) 86:396, 1936.
7. Floyd, W. F., and Walls, E. W.: Electromyography of the sphincter ani externus in man, J. Physiol. (Lond.) 122:599, 1953.
8. Franksson, C., and Petersen, K.: Electromyographic investigation of disturbances in the striated muscle of the urethral sphincter, Br. J. Urol. 27:154, 1955.
9. Garrett, R. A.: Conservative management of reflux: indications, objectives, technique, follow-up, and results. Proceedings of a workshop on ureteral reflux in children, Washington, D.C., 1967, National Academy of Sciences—National Council, pp. 107, 155.
10. Hinman, F.: The principles and practice of urology, Philadelphia, 1935, W. B. Saunders Co.
11. Kaplan, P. E., and Nanninga, J. B.: Analysis of hyperreflexic neurogenic bladders by bladder electromyography, Electromyogr. Clin. Neurophysiol. 59:297, 1978.
12. Kaplan, P. E., and Nanninga, J. B.: Reduction of bladder contractility after alpha-adrenergic blockade and after ganglionic blockade, Acta Neurol. Scand. 59:172-177, 1979.
13. Kaplan, P. E., Nanninga, J. B., and Lal, S.: Electromyography and cystometry of the neurogenic bladder—a preliminary report, Electromyogr. Clin. Neurophysiol. 16:463, 1976.
14. Kaplan, P. E., Nanninga, J. B., and Lal, S.: Detrusor muscle in spinal cord injured patients: correlations between cystometry and electromyography, Arch. Phys. Med. Rehabil. 58:287, 1977.
15. Kaplan, P. E., Nanninga, J. B., and Lal, S.: Urinary bladder smooth muscle electrical activity: response to atropine and bethanechol, Arch. Phys. Med. Rehabil. 59:454, 1978.
16. Kolesnikov, J. F., Perogov, V. A., and Fotieva, L. V.: Electromyography of the urinary bladder and urethral sphincters, Urol. Nefrol. (Mosk.) 33:34, 1968.
17. LaJoie, W. J., Cosgrove, M. D., and Jones, W. G.: Electromyographic evaluation of human detrusor muscle activity in relation to abdominal muscle activity, Arch. Phys. Med. Rehabil. 57:382, 1976.
18. LaJoie, W. J., Cosgrove, M. D., Jones, W. G., and Kaplan, P. E.: Electromyography of the human bladder, Electromyogr. Clin. Neurophysiol. 15:191, 1975.
19. Lapides, J., Friend, C. R., Ajemian, E. P., and Reus, W. S.: Denervation supersensitivity as a test for neurogenic bladder, Surg. Gynecol. Obstet. 114:241, 1962.
20. Leivin, M. L., Culp, D. A., Flocks, R. H., and Spieer, P. F.: Dynamics of lower urinary tract: a method of study, J. Urol. 96:756, 1966.
21. Mayo Clinic and Mayo Foundation: Clinical examinations in neurology, Philadelphia, 1976, W. B. Saunders Co.
22. Nanninga, J. B., and Kaplan, P. E.: Cystometry and periurethral striated muscle electromyography using cold and room temperature fluid, Urology 13:342-344, 1979.
23. Petersen, I., and Franksson, C.: Electromyographic study of the striated muscles of the male urethra, Br. J. Urol. 27:148, 1955.
24. Porter, N. H.: Megacolon: a physiological study, Proc. R. Soc. Med. 54:1043, 1961.
25. Power, R. M. H.: Embryological development of the levator ani muscles, Am. J. Obstet. Gynecol. 55:367, 1948.

26. Tang, P. C., and Ruch, T. C.: Localization of brain stem and diencephalic areas controlling the micturition reflex, J. Comp. Neurol. **106:**213, 1956.

27. Vereecken, R. L., and Verduyn, H.: The electrical activity of the paraurethral and perineal muscles in normal and pathological conditions, Br. J. Urol. **42:**457, 1970.

28. Waylonis, G. W., and Krueger, K. C.: Anal sphincter electromyography in adults, Arch. Phys. Med. Rehabil. **51:**409, 1970.

29. Winter, C. C.: Application of the scintillation camera in urology, J. Urol. **97:**766, 1967.

30. Zinner, N. R., and Paquin, A. J., Jr.: Clinical urodynamics, J. Urol. **90:**719, 1963.

CHAPTER 13

Radiologic assessment of the urinary system

LEONID CALENOFF, M.D.

The nature of spinal cord injury is such that the effects on the proper functioning of the urinary bladder are not only immediate, but also lasting for a lifetime. It goes without saying that urologic care of a spinal cord injured patient becomes a lifelong task, particularly when the injury is sustained at a young age. Good urologic care is of paramount importance not only for survival, but also for a complication-free life.[10] Sound and meaningful urologic care would be unthinkable without the help of radiology and its various modalities: routine diagnostic procedures, ultrasonography, computed tomography, arteriography, and nuclear medicine. The radiologist practicing in a rehabilitation environment can be of significant help to the physiatrist in the care of spinal cord injured patients. Radiologists involved in the radiologic procedures of the urinary system in spinal cord injured patients are usually fully aware of the particular aspects of spinal cord uroradiology and its underlying pathophysiology and dynamics from the day of injury through the long years of rehabilitation.[59]

The focus of attention after spinal cord injury is certainly the neurogenic bladder, which has to be constantly and thoroughly evaluated clinically and with all testing modalities available, as described in Chapter 12. The neurogenic bladder, however, affects directly or indirectly other components of the urinary system: ureters and kidneys become supravesical problems; the urethra and surrounding structure become infravesical problems. The radiologic problems in the spinal cord injured patient should preferably be assessed in that order: neurogenic bladder, supravesical complications, and infravesical complications. Separate from this approach but not isolated are concomitant injuries of the urinary tract sustained at the time of the spinal cord injury.

CONCOMITANT INJURIES OF THE URINARY SYSTEM

When a spinal cord injury has occurred in a moving accident, such as one involving an automobile or a motorcycle or a fall from a height, injuries of the urinary system can accompany the major injury. At the site of accident or in the emergency room of a hospital, the attention is usually directed to the major injury that has rendered the patient paralyzed. This injury certainly requires all the attention, but it should not distract health care personnel from evaluating other less obviously injured systems such as the organs in the chest (Chapter 8) or in the abdomen (Chapter 9). In addition to the liver and spleen, part of the genitourinary system can sustain minor or major trauma, which if neglected, can lead to grave consequences. A spinal cord injured patient who has lost sensation for pain has no subjective complaints that may attract attention to the urinary system. Therefore hematuria, gross or microscopic, discovered when the urinary catheter is first inserted after the injury, becomes a red flag and calls for further investigation to rule out a concomitant urinary injury. Any difficulties encountered while introducing the catheter should alert health care personnel that

327

there might be a concomitant injury of the urethra.

Concomitant injuries can affect the kidney, ureter, urinary bladder, or urethra. Most of the concomitant injuries can be diagnosed or ruled out by an intravenous urogram. This can be easily performed by injecting or infusing the contrast medium into the IV line placed in the patient immediately after the accident.[63]

Renal trauma

Injury to the kidney can be symptomatic or silent but there always must be significant trauma for injury to occur.[46] In order of gravity, renal trauma can result in (1) contusion, (2) parenchymal laceration with or without tear of the capsule, (3) shattered kidney, or (4) major vessel injury. The first three injuries can be diagnosed by an intravenous urogram, which may show extravasation of the contrast medium from the collecting system, edema with a resulting enlarged kidney (Fig. 13-1), or subcapsular hematoma. When the kidney cannot be visualized on the urogram, it could be related to either massive parenchymal damage or vascular compromise. Arteriography can show damage to minor or major vessels. A neglected injury or a conservatively treated renal injury can result in urinoma formation, hydronephrosis, or renal atrophy. In general, unless there is a major vessel injury, the treatment of concomitant renal trauma is conservative. This is beneficial to the spinal cord injured patient who needs the least number of surgical interventions possible.

Ureteral injury

Concomitant injuries to a ureter are rare. They can occur when a sudden hyperextension of the thoracolumbar spine is accompanied by abrupt deceleration.[46] The rupture of the ureter usually occurs near the ureteropelvic junction. Intravenous urogram will show extravasation of contrast medium, but a retrograde examination may be needed for confirmation.

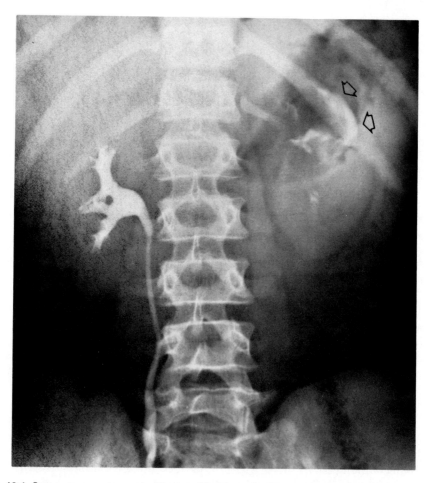

Fig. 13-1. Intravenous urogram in 18-year-old C5 quadriplegic performed shortly after automobile accident, because of hematuria. Left kidney is enlarged, and there is extravasation of contrast medium (*arrows*) in parenchyma of kidney from tear in collecting system. Renal contusion and laceration were treated conservatively.

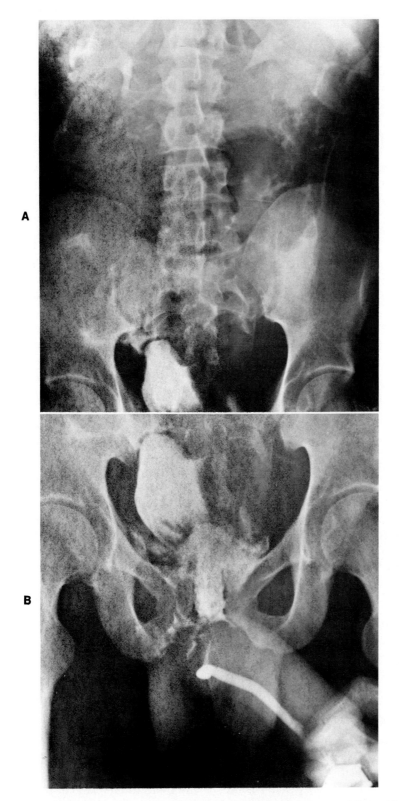

Fig. 13-2. A, Intravenous urogram in 25-year-old man injured in automobile accident who sustained a compression fracture of T4 and injury to pelvis. There is intraperitoneal extravasation of contrast medium, outlining bowel loops. Urinary bladder is displaced to right. **B,** Retrograde urethrogram shows laceration of membranous urethra with extravasation of contrast medium. Urinary bladder is displaced to right by perivesical hematoma.

Trauma to the bladder

If the spinal cord injury is accompanied by trauma to the bony pelvis, in particular if pelvic fractures are present, the urinary bladder might be subject to minor or major injury, with resulting extravasation of urine into the peritoneal space or extraperitoneal structures. When a concomitant urinary bladder injury is suspected, a cystogram should be done first. This is particularly easy if the urinary catheter has been already inserted. The cystogram should be followed by an intravenous urogram.[63] Intraperitoneal ruptures of the bladder are surgically treated. Perivesical hematoma (Fig. 13-2) accompanies pelvic fractures and usually displaces the urinary bladder. If there is no tear, a hematoma can be treated conservatively.

Urethral injury

Concomitant urethral injuries are rare in spinal cord injured patients unless there is severe trauma to the symphysis pubis. The urethra can sustain an iatrogenic injury immediately after spinal cord injury if the Foley catheter is hurriedly or improperly inserted. A retrograde urethrogram is the examination of choice when there is such an injury.

BLADDER CARE AS RELATED TO URORADIOLOGY

Certain aspects of bladder care affect the performance of radiologic procedures, and others influence the radiographic appearance of the urinary tract in spinal cord injured patients. Uroradiologic examinations can look different in the early stages following spinal cord injury, depending on whether the patient has an indwelling catheter, is on intermittent catheterization, or has attained a catheter-free state. A brief review of these terms and related neurogenic bladder function abilities will clarify radiologic manifestations.

Early bladder care

It has become routine to insert a Foley catheter in a spinal cord injured patient immediately on his arrival in the emergency room. The Foley catheter is left in the patient for the entire areflexic state, which lasts about 8 weeks, or until further plans are made for his urologic management. The introduction of the Foley catheter is obviously accompanied by bladder infection, which can plague that patient's management if not eradicated early. To prevent infection, different methods have been advocated. One such method is the closed, aseptically controlled cystostomy method.[37] A percutaneous cystocath[16] is used. A suprapubic cystocath can be used also on an intermittent basis with aspiration of urine done every 6 hours,[21] thus maintaining sterile urine.

Whatever the system of immediate bladder drainage

care, and transition toward permanent bladder care will depend largely on the speed and pattern of bladder recovery in any particular spinal cord injured patient. Such recovery is complex most of the time and does not follow preestablished rules. About 70% of spinal cord injured patients will eventually void spontaneously if properly rehabilitated. Nonetheless, about 30% will require surgery to permit them to pass urine.[7]

Intermittent catheterization

Intermittent catheterization, introduced first in England in 1966, has gained significant popularity. It has its advocates and opponents.[1,33,41,44,55] It is a physiologic trial-of-voiding for establishment of a balanced catheter-free bladder.[44] According to Perkash,[41] catheter-free states can be achieved in 91% of patients after varying periods of intermittent catheterization. An intermittent catheterization program can be judged successful if the patient becomes catheter free, has a low residual urine volume, and a negative urine culture.[55]

Intermittent catheterization can be done via a urinary catheter introduced by the patient himself, by a family member, or by an attendant or via a suprapubic cystocath.[16] The patient's full participation is required because an intermittent catheterization program requires a measured fluid intake and regular catheterization performed initially every 4 hours day and night and later replaced with 6-, 8-, 12-, 24-hour, or postvoiding catheterization. The interval depends on the residual urinary volume found on intermittent catheterization and the progressive ability of the patient to empty the bladder by reflex voiding. Intermittent catheterization can be started soon after injury and can be maintained until reflex voiding develops in upper motor neuron lesions. Reflex voiding may appear as early as 4 to 6 weeks or as late as 2 to 4 months after the injury. In flaccid lower motor neuron areflexic bladders, intermittent catheterization can be continued until the patient becomes able to empty the bladder by Credé's or Valsalva's maneuver. In addition to preventing or minimizing urinary infection, intermittent catheterization has helped to decrease the incidence of periurethritis, periurethral abscess, penoscrotal fistulas, and calculus disease in spinal cord injured patients.[44]

Catheter-free state

As stated earlier, a good number of spinal cord injured patients attain a catheter-free state. In certain individuals this can be achieved easily, whereas in others the route to the catheter-free state is hampered by infection, vesicoureteral reflux, calculi formation, and kidney damage. Some spinal cord injured patients never attain a catheter-free state. This is particularly true for female spinal cord injured patients.[35] Upper motor neuron lesion patients have a better chance to achieve a catheter-free state by emptying the bladder by reflex mechanism. Patients with lower motor neuron lesions have no reflex voiding mechanism and can empty the urinary bladder by other means, such as external pressure or Valsalva's maneuver.

TECHNICAL CONSIDERATIONS

Multiple radiologic procedures are available in the assessment of the urinary tract in spinal cord injured patients. Some of these, such as the KUB film, intravenous urogram, voiding cystourethrograms, and retrograde urethrograms, are used on routine bases. Others, such as tomography, ultrasonography, arteriography, computed tomography, and nuclear medicine, are not as popular, or rather, their use in spinal cord injury has not gained a deserved acceptance. Such an example is ultrasonography, which eventually may substitute for other invasive procedures.

KUB film

The KUB (kidney, ureters, and bladder) film is a plain film of the abdomen taken as a general survey of the urinary tract. It may be a very valuable and simple examination in non–spinal cord injured patients in whom kidney outline can be well seen, calculi can be picked up, and a distended urinary bladder can be well made out. In spinal cord injured patients, however, this type of plain film of the abdomen becomes worthless (Fig. 13-3). Spinal cord injured patients notoriously have a gassy abdomen (Chapter 9), and their colon usually contains excessive amounts of fecal material. As a result, kidney detail will be obscured and calculi are almost impossible to diagnose. This is particularly true for the urinary bladder, where overlying rectal fecal material can make the detection of calculi virtually impossible. The KUB film, however, should be included as a preliminary film on an intravenous urogram, a cystogram, or a retrograde examination.

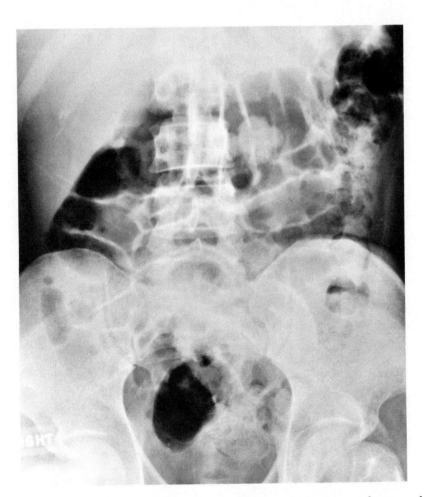

Fig. 13-3. Plain film of abdomen (KUB) in 36-year-old C5 quadriplegic man taken to evaluate for renal calculi. Because of large amount of fecal material and gas in bowel, detail is totally obscured. Note ectopic bone at left hip.

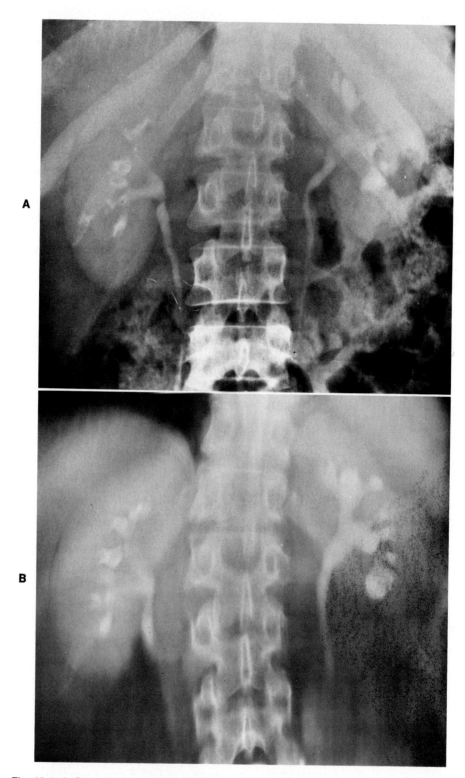

Fig. 13-4. A, Intravenous urogram in 38-year-old T2 paraplegic man with long-standing urinary tract infection. There is bilateral function, but renal outline is obscured by left eleventh rib. **B,** Tomographic cut taken as part of same examination demonstrates smaller-size left kidney with clubbed upper and lower calices and loss of cortex, clear signs of chronic pyelonephritis.

Intravenous urogram

The intravenous urogram is the most frequently performed examination of the urinary system in spinal cord injured patients. Normally a precondition for the performance of a good intravenous urogram is proper bowel preparation. In spinal cord injured patients, however, a bowel preparation can unbalance a well-regulated bowel function. We have eliminated totally bowel preparation for intravenous urograms at the Rehabilitation Institute of Chicago. For 3 years, instead of injecting the standard amount of 50 to 100 ml of contrast medium (Renografin-60 or Hypaque), we were using a 30%, 300 ml infusion of the same product, thus obtaining a better visualization of the collecting system and ureters. Kidney outline and particularly kidney size were difficult to ascertain. The lack of bowel preparation in spinal cord injured patients can be compensated for if tomography is added to the intravenous urogram routine.[24] Modern x-ray machines permit tomography to be done without moving the patient from the usual radiographic table to a specialized tomographic unit. We have been using such a machine for the past 3 years. Tomographic cuts are taken immediately on completion of a bolus intravenous injection of 100 ml of contrast medium. The nephrogram obtained permits adequate kidney measurement. Additional cuts are taken at 5 minutes, when the collecting system is well visualized (Fig. 13-4). The examination is completed with supine and oblique plain films to include the ureters and the bladder and a postvoiding film when the patient has no catheter. The postvoiding film will permit a rough estimate of the bladder residual. If the patient has a Foley catheter, a postdrainage film is taken, which will indicate proper function of the Foley catheter.

The intravenous urogram offers numerous diagnostic possibilities, some of which are evaluation of renal function, anatomic status of the collecting system, and calculi formation and detection of ureterectasis, hydronephrosis, renal atrophy, and neoplastic processes involving the kidneys. The urinary bladder can be roughly estimated as to capacity, size and shape, diverticula, displacement, postvoiding residual, and calculi.

Reactions to urographic contrast media

There is some risk involved in the injection of contrast medium into the patient's system. Reactions vary from the minor, such as nausea and vomiting, flushing, and a few hives, to the more serious, such as hypotension and pulmonary congestion. Very serious complications, although rare, are syncope, shock, bronchospasm, laryngeal edema, and grand mal epileptic seizure.[61] To prevent some of these reactions, it is important not to restrict the patient's fluid intake overnight.

Overnight restriction of fluids prior to an intravenous urogram is an old habit based on the belief that such restriction will enhance the concentration of contrast medium in the collecting system. Such restriction of fluid is not only unnecessary but also dangerous because it may cause dehydration, oliguria, and precipitation of small aggregates and viscid casts that may plug distal tubules, with resulting short- or long-term renal failure. Therefore there should be no restriction of fluid, but solid breakfast should be withheld in order to prevent aspiration in case the patient vomits after the injection of the contrast medium.

Minor reactions to contrast medium do not require treatment; moderate reactions are treated by intramuscular or intravenous injection of an antihistamine. Serious reactions should be treated as any other cardiovascular or respiratory emergency.

Voiding cystourethrography

The next most common radiologic examination of spinal cord injured patients is the voiding cystourethrogram. The purposes of this examination are (1) to evaluate the capacity of the urinary bladder, (2) to detect anatomic abnormalities, (3) to determine the presence of vesicoureteral reflux, (4) to evaluate the voiding capability of the patient, and (5) to evaluate the male urethra for iatrogenic abnormalities.

No preparation is needed for a voiding cystourethrogram except the insertion of a Foley catheter in case one is not already present. If the voiding cystourethrogram is done in a dynamic retrograde fashion,[34] no Foley catheter need be inserted. A cystogram without the voiding part is not advised because vesicoureteral reflex is often seen only during voiding. A voiding cystourethrogram should precede an intravenous urogram. An intravenous urogram can be done immediately after the voiding cystourethrogram if the patient is unavailable for a next-day examination, provided there was no vesicoureteral reflux demonstrated and that the urinary bladder was completely emptied or drained prior to the intravenous urogram. Vesicoureteral reflux can mask a nonfunctioning kidney, and a full urinary bladder can produce a nonexistent ureterectasis on the urogram. A voiding cystourethrogram can be done in an antegrade[13] or retrograde fashion.[34] Contrast medium is usually instilled into the urinary bladder at room temperature, but iced contrast media have been tried to test bladder neck and external sphincters.[38] Fluoroscopy can be used,[34,56] or rapid sequence filming with a 100mm or a 105mm camera can be substituted for fluoroscopy.

Reactions to the contrast medium used in cystography are extremely rare but can occur if the contrast medium refluxes into the collecting system or gets absorbed.[60]

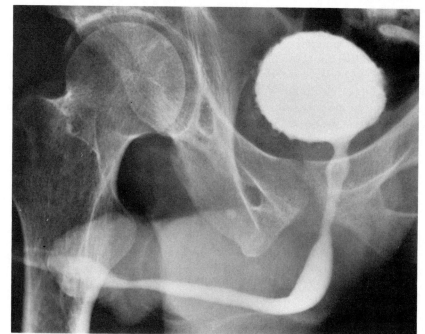

Fig. 13-5. Normal voiding cystourethrogram in 19-year-old C4 incomplete quadriplegic. Reflex voiding started on removal of catheter and stroking thigh.

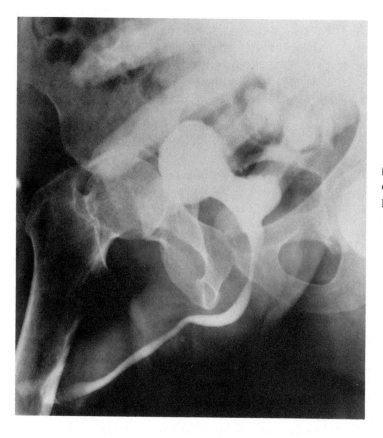

Fig. 13-6. Normal voiding cystourethrogram in 40-year-old T11 paraplegic for past 8 years. Note patient's hand pressing on urinary bladder (Credé's method).

The voiding cystourethrograms are done in our institution in the following manner. After a preliminary film of the abdomen is taken, 30% iodinated contrast medium (Cystografin) is infused through the Foley catheter in the empty urinary bladder. The infusion is not watched fluoroscopically. The infusion is stopped when the contrast medium stops dripping. The amount of contrast medium is recorded, giving an indication about the capacity of the urinary bladder, and a film of the abdomen is taken. This film should include the bladder and the kidney areas. The patient is then turned 45° to the right side and instructed to trigger his voiding mechanism, if he uses such trigger, exactly at the time the catheter will be removed. Regardless of whether the patient uses a trigger or not, a film is taken immediately on the removal of the catheter and usually there is visualization of the entire male urethra (Fig. 13-5). The same can be done with female patients. If the patient continues to void, another film is taken in the same position. On termination of urination, a postvoiding film is taken, which will indicate the degree of emptying. Triggers used are stroking the thigh, tapping the suprapubic area, and insertion of a finger in the rectum[15] in patients with a spastic bladder. Manual pressure (Credé's method) is applied on the urinary bladder in patients with flaccid bladders (Fig 13-6).

If the patient has a suprapubic catheter, the contrast medium is instilled through this catheter. Vesicoureteral reflux can be demonstrated, and often the urethra will be seen and will show anatomic details (Fig. 13-7).

McCallum[34] and Damanski[13] use retrograde techniques to perform voiding cystourethrography. McCallum inserts a size 14 Foley catheter about 2 cm into the penis. One or 2 ml of saline is injected into the balloon of the Foley catheter, and the partially dilated balloon is fixed in the fossa navicularis. With the use of a 50 ml syringe connected to the catheter, contrast medium is injected retrogradely and the urethra is visualized under fluoroscopy. Films are obtained during the retrograde injection. The bladder is then filled through the same catheter, and a voiding study is obtained. The catheter may be either removed for the voiding study

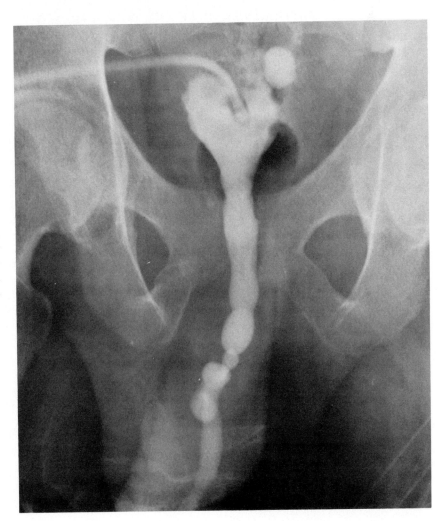

Fig. 13-7. Suprapubic cystourethrogram in 45-year-old who has been quadriplegic for past 7 years. Small-capacity urinary bladder has a diverticulum. Urethra filled spontaneously with contrast medium and demonstrated multiple strictures.

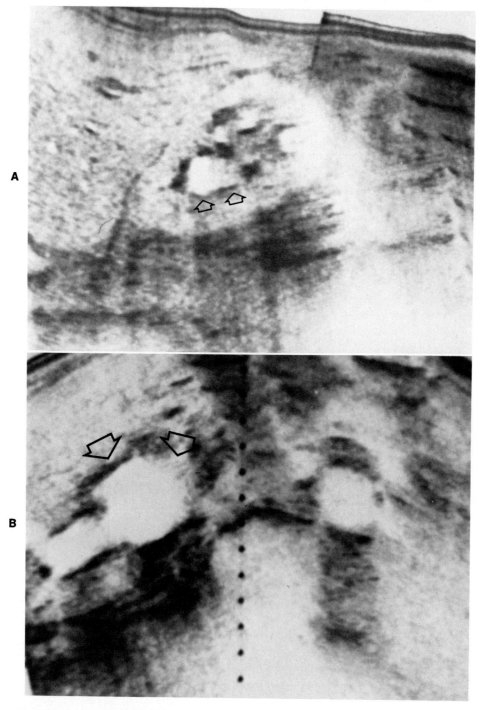

Fig. 13-8. A, Longitudinal and, **B,** transverse sonograms show hydronephrotic right kidney. Dilated renal pelvis *(arrows)* is twice the size of the normal left renal pelvis.

or a choke voiding urethrogram may be obtained by leaving the catheter and syringe in place while the patient voids against pressure.

Regardless of the mode used in cystourethrography, if the patient has a history of autonomic dysreflexia, the filling of the bladder has to be slow. If signs of dysreflexia develop, the bladder is emptied immediately (see Chapter 20).[2]

Retrograde urethrogram

A nondynamic retrograde urethrogram is generally done to evaluate a damaged urethra. Such urethral damage may have occurred as a concomitant injury to the spinal cord injury or may have been inflicted even during the first catheterization at the scene of the accident or shortly thereafter. In most instances iatrogenic changes follow numerous catheterizations.

Nuclear studies

Nuclear medicine study can be used to ascertain renal function, renal size, extravasation of the contrast medium, and vesicoureteral reflux. Details are described in Chapter 19.

Ultrasonography

Ultrasonography is becoming increasingly popular in the evaluation of the urinary system in general. It has no specific applications in spinal cord injury, but it is anticipated that it might in the future complement or even substitute for some of the routine radiologic examinations performed so often in spinal cord injured patients.

In addition to detection of renal masses such as cysts or tumors, ultrasonography has become valuable in demonstrating the parenchymal anatomy of the kidney with its cortex, medulla, and arcuate vessels.[48] Chronic atrophic pyelonephritis has ultrasonic characteristics and can show foci of parenchymal loss.[30] Hydronephrosis and hydroureter are readily diagnosed by ultrasonography (Fig. 13-8) and can be easily observed without the necessity of injecting contrast medium into the patient. The urinary bladder can be well demonstrated by ultrasonography (Fig. 13-9). Bladder volume can be calculated if the width of the bladder is obtained from the transverse scan and the length and the depth from the longitudinal scan. The bladder volume can then be easily shown before and after voiding.[36] Residual urine can also be calculated from a sonogram. Very small bladder volume may be difficult to show but a postvoiding residual will usually be demonstrated by ultrasonography.[39] Ultrasonography is definitely used to detect and evaluate renal and urinary bladder calculi (Fig. 13-10). Renal calculi are difficult to evaluate on plain films of the abdomen, intravenous urogram, or other radio-

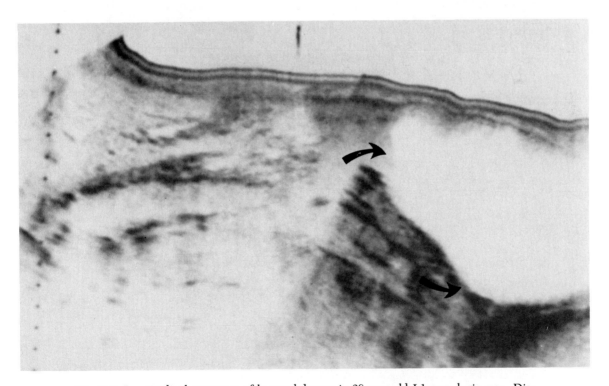

Fig. 13-9. Longitudinal sonogram of lower abdomen in 38-year-old L1 paraplegic man. Distended flaccid urinary bladder *(arrows)* almost reached umbilicus (marker). Bladder volume (full and residual) can be calculated by obtaining bidirectional sonograms.

graphic means. Ultrasonography, however, can pick up very small acoustic shadows produced on the sonogram by calculi in the renal collecting system.[18,45]

Computed tomography

Computed tomography (CT) is not used as a routine procedure in the radiologic assessment of the urinary system in the spinal cord injured patient. In specific instances, however, it can be a very valuable examination.[25] When concomitant renal damage is suspected and the patient is undergoing CT to evaluate the spinal canal or spinal cord, it will require very little additional effort to visualize the kidneys, particularly if contrast medium has already been infused for the evaluation of the spinal cord structures.

In spinal cord injured patients, particularly in the chronic stages of rehabilitation, CT can be useful in the evaluation of renal atrophy, renal calcifications, or hydronephrosis (Fig. 13-11). Suspected or unsuspected renal masses are most readily diagnosed by CT.

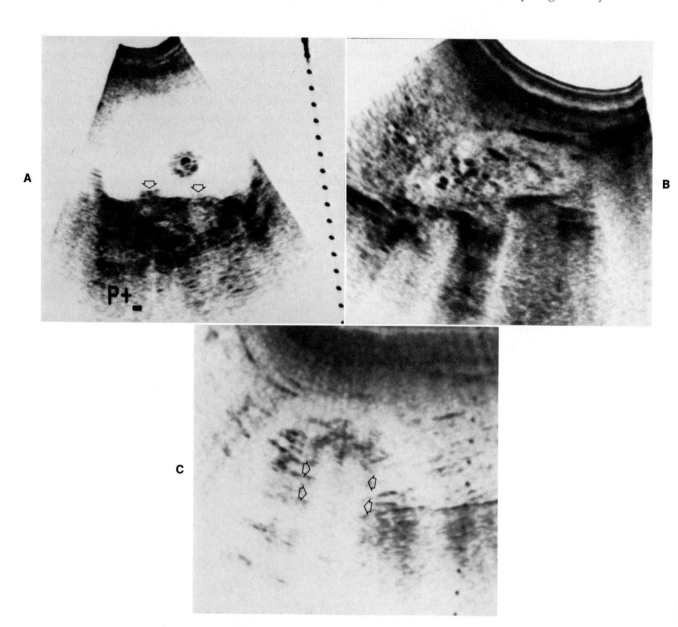

Fig. 13-10. A, Transverse sonogram of urinary bladder in 31-year-old T3 paraplegic woman. Opaque calculi are seen *(arrows).* Note Foley catheter in center. **B,** Sonogram of right kidney of same patient shows about five opaque calculi, which were not detected on urogram. **C,** Longitudinal sonogram of kidney in 25-year-old C5 paraplegic shows two nonopaque calculi in collecting system. Note acoustic shadows *(arrows).*

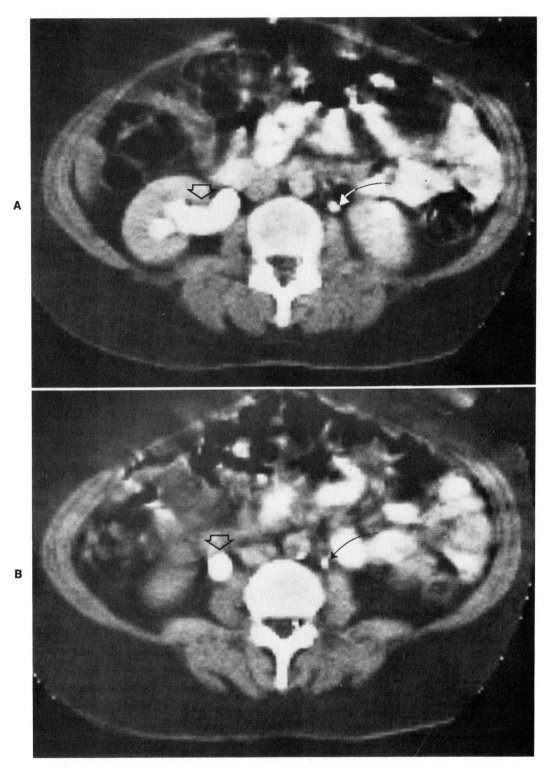

Fig. 13-11. CT scans at level of kidneys, **A,** and at level of L5, **B,** show right-sided hydronephrosis with distended renal pelvis *(arrow* in **A).** Right-sided hydroureter is well seen on
lower level cut *(arrow* in **B).** Note normal-size left ureter *(long arrows).*

NEUROGENIC BLADDER

As stated earlier, the cause for pathophysiologic and morphologic changes in the urinary system in spinal cord injury is the neurogenic bladder. A normal urinary bladder becomes a "neurogenic bladder" at the time of the spinal cord injury. The neurogenic bladder status is dynamic in nature and thus creates a wide spectrum of radiologic manifestations. The applied physiology and the clinical evaluation of the neurogenic bladder are given in detail in Chapter 12. Although not always easy to perform or interpret, a radiologic evaluation should be made in order to determine if one is dealing with a reflex or a flaccid bladder.

Spastic bladder

If the spinal cord injury is above the micturition center located in the conus medullaris at the level of T12-L1 vertebral bodies, neurologic pathways to the brain are interrupted and voluntary control of micturition becomes nonexistent (Fig. 13-12). After the initial "spinal shock," there is a progressive return of somatic and visceral reflex activity to the bladder area controlled by the powerful spinal reflex center. Reflex activity returns first to the striated muscle of the pelvic floor (pudendal nerve) and then to the detrusor, the smooth muscle of the bladder (pelvic splanchnic nerves). In the early stages after injury, the contractions of the detrusor are not strong enough to open the bladder neck. Gradually, however, contractions of the detrusor become more powerful and spinal reflex micturition develops. As stated earlier, this visceral process may take weeks or months. Simultaneously, there is development of the somatic reflex mechanism concerning the external sphincter located distal to the bladder neck at the level of the membranous urethra. When total reflex voiding is achieved, the reflex action should open the external sphincters simultaneously with the contraction of the detrusor. This is not always the case, and some bladders remain typically "neurogenic" (Fig. 13-13).

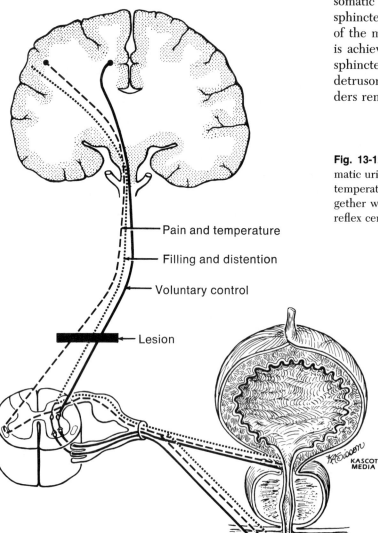

Pain and temperature

Filling and distention

Voluntary control

Lesion

Fig. 13-12. Schematic illustration of reflex, spastic, or automatic urinary bladder with site of lesion. The feeling for pain, temperature, and bladder distention is usually destroyed together with important voluntary bladder control. S2-4 spinal reflex center remains intact.

Fig. 13-13. Spastic bladder in 29-year-old T9 paraplegic woman injured in gunshot accident 2 years earlier. Cystogram shows hourglass deformity, trabeculations, and bilateral vesicoureteral reflux. Patient has never been without Foley catheter since her injury.

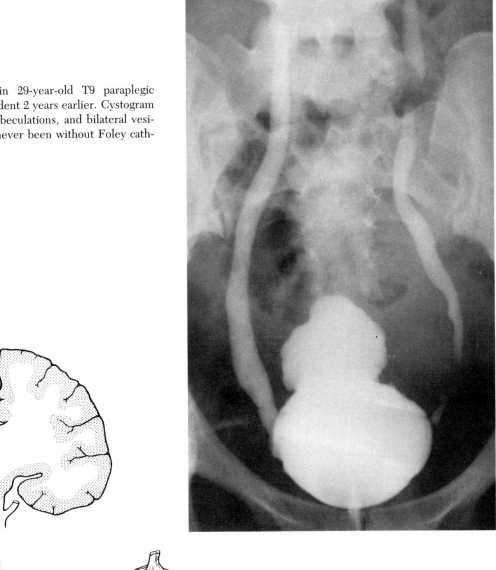

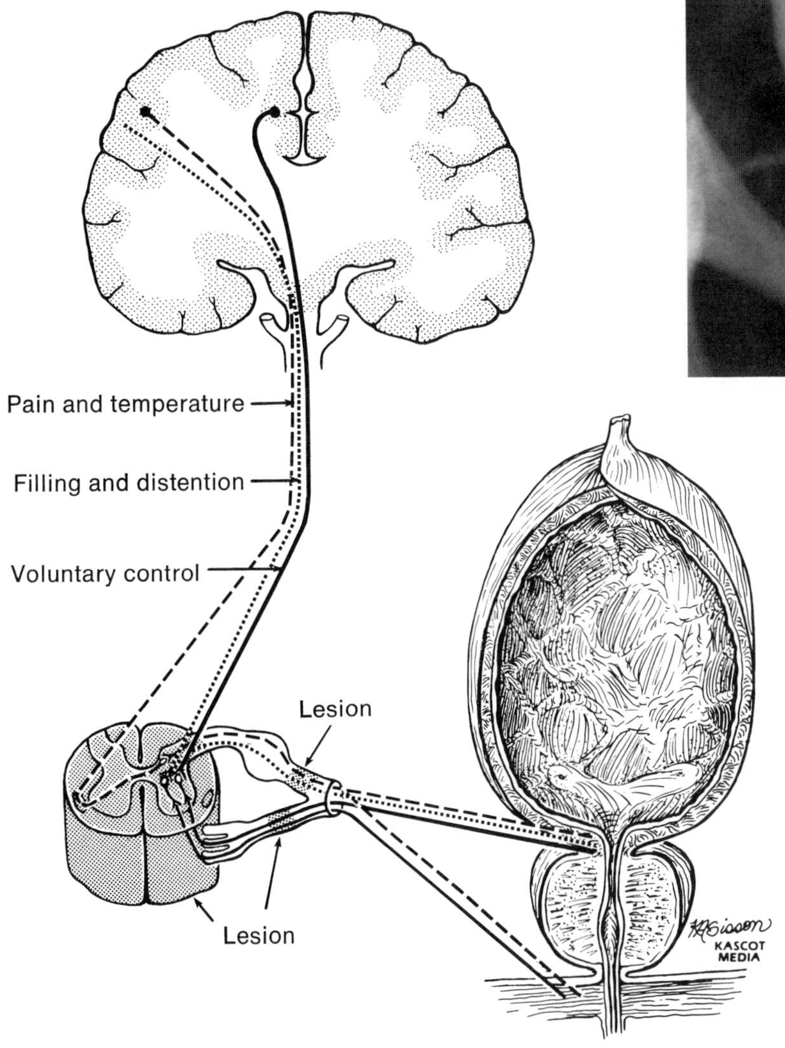

Pain and temperature

Filling and distention

Voluntary control

Lesion

Lesion

KASCOT
MEDIA

Fig. 13-14. Schematic illustration of atonic, nonreflex, autonomous, or flaccid urinary bladder, caused by lesions at or below micturition center of S2-4. Voluntary control and spinal reflex center are destroyed.

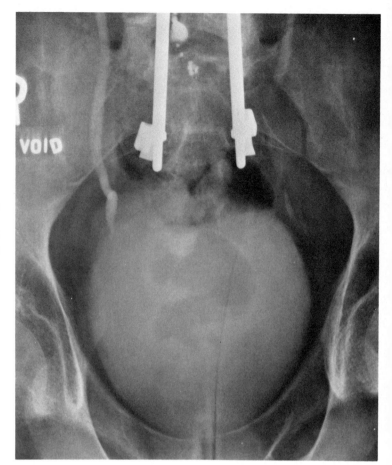

Fig. 13-15. Flaccid bladder in 20-year-old man with fracture of L3 and incomplete lesion of cauda equina, demonstrated on this intravenous urogram. He is catheter free and uses external pressure (Credé's method). Note Harrington rods.

Flaccid bladder

If the micturition center is destroyed or the lesion is below the center, a lower motor neuron bladder is produced. When this situation arises, reflex voiding becomes impossible and the result is a flaccid, atonic, nonreflex or autonomous bladder (Fig. 13-14). After the initial "spinal shock," there is complete urinary retention and closure of the bladder neck. If immediate catheterization does not take place, the overdistention of the bladder will damage sensitive neural elements in the detrusor. In about 2 to 4 weeks if the bladder muscle has not been severely damaged, the bladder can be emptied by pressure: straining with the unparalyzed abdominal muscles or diaphragm or by external pressure (Credé's method). The flaccid bladder is usually of large capacity (Figs. 13-15 and 13-16).

Bladder sphincters

As already mentioned there is dual innervation of the bladder sphincters (Fig. 13-17): splanchnic innervation for the *internal sphincter* made out of smooth muscle fibers, located at the most proximal part of the prostatic urethra, namely, the bladder neck, and for the *intrinsic sphincter* also made of smooth muscle fibers applied to the urethra at the membranous portion; and pudendal innervation for the important *external sphincter* made of striated muscle and located also at the membranous portion of the urethra. This external sphincter is voluntarily controlled before the spinal cord injury. If all functions well, when the detrusor muscle of the bladder contracts, all sphincters should simultaneously relax to permit voiding. This not always being the case, spasm of one or more sphincters occurs with a resulting sphincter dyssynergia.[42,59]

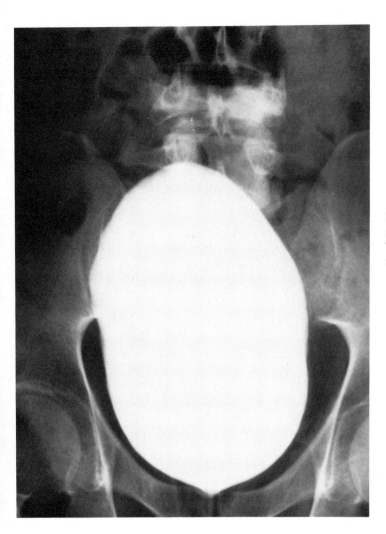

Fig. 13-16. Flaccid, large-capacity urinary bladder filled with 500 ml of contrast medium on cystography. This 23-year-old man was paraplegic as a result of a fracture of L4.

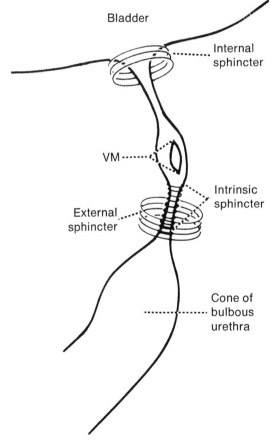

Fig. 13-17. Schematic illustration of urinary bladder sphincters. *Internal sphincter* made of smooth muscle fibers is located at most proximal part of prostatic urethra at bladder neck. *External sphincter* made of striated muscle is located at membranous portion of urethra. *Intrinsic sphincter* made of smooth muscle fibers applied to urethra is also at membranous portion. *VM*, Verumontanum. (From McCallum, R.W.: Radiol. Clin. North Am. **17:**227-244, 1979.)

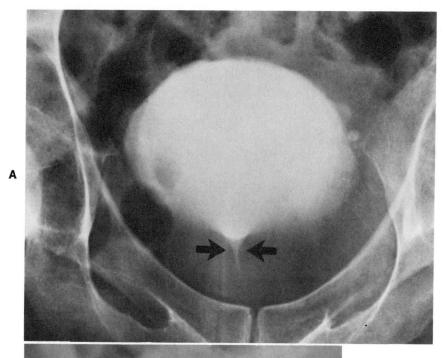

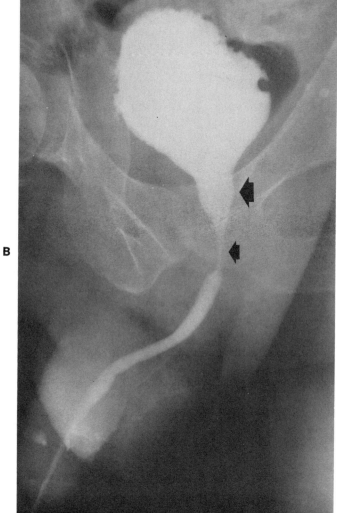

Fig. 13-18. Bladder neck spasm in 26-year-old C6 quadriplegic injured while diving into Lake Michigan. **A,** Baseline voiding cystourethrogram done 1 month after injury shows failure of bladder neck to open *(arrows).* **B,** Same examination 2 years later shows normal reflex voiding. Bladder neck is indicated by large arrow. External sphincter is indicated by small arrow.

Bladder neck spasm

In early reflex activity following an upper motor neuron lesion there may be insufficient activity of the detrusor to pull the bladder neck open and produce voiding.[59] When the bladder neck is not open, the intravenous urogram (Fig. 13-18) or the voiding cystourethrogram (Fig. 13-19) will demonstrate bladder neck spasm.

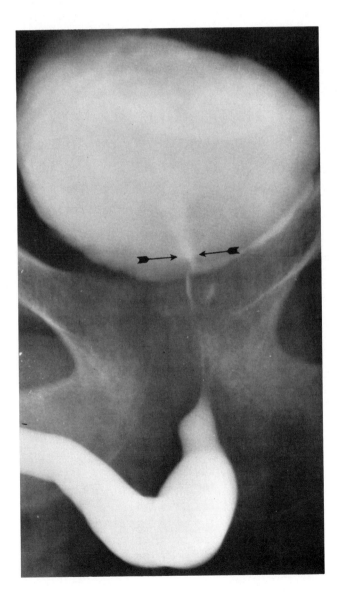

Fig. 13-19. Bladder neck spasm demonstrated on dynamic retrograde urethrogram in 16-year-old quadriplegic. Bladder neck *(arrows)* is closed, but contrast medium jets into bladder by force of the retrograde injection. (Courtesy R. W. McCallum, M.B., F.R.C.P.(C), University of Toronto.)

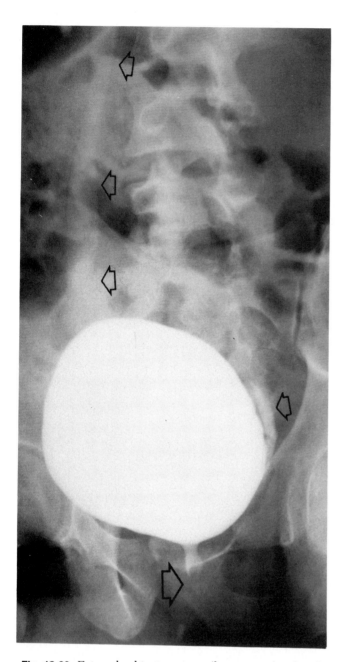

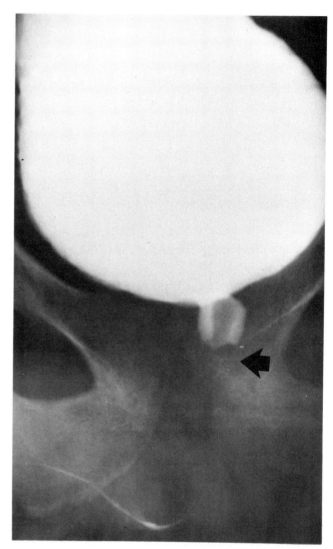

Fig. 13-20. External sphincter spasm *(large arrow)* and early bilateral vesicoureteral reflux *(small arrows)* in 21-year-old C5 quadriplegic injured when diving into shallow water, demonstrated on voiding cystourethrogram done 2 months after injury.

Fig. 13-21. External sphincter spasm *(arrow)* demonstrated on dynamic retrograde urethrogram. The 350 ml of contrast medium injected into bladder stimulated detrusor, opening bladder neck. As a result, prostatic urethra is filled with contrast material, but none enters membranous urethra. This is caused by sphincter dyssynergia. (Courtesy R. W. McCallum, M.B., F.R.C.P.(C), University of Toronto.)

External sphincter spasm

Spasm of the external sphincter is a failure of relaxation of the striated muscle with resulting functional obstruction to the urine flow.[43] Spasm of the external sphincter is best demonstrated during a voiding cystourethrogram (Fig. 13-20) or by a dynamic retrograde urethrogram (Fig. 13-21). On occasion a retrograde urethrogram has to be done because of inability to pass a catheter (Fig. 13-22). Management of dyssynergia, particularly due to external sphincter spasm, can be medical[15] or surgical.[43] (See Chapter 14.)

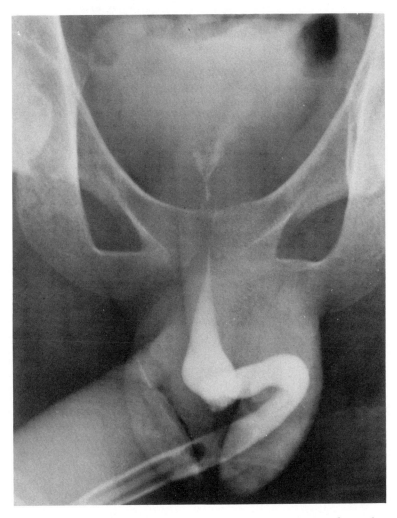

Fig. 13-22. Severe spasm of external sphincter demonstrated on retrograde urethrogram on 18 year-old paraplegic accidentally shot 6 months prior to examination. Placed on intermittent catheterization, he suddenly could not pass the catheter. Cystoscopy revealed swelling of external sphincter.

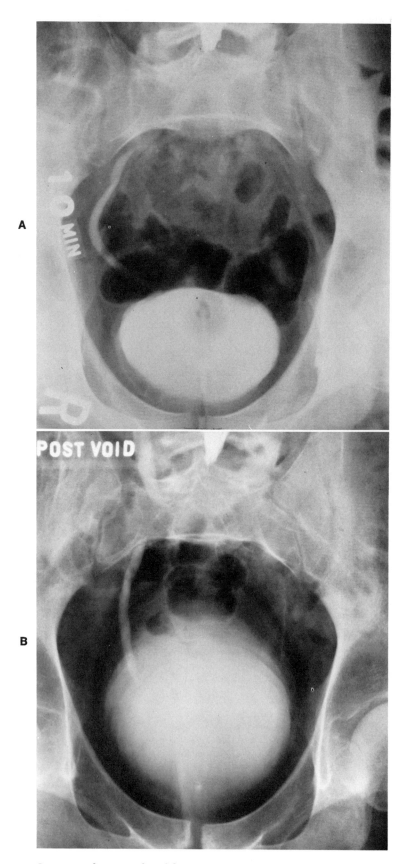

Fig. 13-23. Concentric hypertrophy of detrusor seen in 19-year-old quadriplegic injured from diving into a pile of hay. **A,** Urogram 4 months after injury. **B,** Urogram 18 months later shows concentric hypertrophy of detrusor related to detrusor-sphincter imbalance.

Detrusor hypertrophy

Long-standing detrusor-sphincter dyssynergia and also dyssynergia following long attempts to become catheter free may result in hypertrophy of the detrusor, which is manifested radiographically as concentric layers seen in a contrast medium–filled urinary bladder (Figs. 13-23 and 13-24).

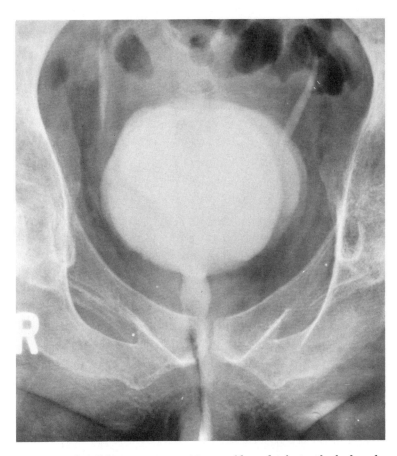

Fig. 13-24. Hypertrophy of detrusor seen in 22-year-old quadriplegic who had made repeated attempts to become catheter free.

SUPRAVESICAL COMPLICATIONS

The ureters and the entire upper urinary tract are always affected by the neurogenic bladder functions and malfunctions. The degree and time of involvement of the upper urinary tract in spinal cord injured patients have no definite correlation with the level of injury or its duration.[27]

A complete obstruction of the bladder neck will pro- duce hydronephrosis, an extreme dilatation of the up- per urinary tract. Spinal cord injured patients are sel- dom neglected in today's rehabilitation setting; there- fore an obstruction is the result of poor home care or the patient's negligence. In most instances there is only a nonobstructive dilatation of the upper urinary tract, which results directly from distention or poor drainage of the neurogenic bladder.[3,52]

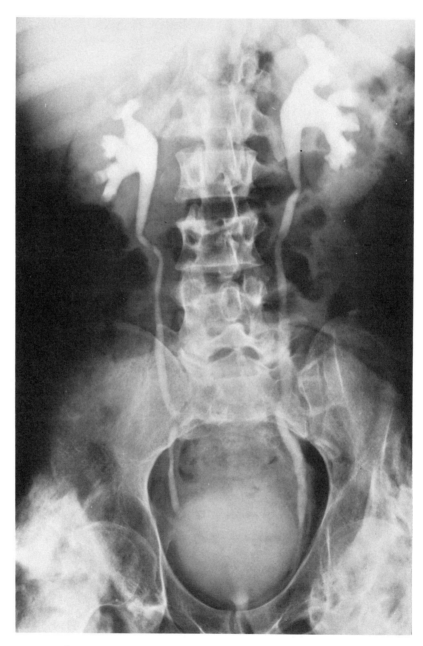

Fig. 13-25. Nonobstructive ureterectasis in 25-year-old T2 paraplegic diagnosed on routine yearly intravenous urogram. Catheter free for 2 years, he apparently had not been able to empty bladder adequately, resulting in distention. Note bilateral severe hip ectopic bone.

Nonobstructive ureterectasis

A nonobstructive ureterectasis is distention of the ureters without obstruction and hydronephrosis (Figs. 13-25 and 13-26). The distinction between nonobstructive ureterectasis and obstructive hydronephrosis is made clinically based on the ability of the patient to pass urine. It has been shown experimentally and verified by fluoroscopy[6] that if the intravesical pressure increases and the urinary bladder becomes distended, the ureters become dilated and ureteral peristalsis diminishes. Ureteral peristalsis ceases completely in patients with upper motor neuron lesions, in whom the maximal intravesical pressure exceeded 37 mm Hg. The same is true for lower motor neuron lesion bladders where the same pressure is induced by Credé's method.

Nonobstructive ureterectasis is usually clinically silent[47] and is commonly discovered on intravenous urography in patients who are catheter free but are unable to empty the bladder satisfactorily. The condition is easily reversible by instituting proper bladder drainage with a well-programmed intermittent catheterization.

One should be careful, however, not to diagnose nonobstructive ureterectasis when the intravenous urogram follows a voiding cystourethrogram with a remaining undrained bladder. Also a significant vesicoureteral reflux will cause ureteral dilatation. Infection can also affect ureteral peristalsis and will show ureterectasis on the urogram.

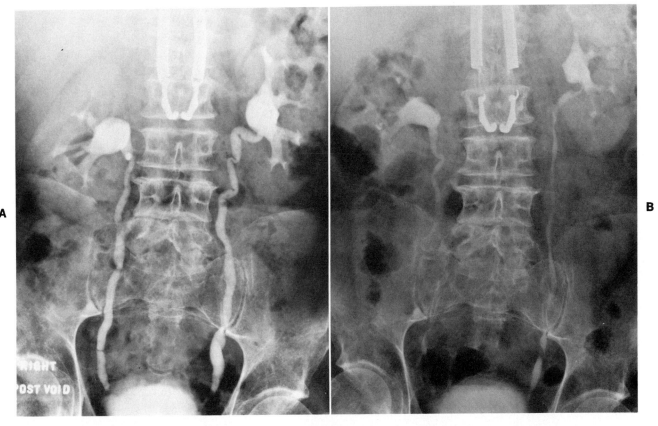

Fig. 13-26. Nonobstructive ureterectasis in 56-year-old T12 paraplegic, catheter free for 18 months. **A,** Both ureters and renal pelvis are dilated. **B,** Placed again on intermittent catheterization, ureters became normal on next 6-month checkup intravenous urogram. Note broken Weiss springs in **B.**

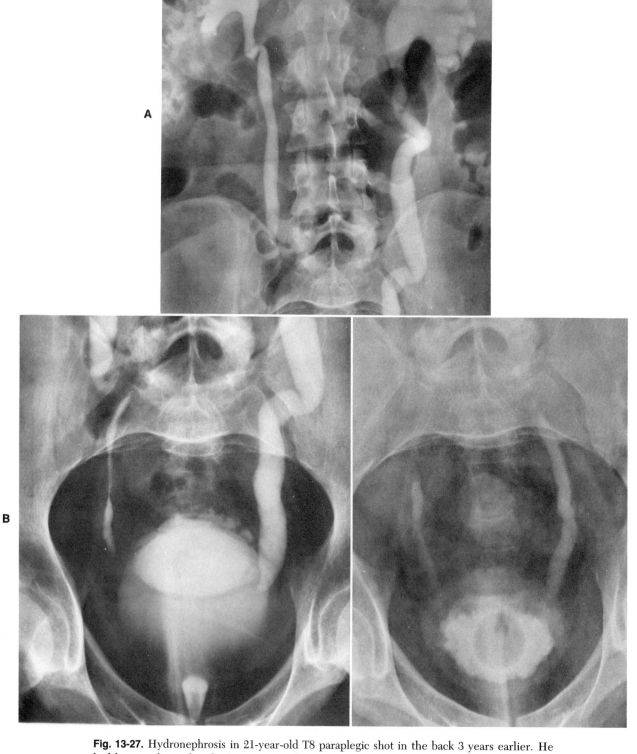

Fig. 13-27. Hydronephrosis in 21-year-old T8 paraplegic shot in the back 3 years earlier. He had been catheter free for 2 years. **A** and **B,** Intravenous urogram done after excessive beer drinking followed by complete urinary retention shows distended urinary bladder and hydronephrotic changes involving ureters, pelvis, and calices. **C,** One week later after introduction of Foley catheter, hydronephrosis had subsided. Note considerable thickening of bladder wall.

Hydronephrosis

True hydronephrosis will occur when there is bladder outlet obstruction, either mechanical or from significant overdistention (Fig. 13-27), a blocked Foley catheter, or a long-lasting spasm of the external sphincter. If not treated properly by institution of bladder drainage, urinary tract infection supervenes. Hydronephrosis can be easily diagnosed by ultrasonography[50] and CT scanning[20] (Figs. 13-8 and 13-11). The ultrasonogram can demonstrate the degree and level of obstruc-

tion. One has to be cautious not to diagnose ureterectasis if the urinary bladder has not been properly drained. To prevent pitfalls, the ultrasonographic examination should always include the urinary bladder and the examination should be done after the patient attempts to empty the bladder.

Vesicoureteral reflux

Vesicoureteral reflux can occur in the early stages following spinal cord injury, or it can be a late phenomenon in a long-standing neurogenic bladder. It is generally related to altered ureterovesical anatomy accompanied but not necessarily produced by infection.[57] Vesicoureteral reflux has to be ruled out before intermittent catheterization is initiated or before the patient is left in a catheter-free state. Vesicoureteral reflux can be seen in spastic and flaccid bladders alike, and it can be unilateral (Fig. 13-28) or bilateral (Fig. 13-29). It is a good idea to grade vesicoureteral reflux as seen on voiding cystourethrography[22]: grade I—reflux into the

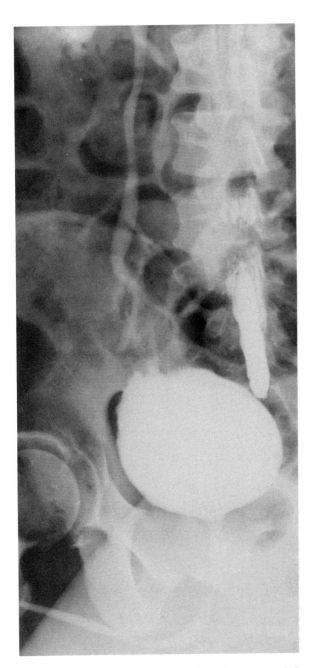

Fig. 13-28. Unilateral vesicoureteral reflux demonstrated during voiding in 46-year-old C5 quadriplegic.

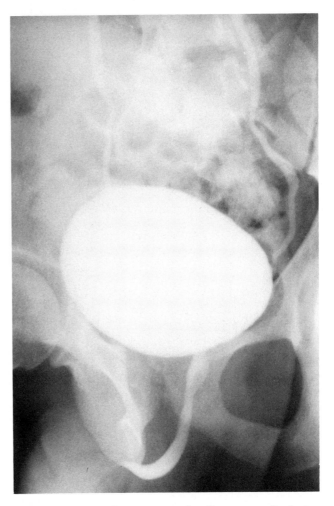

Fig. 13-29. Bilateral vesicoureteral reflux seen only during voiding in 20-year-old C4 quadriplegic.

ureter only; grade II—reflux reaching the renal pelvis; and grade III—reflux extending into the collecting system and causing dilatation (Fig. 13-30).

Hutch[26] associated vesicoureteral reflux to the makeup of a long-standing neurogenic bladder (Fig. 13-31). Such a bladder is small, heavily trabeculated, and numerous saccules or small diverticula are present.

Such a diverticulum can interfere with the detrusor muscle at the vesicoureteral junction, weakening or destroying the normal antireflux mechanism of the intramural segment of the ureter. Reflux, however, can occur in the urinary bladder that radiographically does not look like the typical neurogenic bladder described by Hutch. A long-standing vesicoureteral reflux can cause changes in the ureters detectable on the urogram: ureteral dilatation, mucosal striation, and ureteral calculi formation.[4]

Treatment of long-standing vesicoureteral reflux varies from reinstatement of intermittent catheterization to continuous bladder drainage, bladder neck resection, or external sphincterotomy. An ileal conduit or antireflux procedures are ultimate measures if all else fails.[57]

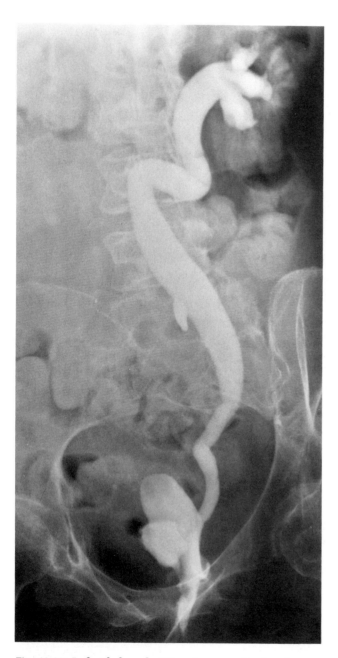

Fig. 13-30. Left-sided grade III vesicoureteral reflux demonstrated on voiding cystourethrogram in 44-year-old C6 quadriplegic woman. There is marked dilatation of left ureter and clubbing of calices. Note reflux into vagina.

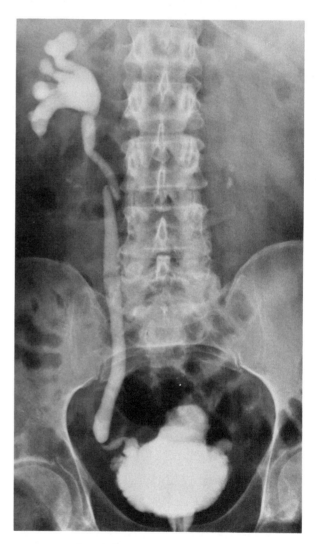

Fig. 13-31. Right-sided grade III vesicoureteral reflux in 56-year-old patient with long-standing neurogenic bladder. Note multiple diverticula, particularly one near ureteral orifice (Hutch diverticulum).

Renal damage

Long-standing vesicoureteral reflux coupled with urinary tract infection can result in acute pyelonephritis or chronic atrophic pyelonephritis (Figs. 13-32 and 13-33). Acute pyelonephritis can be unilateral or bilateral in nature depending on the vesicoureteral reflux.

The diagnosis of acute pyelonephritis in a normal population is seldom done by intravenous urography because the urogram is usually not performed during an acute episode. In spinal cord injured patients, however, intravenous urograms are done at fixed intervals of 3 or 6 months and an acute pyelonephritis may be detected. In three fourths of the cases of acute pyelonephritis, the intravenous urogram will show no abnormalities.[53] In the remaining one fourth the most common findings are renal enlargement, decreased density of the contrast medium, delayed appearance of the calices, and dilatation of the collecting system. The radiologic signs of acute pyelonephritis become more obvious if only one kidney is involved.[58] If both kidneys

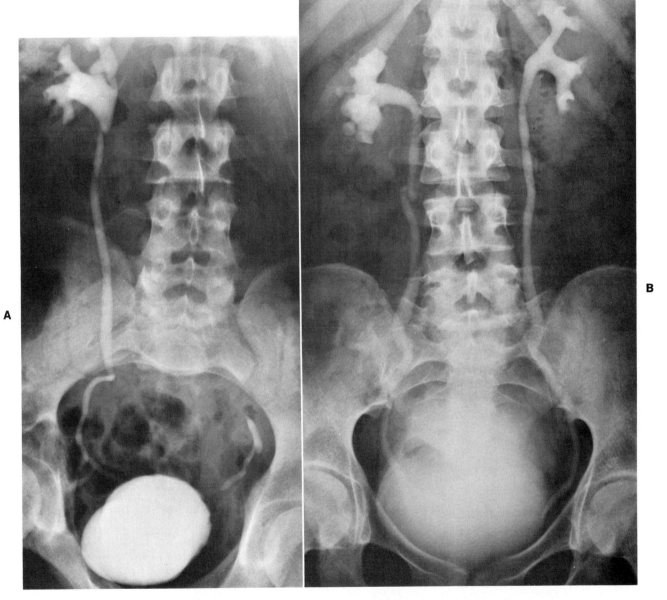

Fig. 13-32. A, Bilateral vesicoureteral reflux demonstrated on voiding cystourethrogram in 20-year-old T11 paraplegic from gunshot injury. Reflux is grade III on right side and minimal on left. **B,** Intravenous urogram done on next day shows clubbing of right upper calices and loss of cortex at upper pole. Note also ureterectasis and hypertrophy of detrusor.

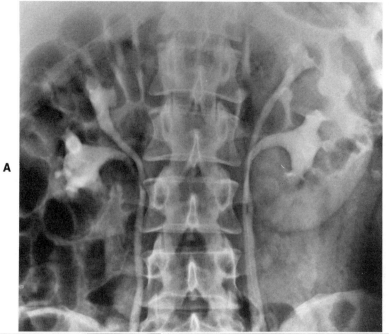

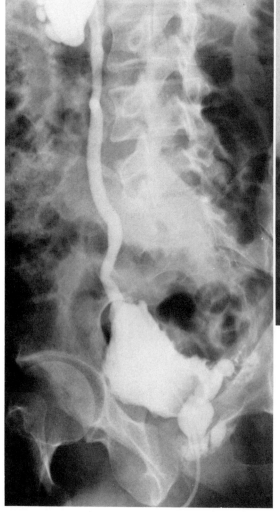

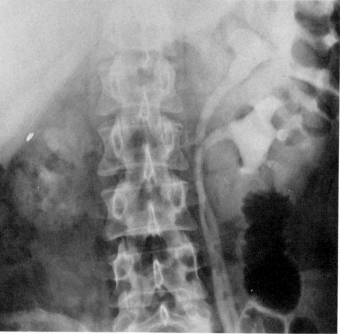

Fig. 13-33. Unilateral vesicoureteral reflux and severe renal damage occurring in slightly over a year in 29-year-old T10 paraplegic injured by 38-caliber bullet. **A,** Intravenous urogram 1 year after injury shows normal kidneys bilaterally. Duplication of left collecting system and ureters is seen. **B,** Voiding cystourethrogram done 14 months later shows right-sided vesicoureteral reflux. There is also refluxed contrast in prostatic ducts and in vas deferens. **C,** Intravenous urogram done on next day shows significant atrophy of right kidney because of chronic pyelonephritis (reflux nephropathy).

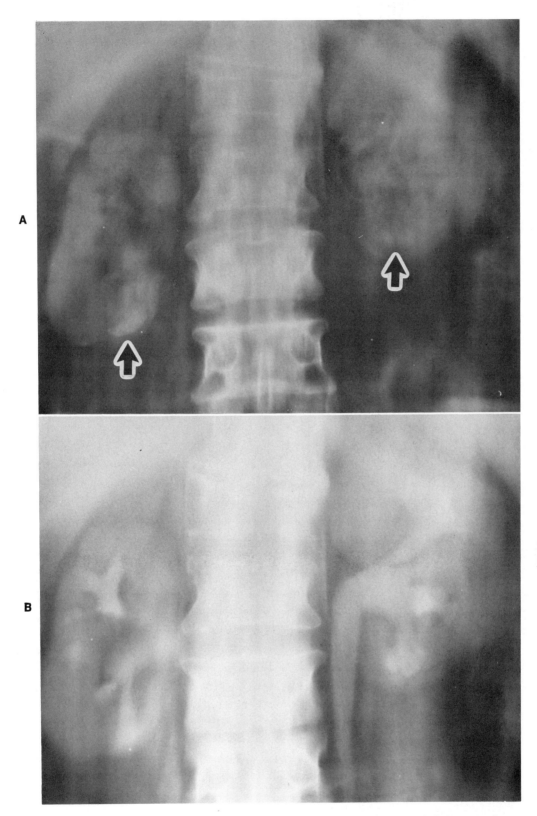

Fig. 13-34. Bilateral chronic pyelonephritis in 39-year-old L1 paraplegic with long-standing bilateral vesicoureteral reflux. **A,** Tomographic cut 30 seconds following injection of contrast medium shows lumpy small kidneys with calculi in both lower poles *(arrows)*. **B,** Five minutes later, clubbed calices and loss of renal cortex are seen.

are affected, some of the above signs could be attributed to other factors.

When the intravenous urogram shows a nonfunctioning edematous kidney and the ultrasonogram rules out hydronephrosis, an arteriogram can rule out acute renal vein thrombosis. The same arteriogram can then establish the diagnosis of acute pyelonephritis,[58] namely, an enlarged kidney with stretched, elongated, and attenuated vessels. The appearance of the vessels reflects the diffuse inflammatory edema of the kidney.

Chronic pyelonephritis is easily diagnosed on the intravenous urogram where it shows a small-size kidney or kidneys with lumpy borders and sometimes calculi formation, diminished cortex, and clubbed calices (Fig. 13-34). The loss of cortex is a most significant finding and accounts for the decrease in renal size. If an arteriogram is performed, it will show, in addition to the severe loss of cortex, a "winter tree" appearance of the vessels with only major branches remaining functional (Fig. 13-35).

Chronic atrophic pyelonephritis can also be diagnosed by ultrasonography. The findings are loss of renal parenchyma, retraction of calices, decrease in renal size, and increased echoes from fibrosis.[30] The ultrasonogram becomes an important examination when renal function is severely impaired or an intravenous urogram is not indicated because of failing renal function.

Death from renal damage in spinal cord injured patients is less prevalent today than it formerly was, and this is probably related to proper urologic care. Statistics from World War II spinal cord injured patients revealed that 20.3% of deaths were from renal disease, including renal amyloidosis.[14,19]

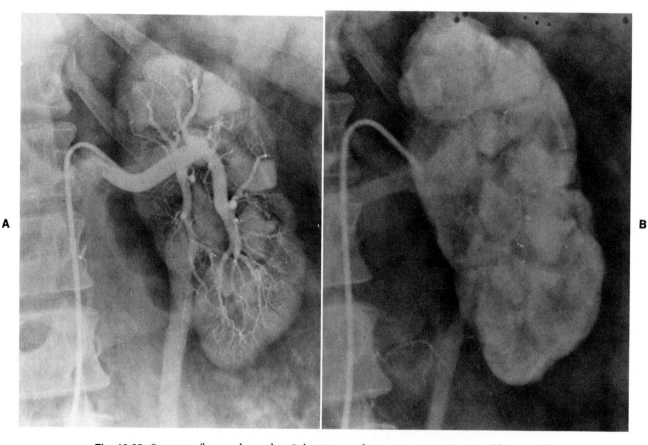

Fig. 13-35. Severe reflux nephropathy. Selective renal arteriogram in 29-year-old man with long-standing vesicoureteral reflux. **A,** Arterial phase shows severe changes in upper pole: "winter tree" appearance and pruning of vessels with only major branches remaining. Lower pole shows moderate changes with no arcuate branches seen. **B,** Late film shows marked dilatation and clubbing of calices and complete loss of renal cortex at upper pole.

INFRAVESICAL COMPLICATIONS

Infravesical complications pertain mainly to the male urethra, which is subject to countless episodes of minor and major trauma since day 1 of spinal cord injury. Minor trauma is usually the result of catheterization, and major trauma can result from instrumentation or surgery, such as cystoscopy, cystolithoplexy, sphincterotomy, or sphincterectomy. In females the urethra is very short and seldom causes serious problems.

Normal male urethra

The normal male urethra, as seen on voiding cystourethrography (Figs. 13-36 and 13-37), is divided into two segments. The *anterior urethra* consists of penile and bulbous segments with the penoscrotal junction in between. The *posterior urethra* consists of the membranous urethra and the prostatic urethra. The external sphincter is located at the membranous segment of the urethra.

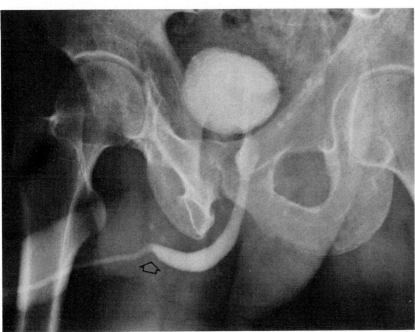

Fig. 13-36. Normal male urethra as seen on voiding cystourethrogram in 45-year-old quadriplegic. Note penoscrotal junction *(arrow)*.

Fig. 13-37. Schematic illustration of normal voiding cystourethrogram with anatomic landmarks. *Anterior urethra:* penile and bulbous segments with penoscrotal junction in between. *Posterior urethra:* membranous and prostatic segments. *VM,* Verumontanum. (From McCallum, R. W.: Radiol. Clin. North Am. **17:**227-244, 1979.)

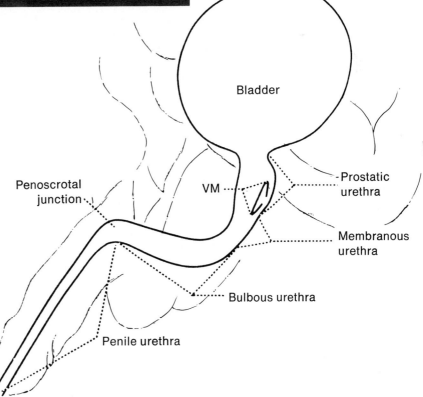

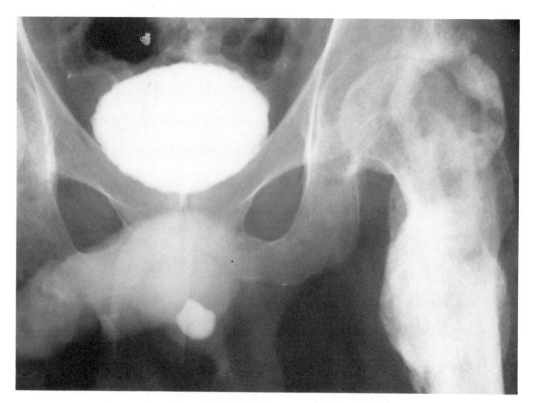

Fig. 13-38. Diverticulum of bulbous urethra in 20-year-old C5 incomplete quadriplegic. Note ectopic bone at left hip.

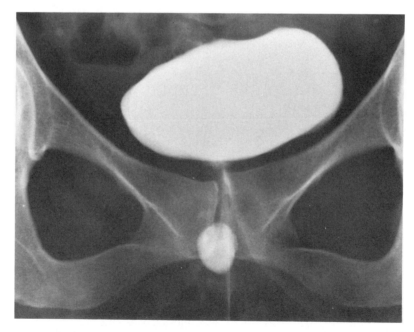

Fig. 13-39. Urethral diverticulum probably iatrogenic in nature in 23-year-old C5 quadriplegic woman seen on voiding cystourethrogram.

Evaluation techniques

The male urethra is evaluated radiographically by two methods: antegrade and retrograde. An antegrade urethrogram is part of the voiding cystourethrogram already described. For a retrograde urethrogram a catheter is introduced into the distal urethra and contrast medium is injected retrogradely. As stated earlier, a carefully performed voiding cystourethrogram can yield a great deal of information about the status of the male urethra.[8,9]

Diverticula

It should be noted that congenital diverticula are-lined with epithelium, whereas acquired posttraumatic or postinfection diverticula are not.[62] Diverticula are seen on voiding cystourethrograms as collections of contrast medium in an outpouching or concentric dilatation of the urethra in the membranous portion or penoscrotal junction (Figs. 13-38 to 13-41). They are most often the result of improper catheterization, when the urethra is punctured once or repeatedly at a specific location. Diverticula are usually asymptomatic and are discovered incidently during a radiologic examination. A small diverticulum is sometimes seen at the fossa navicularis (Fig. 13-42) and should not be confused with the fossa itself.

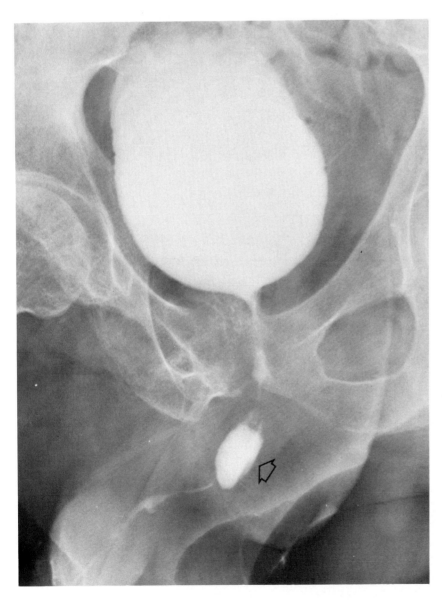

Fig. 13-40. Diverticulum of membranous urethra *(arrow)* resulting from prior cysto-lithoplexy in 20-year-old C5 quadriplegic. Note concentric hypertrophy of detrusor.

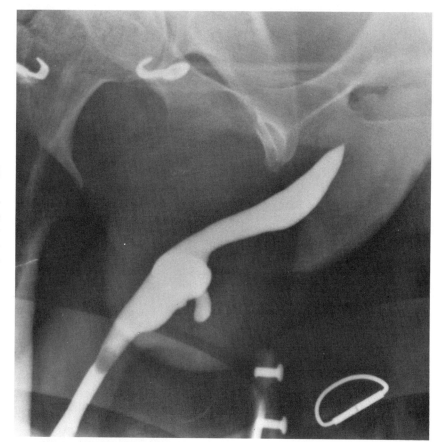

Fig. 13-41. Diverticulum of penoscrotal junction in 20-year-old C5 quadriplegic. Diverticulum was demonstrated on retrograde examination, which produced a severe spasm in area of external sphincter. Note bilateral ischiectomies. Diverticulum is posttraumatic or related to ischiectomy. (See also Fig. 13-64.)

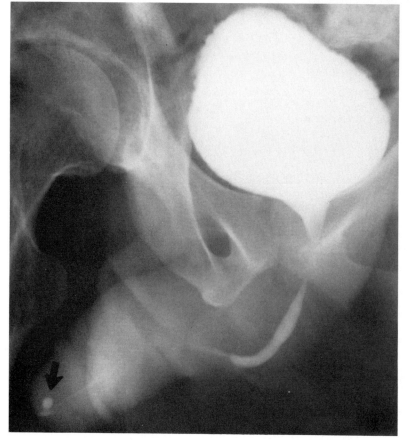

Fig. 13-42. Diverticulum of fossa navicularis (*arrow*) in 22-year-old T11 complete paraplegic.

Strictures

Postinflammatory strictures are rare in spinal cord injured patients. When they occur, they are usually secondary to an abscess resulting from an iatrogenic injury. Strictures seldom develop from a diverticulum. They are localized at the urethral meatus or in the penoscrotal junction and are well demonstrated by a retrograde urethrogram.[31] A voiding cystourethrogram is obtained with difficulty in patients with strictures because of the inability to introduce a catheter. A small-size catheter can sometimes produce a good voiding urethrogram (Fig. 13-43).

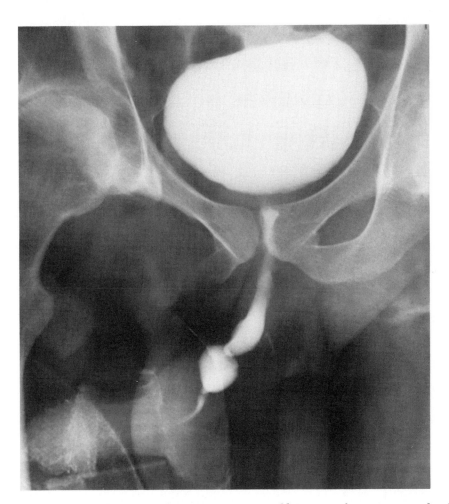

Fig. 13-43. Stricture of penoscrotal junction in 31-year-old T12 paraplegic. Stricture developed as a result of urethral abscess excised 8 years earlier.

False passage, intravasation, blowout

False passages are produced more often than clinically suspected. They are diagnosed if the voiding cystourethrogram is part of the routine urologic workup (Figs. 13-44 and 13-45). When intravasation has resulted from an iatrogenic injury, venous structures and the venous plexus are demonstrated on antegrade or retrograde examinations (Fig. 13-46). Blowout of the urethra is a severe and fortunately rare iatrogenic injury that can occur if the Foley catheter balloon has been placed in the urethra instead of the urinary bladder and has been fully inflated. The injury can be detected clinically since there is an instant swelling of the penis. To assess the damage, a retrograde urethrogram is done showing intravasation in venous plexuses or corpora cavernosa or surrounding soft tissue edema (Fig. 13-47).

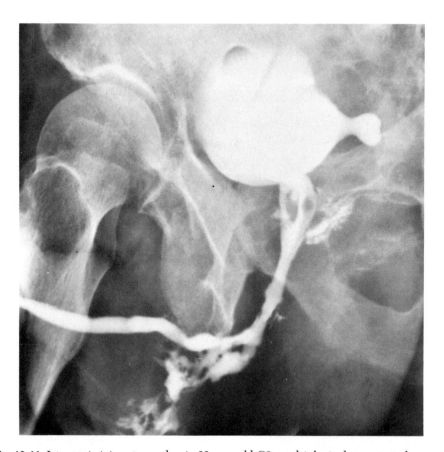

Fig. 13-44. Iatrogenic injury to urethra in 32-year-old C6 quadriplegic demonstrated on voiding cystourethrogram. There is a small-capacity urinary bladder with diverticulum. Extravasation of contrast medium originates at penoscrotal junction.

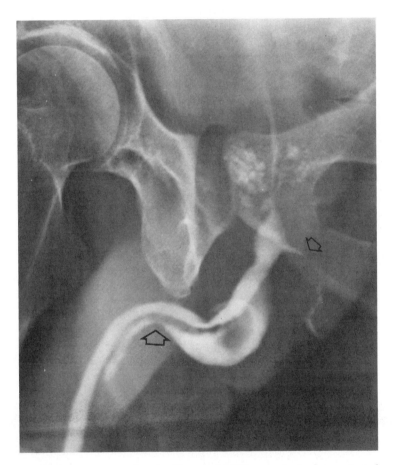

Fig. 13-45. False passage in urethra in 20-year-old T11 paraplegic demonstrated on retrograde urethrogram. Point of injury is penoscrotal junction *(large arrow)*. There is also a small track of extravasation originating at membranous urethra *(small arrow)*. Prostatic ducts are filled.

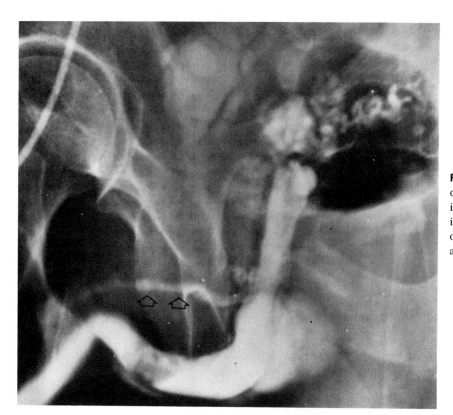

Fig. 13-46. Intravasation in venous plexuses demonstrated by retrograde urethrogram in 22-year-old T4 paraplegic. Urethra was injured by improper catheterization. Note dorsal penile vein *(arrows)* and prostatic and seminal vesical plexuses.

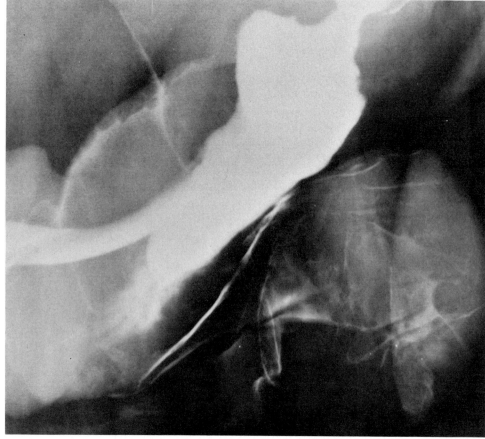

Fig. 13-47. Urethral blowout in 56-year-old T8 complete paraplegic. Foley catheter balloon was erroneously inflated in penile urethra. Retrograde urethrogram shows contrast medium in corpora cavernosa. Penis is markedly edematous. Patient developed a gram-negative sepsis but subsequently recovered completely.

Pressure necrosis of urethra and penoscrotal fistula

Improper wear of the Foley catheter can result in pressure necrosis of the urethra, periurethral abscess, and fistula. A Foley catheter not taped to the thigh or lower abdomen will exert constant pressure on the inferior aspect of the urethra in the penoscrotal junction and produce pressure necrosis (Fig. 13-48).[54] Such a pressure necrosis may be followed by an abscess formation (Fig. 13-49). The abscess can result in a penoscrotal fistula (Fig. 13-50).[40] Such a fistula can be demonstrated on antegrade or retrograde urethrograms or via a fistulogram when contrast medium is injected directly into the fistula opening.

Management of penoscrotal fistula is difficult. To properly treat such a fistula the patient has to be catheter free or no attempt at drainage or plastic surgery in the area can be done. The ultimate solution for intractable penoscrotal fistula is urinary diversion.[11]

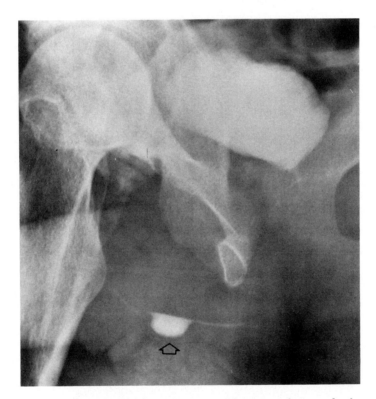

Fig. 13-48. Pressure necrosis of urethra in 17-year-old C4 complete quadriplegic from improper wear of Foley catheter. The diverticulum-like collection of contrast is located on the undersurface of the urethra *(arrow)*.

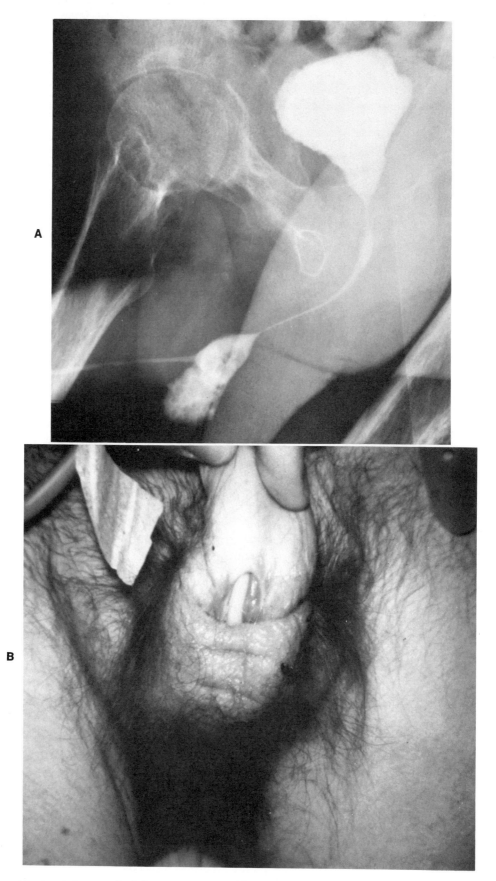

Fig. 13-49. Peri-urethral abscess in 20-year-old C5 quadriplegic, secondary to pressure necrosis of urethra. **A,** Voiding cystourethrogram was performed to evaluate chronic drainage of mucus around Foley catheter and gram-negative sepsis. **B,** A few months later a scrotal fistula developed followed by breakdown of tissue. Catheter can now be seen through soft tissue defect on undersurface of penis.

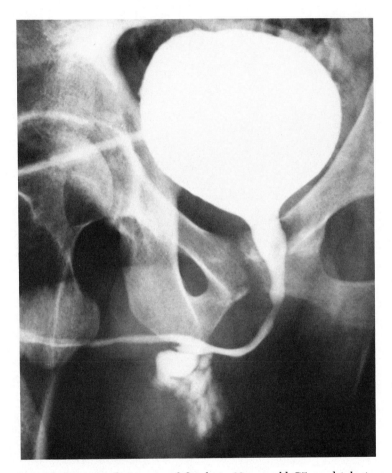

Fig. 13-50. Scrotal abscess and penoscrotal fistula in 23-year-old C5 quadriplegic secondary to pressure necrosis of urethra.

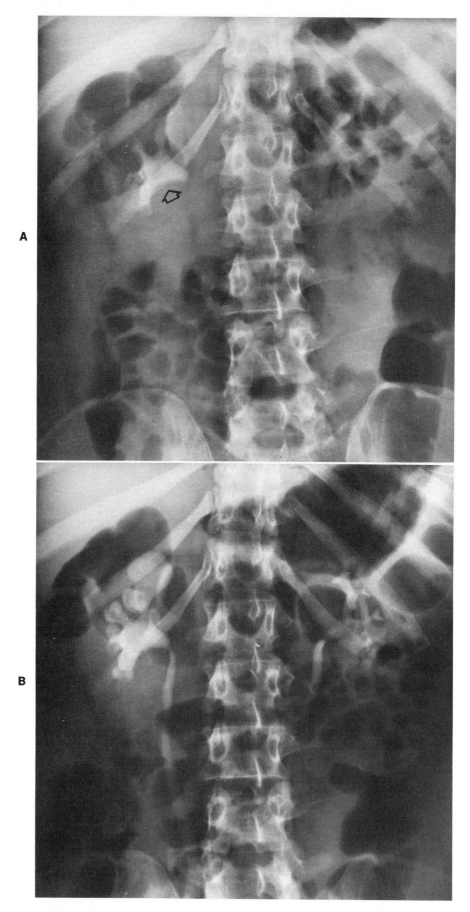

Fig. 13-51. Staghorn calculus and pyelonephritis in 17-year-old girl who has been a C5 quadriplegic for past 5 years. **A,** Staghorn calculus is seen on preliminary film *(arrow)*. **B,** Intravenous urogram shows preserved function but clubbing of right calices.

URINARY CALCULI

Urinary calculi in spinal cord injured patients can be suspected clinically, but radiologic confirmation is needed. In order to visualize calculi on plain radiographs, they have to contain calcium. Non–calcium containing calculi are nonopaque and may become visible only as filling defects in contrast-containing components of the urinary system. But even calcium-containing calculi are difficult to detect when they are small or they are obscured by other structures in the abdomen. Tomography of the kidney can accurately detect calcium-containing calculi (Fig. 13-34, *A*). Nonopaque calculi in general are demonstrated easily by ultrasonography (Fig. 13-10).

Etiology and composition

Two factors play an important role in calculi formation in spinal cord injured patients: hypercalciuria and infection.[12] Injury to the spinal cord is followed by a period of increased urinary calcium excretion, which becomes less prominent when the patient ambulates. Urinary stasis, infection, and the presence of a Foley catheter predispose to urinary calculi formation. How often is urinary infection present in spinal cord injured patients? In 116 such patients admitted within the Midwest Regional Spinal Cord Injury Care System in 1978 a total of 99 patients, or 85%, had a urinary tract infection (urine bacterial count of 100,000/ml or greater).

The primary cause for infection-induced urinary calculi is urease producing bacteria.[23] The enzyme urease is present in certain urinary pathogens: *Proteus* species, *Klebsiella*, and occasionally *Pseudomonas* and *Staphylococcus*.

Urease alkalizes the urine by hydrolyzing urea to ammonia.[51] This leads to supersaturation, a decrease in solubility of magnesium and calcium phosphate, and formation of stones composed of *struvite* and *apatite*. Struvite calculi are of a radiolucent nature. Apatite calculi, which form at the onset of paraplegia or in patients in whom hypercalciuria has not been controlled, contain 98% calcium phosphate and 2% calcium oxalate, thus becoming radiopaque.[5] In short, the *apatite* content in stones in spinal cord injured patients will depend on the pH and calcium content in the urine, and the *struvite* content will reflect the presence of urea-splitting organisms. Struvite, or magnesium ammonium phosphate, calculi do not contain calcium initially, but they may serve as a nidus for future calcium deposits. In general, the composition and site of occurrence of stones are not related to the level of spinal cord injury, sex of the patient, or therapy with acidifying drugs.[5]

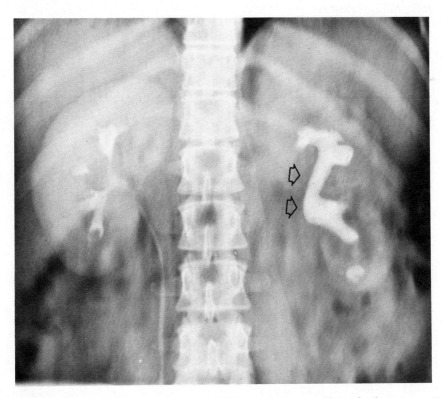

Fig. 13-52. Staghorn calculus *(arrows)* in left kidney of 36-year-old quadriplegic man. Urogram shows normal right collecting system but no nephrogram and no function on left side.

Radiologic manifestations

Renal calculi can grow in size and affect one or both kidneys alike. When left untreated, a staghorn calculus can occupy the entire collecting system and result in pyelonephritis (Fig. 13-51). The presence of a staghorn calculus will eventually cause mechanical obstruction with hydronephrosis and/or impairment of renal function (Fig. 13-52). There are instances, however, in which, despite the presence of numerous calculi, no visible renal damage may be detected (Fig. 13-53).

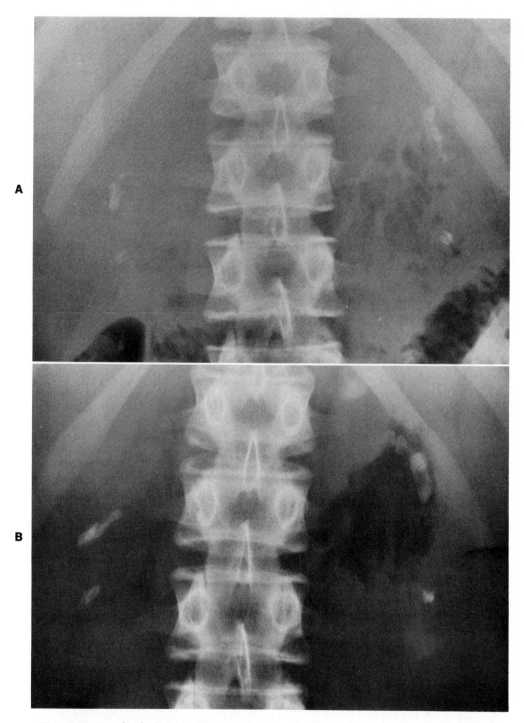

Fig. 13-53. Renal calculosis in 20-year-old C6 quadriplegic woman. **A,** Renal calculi were diagnosed 6 months after injury. **B,** Six months later, calculi on both sides have increased in size and number.

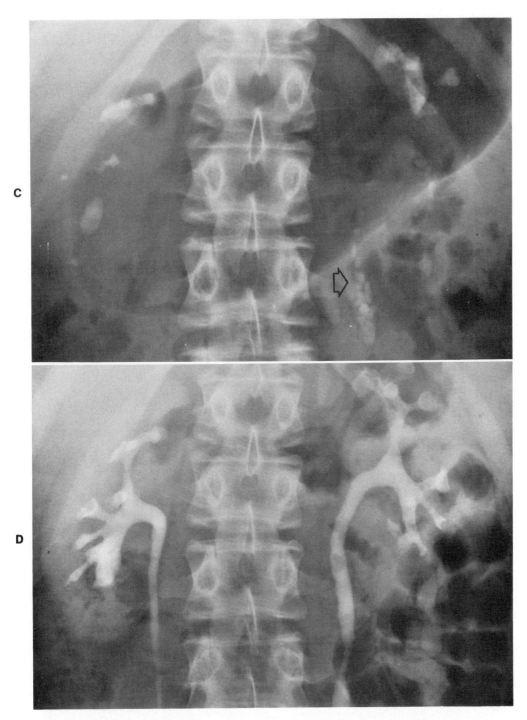

Fig. 13-53, cont'd. C, In another 10 months, calculi have filled renal collecting system on both sides and are also seen in left upper ureter *(arrow).* **D,** Intravenous urogram shows bilateral function and no visible renal damage.

Most of the calculi in the urinary bladder are related to the presence of the Foley catheter coupled with infection. Nonopaque concretions can form around or at the tip of the Foley catheter (Fig. 13-54). The typical bladder calculi form around the Foley catheter (Fig. 13-55). These eggshell crusts fall off into the bladder and become a nidus for calculi formation.[12] As a result the typical bladder calculi of spinal cord injured patients have a very specific semilunar shape, regardless of the size they attain (Fig. 13-56). Bladder calculi usually enlarge slowly. The fact of size increase usually indicates persistence of organisms (Fig. 13-57).

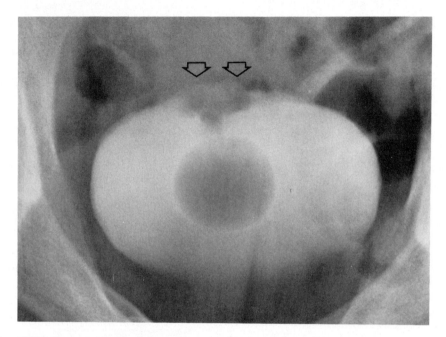

Fig. 13-54. Nonopaque calculi formed at tip of Foley catheter *(arrows)* in 22-year-old C5 quadriplegic woman.

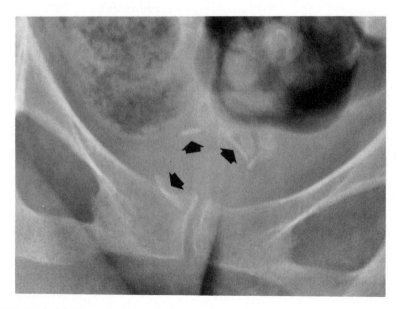

Fig. 13-55. Early bladder calculi (eggshell crusts) formed around Foley catheter *(arrows)* in 36-year-old man who became quadriplegic in a fall from a porch.

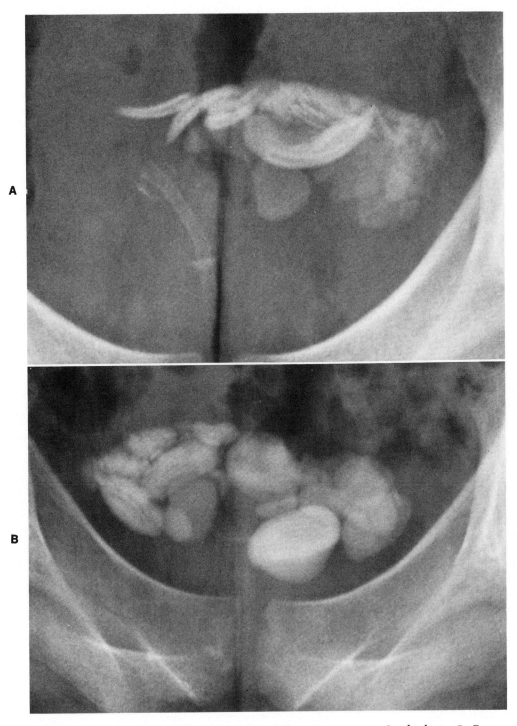

Fig. 13-56. Semilunar bladder calculi in two different patients. **A,** Quadriplegic. **B,** Para-plegic.

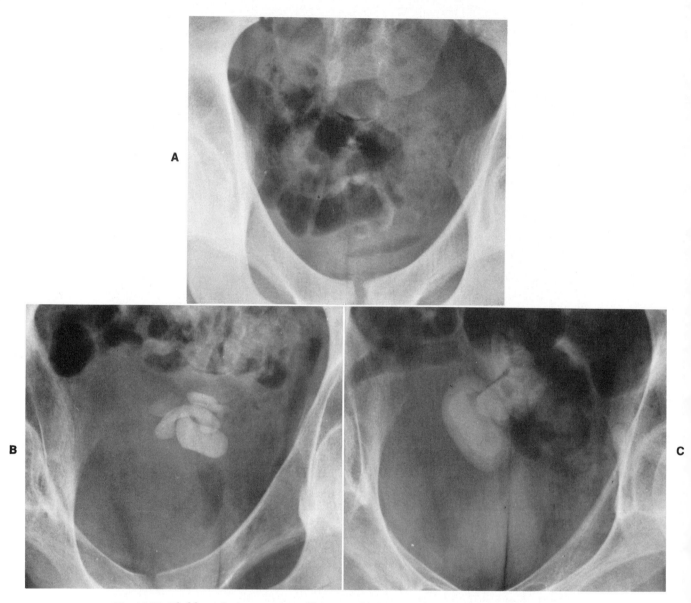

Fig. 13-57. Bladder calculi in 20-year-old C6 quadriplegic man. Calculi were diagnosed but were never treated. **A,** 1974. **B,** 1976. **C,** 1978.

Ultrasonography

Ultrasonography is particularly valuable in detecting renal calculi (Fig. 13-10). A renal calculus completely reflects sound waves and casts a sonic or acoustic shadow behind the stone. Ultrasonography can detect both radiopaque and radiolucent stones and may even offer a relative indication as to their composition.[9] Ultrasonography can detect matrix stones that cannot be visualized on routine radiography. Calculi as small as 1.5 cm in size can be diagnosed by ultrasonography.[45]

POSTSURGICAL APPEARANCE OF URINARY TRACT

The radiologic appearance of the neurogenic bladder after surgical procedures may be very straightforward, indicating the nature of the procedure performed. In some instances, however, it is confusing and surgical protocol information is needed.

Vesicostomy is seldom performed today. It is a permanent opening in the urinary bladder, and the patient wears a vesicostomy bag. The bladder empties by overflow, which is not very effective in patients who are most of the time in a recumbent position and may lead to urinary bladder distention and ureterectasis (Fig. 13-58).

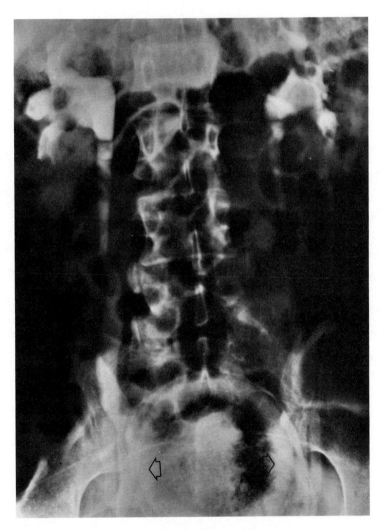

Fig. 13-58. Vesicostomy in 30-year-old C5 quadriplegic. This intravenous urogram shows bilateral nonobstructive ureterectasis and vesicostomy bag *(arrows)*. Bladder always showed large residual volume.

When transureteral resection of bladder neck and external sphincter have been performed, the membranous urethra appears wide on the voiding cystourethrogram. On occasion the membranous urethra becomes dilated to the point that it can trap an inflated Foley catheter balloon (Figs. 13-59 and 13-60). When external sphincterotomy alone is done, the membranous urethra may have a normal physiologic appearance or become wide (Fig. 13-61).

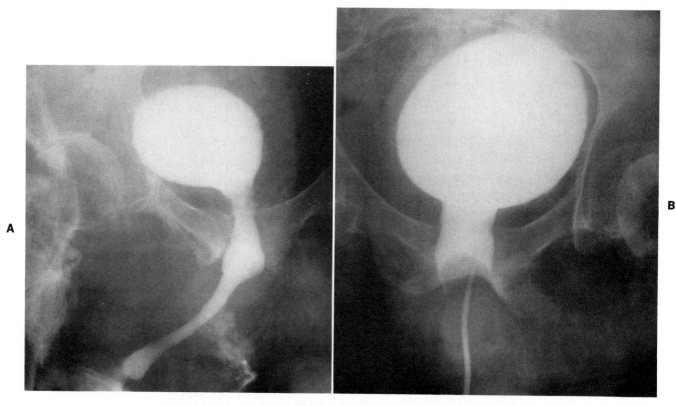

Fig. 13-59. Transurethral resection of bladder neck and external sphincter in 40-year-old C5 complete paraplegic done 10 years prior to this voiding cystourethrogram. **A,** Bladder neck and external sphincter are well relaxed during voiding. **B,** On one occasion Foley catheter balloon was inflated in dilated membranous urethra. Note ectopic bone, subluxated hips, and bilateral ischiectomy.

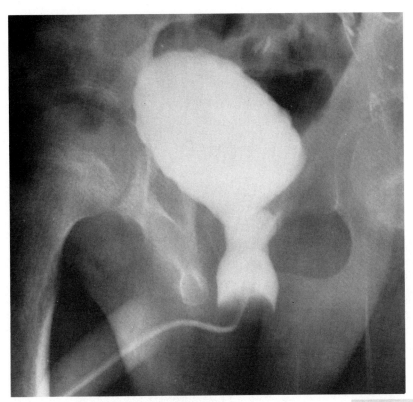

Fig. 13-60. Post–external sphincterotomy cystogram in 26-year-old T4 paraplegic. Foley catheter balloon is inflated in membranous urethra.

Fig. 13-61. Postsphincterotomy dynamic retrograde urethrogram shows wide area of external sphincter. On this examination, bladder emptied completely. (Courtesy R. W. McCallum, M.B., F.R.C.P.(C), University of Toronto.)

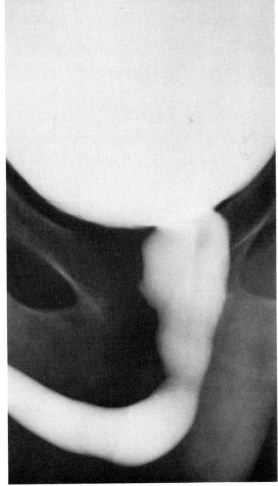

Patients with bladder neck resection can still manifest external sphincter spasm (Fig. 13-62), and patients with external sphincterotomy can still on occasion show spasm of the bladder neck. Following external sphincterotomy and particularly following total cleanup, in which bladder neck, prostate, and external sphincter are resected (Fig. 13-63), there is always a certain degree of incontinence, which sometimes may be very troublesome for the patient.[42]

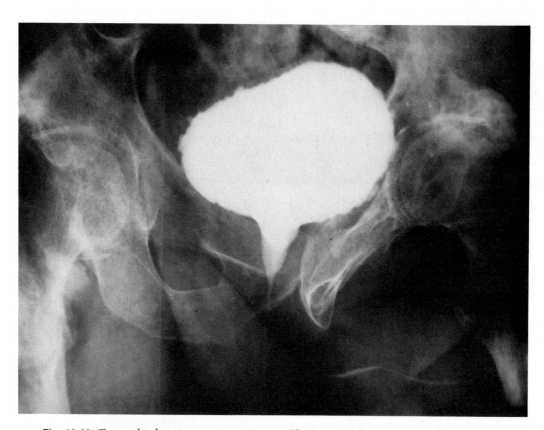

Fig. 13-62. External sphincter spasm in 41-year-old C5 quadriplegic who had bladder neck resection without improvement of voiding. Note left ischiectomy for pressure sore and bilateral ectopic bone.

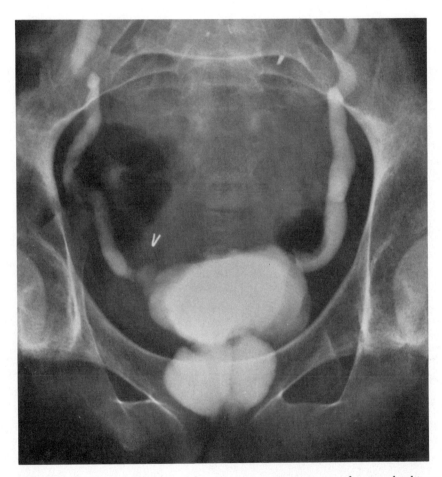

Fig. 13-63. "Total cleanup": bladder neck resection, prostatectomy, and external sphincterotomy in 22-year-old T12 paraplegic secondary to gunshot wound. This intravenous urogram shows small-capacity urinary bladder, bilateral ureterectasis, and prostatic bed filled with contrast medium. As a result of procedure, patient became incontinent.

When a patient undergoes bilateral ischiectomy for serious pressure sores, a perineal urethral diverticulum can develop in the penoscrotal junction (Figs. 13-41 and 13-64). This is a direct result of the surgical severance of the triangular ligament attached to the inferior pubic rami, thus subjecting the nonprotected urethra to direct weight bearing.[10] This diverticulum should not be confused with an abscess or extension of a pressure sore into the periurethral structures.

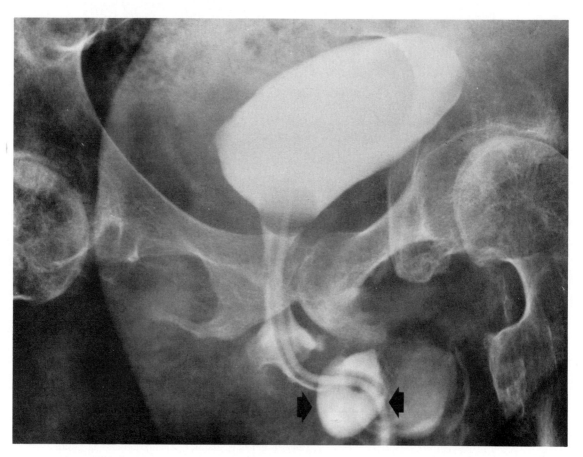

Fig. 13-64. Postischiectomy perineal urethral diverticulum *(arrows)* in 36-year-old quadriplegic injured in automobile accident 20 years prior to this cystogram. He has had also an external sphincterectomy. Note atrophy of right hip, subluxation of left hip, and bilateral ischiectomy.

Urinary diversion is done when everything else has failed to control reflux and infection. The most popular method is the ileal bladder (Fig. 13-65), which if well done, can give very satisfactory results.[32]

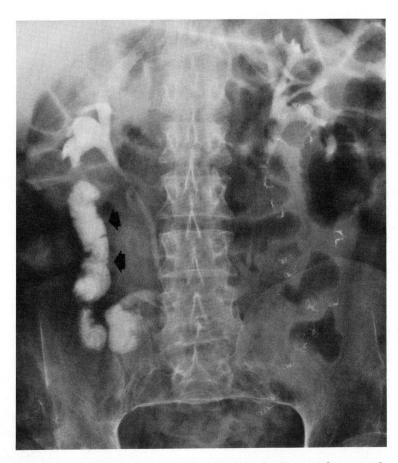

Fig. 13-65. Ileal bladder *(arrows)* in 31-year-old C5 quadriplegic. Kidneys are functioning well, and there is no ureterectasis.

BLADDER CANCER

It is not surprising that prolonged wearing of a Foley catheter will cause pathologic changes in the urinary bladder mucosa, ranging from squamous metaplasia to frank bladder cancer formation. In a study performed by Kaufman and co-workers[28] 42% of patients with indwelling catheters from 6 months to 10 years and 80% of patients with an indwelling catheter for more than 10 years showed squamous metaplasia of the bladder mucosa. Ten percent of a group of 62 spinal cord injured patients had developed bladder cancer. In another group of 1600 patients studied by Kawaichi,[29] four had developed carcinoma of the bladder (Fig. 13-66). Spinal cord injured patients who have developed bladder cancer have gross or microscopic hematuria. The radiologic manifestation is a filling defect in the urinary bladder. If the cancer spreads toward a ureteral orifice, the orifice is blocked and hydronephrosis develops with eventual loss of renal function.

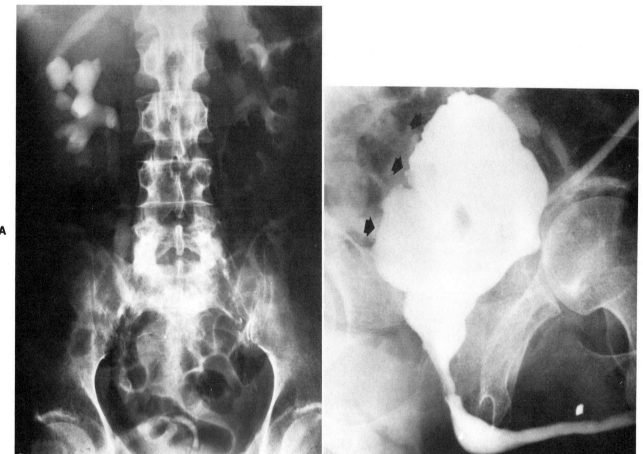

Fig. 13-66. Carcinoma of urinary bladder developed in 51-year-old C5 quadriplegic who has been wearing a urethral Foley catheter for past 30 years, replaced subsequently with a suprapubic catheter. **A,** Intravenous urogram shows right-sided hydronephrosis and cortical atrophy of kidney. **B,** Voiding cystourethrogram shows contour defect *(arrows)* on right side of urinary bladder. Histologic examination showed poorly differentiated invasive, transitional, and squamous cell carcinoma. (From Kaufman, J. M., et al.: J. Urol. **118**:967, 1977. © 1977 The Williams & Wilkins Co., Baltimore.)

REFERENCES

1. Abramson, A. S.: Management of the neurogenic bladder in perspective, Arch. Phys. Med. Rehabil. **57**:197-201, 1976.
2. Barbaric, Z. L.: Autonomic dysreflexia in patients with spinal cord lesions: complication of voiding cystoure-thrography and ileal loopography, Am. J. Roentgenol. **127**:293-295, 1976.
3. Berdon, W. E., and Baker, D. H.: The significance of a distended bladder in the interpretation of intravenous pyelograms obtained on patients with "hydronephrosis," Am. J. Roentgenol. **120**:402-409, 1974.
4. Berquist, T. H., Hattery, R. R., Hartman, G. W., et al.: Vesicoureteral reflux in adults, Am. J. Roentgenol. **125**:314-321, 1975.
5. Burr, R. G.: Urinary calculi composition in patients with spinal cord lesions, Arch. Phys. Med. Rehabil. **59**:84-88, 1978.
6. Butler, E. D., Jr., Friedland, G. W., and Govan, D. E.: A radiological study of the effect of elevated intravesical pressures on ureteral calibre and peristalsis in patients with neurogenic bladder dysfunction, Clin. Radiol. **22**:198-204, 1971.
7. Butler, M. R.: Patterns of bladder recovery in spinal injury evaluated by serial urodynamic observations, Urology **11**:308-314, 1978.
8. Calenoff, L., Arkema, K. K., Miller, J., and Rogers, L. F.: Radiological considerations in rehabilitation medicine. Presentation at the Sixty-third Scientific Assembly and Annual Meeting of the Radiological Society of North America, Nov. 28, 1977.
9. Calenoff, L., Putnam, T., and Betts, H. B.: Iatrogenic changes of the male urethra in spinal cord injury patients. Presentation at the Fifty-fifth Annual Session of the American Congress of Rehabilitation Medicine, Nov. 14, 1978.
10. Comarr, A. E.: The practical urological management of the patient with spinal cord injury, Br. J. Urol. **31**:1-46, 1959.
11. Comarr, A. E.: Management of peno-scrotal fistulae and/or diverticula. Clinical spinal cord injury conference, 1961, pp. 83-86.
12. Comarr, A. E., Kawaichi, G. K., and Bors, E.: Renal calculosis of patients with traumatic cord lesions, J. Urol. **87**:647-656, 1962.
13. Damanski, M.: Cystourethrography in paraplegia as a guide to catheter free life: 17 years experience of a paraplegic center, J. Urol. **93**:466-471, 1965.
14. Dietrick, R. B., and Russi, S.: Tabulation and review of autopsy findings in fifty-five paraplegics, J.A.M.A. **166**:41-44, 1958.
15. Donovan, W. H., Clowers, D. E., Kiviat, M. D., and Macri, D.: Anal sphincter stretch: a technique to overcome detrusor-sphincter dyssynergia, Arch. Phys. Med. Rehabil. **58**:320-324, 1977.
16. Donovan, W. H., Kiviat, M. D., and Clowers, D. E.: Intermittent bladder emptying via urethral catheterization or suprapubic cystocath: a comparison study, Arch. Phys. Med. Rehabil. **58**:291-296, 1977.
17. Dure-Smith, P.: Fluid restriction before excretory urography, Radiology **118**:487-489, 1976.
18. Edell, S., and Zegel, H.: Ultrasonic evaluation of renal calculi, Am. J. Roentgenol. **130**:261-263, 1978.
19. Ekelund, L.: Radiologic findings in renal amyloidosis, Am. J. Roentgenol. **129**:851-853, 1977.
20. Ellenbogen, P. H., Scheible, F. W., Talner, L. B., and Leopold, G. R.: Sensitivity of gray scale ultrasound in detecting urinary tract obstruction, Am. J. Roentgenol. **130**:731-733, 1978.
21. Fam, B. A., Rossier, A. B., Blunt, K., et al.: Experience in the urologic management of 120 early spinal cord injury patients, J. Urol. **119**:485-487, 1978.
22. Fellows, G. J., and Silver, J. R.: Long-term follow-up of paraplegic patients with vesico-ureteric reflux, Paraplegia **14**:130-134, 1976.
23. Griffith, D. P., Musher, D. M., and Itin, C.: Urease. The primary cause of infection induced urinary stones, Invest. Urol. **13**:346-350, 1976.
24. Hattery, R. R., Williamson, B., Jr., and Hartman, G. W.: Urinary tract tomography, Radiol. Clin. North Am. **14**:23-49, 1976.
25. Hattery, R. R., Williamson, B., Jr., Stephens, D. H., et al.: Computed tomography of renal abnormalities, Radiol. Clin. North Am. **15**:401-418, 1977.
26. Hutch, J. A.: Vesico-ureteral reflux in the paraplegic: cause and correction, J. Urol. **68**:457-467, 1952.
27. Irvine, A. H.: Upper urinary tract dilatation in paraplegia, Br. J. Urol. **31**:47-52, 1959.
28. Kaufman, J. M., Fam, B., Jacobs, S. C., et al.: Bladder cancer and squamous metaplasia in spinal cord injury patients, J. Urol. **118**:967-971, 1977.
29. Kawaichi, G. K.: GU tumors in patients with spinal cord injuries. Clinical spinal cord injury conference, 1960, pp. 104-109.
30. Kay, C. J., Rosenfield, A. T., Taylor, K. J. W., and Rosenberg, M. A.: Ultrasonic characteristics of chronic atrophic pyelonephritis, Am. J. Roentgenol. **132**:47-49, 1979.
31. Lapides, J., and Stone, T. E.: Usefulness of retrograde urethrography in diagnosing strictures of the anterior urethra, J. Urol. **100**:747-750, 1968.
32. Lee, I. Y., Ragnarsson, K. T., Sell, G. H., et al.: Transurethral bladder neck surgery in spinal cord injured patients, Arch. Phys. Med. Rehabil. **59**:80-83, 1978.
33. Lindan, R., and Bellomy, V.: Effect of delayed intermittent catheterization on kidney function in spinal cord injury patients—a long-term follow-up study, Paraplegia **13**:49-55, 1975.
34. McCallum, R. W.: The adult male urethra. Normal anatomy, pathology and method of urethrography, Radiol. Clin. North Am. **17**:227-244, 1979.
35. McGuire, E. J., Diddel, G., and Wagner, F., Jr.: Balanced bladder function in spinal cord injury patients, J. Urol. **118**:626-628, 1977.
36. McLean, G. K., and Edell, S. L.: Determination of bladder volumes by gray scale ultrasonography, Radiology **128**:181-182, 1978.
37. Namiki, T., Ito, H., and Yasuda, K.: Management of the

urinary tract by suprapubic cystostomy kept under a closed and aseptic state in the acute stage of patient with spinal cord lesion, J. Urol. **119**:359-362, 1978.

38. Pearman, J. W., Low, A. I., and Fisher, A. A.: The "iced cystogram." A new technique for distinguishing obstruction at the level of the external sphincter from obtruction of the bladder neck, Paraplegia **12**:153-157, 1974.

39. Pedersen, J. F., Bartrum, R. J., Jr., and Grytter, C.: Residual urine determination by ultrasonic scanning, Am. J. Roentgenol. **125**:474-478, 1975.

40. Pennisi, S. A.: Urethroperitoneal fistula. Clinical spinal cord injury conference, 1959, pp. 86-87.

41. Perkash, I.: Intermittent catheterization and bladder rehabilitation in spinal cord injury patients, J. Urol. **114**:230-233, 1975.

42. Perkash, I.: An attempt to understand and to treat voiding dysfunctions during rehabilitation of the bladder in spinal cord injury patients, J. Urol. **115**:36-40, 1976.

43. Perkash, I.: Modified approach to sphincterotomy in spinal cord injury patients. Indications, technique, and results in 32 patients, Paraplegia **13**:247-260, 1976.

44. Perkash, I.: Intermittent catheterization failure and an approach to bladder rehabilitation in spinal cord injury patients, Arch. Phys. Med. Rehabil. **59**:9-17, 1978.

45. Pollack, H. M., Arger, P. H., Goldberg, B. B., and Mulholland, S. G.: Ultrasonic detection of nonopaque calculi, Radiology **127**:233-237, 1978.

46. Richter, M. W., Lytton, B., Myerson, D., and Grnja, V.: Radiology of genitourinary trauma, Radiol. Clin. North Am. **11**:593-631, 1973.

47. Rosen, J. S., Nanninga, J. B., and O'Connor, V. J.: Silent hydronephrosis, a hazard revisited, Paraplegia **14**:124-129, 1976.

48. Rosenfield, A. T., Taylor, K. J. W., Crade, M., and DeGraaf, C. S.: Anatomy and pathology of the kidney by gray scale ultrasound, Radiology **128**:737-744, 1978.

49. Sagel, S. S., Stanley, R. J., Levitt, R. G., and Geisse, G.: Computed tomography of the kidney, Radiology **124**:359-370, 1977.

50. Sanders, R. C., and Bearman, S.: B-scan ultrasound in the diagnosis of hydronephrosis, Radiology **108**:375-378, 1973.

51. Schaeffer, A. J.: Renal infection stones, Ill. Med. J. **156**:105-109, 1979.

52. Sherwood, T.: The dilated upper urinary tract, Radiol. Clin. North Am. **17**:333-340, 1979.

53. Silver, T. M., Kass, E. J., et al.: The radiological spectrum of acute pyelonephritis in adults and adolescents, Radiology **118**:65-71, 1976.

54. Stover, S. L.: Spinal cord injury, Continuing Education **17**:54-58, 1978.

55. Stover, S. L., Lloyd, L. K., Nepomuceno, C. S., and Gale, L. L.: Intermittent catheterization follow-up studies, Paraplegia **15**:38-46, 1978.

56. Talbot, H. S.: Fluoroscopy of the ureters in vesico-ureteral reflux. Clinical spinal cord injury conference, 1955, pp. 33-39.

57. Tarabulcy, E., Morales, P. A., and Sullivan, J. F.: Vesico-ureteral reflux in paraplegia: results of various forms of management. Clinical spinal cord injury conference, 1967, pp. 180-183.

58. Teplick, J. G., Teplick, S. K., Berinson, H., and Haskin, M. E.: Urographic and angiographic changes in acute unilateral pyelonephritis, Clin. Radiol. **30**:59-66, 1978.

59. Thomas, D. G., Smallwood, R., and Graham, D.: Urodynamic observations following spinal trauma, Br. J. Urol. **47**:161-175, 1975.

60. Umakantha, K. V., Rosen, J. S., and Betts, H. B.: Acute oliguria following cystography in spinal cord injury: case report, Arch. Phys. Med. Rehabil. **59**:88-91, 1978.

61. Witten, D. M.: Reactions to urographic contrast media, J.A.M.A. **231**:974-977, 1975.

62. Witten, D. M., Myers, G. H., and Utz, D. C.: Emmett's clinical urography, ed. 4, Philadelphia, 1977, W. B. Saunders Co., pp. 1149-1162, 1849-1854.

63. Zamora-Munoz, S., Sharifi, R., Bush, I. M., et al.: A unified approach to management of genitourinary trauma, Ill. Med. J. **156**:165-170, 1979.

CHAPTER 14

Surgical treatment of neurogenic bladder problems

JOHN B. NANNINGA, M.D.

Surgical treatment of neurogenic bladder dysfunction is based on the type of abnormal bladder function. Generally speaking, after a spinal cord injury, the bladder will recover a detrusor reflex if the sacral nerves S2, S3, and S4 are intact. Probably S3 alone will suffice to induce bladder emptying. If the sacral cord is damaged, then bladder areflexia may result. There are two other factors that must be considered in planning treatment. The presence of a sensation of bladder fullness is important because if the patient retains this, then he will have some warning of impending micturition and will be able to use a receptacle for urination. But if sensation is absent, then the patient, if he is to be catheter free, must wear some type of external collecting device. Thus surgical procedures that may produce incontinence can be advocated when the patient already relies on the external collecting device to collect urine. Another function that must be evaluated is the status of the voluntary striated periurethral (external) sphincter. If the normal relationship between the bladder and external sphincter is maintained, that is, if the sphincter relaxes when the bladder contracts, then the patient will have a relatively unobstructed flow of urine. However, if, on the other hand, the striated sphincter develops spasticity, just as striated muscle does below the level of the lesion, then the spincter will fail to relax during a detrusor contraction,[2,7] In fact, the sphincter may contract vigorously as the bladder is trying to expel its contents. Therefore efforts to promote bladder emptying should be directed at reducing the obstruction at the striated sphincter level.

PRESURGICAL EVALUATION

The complete evaluation of bladder function was discussed in Chapter 12. To review briefly, a cystometrogram will demonstrate whether the bladder will contract. Combining the cystometrogram with sphincter electromyography will demonstrate whether the periurethral striated muscle relaxes during a detrusor contraction.[5,7]

Radiologic studies are also of importance in studying bladder function.[1] Spot voiding films or cine studies should demonstrate the degree to which the sphincter mechanism opens and allows the expulsion of the bladder contents (Fig. 14-1). Also, the voiding cystourethrogram will demonstrate the presence of reflux, diverticula, or other abnormalities. The intravenous urogram will demonstrate the presence of hydronephrosis, an indication that outflow obstruction or retention or both are present (Fig. 14-2).[3,6] Thus once the type of bladder dysfunction has been diagnosed, the necessary corrective surgical procedure can be recommended.

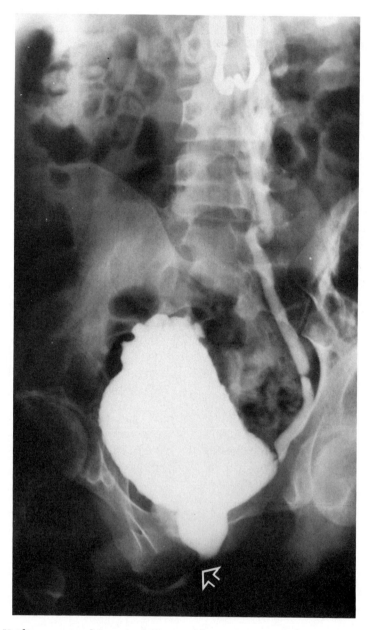

Fig. 14-1. Voiding cystourethrogram of 19-year-old paraplegic demonstrates marked narrowing in region of periurethral striated sphincter just distal to prostatic urethra (arrow). Note also dilatation of prostatic urethra and presence of ureteral reflux.

SURGICAL PROCEDURES

Those patients with a detrusor reflex and relatively normal sphincter function usually do not require any surgical procedure unless some other disease process is present, such as a bladder neck contracture or benign prostatic hyperplasia. Such patients usually have incomplete injuries. However, there are those patients who are bothered by a hyperreflexic bladder, which gives very little warning as to when a bladder contraction will occur. Such patients are quite prone to incontinence and, despite the use of anticholinergic medications, the sudden onset of urination may persist. For such patients, denervation of the bladder can be considered. Both complete denervation and selective denervation have been performed in the past, but surprisingly enough, the bladder tone may return after 1 or 2 years and incontinence may occur again.[8]

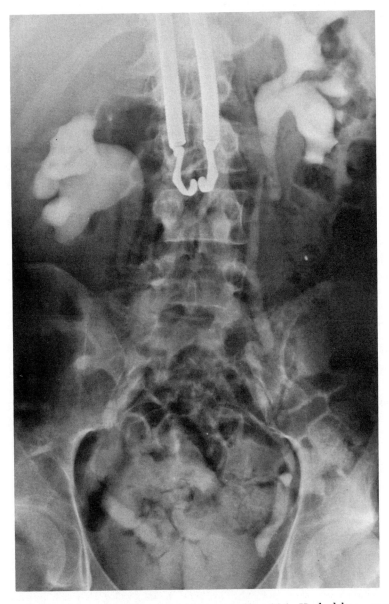

Fig. 14-2. Intravenous urogram in same patient as in Fig. 14-1. He had been successfully decatheterized but because of increasing obstruction at level of striated sphincter, hydronephrosis developed. Patient subsequently was treated by transurethral sphincterotomy.

Sphincterotomy

In those patients with relatively complete spinal injury and evidence of sphincter dysfunction, the goal is to reduce the outflow obstruction.[6] First, drugs that have skeletal muscle relaxing effects can be tried. But if sphincter obstruction persists, then I will recommend sphincterotomy.[5] This is performed transurethrally, using either a standard resectoscope with cutting electrode or a urethrotomy blade. The sphincter is cut anteriorly, which is where the larger number of sphincter fibers are located, and the anterior resection also seems to reduce the occasional occurrence of impotence, which can occur after sphincterotomy. It is my preference to leave the bladder neck alone since this has not been a very frequent site of obstruction in our experience.[5] It also decreases the chance of total incontinence, although many patients will wear an external collecting device so that incontinence is no problem. Documentation of the effectiveness of the sphincterotomy can be determined by voiding cystourethrography.

In female patients with a reflex bladder and sphincter dysynergy, measures to reduce the sphincteric obstruction often result in annoying incontinence, requiring diapers or ineffective collecting devices. In this situation the patient will benefit more by intermittent catheterization and anticholinergic medication to reduce bladder hyperreflexia.

In male patients with an areflexic bladder and outflow obstruction from the bladder neck, a transurethral resection can be performed. The patient may have to wear an external collector afterward to prevent stress incontinence. In female patients, efforts to reduce bladder neck and urethral resistance only accentuate incontinence; consequently it is better to maintain the patient on intermittent catheterization. In fact, with the development of pocket-sized catheter kits, many male patients now prefer to use intermittent catheterization rather than have a transurethral resection performed.

Suprapubic cystotomy

Suprapubic cystotomy has been a useful procedure in the past for bladder drainage. It has been used less frequently in recent years because of the increased use of intermittent catheterization and sphincterotomy. Certainly, suprapubic cystotomy avoids the problems of urethral catheterization in the male. However, unless the patient has a completely areflexic bladder, one of the more annoying complications is the periodic passage of small amounts of urine from the urethra. This problem can be reduced somewhat by anticholinergic medication, but there are still those patients who have to wear some form of external collector or diaper. Also, the suprapubic tube can cause the problems associated with all indwelling tubes, namely, chronic bacteriuria and calculi.

Supravesical diversion

In a rare individual it may be preferable to perform supravesical diversion. Fig. 14-3, A, illustrates the upper tract changes in a patient who had been paraplegic for 15 years. His urogram had been unchanged for 15 years, and renal function was stable. The reason for the rather rapid deterioration in terms of marked calyectasis and some ureterectasis was not totally clear. However, the patient had developed the habit of taping the catheter to his leg under some tension so that the balloon would prevent leakage of urine around the catheter. In doing this, the balloon must have been pulled down gradually into the prostatic urethra so that the catheter drainage opening was at least partially occluded. The cystogram in Fig. 14-3, B and C, reveals reflux and a small, contracted bladder. On cystopic examination the bladder wall appeared fixed and the ureteral orifices were gaping. It was my impression that this bladder could not be rehabilitated so as to provide an expansile reservoir for storage and then to eliminate urine adequately. Also, the results of reimplanting the dilated ureters into a small, trabeculated bladder are much less satisfactory than in a relatively normal bladder.[4] Consequently the patient underwent an ileal conduit procedure. The postoperative improvement in radiographic findings is striking (Fig. 14-3, D). This patient will have to be observed closely in the future because ureteroileal stenosis, stomal skin stenosis, and upper tract calculi are long-term complications.

Fig. 14-3. Thirty-six-year-old man who has been paraplegic for 15 years. **A,** Intravenous urogram demonstrates cortical thinning, calyectasis, and ureterectasis. **B** and **C,** Cystogram shows contrast medium running freely into upper tracts. Bladder capacity is quite limited. **D,** Following urinary diversion, there has been rapid improvement in radiographic appearance of kidneys as evidenced by decrease in calyectasis. There is still some clubbing of lower left calyces. Serum creatinine level is now 1.7.

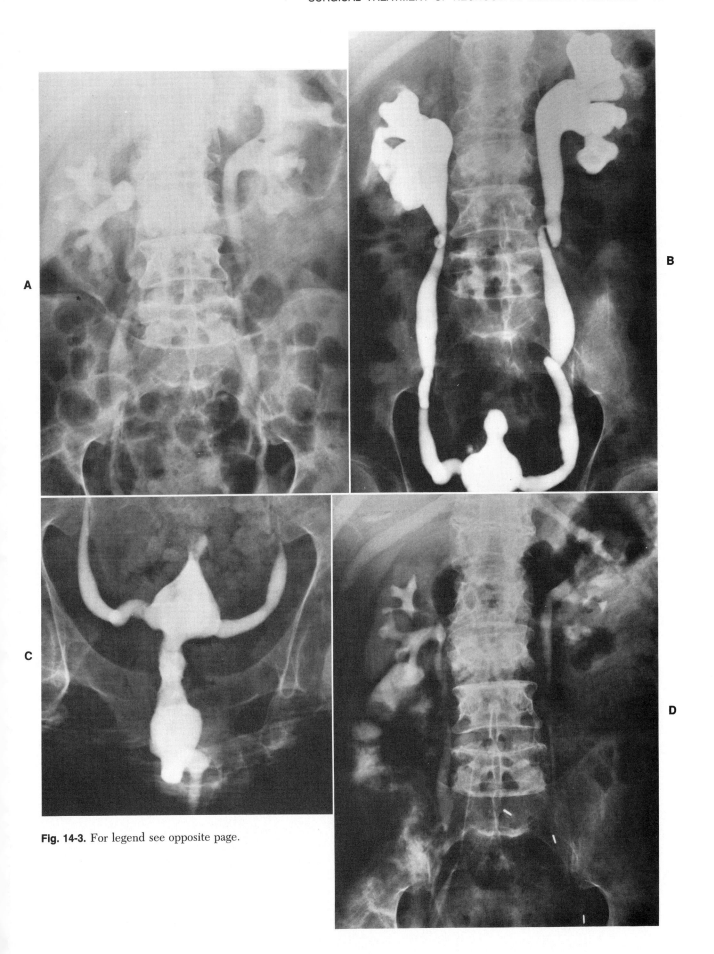

Fig. 14-3. For legend see opposite page.

CALCULI

Renal calculi may develop in patients with spinal cord injury because of immobilization; there may be subsequent hypercalciuria or chronic urinary infection with an organism such as *Proteus*, which is a so-called urea splitter and produces an alkaline urine. I usually recommend that a KUB examination be performed every 6 months for at least the first few years after injury for the purpose of detecting urinary calculi. Renal pelvic calculi should be removed promptly if the patient is a reasonable surgical risk. This can be done by extended pyelotomy or, for larger branched calculi, by nephrotomy. At times, when there is calcific debris in the calyces, a nephrostomy tube may be left in place for the purpose of irrigating the kidney and dissolving the stones with Renacidin. It is helpful to obtain renal tomograms preoperatively and postoperatively to evaluate the extent of the infectious stones because the calcium content varies in these relatively soft stones. When the films are clear, the irrigations are stopped and the nephrostomy tube removed.

By keeping the urinary system draining properly, eliminating infection when feasible, and removing calculi, which can be both a source of obstruction and infection, the patient's renal function can be preserved.

REFERENCES

1. Ascoli, R. R.: Radiological study of the vesical neck in paraplegia secondary to spinal cord injury, Int. J. Paraplegia 4:235, 1967.
2. Butler, M. R.: Patterns of bladder recovery in spinal injury evaluated by serial urodynamic observations, Urology 11:308, 1978.
3. Butler, E. D., Jr., Friendland, G. W., and Govan, D. E.: A radiological study of the effect of elevated intravesical pressures on ureteral calibre and peristalsis in patients with neurogenic bladder dysfunction, Clin. Radiol. 22:198, 1971.
4. Hackler, R. H.: Spinal cord injuries: urology care, Urology 2:13, 1973.
5. Nanninga, J. B., Rosen, J., and O'Conor, V. J., Jr.: Experience with transurethral external sphincterotomy in patients with spinal cord injury, J. Urol. 112:72, 1974.
6. Ross, J. C.: Surgical treatment of hydronephrosis in paraplegia, Int. J. Paraplegia 2:137, 1963.
7. Thomas, D. G., Smallwood, R., and Graham, D.: Urodynamic observations following spinal trauma, Br. J. Urol. 47:161, 1975.
8. Torrens, M., and Hald, T.: Bladder denervation procedures, Urol. Clin. North Am. 6:283, 1979.

CHAPTER 15

Skeletal changes after spinal cord injury

RONALD W. HENDRIX, M.D.

Multiple changes occur within the skeleton after spinal cord injury. They characteristically develop slowly and manifest themselves months or years after the initial cord injury. The loss of bone mass from the denervated portion of the skeleton leads to early bladder stone formation secondary to the resulting hypercalciuria. The loss of bone may continue until the bones become weak and fracture easily. Immobilization of resulting fractures can lead to development of a pressure sore and subsequent extended hospitalization. Bone erosion and osteomyelitis may occur secondary to a pressure sore in adjacent soft tissues. Surgical changes in the bones especially from bone resection as treatment for osteomyelitis or in association with resection of a pressure sore are frequently seen and must be distinguished from bone erosion secondary to a pressure sore. Loss of innervation to the trunk muscles in a growing child or adolescent leads to muscle imbalance and development of scoliosis or other spinal deformity. The paralysis of intercostal muscles leads to resorption of rib margins in some patients with long-standing spinal cord injuries.

The radiologic findings of most of the bone abnormalities resulting from cord injuries are straightforward. Knowledge of the findings and searching for them are usually sufficient to correctly diagnose the problem. Distinguishing the cause of bone erosion secondary to a pressure sore is an exception. Special techniques are helpful as is the knowledge that all bone erosion is not caused by osteomyelitis. A multitude of special techniques are also available for quantitative evaluation of osteoporosis.

OSTEOPOROSIS

Osteoporosis, or bone atrophy, is the state in which bone mass is decreased from normal. This may involve the whole skeleton or a portion of the skeleton. There is a loss of normal bone, which includes loss of organic bone matrix and bone mineral simultaneously. The remaining bone matrix contains a normal amount of bone mineral. The total bone mass has decreased. Osteoporosis must be distinguished from osteomalacia, which is the state of decreased bone mineral with a concomitant increase of organic bone matrix. Osteoporosis and osteomalacia both may lead to a decreased density of the bones as seen on radiographs. This similarity may lead to confusion. The definitive way to distinguish between these processes is by bone biopsy.

Early manifestations

Multiple studies have demonstrated that osteoporosis usually develops in the bones of spinal cord injured patients and occurs below the level of the cord injury.* The first manifestation of this osteoporosis is an increase of urinary excretion of calcium and hydroxyproline.[35,58] This increased excretion is caused by bone resorption occurring significantly faster than bone apposition. From 20% to 60% of the bone mineral must be resorbed before bone loss can be detected using conventional radiographic techniques.[10,91,92] For this reason it may be several months before such findings are detectable on radiographs. The radiologic appearance depends on the time interval since the cord lesion

_____
*References 1, 3, 20, 33-36, 49, 77, 94, 106, 110, 118.

was sustained, the bone mass present at the time the cord injury occurred, and the amount of residual muscle activity.

Pathogenesis

The mechanism causing the bone atrophy is not known, and the importance of contributing factors is in dispute. Mechanical, endocrine, neural, and vascular mechanisms have been suggested as possible causes of the bone rarefaction.* Work has been done in normal, quadriplegic, paraplegic, and poliomyelitis patients and in laboratory animals to identify the important factors causing loss of bone as a result of immobilization or paralysis.[43,45,63,83,110] Although some investigators hold that immobilization and paralysis have an equivalent effect on the skeleton, this is probably not true[35] because immobilization does not eliminate muscle tone and isometric muscle contractions.[3] The role that disuse plays in causing osteoporosis has been considered to be the most important factor by some investigators[63,110] and as almost negligible by others.[26,34]

The contributions of Albright[5-7] have had a profound influence on thinking about osteoporosis. His thesis that osteoblasts lay down new organic matrix because of stress and strain is a refinement of Wolff's law of the transformation of bone.[128] This law states that the internal architecture and the external configuration of a bone reflect its function and that the bone shape changes according to changes in function. Albright emphasized that bone tissue is dynamic and is constantly changing. In a given area osteoclasts are resorbing bone while nearby osteoblasts are laying down organic matrix and calcium salts are being deposited into adjacent organic matrix. A decrease of bone mass may occur from increased bone resorption or decreased bone formation. Decreased bone formation may result from inactivity of osteoblasts or failure of inorganic calcium salt deposition into the organic matrix. The former condition is called osteoporosis, the latter condition osteomalacia.[6]

A spinal cord injured patients is usually an active healthy individual who suddenly loses control of a large portion of his body because of a spinal cord injury. During much of the convalescent and rehabilitation period, the patient is recumbent. As a result disuse plays some part in the demineralization seen in these patients. A definite increase in urine output of calcium is seen in normal patients immobilized in a plaster hip spica cast for several weeks.[45] This increase of urine calcium persists until the patient is remobilized.[45,83,110] Similar findings occurred with astronauts subjected to weightlessness.[35,95] The calcium loss ceased with resumption of mobilization at the same time gravitational

*References 2, 6, 26, 34, 61, 63, 106.

forces were restored. Ambulation and even standing were initially thought to decrease the urine calcium output in spinal cord injured patients.[58,130] More elaborate studies of this point have since failed to demonstrate a decrease in hypercalciuria or its duration with therapeutic mobilization short of the patient walking.[110] The amount and duration of the hypercalciuria are directly related to the degree of paralysis and the amount of immobilization.[49] Further support of the stress and strain theory is supplied by histologic and radiologic study of rabbits with an immobilized hind limb. Electric stimulation causing muscle contraction in the immobilized hind limbs significantly decreased the amount of bone rarefaction as compared to controls.[63] It appears that muscle activity rather than the compressive stress of mere standing or weight bearing is the important source of stress and strain necessary to maintain normal bone mass.[2,110] An average-size man in a standing position exerts approximately 70 pounds of compressive force on each leg; walking greatly increases the amount of stress to each leg.

After spinal cord injury there is a marked increase in the amount of urinary hydroxyproline, a breakdown product of collagen.[89] Within a few weeks after immobilization there follows a significant increase in urinary calcium excretion.[35] The abnormal urinary hydroxyproline excretion can return to normal within a few months but may be elevated even after 2 years. The calcium loss can also remain high for a similar length of time.[113] Calcium turnover studies using ^{45}Ca have demonstrated an active turnover rate in patients during the first year after spinal cord injury. In a group of patients examined several years after injury, there was no longer an active turnover rate. A new calcium equilibrium or steady state had been established.[77] This new steady state occurs in the following manner: The patient's activity decreases with a corresponding decrease of stress and strain on the skeleton. The bone mass decreases to a new steady state that corresponds to the new amount of stress and strain. The rate of bone destruction and bone apposition reaches a new equilibrium state. During the time prior to reaching this state, there is a more rapid breakdown of bone than of bone apposition. The excess bone mineral is excreted, causing hypercalciuria.

The presence of vascular abnormalities is thought to have some influence on bone resorption. The precise mechanism is not known. Early venous return can be demonstrated by angiography in paralyzed areas.[61,113] The presence of arteriovenous shunts has also been demonstrated using radioactive albumin microspheres.[20] The early venous return has its onset at about 2 to 3 months after the cord injury. It regresses with time and disappears by approximately 15 months. It is independent of the cord level or the presence of spasticity or flaccidity.[113] The demonstration of arterialized venous blood in paralyzed areas also supports the angiographic findings.[18,19] It has been suggested that injury to the sympathetic nervous system is probably responsible for these changes.[113] The presence of arteriovenous anastomoses after damage to the sympathetic nervous system has been demonstrated in rabbits.[70] Stimulation of the distal sympathetic nerve trunk led to closure of the anastomoses in the rabbits. When stimulation ceased, the arteriovenous anastomoses reappeared. It has also been suggested that these arteriovenous anastomoses may be related to ectopic bone formation.[113]

Histologic changes

Histologic changes in bone due to immobilization resulting from paralysis have been documented using bone biopsies, a few of which were serial.[106] Osteoclastic resorption reached its maximum at approximately 15 weeks after spinal cord injury. This is coincident with maximal hypercalciuria and hyperhydroxyprolinuria.[20,106] It also approximates the onset of ectopic bone formation. Trabecular bone volume was decreased significantly as early as the fourth week. Tetracycline labeling done prior to the bone biopsies demonstrated that the mineralization rate of the osteoid was extremely low. The volume of osteoid present was also demonstrated to be decreased. These findings reflect a slow rate of laying down new bone. This conclusion is disputed by another investigator on the basis of less convincing evidence.[34]

Bone dynamics

Bone resorption and formation do not necessarily occur at the same rate. Bone atrophy occurs over a period of time when there is a net loss of bone substance because bone destruction is greater than bone formation. The remodeling rate may be increased, decreased, or normal, but net resorption is greater than apposition. Resorption from the cortex can be from the endosteal surface or the periosteal surface, or it can be intracortical from compact bone between these two surfaces.[60] Usually the first place that loss of bone substance due to a generalized process, as in these patients, can be detected is in the trabecular or cancellous bone and not in the cortical bone. This is because the cancellous bone has a significantly greater surface-to-volume ratio with a remodeling rate that is approximately three times that of compact cortical bone.[59]

Complications

Atrophy of the skeleton in spinal cord injured patients is important because of resulting clinical problems. The bones are weakened from a loss of significant bone mass with a susceptibility to fracture. The calcium from resorbed bone is excreted by the kidneys and leads to urinary calculi, which are one of the major chronic problems encountered in these patients.[58] The mobilization of large amounts of calcium from the skeleton has also been implicated in the formation of ectopic bone in the soft tissue.[20,94]

Radiologic findings

A convenient way to conceptually deal with the radiologic changes of osteoporosis in spinal cord injured patients is to arbitrarily divide the findings into early, intermediate, and advanced changes. The early findings fit rather well into a time period covering approximately the first 6 months after a spinal cord injury. These findings are essentially limited to the trabecular bone. The intermediate findings consist of progressive loss of trabecular bone and the onset and progression of changes in cortical compact bone; these latter changes may never occur in many patients[34,73] or may be limited to the diaphyseal area nearest the metaphyseal region when they do occur. The intermediate changes may be seen during a time span from roughly 6 months to many years after a spinal cord injury. Advanced changes represent the end stage of severe cortical and trabecular atrophy. The occasional patient in whom such advanced changes occur is a patient with long-standing paralysis. The advanced changes may be caused by the natural loss of bone seen with increasing age[62] superimposed on the loss from paralysis.

The earliest radiologic findings of osteoporosis occur in cancellous bone. These findings usually become apparent radiographically within 2 to 6 months after a spinal cord injury. The time of appearance is variable because of its relation to the amount of residual motor activity. A large percent of the bone is already gone before any changes can be detected with routine radiographs. In general, osteoporosis will eventually be more severe in patients with complete paralysis rather than partial paralysis.[49] The feet and also the hands and wrists, if the cord level is high enough, are the places to look for the earliest findings of bone loss. The knees, ankles, and calcanei will also demonstrate bone loss at a slightly later time. Radiographs are not frequently obtained in any of these areas because the presence of osteoporosis only rarely affects the patient's management during the first year after injury. The lumbar spine and pelvis contain a much greater amount of cancellous bone than the appendicular bones, but the overlying thick soft tissues make it impossible to detect early loss of bone trabeculae within these bones with routine radiographs. The soft tissues scatter the x-rays, which degrade the radiographic image, causing significant loss of detail and thus preventing detection of early changes with routine technique. More sophisticated

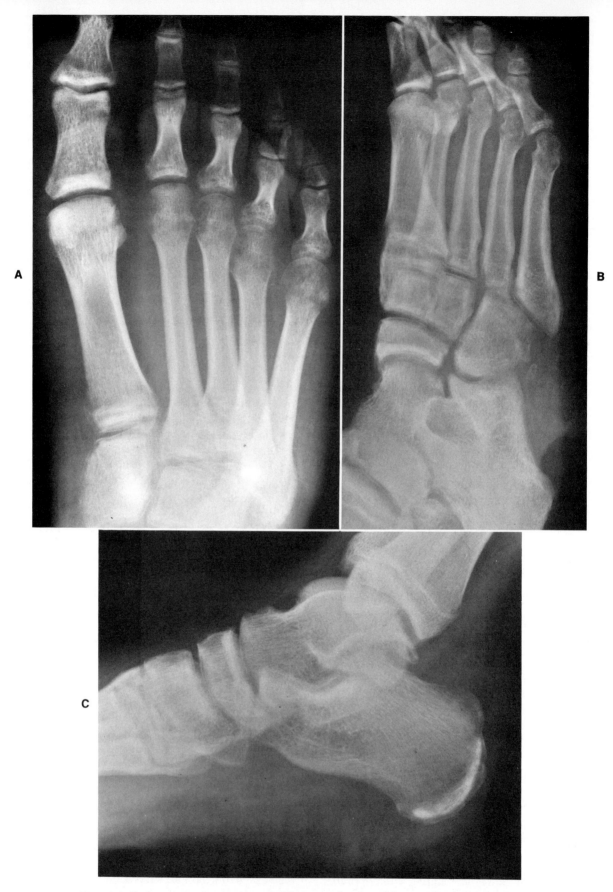

Fig. 15-1. Early osteoporosis in 21-year-old man with T9 cord lesion of 5 months' duration. **A,** Anteroposterior view shows nonuniform distribution of bone resorption in heads of second to fifth metatarsal bones and in base of corresponding proximal phalanges. Bone loss in first metatarsal bone is primarily proximal. **B,** Oblique view demonstrates subcortical bone loss in multiple proximal metatarsal and tarsal bones. **C,** Lateral view shows subcortical bone loss in most of tarsal bones and selective bone loss in calcaneus immediately anterior to dense tuberosity. This typical appearance of bone loss in calcaneus is unrelated to large pressure sore superficial to calcaneal tuberosity.

methods are necessary to evaluate these areas and have only recently been developed. They are discussed later under special techniques. Bone loss may progress at different rates in adjacent bones and in a nonuniform distribution or patchy fashion in a given bone (Fig. 15-1). This patchiness may persist until advanced loss of bone trabeculae and cortical thinning is radiologically evident. The nonuniformity is best seen in the metacarpal and metatarsal bones.

The resorption first appears as a nonuniform patchy loss of bone trabeculae that is generalized in nontubular bones and at the ends of tubular bones. In tubular bones this progresses rapidly and can develop into a well-defined lucent band across the metaphysis or a thin band of subarticular resorption. Either one or both of these findings may be present at the end of a given tubular bone. In the distal femur there is usually loss of subarticular bone in addition to loss in the metaphysis.

In the proximal tibia the metaphysis is more affected than the subarticular area (Fig. 15-2). In nontubular bones a well-defined subarticular band of trabecular resorption develops within several weeks after the onset of patchy resorption (Fig. 15-3). This will occur simultaneously in many, but not in all, carpal and tarsal bones. In the calcaneus a lucent band of bone loss occurs immediately anterior to the thick posterior tuberosity (Fig. 15-1, *C*). The bone loss slows down and plateaus or ceases at some time between 6 months and 2 years after injury.[106] This stabilization may be secondary to increased activity because of rehabilitation with reestablishment of a new calcium equilibrium related to the patient's reduced activity. Also, the bone loss may have reached a lower limit or threshold,[106] below which bone loss will not continue without the presence of factors, in addition to paralysis that predispose the patient to osteoporosis.

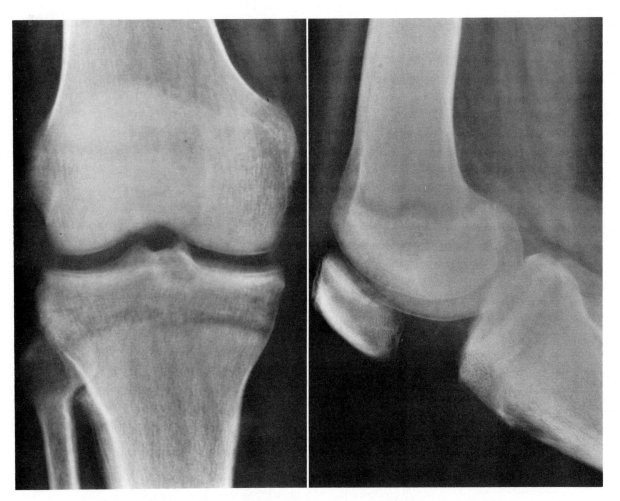

Fig. 15-2. Early osteoporotic changes in C6 complete quadriplegic 20-year-old man 11 months after injury. Most advanced bone loss is in metaphyseal areas of femur and tibia and in subcortical bone of femoral condyles and tibial plateau. Bone loss is progressing more slowly in this patient than is usually seen.

The intermediate radiologic findings are a progression of the early findings. Additional patchy areas of bone resorption will appear in tubular and in nontubular bones. The well-defined lucent metaphyseal and subarticular bands of bone loss become wider and less well defined (Fig. 15-4). This bone loss may extend far into the epiphyseal and diaphyseal areas in tubular bones. In nontubular bones the subcortical bone loss may intensify and spread in a manner similar to that in tubular bones with patchy areas of bone loss becoming confluent with the subcortical lucent area. Endosteal bone resorption of the diaphyseal cortex in long bones may appear, causing a wavy, irregular endosteal margin. Intracortical tunneling may also be seen at the same time and in the same bone. This is seen as long tunnels of bone resorption that cause the diaphyseal cortex to have a porous appearance. The patchy distribution of the bone loss resulting from the summation of these processes may persist for several years. Bone remodeling is slow and may in time reduce the nonuniform distribution of the bone loss (Fig. 15-5).

The advanced changes of osteoporosis are manifested by a thin diaphyseal cortex and a medullary cavity that has a relatively empty appearance because of a marked decrease in the number of bone trabeculae (Figs. 15-5 and 15-6). These findings are usually not seen until many years after a spinal cord injury and are not present in all patients.[73] There is an exception in a few patients who develop severe localized bone loss very rapidly soon after injury with bone changes resembling reflex sympathetic dystrophy (Fig. 15-7).[9,73] In patients with advanced changes, the intermediate finding of patchy bone loss is replaced by an empty-appearing medullary cavity. The irregular endosteal resorption has progressed until the endosteal surface is quite smooth and the diaphyseal cortex is very thin. The cor-

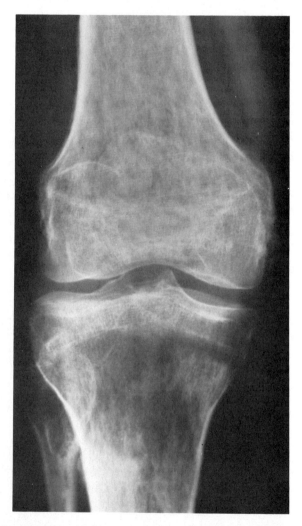

Fig. 15-4. Intermediate osteoporotic changes in 33-year-old complete C6 quadriplegic man 18 months after automobile-pedestrian accident. Nonuniform bone loss is more widespread than that seen in first few months after injury. Many small areas of patchy bone resorption have coalesced into large irregular areas of resorption. Bone loss has progressed from metaphyseal and subcortical areas into epiphyseal and diaphyseal areas of bone.

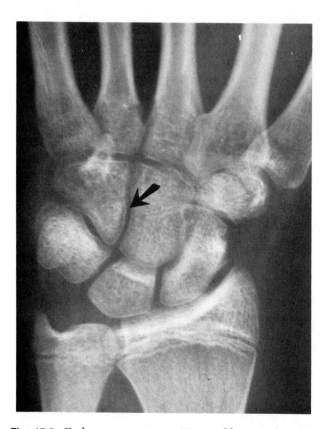

Fig. 15-3. Early osteoporosis in 15-year-old incomplete C6 quadriplegic boy 4½ months after high school football accident. Subcortical bone resorption is best seen in hamate bone (*arrow*).

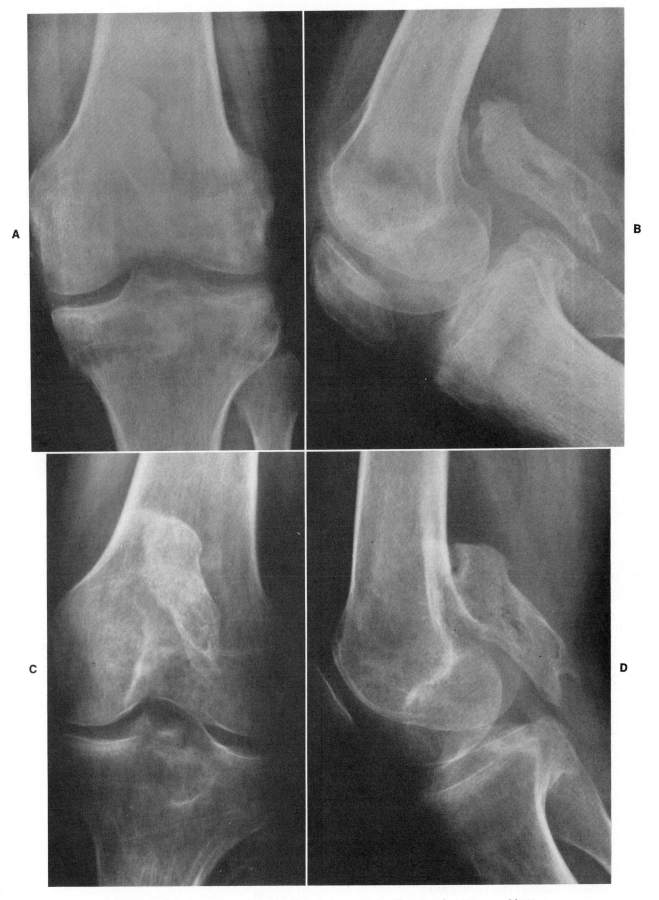

Fig. 15-5. Progression of osteoporotic changes over 34-month interval in 24-year-old T5 complete paraplegic man. **A** and **B,** Extensive subcortical and metaphyseal bone loss is present 16 months after spinal cord injury. Ectopic bone in popliteal fossa is in an unusual position. **C** and **D,** Fifty months after injury. Loss of bone trabeculae is more uniform and diaphyseal cortices of proximal tibia and distal femur are thinner than at 16 months. (See also Fig. 16-12.)

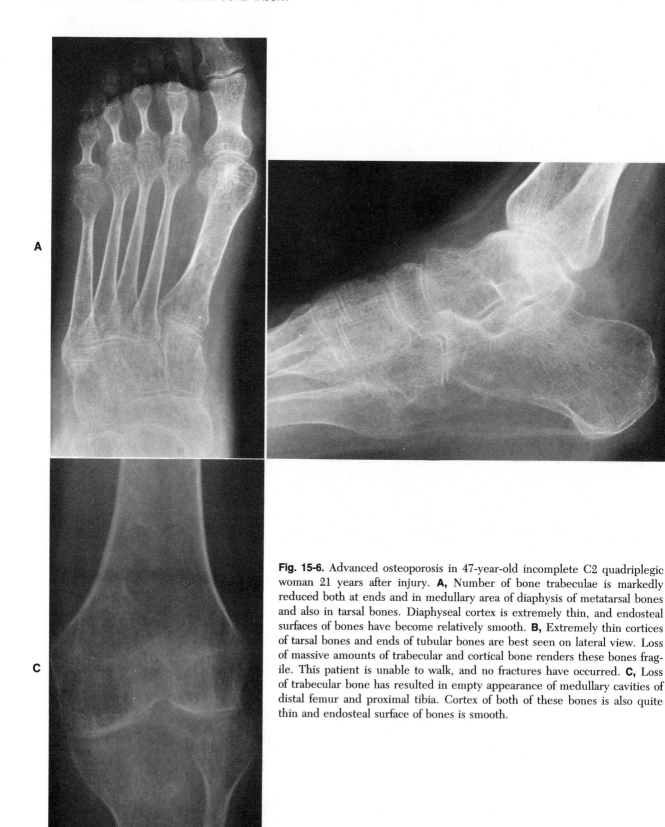

Fig. 15-6. Advanced osteoporosis in 47-year-old incomplete C2 quadriplegic woman 21 years after injury. **A,** Number of bone trabeculae is markedly reduced both at ends and in medullary area of diaphysis of metatarsal bones and also in tarsal bones. Diaphyseal cortex is extremely thin, and endosteal surfaces of bones have become relatively smooth. **B,** Extremely thin cortices of tarsal bones and ends of tubular bones are best seen on lateral view. Loss of massive amounts of trabecular and cortical bone renders these bones fragile. This patient is unable to walk, and no fractures have occurred. **C,** Loss of trabecular bone has resulted in empty appearance of medullary cavities of distal femur and proximal tibia. Cortex of both of these bones is also quite thin and endosteal surface of bones is smooth.

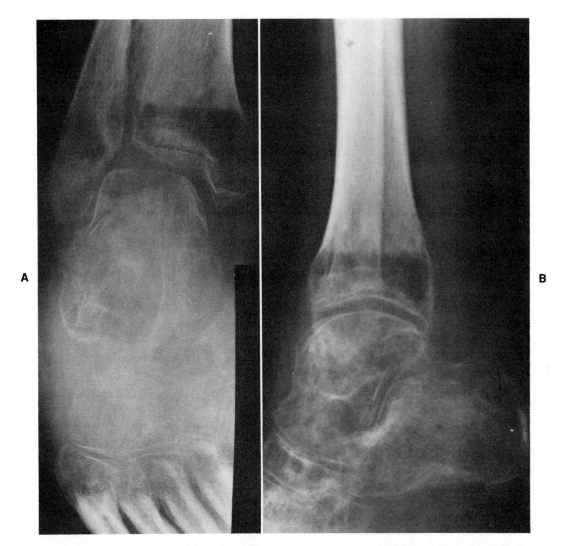

Fig. 15-7. Changes resembling reflex sympathetic dystrophy or Sudeck's atrophy in 27-year-old T5 paraplegic man 11 months after motorcycle accident. **A,** Oblique view. **B,** Lateral view. Intense local loss of bone has occurred in all tarsal bones and in distal metaphyseal and epiphyseal areas of tibia.

tex in the ends of tubular bones is normally thin but becomes even thinner and can decrease in thickness by about 50% of its normal dimension.[118] The findings in the tarsal and carpal bones are similar to those in the ends of the long bones (Fig. 15-6). The number of trabeculae that support the articular cortex is markedly reduced, leaving the articular surfaces greatly weakened. Normally the patients in whom such advanced bone loss occurs are not bearing weight on these bones so the number of complications are relatively few. Nevertheless, the bones may fracture easily with minor trauma. Depending on the amount of spasticity, the patient's activity, and the completeness of the cord lesion, the loss of bone will be arrested at some point between normal bone mass present prior to injury and

severe osteoporosis. The cortex of a given bone will remain dense and well defined, even though it becomes extremely thin from severe bone loss (Figs. 15-6 and 15-7).

Special radiologic procedures

Several definitions must be made in order to understand most of the important radiologic procedures used to determine the amount of bone present. The first is *bone density*, which is defined as mass per unit volume. Although this appears to be a straightforward definition, problems arise because bone is not a completely uniform tissue. There are areas, such as the diaphysis of a long bone, where the bone mineral is very compactly laid down. In the medullary cavity and at the ends of long bones, there are large spaces between the bone trabeculae. As a result the bone density will vary from point to point. The point that one speaks of must be specified in order not to be confusing. When the density of a relatively large volume of bone is considered, this is understood to be an average density. A large volume of bone will ordinarily contain both compact and trabecular bone. This is especially important when dealing with scanning methods that use a cross-sectional area of the diaphysis where the medullary cavity is included in the slice. *Bone mineral content* is another concept that is frequently used. It is defined as the mass of mineral content of a piece of bone 1 cm long. It is also defined mathematically as the bone density times the axial cross-sectional area of a bone.[86] *Bone mass* is another concept in frequent use; it is defined as the amount of bone present without reference to volume. This is usually used with reference to the entire mass of bone present in the skeleton. In an osteoporotic state bone density is normal and unchanged but the total mass of bone in the skeleton is decreased and the mineral content of a given bone is also decreased.

The concept of bone density can be confusing unless one specifies the point of reference. Loss of trabecular or cortical bone in osteoporosis leads to a reduction of the density of the bone considered as a whole. At the same time there is no change in the density of the remaining bone tissue; there is merely less of it. The remaining bone retains the normal amount of mineralization per unit of organic matrix.[14] A radiograph of a bone will demonstrate the distribution of the bone mineral and the morphology of the bone. Some areas within the bone contain more mineral and attenuate more x-rays passing through than do less dense areas. The former areas appear whiter on the radiograph than the latter areas. The in vivo measurements of bone density or bone mineral content are used as reflectors of total skeletal mass. If the process affecting bone is generalized, any change seen in one bone is taken to uniformly reflect that which is occurring in other bones and in the entire skeleton. In spinal cord injured patients, this is usually restricted to the skeleton in the paralyzed areas although this has been questioned by one investigator.[73,74] Cancellous bone has a greater surface-to-volume ratio than does cortical bone. Therefore loss of bone occurs earlier and changes can be detected in the trabecular bone in metabolic disorders, including osteoporosis, earlier than in cortical bone. It is important in a long bone to know whether a measurement was taken through the diaphysis or at the end of the bone. Flat bones such as those of the pelvis or the vertebral bodies in the spine have a much greater number of bone trabeculae than long bones. It would be ideal to measure bone mineral content in these bones,

but they are difficult to evaluate with the available methods.

The *in vivo measurement* of bone mineral content has been made using many different techniques, most of which measure the attenuation of x-rays or photons in bone. The earliest methods were subjective estimates of bone loss determined from visual inspection of a radiograph of a given bone or bones.[47] These are inaccurate modes of determining bone density.[10,47,91,92] The next most simple method is the measurement of the cortical thickness of a bone.[102,103] This is obtained by measuring the external diameter or width of the diaphysis and the transverse width of the medullary cavity at the same point in a bone. The latter measurement is subtracted from the former, giving the combined cortical thickness (CCT) of the bone. Tables of standard values according to age and sex are available for many bones.[125] The CCT primarily reflects endosteal bone resorption. It ignores intracortical and trabecular bone resorption.[65]

Photodensitometry uses a known standard wedge of metal or ivory that is radiographed alongside the bone of interest.[84,104] A densitometer is used to scan the bone and the standard stepwedge on the resulting radiograph. Because the stepwedge is of known density, a density can be assigned to the bone of interest and the bone mineral content can be inferred.

A much more accurate method is *photon absorptiometry*.[28,29] A scanner using a well-collimated ^{125}I source scans across the bone of interest, which may be a radius, ulna, carpal, metacarpal, or metatarsal bone. A sodium iodide scintillation detector on the opposite side of the bone detects the amount of radiation transmitted through the bone. This information is electronically processed and gives an instantaneous readout of the bone mineral content. This method is primarily useful in measuring cortical bone. Positioning is critical with this method and becomes difficult in the metaphyseal area of a bone where there is a proportionately greater amount of trabecular bone.[65]

Computed tomography (CT) has been used recently to determine bone density and bone mineral content.[65,66] This method has a reproducibility similar to that of photon absorptiometry and can be used more easily for measurement of density in bones with a great amount of cancellous bone. Flat bones of the pelvis and vertebrae can be evaluated with this method. The bone density at any point on the CT cross-sectional display can be determined because of the nature of the information available. There are still some flaws in this system so that it is not in general use at this time. One modification of this system has been the use of a low-energy source such as ^{125}I coupled with a CT scanner. This technique is superior for bone density as compared to commercially available CT scanners for peripheral small bones.[114]

OSTEOMYELITIS

Osteomyelitis occurs relatively infrequently in patients after spinal cord injury. Osteomyelitis can occur by hematogenous spread most often originating from a skin infection usually caused by *Staphylococcus*.[127] The spine can become infected secondary to pyelonephritis, which spreads by way of Batson's plexus from the urinary tract to the spine.[15,32,44] Osteomyelitis from skin infection or pyelonephritis is negligible in spinal cord injured patients in comparison to the number of occurrences secondary to pressure sores. Excessive pressure over a bony prominence for as little as 2 to 12 hours leads to ischemia and necrosis of the soft tissues.[81] Either slough or débridement of the necrotic soft tissue results in a pressure sore, which inevitably becomes infected. The infection hastens additional soft tissue necrosis. Pressure sores tend to be self-perpetuating. Continued pressure from lying on a superficial pressure sore causes ischemia of remaining viable soft tissues over the bony prominence. Eventually the bony prominence will become exposed due to necrosis of all the overlying soft tissues if proper treatment is not instituted (see Chapter 16). Once the bony prominence is exposed and becomes continuous with the infected pressure sore, it may become infected. It can also become infected if contiguous soft tissues are infected. Any bone in the paralyzed portion of the body can potentially become infected if a pressure sore develops in the adjacent soft tissues. By far the most common sites of osteomyelitis are the ischia, the greater trochanters, and the sacrum.

Pathogenesis

The mechanisms accounting for spread of infection to bone can be divided into three categories: hematogenous, penetrating trauma, and a contiguous focus of infection. The pathogenesis of hematogenous osteomyelitis of long bones has been well detailed by Trueta.[124] He described the different manifestations seen in infants, children, and adults and demonstrated the anatomic reasons for these differences. Osteomyelitis involving flat bones has not been as rigorously studied as that occurring in long bones. This may be because the lack of a thick diaphyseal cortex makes the pathologic process and the radiologic appearance less complicated, less dramatic,[12,64,131] and usually easier to treat.

Osteomyelitis occurring in flat bones is similar in some ways and dissimilar in other respects from that seen in long bones. Both flat and long bones may become infected by any one of the three routes mentioned; but only osteomyelitis resulting from contiguous

infection is important when a pressure sore is the origin. Probably the most important difference between osteomyelitis in the two types of bones is due to the thick diaphyseal cortex of the long bone. This cortex offers a barrier to a contiguous infection originating in the soft tissues. It also forms a barrier preventing easy spread of established hematogenous osteomyelitis from the medullary cavity into the adjacent soft tissues. The thick cortex delays such spread, preventing expansion and egress of dead cells and debris. The debris collects in the medullary cavity resulting in increased medullary pressure. This eventually exceeds the pressure in the medullary vessels with subsequent avascular necrosis of the inner half of the cortex. Sequestration is formed from the dead cortex. The outer half of the cortex receives its blood supply from periosteal vessels[85] and remains viable. The infection may eventually penetrate the cortex and periosteum and form an abscess in the soft tissues.[124] A different situation occurs with flat bones where the cortex is quite thin. The cortex offers relatively little resistance to penetration from infection originating either within the bone or in adjacent soft tissues in comparison to that offered by the diaphysis of a long bone. Because of its thin cortex, the greater trochanter of the femur acts similarly to the flat bones in this respect. The blood supply to flat bones comes both from nutrient and periosteal arteries. The bone can usually survive on the vascular supply of only one of these sources.[12] Because of the redundant blood supply, sequestration is relatively uncommon in the flat bones of the pelvis.

Bone erosion without osteomyelitis

The body attempts to heal any pressure sore with granulation tissue.[42,81,82] Granulation tissue is a highly vascular young connective tissue. Wherever it comes in contact with cartilage or bone, they both appear to melt away before it.[4] This hyperemic tissue covers the viable soft tissue that forms the inner surface of the pressure sore. It is resistant to infection because it contains a large number of mononuclear phagocytes.[8] If an underlying bone is exposed at the base of a pressure sore, the granulation tissue gradually covers the bony prominence. It is thought that the granulation tissue releases enzymes[117] that cause demineralization of the adjacent bone.

The pathologic interpretation by Jaffe of bone biopsies from exposed bone at the base of ten pressure sores from material of Heilbrun and Kuhn[78] appears to be compatible with a thesis of granulation tissue causing some of the bone erosions associated with pressure sores. In his material there was a spectrum that included osteomyelitis at one extreme and infection of the adjacent soft tissues without osteomyelitis in the underlying bone at the opposite extreme. Erosion of underlying bone was seen in both situations. The frequent observation at our institution of cortical erosion of a bone adjacent to a deep pressure sore with no demonstrable osteomyelitis in the underlying bone as determined by microscopic and microbiologic examination of biopsies of the involved bone[93] led us to seek an explanation other than osteomyelitis to account for the bone erosions. It is well known that granulation tissue forms a lining for the pressure sore, and it is also known that granulation tissue will erode bone.[98,99] The synthesis of this information accounting for erosion of bone adjacent to some pressure sores has not been suggested and appears to us to possibly account for the radiologic and clinical findings. Granulation tissue at the base of a pressure sore will eventually mature and form a very thick fibrous scar that is relatively avascular. It prevents the pressure sore from healing and is always infected. Between this scar and the underlying bone, there may persist a layer of hypervascular immature connective tissue or granulation tissue that will erode bone if it remains undisturbed. Eventually even this layer matures, forming a scar that will become adherent to the bony prominence. We suggest that erosion from granulation tissue appears to account for the majority of cases of bone destruction adjacent to pressure sores in our patients. We initially made the mistake of interpreting these erosions as osteomyelitis. The confusion occurred because osteomyelitis also may present with erosion of the cortex and the underlying bony trabeculae. The erosions caused by what we suspect is granulation tissue occurred more frequently and were more limited in size, whereas osteomyelitis caused progressive bone destruction or reactive bone. So far, we have not seen reactive bone causing sclerosis of the margin of erosions thought to be caused by granulation tissue.

Osteomyelitis secondary to a pressure sore except in cases of fistula formation allows free drainage. Drainage has been a long-prescribed treatment for osteomyelitis. This may be the reason for the relatively infrequent occurrence of osteomyelitis in spite of the almost ubiquitous presence of pressure sores in spinal cord injured patients. Ordinarily the bone vascular supply is also maintained, which is not the case with hematogenous osteomyelitis in long bones. This is an important reason why the latter progresses rapidly and resists therapy. Good circulation is considered the best defense of contaminated tissue against infection.[24] The maintenance of adequate bone blood flow and local drainage of the pressure sore probably account for the rarity of osteomyelitis seen in association with pressure sores. No evidence of osteomyelitis was demonstrated in 36 of 38 bony prominences, including sacra, ischia, and trochanters, resected along with an adjacent pressure sore at our institution.[93]

Clinical findings

Clinical findings may be useful in distinguishing some patients with osteomyelitis from those who have bone erosions simply from granulation tissue. Fever and malaise, as well as the patient appearing toxic, have been seen in those patients with osteomyelitis. Unfortunately the symptoms are usually interpreted as being caused by an urinary tract infection. Patients with erosions from granulation tissue appear to be well and complain of no systemic symptoms resulting from the erosions.

Periostitis

Periostitis can occur from an infection in the adjacent soft tissues secondary to a superficial pressure sore (Fig. 15-8). In such cases the bone is not infected.[119] An underlying bony prominence may develop osteomyelitis either secondary to spread of infection from an adjacent infected periosteum or because the bone is exposed due to necrosis of all the overlying soft tissues. In the latter case the periosteum is absent, rendering the bone incapable of periosteal new bone formation in the area of the bone exposed by the pressure sore. In the former case where the periosteum is infected, the periosteum probably becomes necrotic from pressure before periosteal new bone formation has time to occur. It has been our observation that periosteal new bone formation does not occur in the area immediately adjacent to the pressure sore in cases when the underlying bony prominence has or eventually does become infected or in cases where bare bone is exposed. In the former cases, periosteal new bone formation may be seen at sites removed from the area where the infection was introduced from the pressure sore. The presence of periostitis does not indicate the presence of osteomyelitis but rather suggests the lack of it when it is seen adjacent to the base of a pressure sore. These findings are somewhat the reverse process of hematogenous osteomyelitis, which begins inside the bone and works its way outward with eventual elevation or irritation of the periosteum causing periosteal new bone formation. Osteomyelitis occurring from a contiguous site can penetrate into the medullary cavity of a bone. Once the infection is established in the medullary cavity, it acts much like that from hematogenous spread. Periosteal new bone formation may then occur but in areas distant or removed from the portion of the bone exposed by the pressure sore where the periosteum is absent.

Radiologic findings

The radiologic findings are most dependent on the amount of time that has elapsed since the infection started, the virulence of the infecting organism, and whether the infected bone is a flat or a long bone. The radiologic findings will proceed more quickly with a

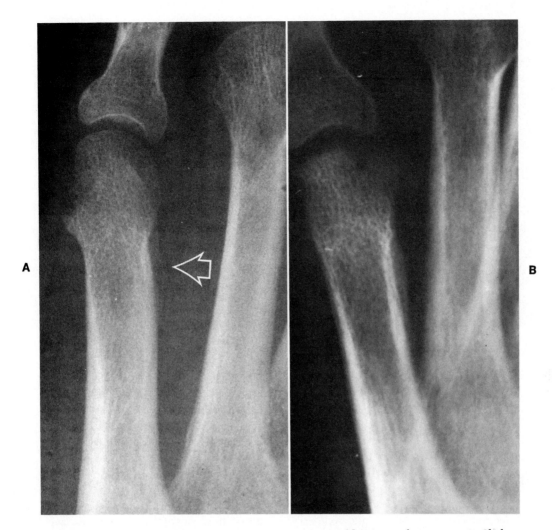

Fig. 15-8. Periostitis of fifth metatarsal bone in 21-year-old T5 paraplegic man. **A,** Slight irregularity of soft tissues overlying distal end of fifth metatarsal head is caused by a pressure sore, and erosion of lateral aspect of metatarsal head has occurred. Early periosteal new bone formation is present *(arrow)*. Periostitis has appeared remote from site of pressure sore, which is typical of osteomyelitis originating from a pressure sore. **B,** Five months later, deformity of fifth metatarsal head has occurred. Periosteal new bone along medial shaft of bone has increased and matured.

more virulent organism. Necrosis and sequestration are more likely to occur in a long bone than in a flat bone. Normally a long bone becomes infected from a contiguous infection at one of its ends through a region where the cortex is thin. In this way it responds similarly to a flat bone. Subsequently the infection can spread to the shaft of the bone and then findings similar to those in any other long bone may be present.

A sequence of events is radiographically discernible. A radiograph is a static record of what has collectively happened in the bone up to the time of the examination. The radiograph may record the findings at any point along the continuum of events that begins with a normal bone and terminates with chronic osteomyelitis. In most patients the bone infection is not identified until the chronic stage of osteomyelitis has been reached.

The earliest finding is that of demineralization of the bone. This is followed by destruction of the cortex and some of the underlying trabeculae. The underlying trabeculae are randomly destroyed with a resulting irregular margin that radiographically appears fuzzy or indistinct. Because of the redundant blood supply and the local drainage by way of the open pressure sore, local necrosis of bone ordinarily does not occur. The infection may spread extensively throughout the medullary cavity of the bone. Even with extensive involvement of the medullary cavity there may not be resulting osteonecrosis, presumably because of the available drainage and lack of resultant pressure buildup in the medullary

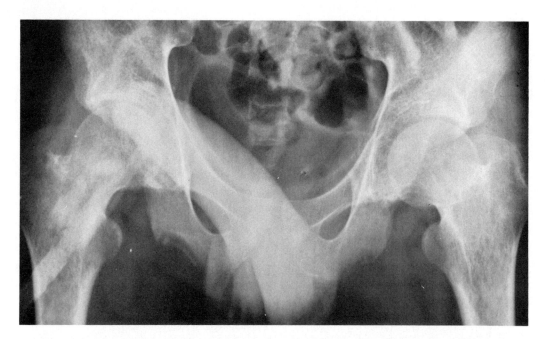

Fig. 15-9. Osteomyelitis of right ischium in 17-year-old boy with complete C7 spastic quadriplegia from 2.5 m (8 ft) fall from a window. Erosions of both ischial bones have occurred. Margin of right ischial erosion is sclerotic, indicating reaction of bone to infection. No bone reaction is associated with left ischial erosion. Biopsies of both bones were cultured and examined microscopically. Osteomyelitis was present in right but not in left ischium.

cavity. The bone reacts to the infection with osteoblastic activity. Bone destruction is seen first and may be the only finding but with enough time bone sclerosis occurs. In most patients radiographs are not obtained in an early stage. Chronic changes of sclerosis of the margin of the eroded area or a dense sclerotic bone are seen more often radiographically (Figs. 15-9 and 15-10). It is possible for infection to spread from the greater trochanter into the proximal shaft of the femur where it will resemble the hematogenous spread of osteomyelitis (Fig. 15-11). In this situation, osteonecrosis may occur in the diaphysis with sequestration formation. The infection may also penetrate the thick diaphyseal cortex, causing periosteal new bone formation. After the extensive spread of osteomyelitis through a flat bone, such as the ischium, it is possible for periosteal new bone to form. This will not form in the area of the bone exposed by the pressure sore but rather at a site removed from this area where the periosteum is still intact (Fig. 15-10).

Magnification and fine detail radiography

Bone detail in a thick part of the body using conventional, routine radiologic technique is not optimal. The thick overlying soft tissues scatter the x-rays, which degrades the detail in the resulting radiologic image. The clinician frequently wishes to know the status of the cortex of the underlying bone in the presence of a sa-

cral, ischial, or trochanteric pressure sore. Magnification radiography is the most accurate available technique for determining bone detail in a thick body part.[68] This technique uses a special x-ray tube with a focal spot measuring 0.1 mm diameter or less as opposed to a conventional tube with a 1.2 mm focal spot size. The part being radiographed is placed close to the x-ray tube and relatively far from the radiographic film (Fig. 15-12, *B*). This is in contrast to normal technique, in which the part being radiographed is placed as close to the film as possible (Fig. 15-12, *A*). The placement far from the film results in a magnification of two to four times. Magnification radiography may be used for thin as well as thick body parts when optimal bone detail is necessary (Fig. 15-13). Excellent bone detail similar to that obtained with the magnification technique can also be obtained using *fine detail radiography*. The problems with scattered radiation and excessive radiation dose to the patient limit the usefulness of this technique to thin body parts such as the hands and feet. This technique uses a fine grain film without a screen.[67] Recently this technique has been adapted using certain single emulsion films with single screens with a 20-fold decrease of patient radiation exposure.[80] An x-ray tube with a 0.3 mm focal spot size, which is available in most large radiology departments, is used for this latter technique. The bones on the film obtained are viewed with optical magnification using a 4 to 8 power hand lens.

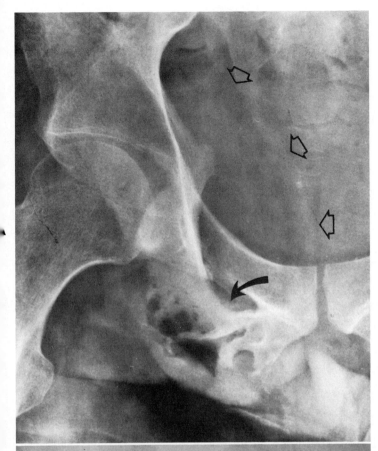

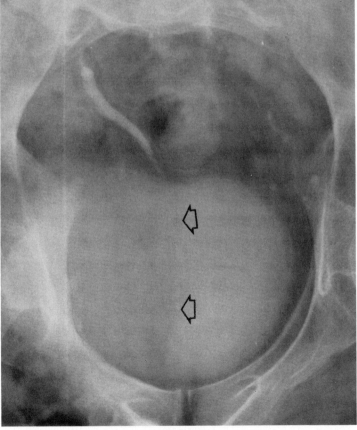

Fig. 15-10. Osteomyelitis of right ischium in 29-year-old complete L1 flaccid paraplegic man. **A,** Ischium and inferior pubic ramus are sclerotic and eroded from chronic infection. Air in pressure sore is superimposed on ischium. Periosteal new bone is present on opposite side of pressure sore *(curved arrow).* Pelvic soft tissue mass caused by an abscess is faintly visible *(open arrows).* Its origin is probably from pressure sore, but it could have originated from ischial osteomyelitis penetrating into soft tissues. **B,** Pelvic abscess is better seen from this intravenous urogram. Bladder is displaced *(arrows)* as is ureter.

Differential diagnosis

There are several points of differential diagnosis that may be helpful to distinguish between osteomyelitis and erosions presumably caused by granulation tissue. The latter erosions are more common than osteomyelitis. They do not incite periosteal reaction. Periosteal new bone formation is frequently seen with osteomye-litis at sites removed or distant from the pressure sore (Figs. 15-8 and 15-10). Reactive sclerosis is seen in some of the infected bones but not in association with erosions from granulation tissue. The latter erosions never cause as much bone destruction as that resulting from osteomyelitis.

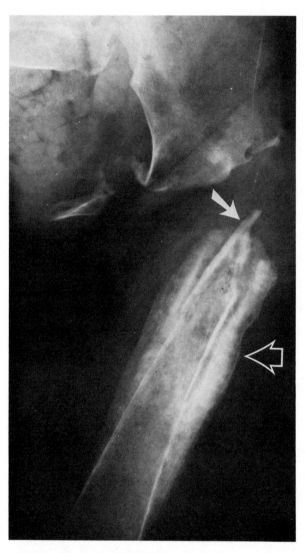

Fig. 15-11. Chronic osteomyelitis of left femur in 35-year-old woman with T6 paraplegia for 18 years. Resections of both femoral heads and necks, ischia, pubic bones, acetabulae, coccyx, and part of sacrum were done. Well-formed involu-crum *(horizontal arrow)* and large sequestration *(slanted arrow)* from chronic osteomyelitis indicate lack of successful treatment in left femur. Identical findings were present in right femur. Bilateral drainage from hips began 6 years after resection of femoral heads and necks and has continued for 7 years. Successful treatment on left necessitated amputation of left lower extremity. (See also Fig. 16-26.)

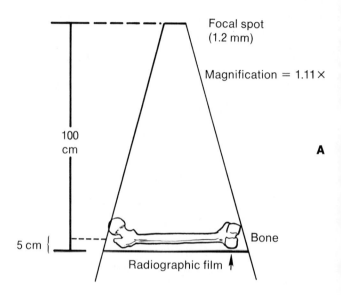

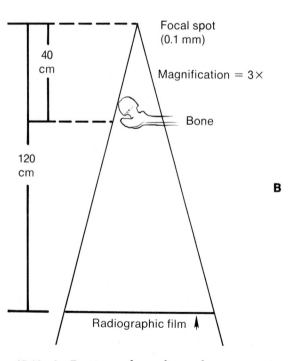

Fig. 15-12. A, Routine radiographic technique. **B,** Direct magnification radiographic technique. Magnification 2.5 to 4 times can be obtained with this technique.

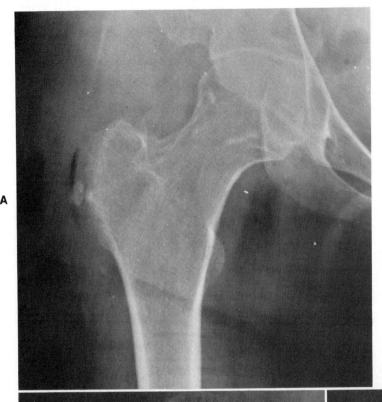

Fig. 15-13. Comparison of routine and magnification techniques in 24-year-old paraplegic woman. **A,** Routine technique. Air outlines pressure sore over greater trochanter, and ectopic bone is present in soft tissues adjacent to trochanter. Normal cortical margin of trochanter is poorly visualized and may be missing. **B,** Direct radiographic magnification (3×) of same hip. Normal thin cortical margin of greater trochanter is definitely absent. It has been eroded by granulation tissue lining pressure sore. **C,** Direct magnification view of hip in normal patient for comparison. Cortical margin of greater trochanter is intact and normal in this patient. Note thin sclerotic line that is normally present over this area.

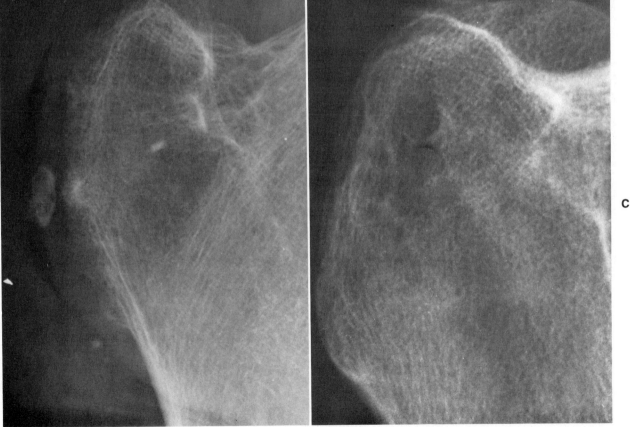

FRACTURES

The many changes and improvements made in the management of the spinal cord injured patient in the past 30 years have greatly increased the life expectancy as well as the self-reliance of these patients. Rehabilitation programs have been developed to teach these people to care for themselves, to drive automobiles, and to compete in sports, as well as to teach them the necessary occupational skills for self-support. In short, they are taught how to be maximally active and to enjoy as normal an existence as possible. Because of this training they are able to function in society. The self-reliance and freedom attained expose them to the ordinary hazards of daily living with a certain amount of inevitable trauma. Sometimes the trauma is sufficient to result in a fracture. With respect to the time sustained, fractures in the spinal cord injured patient can be divided into two categories. The first category is a group of fractures that occurs at the same time as the spinal cord injury. A second group of fractures occurs

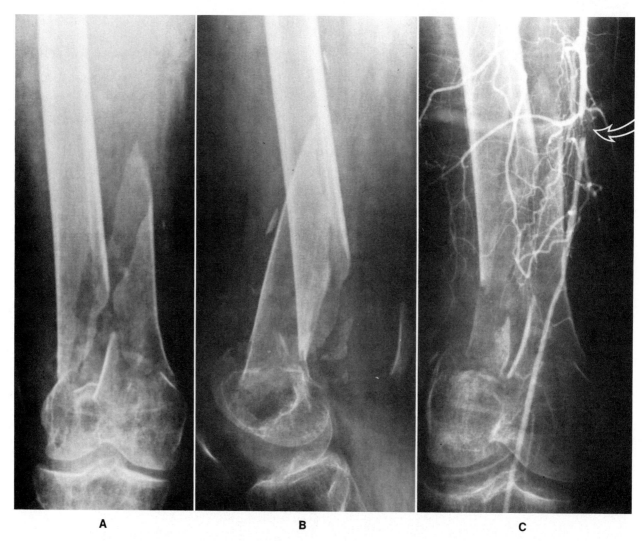

A   B   C

Fig. 15-14. Comminuted supracondylar fracture in 49-year-old woman with flaccid paraplegia for 7 years, a wheelchair user. Radiographs were obtained because of swelling and erythema above knee; there was no history of trauma. Fracture shows relatively good alignment and apposition of fragments on frontal view, **A,** but clearly not in lateral projection, **B.** Note thin cortex of distal femoral shaft resulting from bone resorption for 7 years. Patient's leg was noted to be cold and dusky 1 day after admission. **C,** Arteriogram demonstrates occlusion of femoral artery *(arrow)* adjacent to sharp edge of large bone fragment. Artery was lacerated by bone fragment. Collateral circulation, seen bypassing occlusion, indicated subacute occlusion, which most likely occurred prior to detection of fracture. A surgical bypass graft was required.

at a time remote from the time of cord injury—usually more than 2 years after the initial injury.[57] The early group of fractures are due to high energy forces. The later fractures may be due to a high energy injury from a motor vehicle accident or a fall that has sufficient energy even to fracture a normal bone. However, a larger percentage of the late fractures are due to low energy injuries secondary to an innocuous activity such as changing position.[101]

By far the most common source of trauma that results

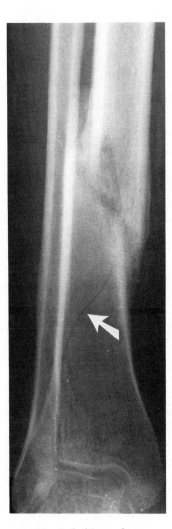

Fig. 15-15. Acute and healed oblique fractures are seen in this 24-year-old woman with flaccid paraplegia for 8 years. Patient can ambulate with braces and crutches. She fell 3 days prior to the present examination. Radiographs were obtained because of local swelling and skin discoloration. An acute oblique fracture of distal tibial shaft *(arrow)* extends through a portion of a healed earlier fracture. This patient has sustained multiple fractures in a serial fashion during the past 3 years.

in a late fracture occurs from a fall while transferring from wheelchair to bed, to car, to bath or vice versa.[57] This is a particular clumsy time with the patient assuming somewhat awkward positions. The inertia of the paralyzed limbs or trunk or both merely complicates the precarious position. Trauma caused by falls from bed or from a wheelchair, auto accidents, or an apparently insignificant source (e.g., twisting, bending over, reaching for an object) is the other common source of fracture.[40] Overzealous range-of-motion exercises during physical therapy may result in occasional fractures.[27]

Almost all of the late fractures occur in the lower extremity (Figs. 15-14 to 15-18),[50,52,57] usually in the tibia or femur and rarely in the ankle or foot. The most frequent site is in the supracondylar portion of the distal femur (Figs. 15-14 and 15-19).[40] The findings from four reported series[17,40,52,57] with a combined total of nearly 3000 patients included 211 fractures in the lower extremities and 12 in the upper extremities. These fractures usually occurred more than 2 years after the onset of paralysis. Bone atrophy from disuse osteoporosis in the paralyzed area where the fractures occurred was thought to be the most significant predisposing factor. In a majority of the fractures, the precipitating trauma was insignificant. The fractures occur approximately three times as frequently in patients with flaccid paralysis as in patients with spastic paralysis.[40,57] It is thought that spasticity provides some stress and strain on the bones, resulting in less disuse bone atrophy and hence stronger bones. In most patients only one fracture occurred at a given time. Frequently the same patient sustained multiple fractures in a serial fashion over a period of several years (Fig. 15-15).[57]

Radiologic findings

The radiologic appearance of fractures sustained by spinal cord injured patients is no different from that seen in the remainder of the population. The fractures may be spiral, transverse, or oblique; simple or comminuted; and closed or open. The fractures are almost always closed, although an occasional open fracture does occur.[40] Clinical diagnosis of a fracture is often difficult because of the lack of pain and because the traumatic incident may be insignificant.[40,55] The patient may have an area of local swelling, erythema, and warmth, which when radiographed, may demonstrate a spectacular fracture (Fig. 15-14). In other patients the fracture may be subtle, and multiple views or special techniques such as tomography and magnification technique may be necessary to demonstrate the fracture (Figs. 15-17 and 15-18). If the fracture occurs near a joint, it may be clinically mistaken for joint sepsis. In the tibia or femur it may be mistaken clinically for thrombophlebitis. As with any fracture the alignment and the apposition of

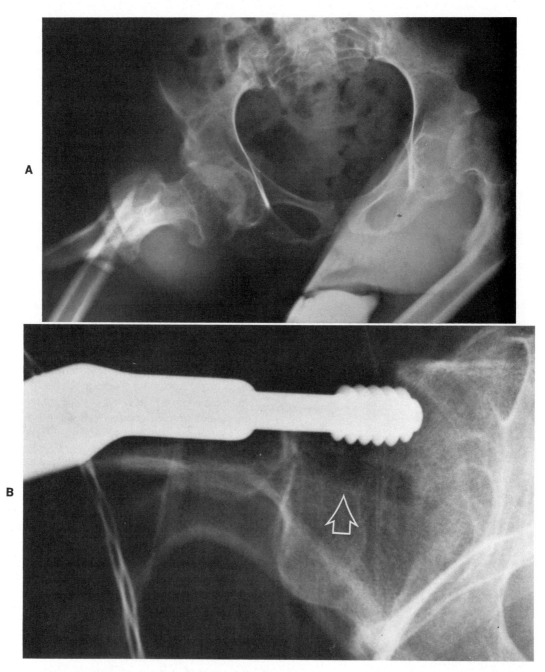

Fig. 15-16. A, Subtrochanteric fracture in 17-year-old boy with C7 quadriplegia after falling from a six-story window at age 7. Present fracture occurred during a transfer from a wheelchair to bed. A tug by the patient on his trouser leg when his leg became stuck during transfer resulted in fracture. Note hip flexion contractures and pelvic tilt. **B,** Cross-table lateral view of same hip during internal fixation of fracture using a Richard's screw and plate. Screw pulled through osteoporotic bone at end of procedure. Its original position can be seen from track *(arrow)* it has left in femoral head and neck.

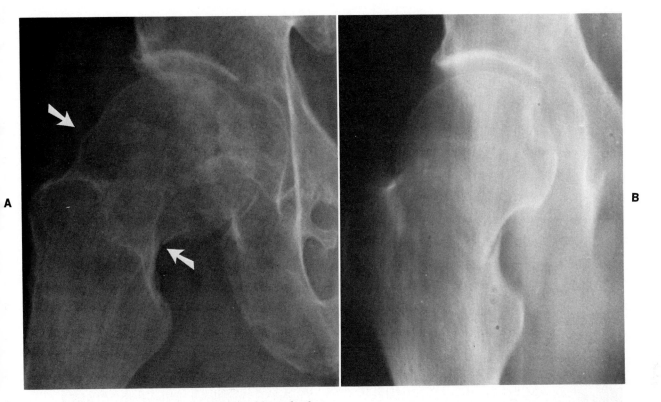

Fig. 15-17. Femoral neck fracture in 58-year-old quadriplegic man. **A,** Fracture is not optimally seen on routine film *(arrows)*. **B,** Tomography demonstrates fracture more clearly.

the bone fragments must be determined by obtaining a minimum of two radiographs taken at right angles (90°) to one another (Fig. 15-14).

Abundant callus formation and rapid healing occur in fractures in spinal cord injured patients below the cord level[17] even with little or no immobilization.[52] Healing occurs more rapidly than in normal patients.[55] Abundant callus formation at the fracture site is probably related to an accompanying large hematoma. The loss of local vascular tone, the incomplete immobilization, and the atrophy and loss of tone in the adjacent muscles predispose the patient to formation of a large hematoma,[52] which may calcify (Figs. 15-19 and 15-20). The hematoma may be large enough even to render the patient anemic.[52] Angulation and displacement of the fracture and some motion at the fracture site while healing also account for a greater than normal amount of callus

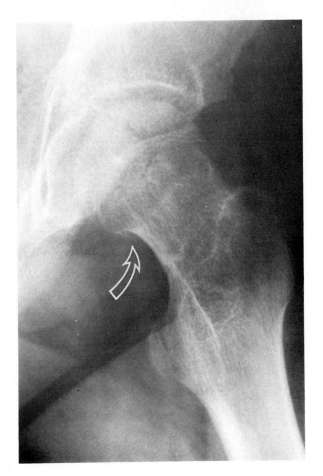

Fig. 15-18. Subtle femoral neck fracture *(arrow)* in 15-year-old incomplete paraplegic girl due to range-of-motion exercises. Patient complained of pain for 4 days prior to radiologic examination. Few fractures in spinal cord injured patients are this subtle, but they can occur.

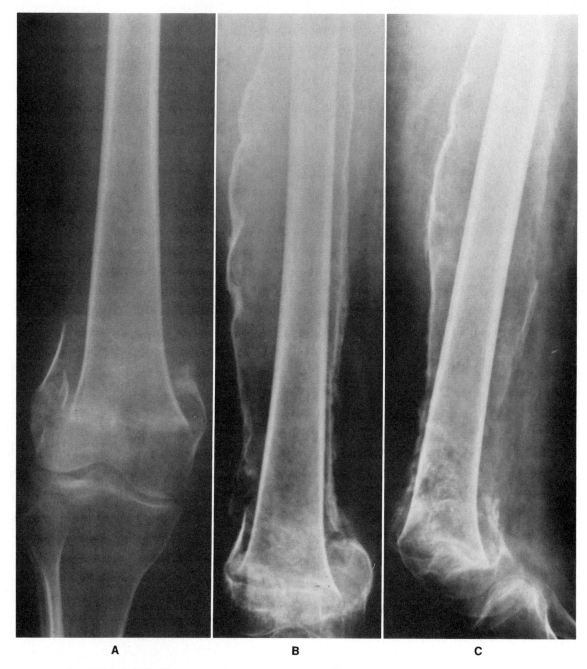

A   **B**   **C**

Fig. 15-19. Calcified hematoma formation in 21-year-old woman with flaccid paraplegia for 5 years. **A,** Impacted supracondylar fracture, most common site of late fractures in spinal cord injured patients. **B** and **C,** Two months later an extensive calcified hematoma surrounds femur. Large hematomas characteristically occur in spinal cord injured patients in association with fractures but usually do not calcify. Fracture is healing with excellent position.

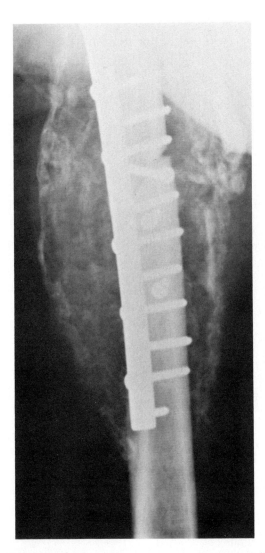

Fig. 15-20. AO plate and screws were used to internally fix this femoral shaft fracture. Extensive soft tissue calcification indicates extent of local postsurgical soft tissue hemorrhage.

formation. Many times a long bone fracture will go undetected clinically, and a healed result (Fig. 15-21) with deformity will be seen coincidently on a radiograph obtained for another reason. An untreated femoral neck fracture may lead to resorption of the neck and nonunion (Fig. 15-21, *B*). Sometimes the head is also resorbed. In other patients the fracture will heal with immobilization. Patients who cannot walk and either remain recumbent or sit rarely have problems even if a fracture nonunion occurs.[40,55,57] The nonunion is acceptable because it does not change the patient's functional status.[57] Patients who are able to walk tend to retain enough bone mineral so that they usually do not sustain spontaneous fractures.[101] If they do fracture a bone, near anatomic reduction is necessary.

Difficulties with radiologic interpretation may occur particularly in children. Fractures through the growth plate may resemble osteomyelitis, and abundant callus formation has been mistaken for an osteosarcoma.[48]

Management

The goals for management of these fractures are for a prompt return to activity, to return the patient to the same functional capacity present prior to the fracture, and most importantly to avoid complications during the healing process.[52,57] Complications secondary to a long bone fracture can be life threatening. Immobilization of the patient inevitably leads to pressure sores unless there is some way the patient can be turned at least every 2 hours.[105] Use of a Stryker or other turning frame to turn the patient prevents such formation of pressure sores.[57] Osteomyelitis has been reported frequently when skeletal traction or open reduction of a fracture was performed.[52,55] As more experience with open reduction techniques has accumulated, the complication rate has markedly decreased.[40,57,101,105] The use of open techniques has been most successful in those fractures sustained at the same time as the cord injury.[101] The late fractures that occur in osteoporotic atrophic bone are a type of pathologic fracture. Care must be exercised in selecting which of these patients are likely to benefit from internal fixation of the fracture. The osteoporotic bone and the frequent presence of a low-grade infection from a pressure sore or urinary tract infection are the material for potential complications if surgery is performed.[101] Also, a prosthesis or fixation device may break through or pull out of the atrophic bone (Fig. 15-16).

Treatment

The treatment of early fractures acquired at the time of spinal cord injury presents several problems. The treatment must be performed in a severely ill, recumbent patient who must be frequently moved and in whom the degree of neurologic recovery is uncertain. Until the cord level is determined to be permanent, fractures should be treated with the intention that the result will allow the patient to function as a normal person. Early fractures are not emergencies unless they are open. Therefore they need only be immobilized to maintain position until the patient is sufficiently stable to allow more definitive treatment.[57]

Multiple methods have been employed to treat fractures in spinal cord injured patients. These methods have included skin traction, skeletal traction, splinting with plaster molds, pillow splints, sandbag immobilization, plaster casts, open reduction using plates, screws, pins, and wires, and amputation. Skin traction leads to sloughing of the skin and should be avoided.[52] Infection

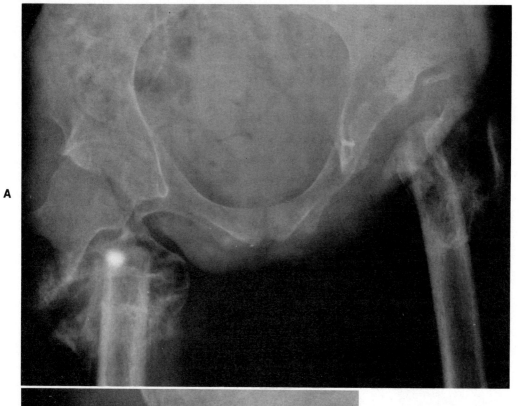

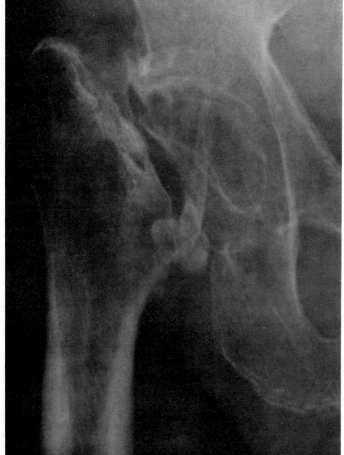

Fig. 15-21. **A,** Undetected right hip fracture in 56-year-old paraplegic man with spontaneous healing and deformity. This fracture was first detected coincidently on an urogram preliminary film. Deformity is acceptable because it did not affect patient's functional status of wheelchair mobility. Girdlestone procedure has been performed on left. **B,** Resorption of femoral neck has occurred in this 76-year-old paraplegic man after an undetected femoral neck fracture.

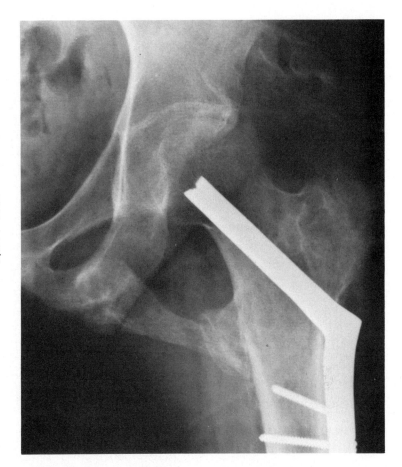

Fig. 15-22. Successful use of a Jewett hip nail and plate for an intertrochanteric fracture in 25-year-old male 3 years after complete T5 cord lesion. Extensive ectopic bone unrelated to fracture has formed adjacent to hip joint, restricting motion. In spite of this, patient can flex hip enough to sit.

of the pin tracks with skeletal traction has occurred,[52] but this is not unique to spinal cord injured patients and is a hazard of this method in any patient. Plaster casts, unless padded extremely well, cause pressure sores at multiple points.[55,105] Open reduction in some hands has frequently led to osteomyelitis and draining sinuses.[52,55,57] In other hands, particularly as more experience with these techniques has accumulated, open reduction has been especially useful in fractures sustained at the time of initial cord injury,[101,105] in patients with the ability to walk, and in patients with massive reflex spasm.[57,105] Open reduction allows rapid mobilization of the patient, which is particularly desirable to prevent development of pressure sores. If immature ectopic bone is present adjacent to a fracture (Fig. 15-22), surgery through this area is expected to result postoperatively in a significantly greater formation of ectopic bone than was present prior to surgery. This is not a frequent problem because most fractures either occur before the formation of ectopic bone or after it has matured. After internal fixation of a fracture, a hematoma may form in the adjacent soft tissues and eventually calcify. Clinically it may be detected as a large mass (Fig. 15-20).

Fracture treatment in a given spinal cord injured patient depends on the patient's motor capacity. If he can walk, a near anatomic reduction is needed. If he cannot walk and will never be able to walk, significant deformity and shortening may be tolerable (Fig. 15-23).[57] The position achieved by reduction must give a result such that undue pressure is not exerted on the skin during any of the routine activities in which the patient engages. In addition, a joint must not be fused or otherwise rendered nonfunctional so that the patient cannot sit or return to the previous function he was capable of prior to the fracture.

PARALYTIC SCOLIOSIS AND SPINE DEFORMITY

Most of the experience with paralytic scoliosis has been in patients with poliomyelitis, meningomyelocele, spinal cord tumors, or spinal infection.[88,108,109] In recent years the survival of spinal cord injured patients has increased with paralytic scoliosis seen in increasing frequency.[88] Children are much more likely to be affected than adults because they still have a period of growth. Juveniles under 11 years of age with partial or complete paralysis above T10 and no spinal deformity resulting

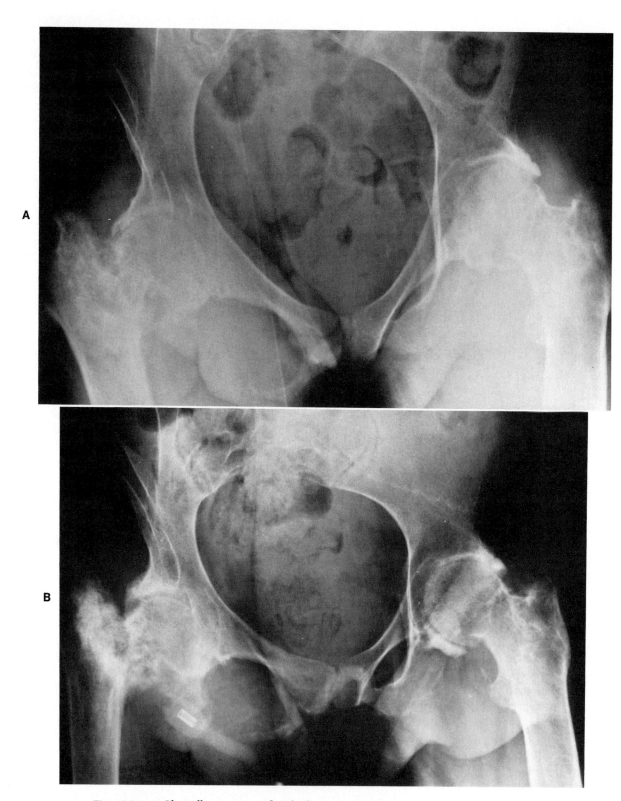

Fig. 15-23. A, Clinically unsuspected right femoral neck fracture in 41-year-old woman with C6 quadriplegia for 20 years. Varus deformity has occurred but is tolerable because of non-walking status of patient. Surgical excision of right ischium was part of treatment for ischial pressure sore. **B,** Two years later an increase of varus deformity is seen. Fracture has healed without surgical intervention.

from a fracture will inevitably develop scoliosis.[16] Marked spinal deformity can also result from the spinal fracture that caused the patient's cord injury. This may lead to difficulties with sitting or standing because of scoliosis or abnormal kyphosis or lordosis resulting from the fracture deformity.

Pathogenesis

Paralysis leads to muscle imbalance of the adductors and abductors of the hip, spasticity, flexion deformities of the hip, hip dislocation, or muscle imbalance in the trunk muscles.[100,108] Any one or a combination of these abnormalities leads to abnormal posture. The spine compensates over a period of time by curving in the opposite direction to maintain balance. The center of gravity must be maintained over the feet or between the ischial tuberosities or nearly so in order to maintain the ability to walk or sit unassisted. The patient loses balance when the center of gravity falls lateral to the ischial tuberosities when sitting or lateral to or in front of the feet when standing. Crutches can be used to compensate for the less severe imbalance but not in the severely affected patient.[88] In the growing spine the portion of the vertebra on the concave side of the curve ceases to grow. It is thought that this is secondary to increased pressure on the epiphyseal end-plates of the vertebral bodies on the concave side of the curve.[11,111] Initially the scoliotic curve can be reduced. With time there is a change in the vertebrae because of asymmetric growth of the vertebral bodies, and the curve becomes fixed.[11,109] Scoliosis progresses until growth ceases. Scoliosis is clinically important because it impairs breathing, circulation, intestinal activity, and kidney and bladder function.[13,16] When a spinal cord injured patient develops scoliosis, there is usually an associated decline of the patient's overall medical status.[13] Often a fixed pelvic obliquity develops in association with the scoliosis, causing an asymmetric pressure distribution during sitting. This leads to the formation of an ischial pressure sore.[13]

Radiologic technique and findings

A routine radiologic study of scoliosis includes upright anterior-posterior (AP) and lateral projections plus supine views with the patient bending maximally to the right and to the left (Fig. 15-24). Upright films are obtained with the patient standing if possible or sitting if he is unable to stand. An upright film may be quite difficult to obtain in patients with paralysis. A supine film must suffice if the patient is unable to sit or stand. The upright films are obtained with a 1.8 m (6 ft) source-to-image distance (SID). A 14 in × 17 in film is used for smaller patients and a 14 in × 36 in film is used for older children and adults. Because the thorax is less

radiodense than the abdomen, compensation must be made for this difference when radiographing the thoracic and lumbar spine with a single exposure. Otherwise, the lumbar spine will be too light if the thoracic spine is properly exposed or the thoracic spine will be grossly overexposed if the lumbar spine is properly exposed. An aluminum wedge filter is attached to the x-ray tube for the necessary compensation. The filter is thickest in the thoracic region and absorbs part of the radiation to this area. This allows enough radiation to be used to penetrate the abdomen so proper exposure of the lumbar spine occurs but without burning out the thoracic spine so that it cannot be interpreted. The AP view is positioned so the top of the 14 in × 36 in cassette is at the level of the external auditory meatus and the pelvis and hip joints are included inferiorly.[107] Obviously the hips cannot be included if the patient is sitting, but it is possible to obtain them with a supine film. Lateral radiographs are taken with the arms held at 90° extended in front of the patient. Even though an upright AP view is obtained, a supine AP view may be desirable. The difference between the upright and supine views reflects the influence of gravity, as well as indicating the functional state of the spine when the patient sits or stands. This difference can be quite striking in a patient with a flaccid spine, sometimes also called a *collapsing, ropelike,* or *spaghetti* spine. This typically occurs in a young paraplegic patient with a high thoracic cord lesion. Such a flaccid spine occurs soon after the onset of paralysis before a fixed deformity develops.[75]

The AP view of the spine demonstrates the position and the amount of scoliosis, the number of curves, and the presence or absence of pelvic obliquity. The lateral bending films demonstrate the flexibility of the curves. Bending toward the convex side of a curve reduces the amount of curve. The remaining curve represents the amount of fixed deformity. Bending toward the concave side of a curve accentuates the curve. Most patients with paralytic scoliosis will have a long C-shaped curve (Figs. 15-24 and 15-29). There will sometimes be a primary curve and one or more secondary curves to compensate for the primary curve (Fig. 15-25). As a result the side bending views in both directions are needed to determine the amount of fixed deformity of the curves that are present. The lateral view is used to determine the site and extent of kyphosis or lordosis of the spine.

There are two popular methods of measuring scoliotic curves from a radiograph. These are the Cobb and the Ferguson methods (Fig. 15-26). The measurements for both methods are taken from the AP thoracolumbar spine radiograph. The transitional vertebrae at each end of the curve are determined. The transitional vertebrae mark the change in direction of the curve. They

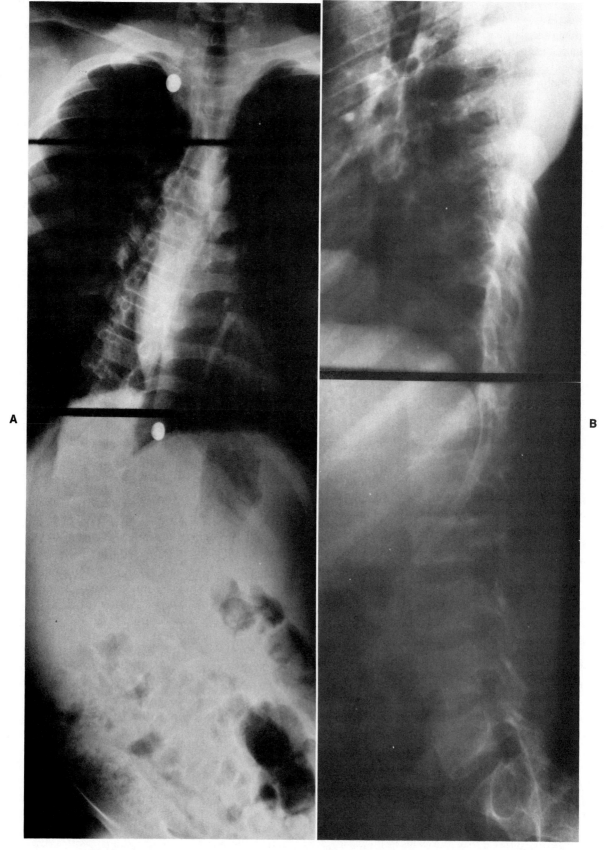

Fig. 15-24. Paralytic scoliosis in 17-year-old quadriplegic boy. A long C-shaped curve, characteristic of scoliosis secondary to paralysis, is seen. Films represent typical scoliosis series. Left lateral bending film was not necessary in this patient because of single right curve. The 30° difference in curve between AP and right lateral bending films is amount of flexibility in curve. **A,** AP view sitting. **B,** Lateral view sitting.

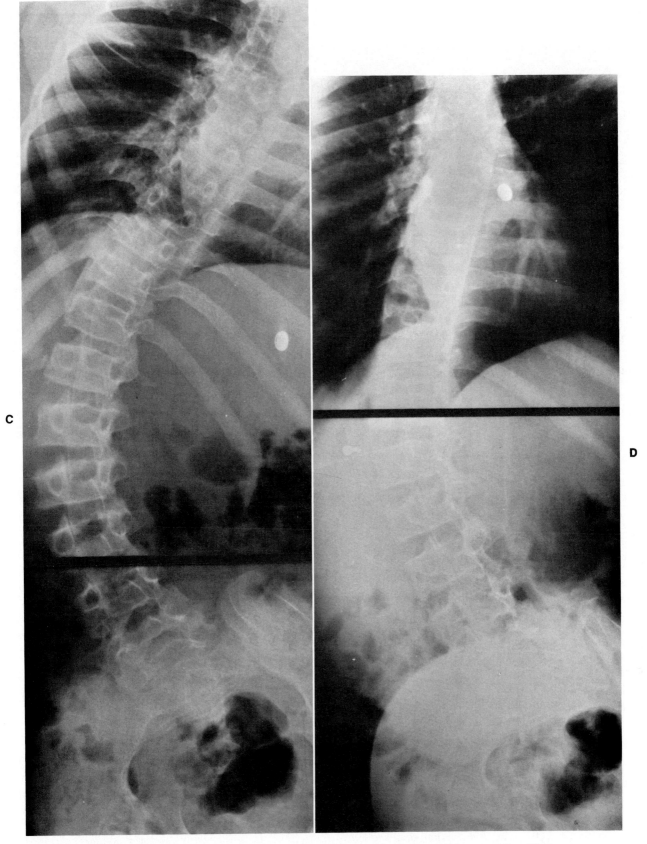

Fig. 15-24, cont'd. C, AP view supine. **D,** Right lateral bending supine view. (Fig. 15-28 shows treatment.)

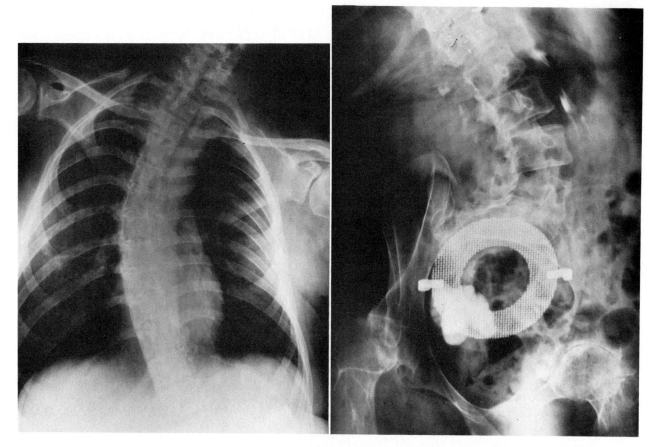

Fig. 15-25. Scoliosis in 20-year-old woman with C6 quadriplegia for 5 years. A double curve as seen here is less frequent than a single long C-shaped curve. Scoliosis occurred after the cord lesion because a period of growth still remained. Pelvis participates in this scoliosis. Pelvic tilt has resulted in subluxation of right hip. Narrowing of both hip joints is present. Contrast agent in kidneys and ileal bladder is from urogram. Partial ischiectomy has been performed.

are the last vertebrae that participate or tilt into the concavity of the curve being measured. The next vertebra tilts away from this concavity. The disc spaces are narrower on the concave than on the convex side of the curve. With the Cobb method the superior end-plate of the cranial transitional vertebra and likewise the inferior end-plate of the caudal transitional vertebra are extended. A perpendicular line is drawn to each of these resultant lines (Fig. 15-26). The angle formed where these two perpendicular lines cross measures the magnitude of the scoliotic curve.[37] With the Ferguson method the centers of the two transitional vertebrae and the apical vertebra of the curve are marked. The apical vertebra is that vertebra farthest from the median plane of the body and is at the apex of the curve. The center of each of the three vertebrae is obtained by drawing diagonal lines connecting the opposite corners of the vertebral body. The intersection of these two lines is the center of the vertebra. Two lines are drawn

joining the centers of the three vertebrae. The resultant angle is the measure of the scoliotic curve and is usually smaller than that obtained with the Cobb method.[53,97] More than one curve may be present, but each curve is measured in the same manner. A curve is designated by the number of degrees, the superior and inferior transitional vertebrae, and the side of the patient on which the curve apex is located. The curve in Fig. 15-24 is described as a 65° T5-L5 right-sided or right thoracolumbar curve.

Measurement of a kyphotic or lordotic curve is done in an analogous manner to the methods of measuring scoliosis. The only difference is that the lateral projection of the spine instead of the AP view is used for this measurement. The transitional vertebrae at each end of the curve are selected and treated in the same manner as for scoliosis measurement (Fig. 15-26). The Cobb method is ordinarily used for a kyphosis or lordosis measurement. The thoracic spine has a normal kyphotic cause the normal lumbar spine has a lordotic curve and the normal thoracic spine has a kyphotic curve. Lordosis is abnormal if it is located in a normally kyphotic area of the spine as in the thoracic area or if it is markedly increased. A high lordosis extends above the second lumbar vertebra and may include the lower thoracic spine. This is always abnormal. A kyphosis at or below the third lumbar vertebra is also abnormal. In practical terms, irrespective of the measurements, a significantly abnormal lordosis is determined functionally by whether the patient's balance is disturbed.[88] The compensations for an exaggerated lordosis take the form of hip flexion below and increased thoracic kyphosis above in order to maintain balance with the center of gravity over the feet or between the ischial bones.[88]

Abnormal kyphosis may be due to accentuation of the normal thoracic kyphosis or kyphosis occurring in the normally lordotic region of the lumbar spine. Compensation for the kyphosis takes the form of a lordosis both above and below the abnormal curve. If there is an insufficient amount of spine below the kyphosis to form a lordotic compensation, this compensation occurs by hyperextension of the hips.

A curve may occur in the growing spine of a spinal cord injured patient below the level of the spinal cord lesion because of the mechanisms mentioned previously. The curve can occur as compensation for pelvic obliquity or because of muscle imbalance with a level pelvis.[88,112] Additional curves may occur above or below an original curve as a compensatory mechanism to maintain the patient's balance. On the radiographs obtained with side bending, compensatory curves can frequently be completely straightened whereas the original curve will almost always have at least some element of fixed deformity. This latter curve is designated the primary or structural curve and the other curves are secondary or compensatory curves.[70] Patients with a flaccid collapsing spine may not have any fixed deformity and are an exception. The primary curve will have a larger measurement than that of the compensatory curve. The pelvis can participate in the scoliosis, becoming oblique and rotating along with the lumbar curve in some patients (Fig. 15-25, *B*). The hips rotate in the opposite direction under the patient to maintain balance with the hip on the convex side of the curve in abduction and the other hip in adduction. With increasing obliquity the adducted hip eventually dislocates (Fig. 15-27). Curves can extend above the level of the cord lesion. They may compensate for a more distal scoliosis, lordosis, or kyphosis. In the case of scoliosis the normal muscles compensate more effectively above the lesion level than do those muscles in the paralytic area. Accentuation of the normal thoracic kyphosis to compensate for an abnormal lumbar lordosis occurs

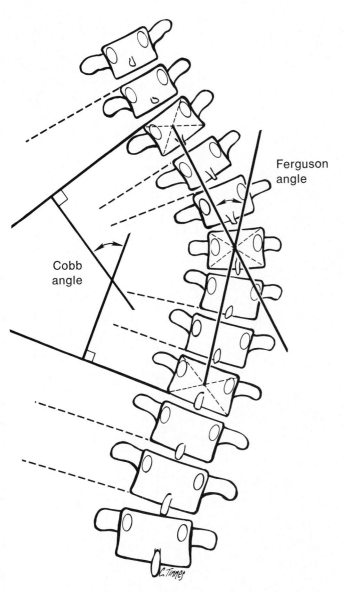

Fig. 15-26. Cobb and Ferguson methods for measuring scoliotic curve. Cobb method[70] is preferred. Most important decision with each technique is determining transitional vertebra at each end of curve. They are last vertebrae that tilt into curve. Extension of end-plate of multiple vertebrae is easiest way to visualize which vertebrae tilt into a curve. Cobb method is also used with lateral view of spine to measure kyphotic or lordotic curves.

curve that measures 20° to 40° using the Cobb method.[112] Any kyphotic curve in the cervical or lumbar spine is always abnormal. The lumbar spine lordosis normally measures 40° to 60°.[107]

Scoliosis, kyphosis, or lordosis may be identified singly or in combination. In a healthy patient the spine is straight on the AP view of the thoracolumbar spine and any lateral curve is designated as scoliosis. The situation is not as straightforward with lordosis and kyphosis be-

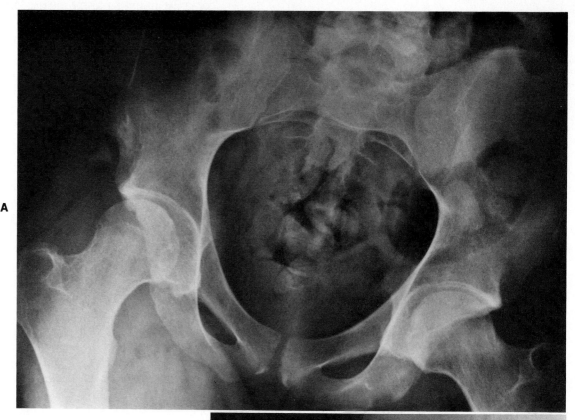

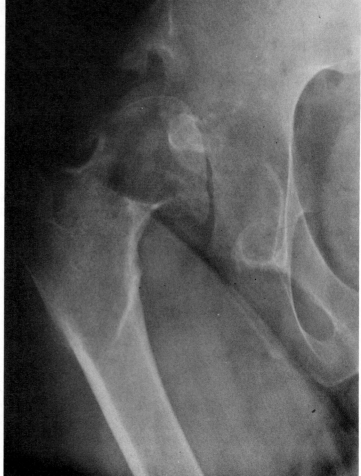

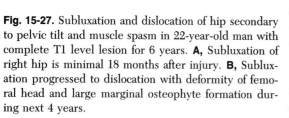

Fig. 15-27. Subluxation and dislocation of hip secondary to pelvic tilt and muscle spasm in 22-year-old man with complete T1 level lesion for 6 years. **A,** Subluxation of right hip is minimal 18 months after injury. **B,** Subluxation progressed to dislocation with deformity of femoral head and large marginal osteophyte formation during next 4 years.

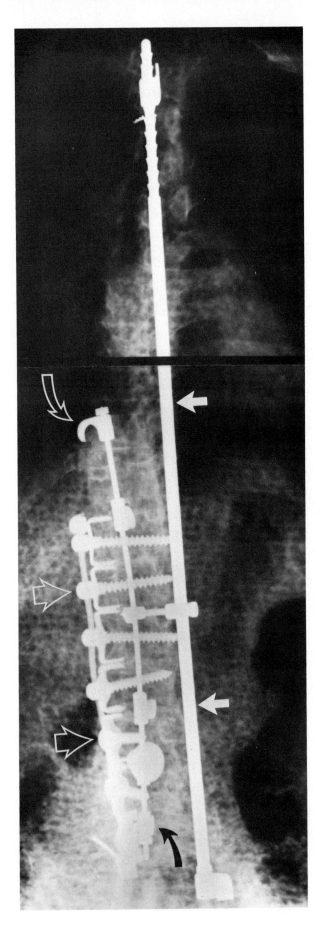

readily. The capacity of the thoracic spine to become lordotic to compensate for a lumbar kyphosis is more limited than is its ability to compensate for scoliosis or kyphosis in the distal spine.[88]

Treatment

The most successful surgical method used to treat paralytic scoliosis has been instrumentation using the Dwyer apparatus,[50,51,121] Harrington rods,[46,76] or a combination of both procedures.[23,109] The Dwyer procedure uses an anterolateral approach along the convexity of the scoliotic curve (Fig. 15-28). The intervertebral discs and vertebral end-plates are removed and the vertebral bodies are approximated by a cable threaded through a large cannulated screw inserted into each vertebra in the exposed portion of the curve. A tensioning device exerts the force needed to shorten the distance between each screw by increasing the cable tension. The chest is opened during the operation and the hemidiaphragm along the convexity of the curve is divided, allowing access to the vertebrae. A rib resected at the upper end of the curve for better exposure is used for bone grafting between the vertebral bodies. An anterior fusion is performed. Dwyer instrumentation is usually not employed above T10 and can extend distally to L5. Using this apparatus above the T10 level is technically difficult because of the necessary surgical exposure, although it can be employed up to the T5 level. The smaller thoracic vertebrae also do not allow exertion of as much tension on the curve as in the lumbar spine. This results in less correction of the curve than is achieved in the lumbar area. Pulmonary complications occur frequently after this procedure because the chest has been opened.[79]

Harrington rods are inserted using a posterior approach and can be applied anywhere between T1 and the sacrum. Stainless steel rods are attached to the laminae, articular processes, or transverse processes of the vertebrae via hooks at the ends of the rods. Two different types of rods are used. Distraction rods are used on the concave side of the curve. After the distraction rod is in place, force is applied to the upper hook, which slides it along a ratchet device on the rod. This pushes the two ends of the curve apart on the concave side straightening the curve. A Harrington compression rod

Fig. 15-28. Radiograph taken after instrumentation for scoliosis. Dwyer apparatus *(open straight arrows)* and Harrington distraction *(closed white arrows)* and compression *(curved arrows)* rods were employed for correction of scoliosis. Preoperative radiographs of this patient are shown in Fig. 15-24. Radiograph was taken through Risser hexalite body cast.

is usually applied for correction of abnormal kyphosis, although it is infrequently used on the convex side of a scoliotic curve in addition to a distraction rod on the concave side.[79] A compression rod is threaded for hexagonal nuts which are tightened against multiple hooks on it, providing the force to straighten the kyphosis (Fig. 15-28). Bone grafting is done posteriorly.

Fusion must extend across the entire portion of the thoracolumbar spine that lacks adequate voluntary muscle strength for stability when sitting or standing. It also must include any thoracic compensatory curve, if one is present, even if it is in a normally innervated area. Inferiorly the fusion must extend to the sacrum (Fig. 15-28). If instrumentation of a shorter extent of the spine is done, the curve will extend beyond the ends of the surgery and recur (Fig. 15-29).[23] Bone grafting is always done concomitantly with the Harrington or Dwyer instrumentation because the metal will eventually fatigue and fracture. Fusion limits the mobility of the spine, but the alternative is cardiovascular and respiratory em-

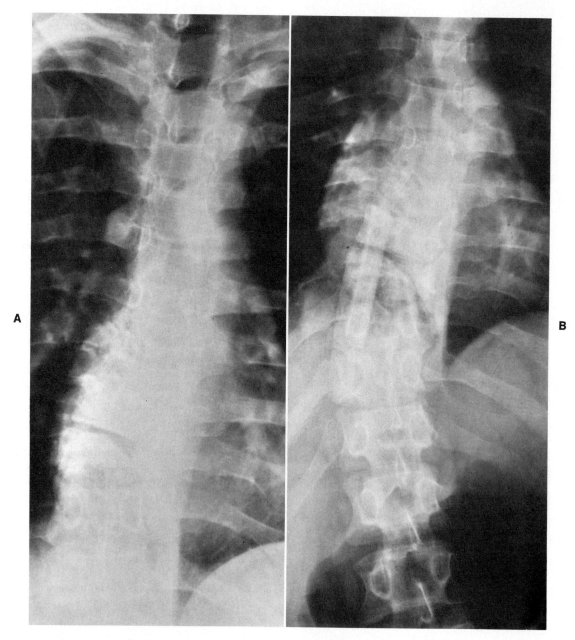

Fig. 15-29. Scoliosis in 20-year-old man with complete T7 paraplegia for 3 years. **A,** Fracture deformity at T9 is present with resulting scoliosis. **B,** Bone grafting was done, but scoliosis and a pelvic tilt developed below level of fusion.

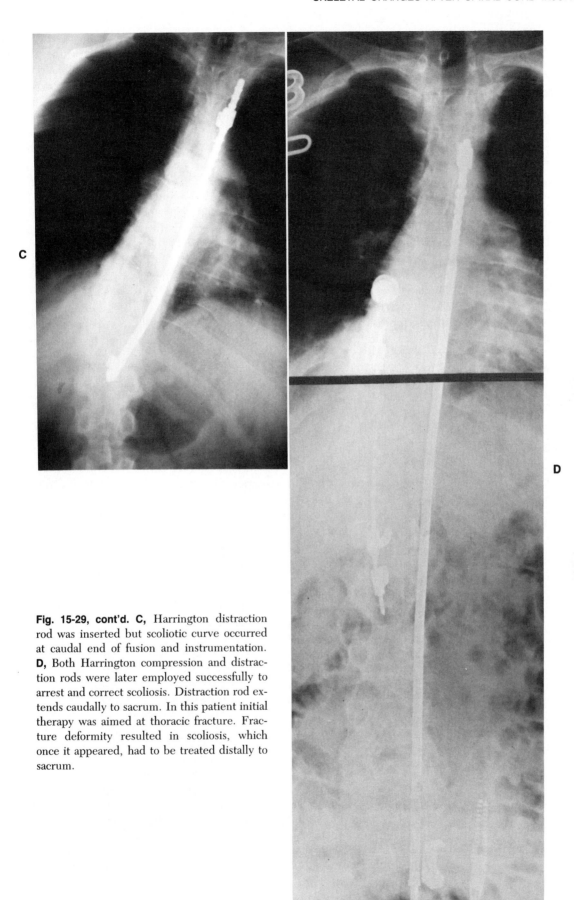

Fig. 15-29, cont'd. C, Harrington distraction rod was inserted but scoliotic curve occurred at caudal end of fusion and instrumentation. **D,** Both Harrington compression and distraction rods were later employed successfully to arrest and correct scoliosis. Distraction rod extends caudally to sacrum. In this patient initial therapy was aimed at thoracic fracture. Fracture deformity resulted in scoliosis, which once it appeared, had to be treated distally to sacrum.

barrasment, abdominal bowel difficulties, and increasing pelvic obliquity with balance problems, hip dislocation, and eventually pressures sores.[16,108]

MARGINAL RIB EROSION

Erosions of the superior margin of multiple ribs was first described in patients with paralysis from poliomyelitis.[21] Subsequently such erosions have been identified in quadriplegic patients (Fig. 15-30). More recently rib erosions have also been demonstrated in patients with restricted chest wall motion from decreased compliance of either the chest wall or the lungs.[87] Mechanical stress is necessary to maintain the integrity of any bone. The loss of innervation to the intercostal muscles is followed by muscle atrophy.[126] This muscle atrophy results in a loss of mechanical stress along the superior margin of the ribs where the muscles insert. Bone is a dynamic organ that is constantly being resorbed and laid down again. Stress and strain appear to be the stimuli to lay down bone.[6] When stress and strain are lacking, the rate of bone resorption appears to be unaffected although the rate of new bone formation decreases. The bone along the superior rib margin is resorbed but is not replaced.[115]

Radiologic findings

Resorption of the superior cortex of ribs was seen earliest in quadriplegic patients 10 months after the onset of paralysis.[21,129] The resorption of the superior margin of the ribs most commonly involves the posterior third to sixth ribs but sometimes the seventh and eighth ribs are also involved. Occasionally the inferior rib margin will show resorption.[21] The lateral and anterior aspects of the ribs are not involved. The distribution of erosions tends to be symmetric.[21] The defects in the rib margins begin as small semicircular excavations. With time, they enlarge and extend over a much larger segment of the posterior rib, causing a long flattened margin along the superior aspect of the bone (Fig. 15-30). Half or more of the diameter of the rib can be eroded in dramatic cases. The greatest frequency of rib involvement occurs in the more severely paralyzed patients.[21] In spite of this trend, erosions are not seen in most patients. It is unclear why this phenomenon is seen in a few quadriplegic patients. It is also unclear why only the posterior section of the third to eighth ribs is involved. No clinical signs or symptoms have been reported due to progressive resorption of the posterior ribs in these patients. Care must be exercised not to confuse superior marginal rib erosion with changes as a result of the projection at which the radiograph was obtained. Several of the upper posterior ribs will appear to have a flat superior surface on an AP or lordotic view of the chest. This is especially true of the third posterior rib. These ribs when normal do not appear significantly thinner than adjacent ribs as compared to those that have been eroded. Scalloping of the superior rib margin from erosion is a relatively early

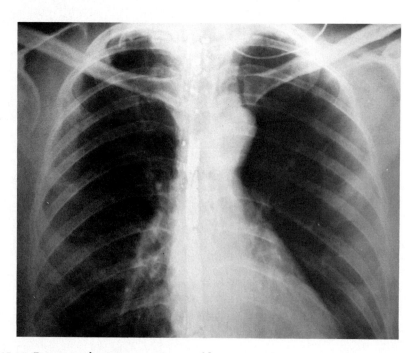

Fig. 15-30. Posterior rib erosions in 41-year-old woman with incomplete C2 quadriplegia for 21 years. Posterior aspect of second to fourth ribs are thin because of erosions. Cervical rib is present on right.

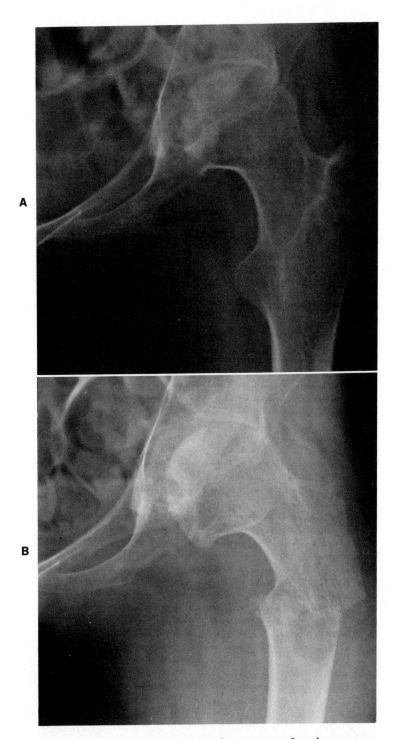

Fig. 15-31. Intertrochanteric fracture 6 weeks after excision of trochanteric pressure sore in 24-year-old woman with C5 quadriplegia from a diving accident 9 years ago. Fracture occurred during physical therapy range-of-motion exercises. **A,** There is erosion of greater trochanter cortical margin due to pressure sore prior to surgery, and there is air in overlying pressure sore. **B,** Pressure sore was excised, and trochanter was trimmed and now is smaller and flattened. Subtrochanteric bone defect presumably occurred during surgical resection of greater trochanter. It simulates a bone erosion. Transverse fracture through weakened bone has appearance of pathologic fracture. No evidence of infection or abnormal bone was seen during subsequent surgery when fracture was reduced and fixed with Jewett hip nail and plate. Fracture healed quickly without any evidence of infection.

finding and can be easily identified and differentiated from a normal rib.

SURGICAL PROCEDURES

Surgical procedures in patients after spinal cord injury fall into three categories. The first group of procedures are those used to treat fractures. This includes fractures of the spine, fractures of other bones sustained at the time of initial cord injury, and fractures occurring at a time remote from the initial cord injury. The second category includes those procedures used to restore function: tendon transfers in the hands or feet, joint fusion in the hands, soft tissue release of joint contractures, and excision of ectopic bone that restricts motion of a joint. The third group of procedures are those performed to deal with pressure sores and their various complications.

Procedures for stabilization of spinal fractures use metal hardware such as Harrington rods (Figs. 15-28 and 15-29) or Weiss springs for early stabilization. Be-

cause metal fatigues and eventually breaks, bone grafts are also performed to maintain long-term stability. In the thoracic and lumbar spine, posterior bone fusions are customarily performed along with Harrington rods or Weiss springs. Occasionally an anterior fusion will accompany these rods or springs for stabilizing a vertebral body fracture. As detailed earlier, routine orthopedic fixtures and hardware may be used in long bones if internal fixation of a fracture is elected (Figs. 15-20 and 15-22).[105]

As described earlier, spinal instrumentation using Harrington rods or the Dwyer apparatus or both is used to correct paralytic scoliosis. A posterior bone fusion is always performed with the Harrington instrumentation, and an anterior bone fusion is used with the Dwyer apparatus.[46,50,51,76] Particularly after Dwyer instrumentation and occasionally after Harrington instrumentation pulmonary complications, such as pleural effusion, pneumothorax, atelectasis pneumonia, and pulmonary infarction, may be seen.[80]

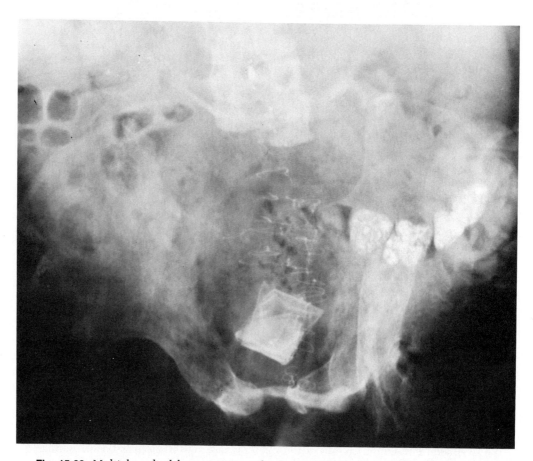

Fig. 15-32. Multiple radical bone resections for uncontrollable osteomyelitis in 24-year-old paraplegic man. Bilateral lower extremity disarticulations and ischiectomies and sacrectomy have been performed. Ectopic bone is superimposed on left acetabulum remnant. Radiodense gauze in midline in pelvis is in a draining sinus. Such extensive surgery is less frequently necessary now than in the past.

As described in detail in Chapter 16, pressure sores occur in areas adjacent to a bony prominence. One of the fundamental surgical concepts used when treating pressure sores is to resect the underlying bony prominence.[22,31,41,71,90] The ischium (Figs. 15-11, 15-21, 15-23, and 15-25), the greater trochanter (Fig. 15-31), the sacrum (Figs. 15-11 and 15-32), and the calcaneus (Fig. 15-33) are the most common bony prominences resected. The surgical procedure consists of complete resection of the pressure sore, excision of the bony prominence, filling in of the resulting soft tissue defect with adjacent muscle and fascia, and finally covering the defect with a full thickness skin flap that is rotated into place.[30,41,72] Radical excision of the underlying bony prominence, such as total ischiectomy, was popular in the past for treatment of pressure sores.[38] The high incidence of resulting posterior urethral diverticula and fistulae and perineal pressure sores led to abandonment of this procedure in favor of a more moderate partial ischiectomy for ischial pressure sores.[39] Radical excision of a bony prominence has been replaced by bone excision with

moderation as surgical therapy of pressure sores at any site.

Amputation of a lower extremity is performed less frequently than in the past, but it is resorted to occasionally even now (Fig. 15-32). There are two indications for this radical surgery. The first is intractable infection of a hip joint or the adjacent proximal femur (Fig. 15-11).[54,56,122] The second indication occurs with a pressure sore that cannot be closed either because of its size or because there have been recurrent pressure sores and surgery in the area with exhaustion of local available skin for a rotational flap. This latter situation is extreme and fortunately does not occur frequently. Amputation can occur either as a hip disarticulation[72,116,122] or as an above-the-knee amputation with the soft tissues distal to the knee used to cover the pressure sore.[25] In less severe cases of osteomyelitis, it may suffice to resect the affected portions of the involved bones. This most frequently occurs in the hip with resection of the femoral head and neck and a portion of the acetabulum.[56,69,123] Extensive osteomyelitis

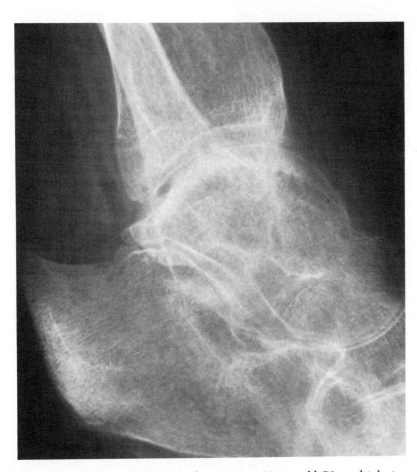

Fig. 15-33. Surgical excision of calcaneal tuberosity in a 20-year-old C6 quadriplegic woman. Pressure sore has recurred and again extends down to bone.

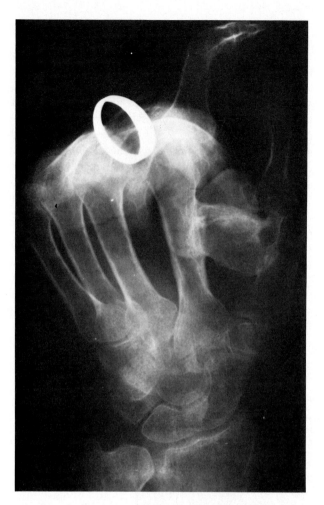

Fig. 15-34. Surgical bone block fusion between first and second metacarpal bones in C6 quadriplegic 39-year-old man. Bone block stabilizes thumb for better grasping and apposition of thumb and other fingers.

involving the sacrum may lead to surgical excision of a large portion of the sacrum (Figs. 15-11 and 15-32).

Surgical procedures involving only the soft tissues usually are performed in the hands, the ankles, the feet, or the hips. In the hands, tendon transfers are performed to improve grasping. Usually accompanying fusion of the greater multangular-first metacarpal joint or a block fusion between the first and second metacarpal bones (Fig. 15-34) is also performed to give greater

stability to the thumb and to provide better apposition of the thumb and remaining digits.[132] In the hips and ankles, soft tissue release of joint contractures is commonly performed. The only radiologic finding that may be evident after these procedures is an improvement of the alignment of the involved joint as seen on subsequent radiographs (see Chapter 17, Fig. 17-6).

COINCIDENTAL BONE PATHOLOGY

The abnormalities discussed in the preceding pages of this chapter represent the bone pathology seen in patients after spinal cord injury. Most of the changes discussed occur at a time relatively remote from the time the spinal cord injury was sustained. It must be remembered that these patients are not exempt from other bone lesions that are seen in the general population. They may have a congenital or an acquired bone lesion that was present prior to sustaining their cord injury. They are also at risk to develop a bone lesion that has no relation to their cord lesion, such as a primary or secondary bone tumor, arthritis, or metabolic bone disease from causes other than disuse atrophy (Fig. 15-35).

Cord lesions may cause complete or incomplete loss of sensation. The lack of normal sensation greatly hinders the early diagnosis of infection, arthritis, fractures, bone tumors, and metabolic bone disease. This is important because pain is a prominent early manifestation of a large number of bone lesions. It calls attention to the presence of the abnormality. In the spinal cord injured patient the first manifestation of a bone abnormality may be soft tissue swelling, a palpable mass, erythema, deformity of an extremity, general symptoms of headache or malaise, or a vague sense that something is wrong. Bone lesions may be advanced when first identified in these patients because of late detection. Many times there will be no clinical findings and the first evidence of a bone lesion is detected on a routine chest radiograph or on films from an urogram or cystogram. Therefore the bones should be closely scrutinized on all studies. Care should be taken to look at all four corners of all radiographs. Because abnormalities are found when they are looked for, systematic inspection of the bones on all radiographs may lead to detection of a surprising amount of silent bone pathology.

Fig. 15-35. Multiple osteochondromas or cartilaginous exostoses in 37-year-old C7 quadriplegic man. Osteochondromas cease growing at same time epiphyses close. Malignant degeneration of an osteochondroma into a chondrosarcoma can occur. Pain is most reliable indication of such a change. This would be impossible to detect in this patient if it occurred. As a result if such malignant degeneration occurred, it probably would not be detected early.

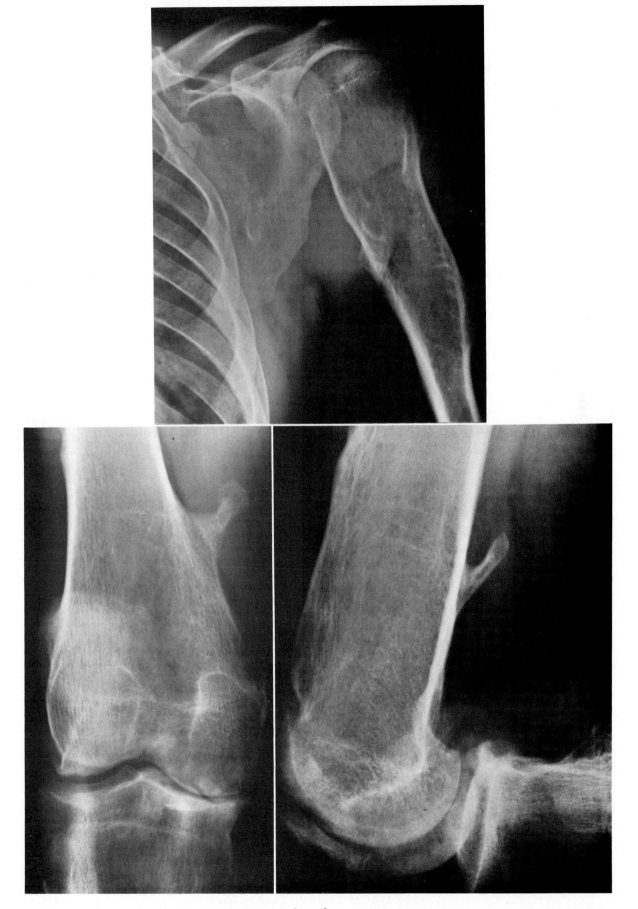

Fig. 15-35. For legend see opposite page.

REFERENCES

1. Abramson, A. S.: Bone disturbances in injuries to spinal cord, and cauda equina (paraplegia): their prevention by ambulation, J. Bone Joint Surg. [Am.] **30:**982, 1948.
2. Abramson, A. S., and Delagi, E. F.: The contribution of physical activity to rehabilitation, Res. Q. **31:**365, 1960.
3. Abramson, A. S., and Delagi, E. F.: Influence of weight-bearing and muscle contraction on disuse osteoporosis, Arch. Phys. Med. Rehabil. **42:**147, 1961.
4. Aegerter, F., and Kirkpatrick, J. A., Jr.: Orthopedic diseases, ed. 4, Philadelphia, 1975, W. B. Saunders Co.
5. Albright, F.: Osteoporosis, Ann. Intern. Med. **27:**861, 1947.
6. Albright, F., Burnett, C. H., Cope, O., and Parson, W.: Acute atrophy of bone (osteoporosis) simulating hyperparathyroidism, J. Clin. Endocrinol. Metab. **1:**711, 1941.
7. Albright, F., and Reifenstein, E. C., Jr.: The parathyroid glands and metabolic bone disease: selected studies, Baltimore, 1948, The Williams & Wilkins Co.
8. Anderson, W. A. D., and Kissane, J. M.: Pathology, ed. 7, St. Louis, 1977, The C. V. Mosby Co.
9. Andrews, L. G., and Armitage, K. J.: Sudeck's atrophy in traumatic quadriplegia, Paraplegia **9:**159, 1971.
10. Ardran, G. M.: Bone destruction not demonstrable by radiography, Br. J. Radiol. **24:**107, 1951.
11. Arkin, A. M.: The mechanism of the structural changes in scoliosis, J. Bone Joint Surg. [Am.] **31:**519, 1949.
12. Badgley, C. E.: Osteomyelitis of the ilium, Arch. Surg. **28:**83, 1934.
13. Banniza von Bazan, U. K., and Paeslack, V.: Scoliotic growth in children with acquired paraplegia, Paraplegia **15:**65, 1977.
14. Barnett, E., and Nordin, B. E. C.: Radiological assessment of bone density, Br. J. Radiol. **34:**683, 1961.
15. Batson, O. V.: The function of the vertebral veins and their role in the spread of metastases, Ann. Surg. **112:**138, 1940.
16. Bedbrook, G. M.: Correction of scoliosis due to paraplegia sustained in paedriatric age-group, Paraplegia **15:**90, 1977.
17. Benassy, J.: Associated fractures of the limbs in traumatic paraplegia and tetraplegia, Paraplegia **5:**209, 1968.
18. Benassy, J., Boissier, J. R., Patte, D., and Diverres, J.: Osteomes des paraplegiques (contribution a l'étude de l'ossification neurogene) [Osteoma in paraplegics (contribution to the study of neurogenic ossification)], Presse Medicale **68:**811, 1960.
19. Benassy, J., Mazabraud, A., and Diverres, J.: L'osteogenese neurogene [Neurogenic osteogenesis], Rev. Chir. Orthop. **49:**95, 1963.
20. Bergmann, P., Heilporn, A., Schoutens, A., et al.: Longitudinal study of calcium and bone metabolism in paraplegic patients, Paraplegia **15:**147, 1977-78.
21. Bernstein, C., Loeser, W. D., and Manning, L. E.: Erosive rib lesions in paralytic poliomyelitis, Radiology **70:**368, 1958.
22. Blocksma, R., Kostrubala, M. D., and Greenley, P. W.: Surgical repair of decubitus ulcers in paraplegics: further observations, Plast. Reconstr. Surg. **4:**123, 1949.
23. Bonnett, C., Brown, J. C., Perry, J., et al.: Evolution of treatment of paralytic scoliosis at Rancho Los Amigos Hospital, J. Bone Joint Surg. [Am.] **57:**206, 1975.
24. Brown, P. W.: The prevention of infection in open wounds, Clin. Orthop. **96:**42, 1973.
25. Burkhardt, B. R.: An alternative to the total-thigh flap for coverage of massive decubitus ulcers, Plast. Reconstr. Surg. **49:**433, 1972.
26. Burkhart, J. M., and Jowsey, J.: Parathyroid and thyroid hormones in development of immobilization osteoporosis, Endocrinology **81:**1053, 1967.
27. Calenoff, L., Geimer, P. C., and Rosen, J. S.: Lumbar fracture-dislocation related to range-of-motion exercises, Arch. Phys. Med. Rehabil. **60:**183, 1979.
28. Cameron, J. R., Mazess, R. B., and Sorenson, J. A.: Precision and accuracy of bone mineral determination by direct photon absorptiometry, Invest. Radiol. **3:**11, 1968.
29. Cameron, J. R., and Sorenson, J.: Measurement of bone mineral in vivo: an improved method, Science **142:**230, 1963.
30. Campbell, R. M.: The surgical management of pressure sores, Surg. Clin. North Am. **39:**509, 1959.
31. Cannon, B., O'Leary, J. J., O'Neil, J. W., and Steinsleck, R.: An approach to the treatment of pressure sores, Ann. Surg. **132:**760, 1950.
32. Carson, H. W.: Acute osteomyelitis of the spine, Br. J. Surg. **18:**400, 1931.
33. Chantraine, A. L.: Clinical investigation of bone metabolism in spinal cord lesions, Paraplegia **8:**253, 1971.
34. Chantraine, A. L.: Actual concept of osteoporosis in paraplegia, Paraplegia **16:**51, 1978.
35. Claus-Walker, J., Singh, J., Leach, C. S., et al.: The urinary excretion of collagen degradation products by quadriplegic patients and during weightlessness, J. Bone Joint Surg. [Am.] **59:**209, 1977.
36. Claus-Walker, J., Spencer, W. A., Carter, R. E., et al.: Bone metabolism in quadriplegia: dissociation between calciuria and hydroxyprolinuria, Arch. Phys. Med. Rehabil. **56:**327, 1975.
37. Cobb, J. R.: Outline in the study of scoliosis. Instructional course lectures, Am. Acad. Orthop. Surg. **5:**261, 1948.
38. Comarr, A. E., and Bors, E.: Radical ischialectomy in decubitus ischial ulcers complicating paraplegia, Ann. West. Med. Surg. **5:**210, 1951.
39. Comarr, A. E., and Bors, E.: Perineal urethral diverticulum—complication of removal of ischium, J.A.M.A. **168:**2000, 1958.
40. Comarr, A. E., Hutchinson, R. H., and Bors, E.: Extremity fractures of patients with spinal cord injuries, Am. J. Surg. **103:**732, 1962.
41. Conway, H., and Griffith, B. H.: Plastic surgery for closure of decubitus ulcers in patients with paraplegia, Am. J. Surg. **91:**946, 1956.
42. Conway, H., Kraissl, C. J., Clifford, R. H., et al.: The plastic surgical closure of decubitus ulcers in patients with paraplegia, Surg. Gynecol. Obstet. **85:**321, 1947.

43. Cuthbertson, D. P.: Influence of prolonged muscular rest on metabolism, Biochem. J. **23**:1328, 1929.

44. DeFeo, E.: Osteomyelitis of the spine following prostatic surgery, Radiology **62**:396, 1954.

45. Deitrich, J. E., Whedon, G. D., and Shorr, E.: Effects of immobilization upon various metabolic and physiologic functions of normal men, Am. J. Med. **4**:3, 1948.

46. Dickson, J. H., and Harrington, P. R.: The evolution of the Harrington instrumentation technique in scoliosis, J. Bone Joint Surg. [Am.] **55**:993, 1973.

47. Doyle, F. H.: An assessment of radiological criteria used in the study of spinal osteoporosis, Br. J. Radiol. **40**:241, 1967.

48. Drennan, J. C., and Freehafer, A. A.: Fractures of the lower extremities in paraplegic children, Clin. Orthop. **77**:211, 1971.

49. Dunning, M. F., and Plum, M.: Hypercalciuria following poliomyelitis: its relationship to site and degree of paralysis, Arch. Intern. Med. **99**:716, 1957.

50. Dwyer, A. F.: Experience of anterior correction of scoliosis, Clin. Orthop. **93**:191, 1973.

51. Dwyer, A. F., and Schafer, M. F.: Anterior approach to scoliosis, J. Bone Joint Surg. [Br.] **56**:218, 1974.

52. Eichenholtz, S. N.: Management of long-bone fractures in paraplegic patients, J. Bone Joint Surg. [Am.] **45**:299, 1963.

53. Ferguson, A. B.: Roentgen diagnosis of the extremities and spine, New York, 1949, Paul B. Hoeber.

54. Freehafer, A. A.: Sepsis of the hip in patients with advanced neurologic disease, Clin. Orthop. **29**:180, 1963.

55. Freehafer, A. A.: Treatment of fractures of the limbs in patients with spinal cord injuries, Proc. Ann. Clin. Spinal Cord Injury Conf. **18**:74, 1971.

56. Freehafer, A. A., and Herndon, C. H.: Infection of the hip as a complication of advanced neurologic disease, Clin. Orthop. **64**:135, 1969.

57. Freehafer, A. A., and Mast, W. A.: Lower extremity fractures in patients with spinal cord injury, J. Bone Joint Surg. [Am.] **47**:683, 1965.

58. Freeman, L. W.: Metabolism of calcium in patients with spinal cord injuries, Ann. Surg. **129**:177, 1949.

59. Frost, H. M.: Bone remodeling dynamics, Springfield, Ill., 1963, Charles C Thomas, Publisher.

60. Frost, H. M.: Bone dynamics in metabolic bone disease, J. Bone Joint Surg. [Am.] **48**:1192, 1966.

61. Galibert, P., Fossati, P., Lopez, C., et al.: Etude angiographique de la circulation des membres inferieurs aux differents stades evolutifs d'une paraplegie, Neurochirurgie **7**:181, 1961.

62. Garn, S. M., Rohmann, C. G., and Wagner, B.: Bone loss as a general phenomenon in man, Fed. Proc. **26**:1729, 1967.

63. Geiser, M., and Trueta, J.: Muscle action, bone rarefaction and bone formation: experimental study, J. Bone Joint Surg. [Br.] **40**:282, 1958.

64. Geist, E. S.: Osteomyelitis of the pelvic bones, J.A.M.A. **77**:1939, 1921.

65. Genant, H. K.: Quantitative bone mineral analysis using computed tomography. In Feldman, F., editor: Radiology, pathology and immunology of bones and joints: a review of current concepts, New York, 1978, Appleton-Century-Crofts, p. 183.

66. Genant, H. K., and Boyd, D.: Quantitative bone mineral analysis using dual energy computerized tomographic scanning, Invest. Radiol. **12**:545, 1977.

67. Genant, H. K., Doi, K., and Mall, J. C.: Comparison of non-screen techniques (medical vs. industrial film) for fine-detail skeletal radiography, Invest. Radiol. **11**:486, 1976.

68. Genant, H. K., Doi, K., Mall, J. C., et al.: Direct radiographic magnification for skeletal radiology, Radiology **123**:47, 1977.

69. Girdlestone, G. R.: Acute pyogenic arthritis of hip: operation giving free access and effective drainage, Lancet **1**:419, 1943.

70. Goldstein, L. S., and Waugh, T. R.: Classification and terminology of scoliosis, Clin. Orthop. **93**:10, 1973.

71. Grant, R. T.: Observations on direct communications between arteries and veins in the rabbit ear, Heart **15**:281, 1929.

72. Griffith, B. H., and Schultz, R. C.: Prevention and surgical treatment of recurrent decubitus ulcers in patients with paraplegia, Plast. Reconstr. Surg. **27**:248, 1961.

73. Griffiths, H. J., Bushueff, B., and Zimmerman, R. E.: Investigation of the loss of bone mineral in patients with spinal cord injury, Paraplegia **14**:207, 1976.

74. Griffiths, H. J., and Zimmerman, R. E.: The use of photon densitometry to evaluate bone mineral in a group of patients with spinal cord injury, Paraplegia **10**:279, 1973.

75. Hamel, A. L., and Moe, J. H.: The collapsing spine, Surgery **56**:364, 1964.

76. Harrington, P. R.: Treatment of scoliosis. Correction and internal fixation by spine instrumentation, J. Bone Joint Surg. [Am.] **44**:591, 1962.

77. Heaney, R. P.: Radiocalcium metabolism in disuse osteoporosis in man, Am. J. Med. **33**:188, 1962.

78. Heilbrun, N., and Kuhn, W. G.: Erosive bone lesions and soft tissue ossifications associated with spinal cord injuries (paraplegia), Radiology **48**:579, 1947.

79. Hendrix, R. W., Matalon, T. S., Calenoff, L., et al.: Pulmonary complications following spinal instrumentation. Scientific exhibit presented at the Seventy-ninth Annual Meeting of the American Roentgen Ray Society, Toronto, March 1979.

80. Hendrix, R. W., Mintzer, R. A., and Lin, P. J.: Efficacy of new film-screen combinations in arthritis. Scientific exhibit presented at the Sixty-fourth Annual Meeting of the Radiologic Society of North America, Chicago, Nov. 27, 1978.

81. Herceg, S. J., and Harding, R. L.: Surgical treatment of pressure sores, Pa. Med. **74**:45, 1971.

82. Herceg, S. J., and Harding, R. L.: Surgical treatment of pressure ulcers, Arch. Phys. Med. Rehabil. **59**:193, 1978.

83. Howard, J. E., Parson, W., and Bigham, R. S., Jr.: Studies on patients convalescent from fracture, urinary

excretion of calcium and phosphorus, Johns Hopkins Med. J. **77**:291, 1945.

84. Hurxthal, L. M., Vose, G. P., and Dotter, W. E.: Densitometric and visual observations of spinal radiographs, Geriatrics **24**:93, 1969.

85. Johnson, R. W.: A physiological study of the blood supply of the diaphysis, J. Bone Joint Surg. **9**:153, 1927.

86. Joseph, P. M.: Bone mineral determinations: methods and techniques to date. In Feldman, F., editor: Radiology, pathology and immunology of bones and joints: a review of current concepts, New York, 1978, Appleton-Century-Crofts, p. 175.

87. Keats, T. E.: Superior marginal rib defects in restrictive lung disease, Am. J. Roentgenol. **124**:449, 1975.

88. Kilfoyle, R. M., Foley, J. J., and Norton, P. L.: Spine and pelvic deformity in childhood and adolescent paraplegia, J. Bone Joint Surg. [Am.] **47**:659, 1965.

89. Klein, L. R., Van Den Noort, S., and Dejak, J. J.: Sequential studies of urinary hydroxyproline and serum alkaline phosphatase in acute paraplegia, Med. Serv. J. Can. **22**:524, 1966.

90. Kostrubala, J. G., and Greeley, P. W.: The problem of decubitus ulcers in paraplegics, Plast. Reconstr. Surg. **2**:403, 1947.

91. Lachmann, E.: Osteoporosis: the potentialities and limitations of its roentgenologic diagnosis, Am. J. Roentgenol. **74**:712, 1955.

92. Lachmann, E., and Whelan, M.: The roentgen diagnosis of osteoporosis and its limitations, Radiology **26**:165, 1936.

93. Lewis, V. L.: Unpublished data.

94. Liberson, M.: Soft tissue calcifications in cord lesions, J.A.M.A. **152**:1010, 1953.

95. Mack, P. B., and Lachance, R. A.: Effects of recumbency and space flight on bone density, Am. J. Clin. Nutr. **20**:1194, 1967.

96. Makin, M.: Spinal problems of childhood paraplegia, Isr. J. Med. Sci. **9**:732, 1972.

97. Marklund, T.: Scoliosis angle, Acta Radiologica [Diagn.] (Stockh.) **19**:78, 1978.

98. Martel, W.: Radiologic manifestations of rheumatoid arthritis with particular reference to the hand, wrist and foot, Med. Clin. North Am. **52**:655, 1968.

99. Martel, W., Hayes, J. T., and Duff, I. F.: The pattern of bone erosion in the hand and wrist in rheumatoid arthritis, Radiology **84**:204, 1965.

100. Mayer, L.: Further studies of fixed paralytic pelvic obliquity, J. Bone Joint Surg. **18**:87, 1936.

101. McMaster, W. C., and Stanffer, E. E.: The management of long bone fractures in the spinal cord injured patient, Clin. Orthop. **112**:44, 1975.

102. Meema, H. E.: Cortical bone atrophy and osteoporosis as a manifestation of aging, Am. J. Roentgenol. **89**:1287, 1963.

103. Meema, H. E.: Recognition of cortical bone resorption in metabolic bone disease in vivo, Skeletal Radiol. **2**:11, 1977.

104. Meema, H. E., Harris, C. K., and Porrette, R. E.: A method for determination of bone-salt content of cortical bone, Radiology **82**:986, 1964.

105. Meinecke, F. W., Rehn, J., and Leitz, G.: Conservative and operative treatment of fractures of the limbs in paraplegia, Proc. Ann. Clin. Spinal Cord Injury Conf. **17**:77, 1967.

106. Minaire, P., Meunier, P., Edouard, C., et al.: Quantitative histological data on disuse osteoporosis, Calcif. Tissue Res. **17**:57, 1974.

107. Moe, J. H., Winter, R. B., Bradford, D. S., and Lonstein, J. E.: Scoliosis and other spinal deformities, Philadelphia, 1978, W. B. Saunders Co.

108. O'Brien, J. P., Dwyer, A. P., and Hodgson, A. R.: Paralytic pelvic obliquity, its prognosis and management and the development of technique for full correction of the deformity, J. Bone Joint Surg. [Am.] **57**:626, 1975.

109. Odom, J., and Jackson, R. W.: Scoliosis in paraplegia, Paraplegia **11**:290, 1974.

110. Plum, F., and Dunning, M. F.: Effect of therapeutic mobilization on hypercalciuria following acute poliomyelitis, Arch. Intern. Med. **101**:528, 1958.

111. Roaf, R.: Vertebral growth and its mechanical control, J. Bone Joint Surg. [Br.] **42**:40, 1960.

112. Roaf, R.: Scoliosis secondary to paraplegia, Paraplegia **8**:42, 1970.

113. Rossier, A. B., Bussat, P. H., Infante, F., et al.: Current facts on para-osteo-arthropathy (POA), Paraplegia **11**:36, 1973.

114. Ruegsegger, P., Elsasser, U., Anliker, M., et al.: Quantification of bone mineralization using computed tomography, Radiology **121**:93, 1976.

115. Sargent, E. N., Turner, A. F., and Jacobson, G.: Superior marginal defects: an etiologic classification, Am. J. Roentgenol. **106**:491, 1969.

116. Shea, J. D.: Pressure sores: classification and management, Clin. Orthop. **112**:89, 1975.

117. Sledge, C. B., and Dingle, J. T.: Activation of lysosomes by oxygen, Nature **205**:140, 1965.

118. Steinbach, H. L.: The roentgen appearance of osteoporosis, Radiol. Clin. North Am. **2**:191, 1964.

119. Steinbach, H. L.: Infections of bones, Semin. Roentgenol. **1**:337, 1966.

120. Stepanek, V., and Stepanek, P.: Changes in the bones and joints of paraplegics, Radiol. Clin. (Basel) **29**:28, 1960.

121. Stephen, J. P., Wilding, K., and Cass, C. A.: The place of Dwyer anterior instrumentation in scoliosis, Med. J. Aust. **1**:206, 1977.

122. Stewart, J. C., and Comarr, A. E.: Disarticulation of lower extremity in spinal cord injury patients, a 25 year review of 2800 patients, Proc. Ann. Clin. Spinal Cord Injury Conf. **18**:70, 1971.

123. Stewart, J. C., and Comarr, A. E.: Resection of head and neck of femur in spinal cord injury patients, a 25 year review, Proc. Ann. Clin. Spinal Cord Injury Conf. **18**:66, 1971.

124. Trueta, J.: The three types of acute hematogenous osteomyelitis, J. Bone Joint Surg. [Br.] **41b**:671, 1959.

125. Virtama, P., and Helela, T.: Radiographic measurements of cortical bone, Acta Radiol. [Suppl.] (Stockh.) **293:**7, 1969.
126. Wakim, K. G.: A review of denervation atrophy with some comment on the results of electric stimulation in humans and in animals, Clin. Orthop. **12:**63, 1958.
127. Waldvogel, F. A., Medoff, G., and Swartz, M. N.: Osteomyelitis: a review of clinical features, therapeutic considerations and unusual aspects, N. Engl. J. Med. **282:**198, 260, 316, 1970.
128. Wolff, J.: Das Gesetz der transformation der Knochen, Berlin, 1892, A. Hirschwald.
129. Woodlief, R. M.: Superior marginal rib defects in traumatic quadriplegia, Radiology **126:**673, 1978.
130. Wyse, D. M., and Pattee, G. J.: Effect of oscillating bed and tilt table on calcium, phosphorus and nitrogen metabolism in paraplegia, Am. J. Med. **17:**645, 1954.
131. Young, F.: Acute osteomyelitis of the ilium, Surg. Gynecol. Obstet. **58:**986, 1934.
132. Zancolli, E.: Surgery for the quadriplegic hand with active strong wrist extension preserved, Clin. Orthop. **112:**101, 1975.

CHAPTER 16

Soft tissue changes after spinal cord injury

RONALD W. HENDRIX, M.D.

Changes in the soft tissues are among the most important chronic problems that develop in spinal cord injured patients. The most significant pathologic process is the almost universal development of pressure sores at some time after a spinal cord injury.[48] Both the physical health and the mental health of the patient are affected by these sores. They occur frequently, cause much discomfort to the patient in the form of restricted activity during treatment, affect the rehabilitation rate and potential of a given patient, and may develop into life-threatening complications and lead to long hospitalization, which is expensive both in terms of money and lost time to the patient. The almost inevitable recurrence of pressure sores and multiple necessary surgical procedures are discouraging both to the patient and physician. Ectopic bone formation is the other major chronic soft tissue pathologic process seen. It may cause motion limitation in one or more joints, which predisposes the patient to pressure sore formation. Other soft tissue changes are relatively unimportant.

ATROPHY OF SOFT TISSUES

Immobilization because of a spinal cord injury results in a decrease of the muscle bulk from disuse.[2] This is not unique to spinal cord injured patients and is also seen in patients immobilized in plaster casts.[21] A qualitatively different type of muscle atrophy is seen in skeletal muscle when paralysis is caused by a lower motor neuron lesion.[77] Skeletal muscle rapidly becomes atrophic after disruption of its nerve supply. This occurs

with a lower motor neuron but not with an upper motor neuron lesion.[11] In the latter situation the sensory and motor neurons of a given skeletal muscle remain intact. The muscle may atrophy from disuse, but its structural and functional integrity is maintained. After a lower motor neuron lesion the skeletal muscle fibers undergo irreversible, qualitative morphologic and chemical changes.[77]

The original spinal cord injury may be a lower motor neuron lesion or an ethanol or phenol block or a rhizotomy for severe spasticity destroying the peripheral nerve roots and converting an upper motor neuron lesion into a lower motor neuron lesion with resulting muscle atrophy and flaccidity.[20] The connective tissue and blood vessels adjacent to atrophic muscles do not demonstrate similar atrophy.[77] In a denervated skeletal muscle 30% of the muscle weight is lost during the first month, 50% to 60% is lost within 60 days, and 60% to 80% is lost within 120 days. The atrophy stabilizes at this point without further progression.

Radiologic findings

Radiologic differentiation cannot be made between muscle atrophy from disuse and that caused by denervation of the muscle. Only a rough idea of the amount of lost muscle bulk can be obtained from a radiograph. Comparison of radiographs obtained soon after injury with those obtained several months later will demonstrate a difference in muscle bulk in most patients. The wrist and forearm, the area proximal to the knee, and

438

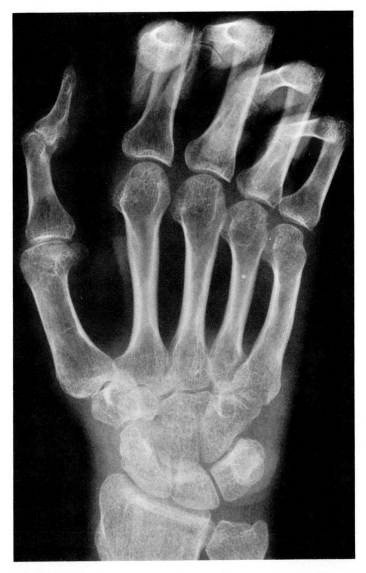

Fig. 16-1. Soft tissue atrophy in 29-year-old C6 quadriplegic man 7 years after gunshot wound to C6 vertebra. Soft tissues of thenar and hypothenar eminences are slightly concave rather than being definitely convex as seen normally. Soft tissues adjacent to distal end of radius and ulna are quite thin, a feature that also can be seen in a very thin healthy individual. There are also flexion contractures of second to fifth digits and demineralization in all visualized bones.

the thenar and hypothenar eminences of the hand are areas where such changes can be readily seen (Fig. 16-1). The amount of atrophy depends on the completeness of the cord lesion, the patient's activity, and the presence of flaccid or spastic paralysis.

ECTOPIC BONE FORMATION

Ectopic bone formation is osteogenesis that occurs in a part of the body where bone does not normally form. Many terms have been used to describe this bone formation, and this has caused considerable confusion.

Myositis ossificans of paraplegia,[54] heterotopic ossification, dystrophic ossification, para-osteo-arthropathy,[22] neurogenic ossification,[19] neurogenic ossifying fibromyopathy,[72] and myositis ossificans circumscripta neurotica are some of the terms used in the literature to describe the same process of ossification in the soft tissues of spinal cord injured patients.

Ectopic bone should be distinguished from myositis ossificans of the traumatic or progressive variety. Neither of these types of ossification is associated with a neurologic deficit. Also, their distribution is not characteristically adjacent to the hips, the medial aspect of the knee, inferior to the shoulder joint, or in close proximity to the elbow, as is usually seen in patients with neurologic deficits.[38,39]

Pathology

Both gross and microscopic features of ectopic bone are helpful in order to understand the radiologic manifestations. Ectopic ossification results from metaplastic osteogenesis with a small amount of associated chondrogenesis.[66] Both cortex and spongiosa are formed of layers of bone substance or lamellae. An occasional haversian system is seen. Bone marrow is present between bony trabeculae and is primarily adipose. Hematopoiesis, if present, is very discrete.

Immature ectopic ossification first appears as edematous connective tissue. Trabeculae of woven bone form in some of this connective tissue and then undergo osteoclastic resorption. They are replaced by appositional bone, which forms a lamellar structure. Some of the woven bone may not be replaced and may be seen on histologic section at the center of trabeculae in mature ectopic bone. The immature bone is not as hard as normal bone[66] and is quite flexible,[73] but it will mature into harder-than-normal bone.[38,66] The immature ectopic ossification is highly vascular especially at its periphery. The vascularity decreases as the bone matures. At maturity it has a cortex approximately 1 mm thick.

The ectopic ossification may develop within the periphery of a muscle, in connective tissue separating muscle masses, in aponeurotic tissue, and in tendons. Although the ectopic bone will sometimes be attached firmly to a joint capsule, it is always extra-articular.[29,66] Muscles and tendons lie in grooves over the surface or occasionally traverse tunnels in a mass of ectopic bone. These grooves and tunnels are lined by part of the immature edematous connective tissue that did not ossify. Sometimes the bone is firmly attached to the adjacent soft tissue structures and at other times there is discrete cleavage between it and adjacent structures.[66] Muscle masses adjacent to ectopic ossification remain well defined without atrophy. A few muscle fibers undergoing atrophy or aponeurotic tissue may be seen in the periphery of immature ectopic bone and occasionally will persist and be seen within mature bone. If ectopic bone arises in the periphery of a muscle, the latter is com-

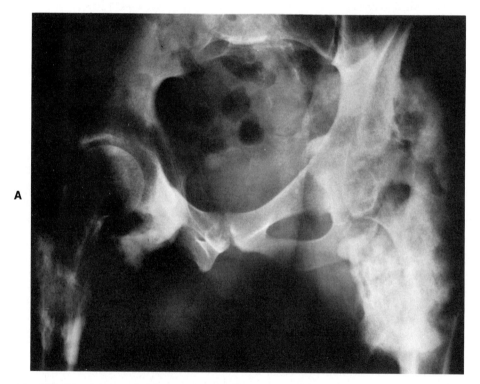

Fig. 16-2. Massive ectopic bone in 33-year-old C8 incomplete quadriplegic man 2 years after a motorcycle accident. **A,** Oblique view of pelvis, demonstrating bilateral ectopic bone formation. On the left there is massive ectopic bone, which extends from anterior margin of iliac wing distally to intertrochanteric area of femur. On the right, ectopic bone has formed between pubic bone and lesser trochanter. Patient has marked restriction of flexion on the left.

pressed by the immature ectopic bone but the compression appears not to persist after the bone matures. The ectopic ossification most frequently is clearly separate from an adjacent skeletal bone but can attach to it. It may be attached directly to the surface of the cortex, leaving the cortex intact, or it may disrupt the normal cortex and merge with the adjacent normal bone. Both osseous structures retain their individual characteristics even though the defined limits between them are lost.[66]

Incidence and onset

The incidence of ectopic bone formation in paraplegic and quadriplegic patients has been reported as any-

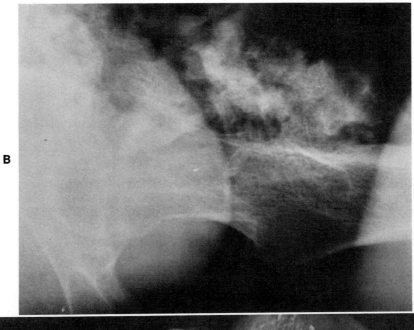

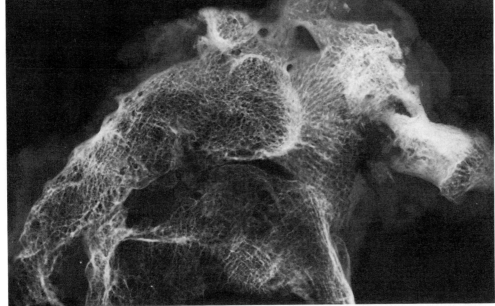

Fig. 16-2, cont'd. B, Cross-table lateral view of left hip. A massive amount of ectopic bone can be seen anterior to proximal femur. No ectopic bone is seen in soft tissues posterior to hip joint. In trochanteric region, ectopic bone appears to have fused with cortex of femur. Patient had virtually no motion in this hip. **C,** Radiograph of a surgically resected specimen of mature ectopic bone. Well-defined, thin cortex and well-developed trabeculae are indistinguishable from normal bone except for random trabecular pattern.

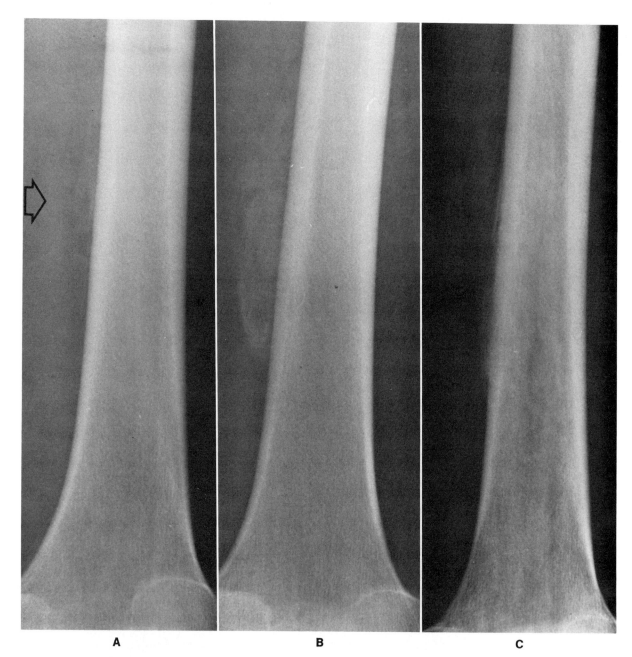

A   B   C

Fig. 16-3. Evolution of ectopic bone formation in 17-year-old complete C5 quadriplegic boy.
A, An amorphous calcific density can be identified along medial aspect of distal femoral shaft
(arrow). No definite cortex or bone trabeculation can be identified yet. This radiograph was
obtained slightly less than 6 weeks after patient's spinal cord injury. **B,** Eight weeks after
injury. There is more extensive amorphous calcification in soft tissues of distal medial thigh.
Ectopic bone characteristically occurs along anteromedial aspect of distal femur. **C,** One
year after injury. Ectopic bone has developed a definite cortical margin and has become
continuous with underlying cortex. Definite bone trabeculae are present within interior of
bone. Volume of bone appears smaller than on previous study because of slightly different
projection.

where from 4%[54] to 49%.[22] No correlation has been established between the level of the cord lesion or the presence of spasticity or flaccidity and the presence of ectopic bone formation.[38,80] Neither could any correlation be made with the presence or absence of passive range-of-motion exercises and ectopic bone.[38,80] The only positive correlation or predisposing factor seems to be the presence of a neurologic deficit.[38] Ectopic bone formation has been reported in paralyzed extremities both with complete and incomplete neurologic deficit, as well as secondary to hemiplegia,[46] poliomyelitis,[17] intracranial tumor, head trauma,[65] and spinal cord injury. Only the latter category is dealt with in the present discussion.

The appearance of ectopic bone formation is almost always within the first year and usually in the first 6 months after a spinal cord injury.[80] The length of time between initial injury and radiologic identification has been as little as 19 or 20 days[38,80] or as long as 18 months or more.[80]

Sites

The areas most frequently affected are adjacent to large joints. In decreasing order of frequency they are the hips, knees, shoulders, elbows, and occasionally the spine.[28,79] The area affected is always below the level of the spinal cord injury,[38,80] and more than one area is affected in most patients.[28] In the hip the ossification is almost always anterior to the joint (Fig. 16-2). In the knee it occurs anteromedially most frequently. An area distant from a large joint may be affected by ectopic bone infrequently (Fig. 16-3). Characteristically ectopic ossification does not occur about the ankles, wrists, fingers, toes, or in the calf or hip extensor muscles.[29]

Etiology

The etiology of ectopic bone formation is uncertain. Some of the proposed mechanisms include calcium mobilization and local pressure,[1] chronic venous insufficiency,[73] infected pressure sores,[38] tissue hypoxia secondary to circulatory stasis,[73] venous shunting,[5,31] and too-vigorous exercise programs resulting in microscopic hemorrhage into the soft tissues.[44,66] The large number of theories reflects in an inverse proportion the amount of certainty about the etiology.

Clinical findings

Ectopic bone formation can frequently be suspected clinically before radiographic manifestations occur. The presentation occurs with soft tissue swelling, edema, erythema, and local warmth near a large joint. There is usually a concomitant sudden decrease in the range of motion in the adjacent joint. These findings are often misinterpreted as resulting from thrombophlebitis, hematoma, septic arthritis, fracture, cellulitis, or a primary sarcoma.[45,79] Two to four weeks or more must elapse after the onset of these clinical symptoms before radiologic evidence of calcification is seen in the soft tissues.[57,66,76] In less florid cases the onset of progressive decreased range of motion of a joint may be confused with increasing spasticity or contracture formation. If range-of-motion exercises are discontinued, there is an even more rapid decrease of motion and ultimate joint ankylosis.[80]

Complications

The importance of ectopic bone arises from the complications that result directly and indirectly from its presence. In the majority of patients no problems result. One third of the patients have a resulting decreased range of motion of the hip joint both to active and passive motion.[80] This limits the patient's daily passive exercises, which are done to prevent joint contractures and may lead to cessation of the exercises altogether with subsequent ankylosis of the joint.[80] It causes increasing difficulty with sitting or transferring from bed to chair. Such a restriction of motion merely limits the patient's already restricted activities even further.

Joint ankylosis occurs in approximately 20% of patients with ectopic bone formation (Fig. 16-2). Of the ankylosed joints approximately 75% involve the hips. The elbows, shoulders, and spine (see Chapter 15), and much less frequently the knee, may be affected.[80] The ankylosis is extra-articular without direct involvement of the joint proper.[19,38] Ankylosis of joints in the upper extremity occurs in the shoulder and less often in the elbow.[80]

A sympathetic joint effusion may occur when ectopic bone is forming in close proximity to a joint. An effusion in the hip or shoulder is identified clinically or radiographically only with difficulty, and the infrequency of elbow ectopic bone makes it unlikely that an effusion will be diagnosed in this joint. Therefore a knee joint effusion is the only effusion likely to be detected in association with early ectopic ossification.

The second major problem stemming from ectopic bone is its contribution to the formation of pressure sores. This occurs in two different ways. In the first way, which involves an indirect effect, ectopic bone causes a decreased range of motion of a joint, particularly a hip joint. This leads to an imbalance of pressure over the opposite ischium during sitting because of a postural change that occurs even with a minimal decrease in the range of motion. Increased pressure on the contralateral ischial soft tissues leads to eventual development of a pressure sore.[39] The second mechanism is directly caused by the presence of ectopic bone

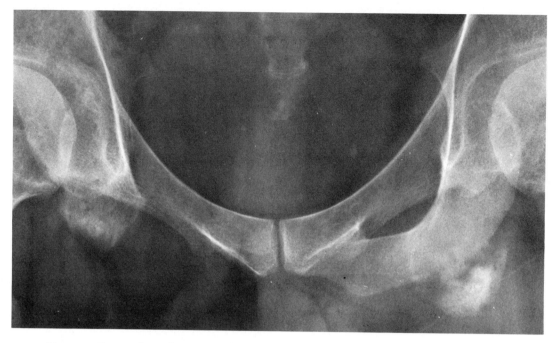

Fig. 16-4. Ectopic bone formation adjacent to ischium. This T5 paraplegic patient has two predisposing factors for pressure sore formation: ectopic bone formation superficial to left ischium and surgical absence of right ischium, removed for pressure sore. Absent right ischium causes increased weight bearing on left.

especially when it is adjacent to the greater trochanters or ischia (Fig. 16-4). This bone functions like a bony prominence. Its presence in the soft tissues reduces the distance between the skin and the usual underlying bony prominence of the area. This decrease of soft tissue between the skin and underlying bone reduces the amount of soft tissue in which to dissipate any external pressure.[70] Tissue ischemia occurs more rapidly than in the absence of the ectopic bone. A pressure sore is therefore more likely to develop over a bony prominence when ectopic bone is present in the adjacent overlying soft tissues.

Maturation

Determining when ectopic bone is mature is important to the management of patients when the ossification has caused some loss of motion or ankylosis of a joint. Surgery performed on immature ectopic ossification results in rapid recurrence of the bone,[4] often in greater quantity than prior to intervention.[75] Excessive bleeding with difficulty maintaining surgical hemostasis and formation of large postoperative hematomas also occurs. Maturation of the ectopic ossification in some patients may take several years. If the patient has an ankylosed hip joint, he must remain recumbent until surgery can be successfully performed.[79] Even under the most favorable circumstances this means waiting months until the ectopic bone is mature. Vigorous range-of-motion exercises have been advocated when ectopic bone first causes any decreased motion in a joint.[80] These exercises fracture and fragment the ectopic ossification but preserve joint motion. However, they may not be possible because of pain in patients with partially intact sensation.

Although it is important to determine the maturity of ectopic bone, the task is not easy. Many different methods have been advocated for this determination. Serum alkaline phosphatase,[29] serum creatine phosphokinase (CPK), and urinary hydroxyproline[66] have been used as indicators of the maturity of ectopic bone. Serum alkaline phosphatase rises within a few days after the onset of clinically detectable soft tissue swelling at the site where ectopic bone is forming. Radiologic evidence of bone mineral will appear only several weeks later. The bone will appear radiographically mature in 3 to 12 months.[18,38] Furman and co-workers[29] found that alkaline phosphatase levels returned to normal at approximately the same time the ectopic bone appeared radiographically mature. Elevated serum alkaline phosphatase levels reflect the presence of growing ectopic bone. However, these levels return to normal in some patients before the ectopic bone is metabolically mature and recurrence of the bone will occur if it is surgically excised.[11,66,76,79,80] Although ectopic bone appears radiographically mature, there can be immature areas and microfractures[66,79] hidden in the depths of the ossification. Serum CPK reflects the amount of striated muscle involved in the development of the ectopic bone. This is variable and is not useful for prediction of bone maturity.[66] Urinary hydroxyproline (UHP) reflects the metabolic activity of connective tissue, which is active during bone formation . UHP may be elevated and parallel alkaline phosphatase elevation during the evolution of ectopic bone formation, but it also may return to normal before the bone has matured.[66] Direct biopsies of ectopic bone[66,79] have been performed but are impractical for determining the serial maturation of this ossification. Serial bone scans are the most reliable means for determining ectopic bone maturity,[39,55,66,75] but a single scan is not reliable for determining maturity. Before surgery can be safely undertaken a continuous decrease of nuclide activity of the ossification should be followed by a steady state documented by two or three consecutive bone scans obtained at 1 month or longer intervals (Fig. 16-5).[75] Some activity will be present in ectopic bone even after maturity because the ossification is normal metabolically active bone. This amount of activity will be similar to that found in adjacent bones of the skeleton. It will be markedly decreased when compared to a scan obtained when the ossification was immature.

Treatment

The treatment of ectopic bone has developed in three diverse directions: drug therapy, physical therapy, and surgery. Clinical trials of diphosphonates have demonstrated that they are effective inhibitors of the formation of ectopic ossification.[67,74] These drugs have not yet been used extensively enough to define the long-term results from their use in treating ectopic bone. However, they are very promising.[74] They may be able to safely eliminate the formation of much or even most of the ectopic ossification. The diphosphonates are similar in structure to inorganic pyrophosphate. The pyrophosphate plays an incompletely understood part in regulation of ossification. The diphosphonates inhibit the precipitation of calcium phosphate in vitro and presumably also in vivo and hence prevent ectopic bone formation. Normal healing of fractures does not appear to be affected by this drug.[74]

Another method of treating ectopic bone formation is the employment of vigorous range-of-motion exercises even in the face of ectopic bone forming around a joint.[73,79] The hip is the area of greatest concern because when its range of motion is reduced, greater disability results than with any other large joint. A further problem is that the area adjacent to the hip is the most common site of ectopic bone formation. Two studies[19,71] have indicated that continued range-of-motion exercises during the formation of ectopic bone caused in-

creased quantity of bone formation. More recent studies[73,79,80] were unable to demonstrate any increase in the amount of ectopic bone formation as a result of vigorous range-of-motion exercises carried out during the acute development of the ossification. These exercises cause fragmentation and fractures of the ectopic bone and formation of a pseudoarthrosis through the ectopic ossification. They must be continued for 12 to 18 months to prevent bony ankylosis.[80] Full joint motion may not be retained with this vigorous physical therapy, but 45° or more of hip flexion can be maintained with the regimen[80]; 45° or more is enough motion to allow the patient to sit even though the position is not optimal. This also allows the individual to transfer from a bed to a wheelchair and vice versa, rather than being confined to a recumbent position because of hip ankylosis. In this manner some of the liability to develop a pressure sore is avoided.

Surgery for ectopic bone formation is a last resort. The most extensive experience has been with procedures in the region of the hip. The specific procedure is determined by the site of the ectopic ossification. In a hip ankylosed in extension by anterior bone the most frequent surgical procedure is a simple wedge resection of bone anterior to the hip joint. Enough ectopic bone is resected to allow flexion of the hip to approximately 90°. A less frequent problem is a hip ankylosed in flexion. A wedge resection of anterior ectopic bone and resection of the femoral head and neck are usually required to restore adequate motion in such a hip. Ankylosis of a hip in extension by lateral and posterior ossification is still less common. A resection osteotomy of the femur at the lesser trochanter level has restored adequate motion.[79] The goal, which is the same no matter what procedure or approach is used, is to restore at least 90° of flexion of the hips so that the patient is able to sit comfortably.[79,80] In some hands complications occur relatively frequently after such surgery,[38,45] whereas in others they occur less often.[79] The most common complication is recurrence of the ectopic bone formation with resulting ankylosis. Every patient has at least a small amount of recurrent ectopic bone postoperatively.[79] This can be minimized by being certain that the ectopic bone is mature before considering surgery.[55,75,76] Other complications include infection, hemorrage,[38] and pressure sores while the patient is recumbent during recuperation from the surgery.[79]

Radiologic findings

The earliest radiologic manifestation of ectopic ossification occurs 1 to 2 days after the first clinical features are evident.[66] The finding consists of soft tissue swelling, which is most frequently seen anterior to the hip in the proximal thigh and less frequently is seen ante-

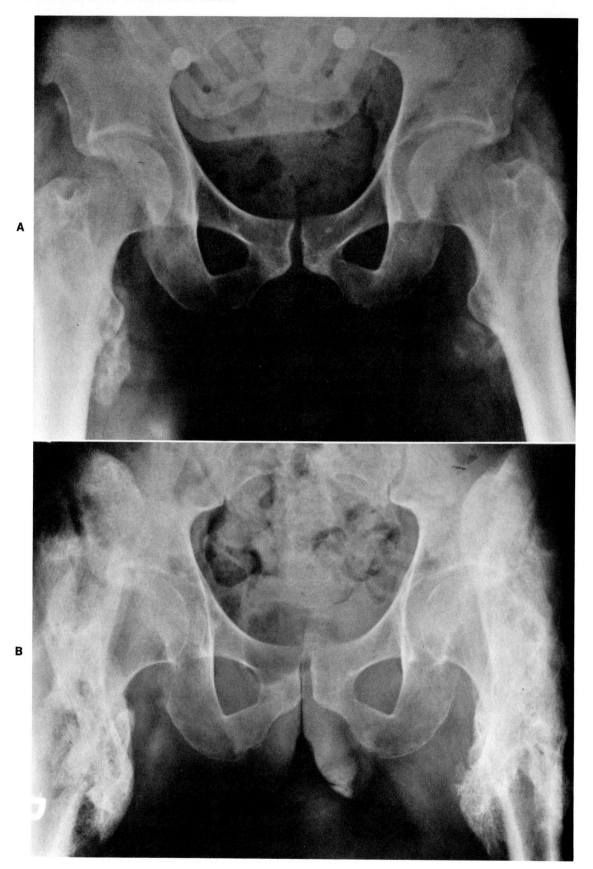

Fig. 16-5. For legend see opposite page.

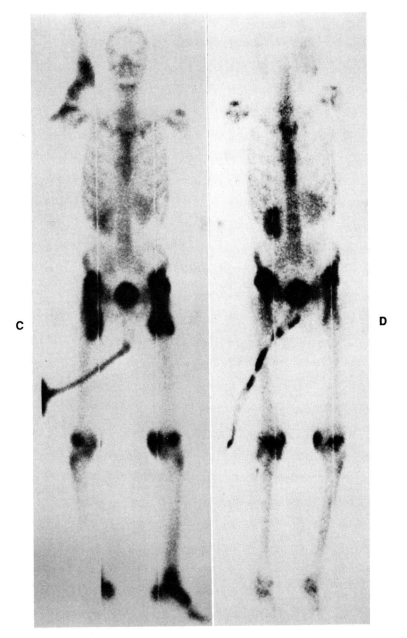

Fig. 16-5. Maturation of ectopic bone in 44-year-old man with complete T8 paraplegia following an industrial accident. **A,** Two months after injury. Ectopic bone formation in an early stage is present medial to both lesser trochanters and lateral and proximal to left greater trochanter. Ectopic bone is amorphous, and no definite cortical margin or discrete trabeculation had developed. **B,** One year after injury. Ectopic bone has matured radiographically. Definite trabeculation can be seen within bone, and its cortical margin is sharply defined. **C,** Five months after injury. Technetium bone scan demonstrates heterogeneous extensive activity from ectopic bone formation adjacent to both hips. Medial aspect of left knee also demonstrates increased activity caused by ectopic bone formation. **D,** Fourteen months after injury. There is significant decrease of activity adjacent to hips. Ectopic bone was resected bilaterally after this scan. Recurrence did not occur until patient's oral diphosphonates were discontinued.

rior and medial to the knee.[80] This soft tissue swelling can only be radiographically appreciated if it is diligently sought. A lateral film is necessary to see it, and comparison with the contralateral side may be the only way to appreciate it. A joint effusion may be detected a few days later if the soft tissue swelling is adjacent to the knee.[29] An effusion will cause loss of definition of the soft tissue planes of the suprapatellar area and an anterior convex bulging of the soft tissues as seen on a lateral view. An effusion in the hip or shoulder is difficult to detect and normally is not appreciated.

The earliest evidence of mineralization of an area where ectopic ossification is forming is a hazy, amorphous area of calcification. At this time the radiodense area has an ill-defined margin and no discernible internal structure (Fig. 16-3). It is at this stage that the ectopic bone is most likely to be mistaken for a tumor, in particular an osteosarcoma. The mineralization of what was previously soft tissue swelling occurs 2 or more weeks after the onset of soft tissue swelling.[73,74] Such mineralization has at times even taken several months before it is radiographically apparent.[76] The area of amorphous calcification increases in size and develops ill-defined trabeculae over the next 3 or 4 months.[28,30] The area of density becomes better defined, but its margins may remain relatively indistinct.[76] Any increase in size of the bony mass or change of the texture of its interior on successive radiographic examinations indicates that the bone is changing and that it is not yet mature.[66]

Eventually the bony mass will demonstrate no changes on multiple successive radiographs. At this point there will be a sharply defined cortical margin that measures approximately 1 mm in thickness. The mass will contain well-defined bone trabeculae that are no longer fuzzy in outline. It may take anywhere from 3 to 18 months or even longer for this appearance to be achieved.[38,79,80] It is very important not to confuse the radiologic mature appearance of this ectopic bone with true maturity. In a large bone mass there can be an immature area that is obscured by overlying bone.[76]

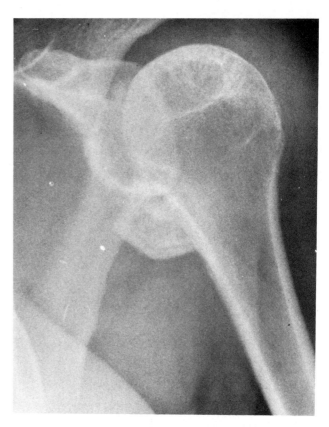

Fig. 16-6. Ectopic bone formation in shoulder of 30-year-old quadriplegic woman. Ectopic bone has formed in a characteristic position inferior to joint. It is continuous with surgical neck of humerus but has not fused with neck of scapula.

The only accurate method available for determining maturity is the employment of serial bone scans.

Patients with ectopic bone formation have been evaluated with bone scans using [85]Sr, [87m]Sr, and, more recently, one of the ^{99m}Tc phosphate complexes. The bone scan is abnormal prior to the appearance of visible mineralization on the radiograph.[45] It has not been documented exactly how early the bone scan becomes abnormal, but it is somewhere between the onset of the soft tissue swelling and the appearance of the hazy,

Fig. 16-7. Ectopic bone formation in 15-year-old incomplete C6 quadriplegic boy. **A,** Eight weeks after injury. Extensive ectopic bone formation is present anterior to elbow joint. Indistinctness of cortical margins and lack of internal trabeculation are characteristics of immaturity of bone. Ectopic bone is definitely in an extracapsular location. **B** and **C,** Fourteen months after injury. Ectopic bone anterior to joint appears to be radiographically mature with a sharp cortical margin and internal trabeculation. Ectopic bone is continuous with cortex of humerus but is not connected to proximal ulna (*arrows*). Patient does have preservation of extension as can be seen from normal appearance of joint on AP view, **C. D,** Eighteen months after injury. Because of marked limitation of flexion, ectopic bone was surgically excised. Satisfactory flexion has been restored.

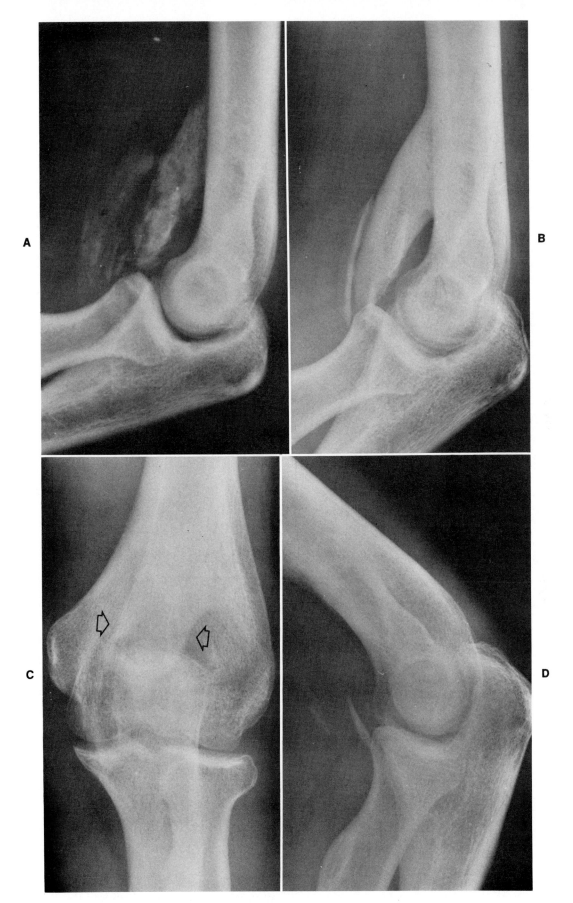

Fig. 16-7. For legend see opposite page.

amorphous calcification on the radiograph. The bone scan is by far the most accurate modality available for determining the metabolic activity and early detection of the ectopic ossification.[55,66,75,76] There has been excellent correlation between the early abnormally active sites demonstrated on bone scan before radiographic evidence of mineralization and eventual formation of ectopic bone at the same site.[29,45] Bone scans demonstrate specific sites of intense activity in the ectopic bone. The metabolic activity within the bone mass is heterogeneous (Fig. 16-5). When serial bone scans are compared, these active sites have been seen to shift from one region to another during the course of maturation.[75] Correlation between the radiograph and bone

scan with respect to maturity of the ectopic bone has not been promising. The bone scan may demonstrate increasing activity on serial scans for months or even years after the radiograph demonstrates no further change.[55] Eventually the activity seen on the scan reaches a plateau, and then at a later time decreasing activity is seen. In most cases the scan eventually returns to normal even though it may take years in a few patients.[76] It must be remembered that mature ectopic bone is mature bone and will demonstrate activity as long as it is present. On scans it will demonstrate normal activity: an amount of activity similar to that of the adjacent skeleton (Fig. 16-5).

In the upper extremity, ectopic bone most frequently occurs between the neck of the scapula and the medial aspect of the proximal humeral shaft including the surgical neck of the humerus (Fig. 16-6). Such ossification can also occur between the proximal humeral shaft and the coracoid process or rarely between the acromion and the proximal end of the humeral shaft.[19,28] Likewise, in the elbow the site of formation of ectopic bone is variable. It can occur anterior (Fig. 16-7) or posterior (Fig. 16-8) to the joint or both. Posteriorly the ectopic bone may surround the ulnar nerve, which makes surgery more difficult if it is attempted.[28]

In the knee the most common site of ectopic ossification is adjacent to the medial femoral condyle and the anteromedial aspect of the distal femoral shaft (Figs. 16-9 and 16-10).[28] The next most likely site to be involved is adjacent to the quadriceps tendon at its insertion into the superior pole of the patella and less frequently adjacent to the patellar ligament where it attaches to the distal pole of the patella (Fig. 16-11).[19] Less likely sites of ossification are adjacent to the medial tibial plateau and along the lateral aspect of the lateral femoral condyle.[19] Occasionally unusual sites such as the popliteal space (Figs. 16-10 and 16-12) are involved.

Multiple sites of ectopic bone occur adjacent to the hip (Figs. 16-13 to 16-15). The most common site is anterior to the joint between the anterior iliac crest and the intertrochanteric area of the femur (Fig. 16-13) or less often between the ischiopubic region and the lesser trochanter. Much less often it occurs laterally in the gluteus medius muscle between the lateral aspect of the iliac wing and the greater trochanter (Fig. 16-14).[19,44] The least frequent site of ossification is posterior to the joint between the ischium and the greater trochanter.[19]

Extra-articular joint fusion is almost exclusively confined to the hip, shoulder, and elbow joints. The hip joint normally fuses in extension but rarely will fuse in flexion (Fig. 16-2).[79] Ankylosis of a shoulder occurs most frequently inferior to the joint with bone between the surgical neck of the humerus and the neck of the scapula or sometimes between the coracoid process and the

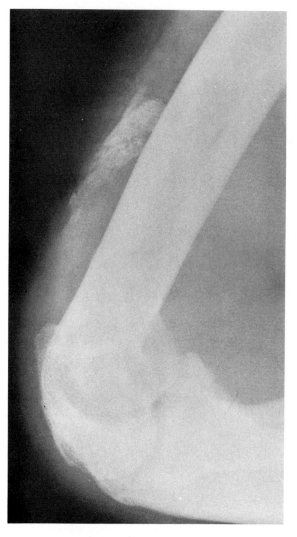

Fig. 16-8. Ectopic bone formation in 31-year-old man with complete C6 quadriplegia for 10 years. Ectopic bone has formed along posterior aspect of distal humeral shaft. In some patients it will form adjacent to joint posteriorly and can cause limitation of extension or extra-articular ankylosis of joint.

proximal humeral shaft.[28] Fusion is much less likely to occur lateral to the joint between the acromion and the proximal humeral shaft. The shoulder fuses with the arm in adduction[19,28] and with partial to almost full internal rotation. Elbow fusion is infrequent and occurs in flexion (Fig. 16-7). Pronation and supination ability may be reduced or eliminated by the fusion. Fusion can occur in the supinated position if the patient spends large amounts of time supine in bed. This is the least useful position of the forearm.

Text continued on p. 460.

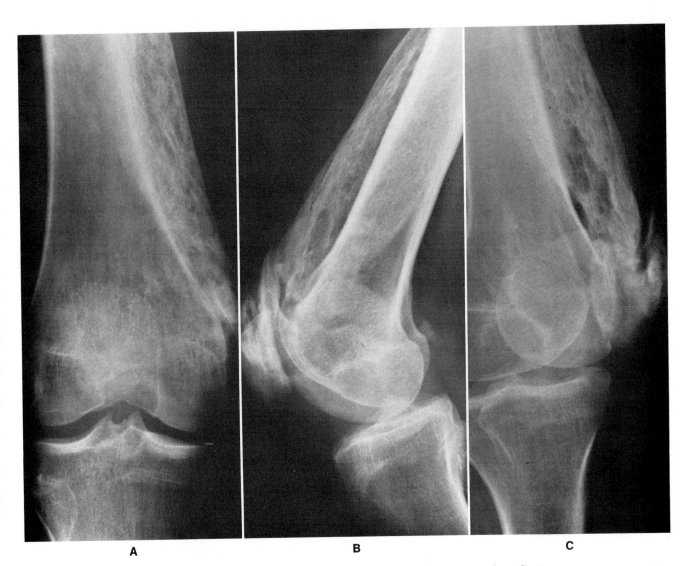

A   **B**   **C**

Fig. 16-9. Ectopic bone in knee of 31-year-old man with complete T11 paraplegia for 3 years. **A** and **B,** AP and lateral views demonstrate anterolateral position of ectopic bone. This is most frequent site of ectopic bone formation adjacent to a knee. **C,** Oblique projection. Cleavage plane can be seen between ectopic bone and adjacent femur. Interior of adjacent knee joint is unaffected by ectopic bone.

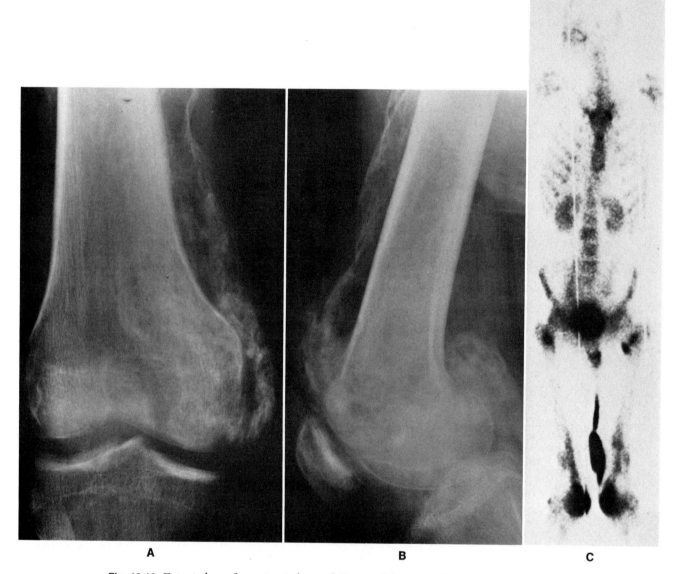

A   B   C

Fig. 16-10. Ectopic bone formation in knee of 18-year-old T4 paraplegic man 4 months after a motorcycle accident. **A,** Ectopic bone is present both medial and lateral to distal femur. **B,** Ectopic bone is forming both anterior and posterior to distal femur. Cortical margins are relatively indistinct as are trabeculae in interior of bone, indicating immaturity. **C,** Technetium bone scan demonstrates abnormal activity adjacent to both distal femurs but also adjacent to both hips. Midline activity between thighs is in tube connecting Foley catheter to drainage bag.

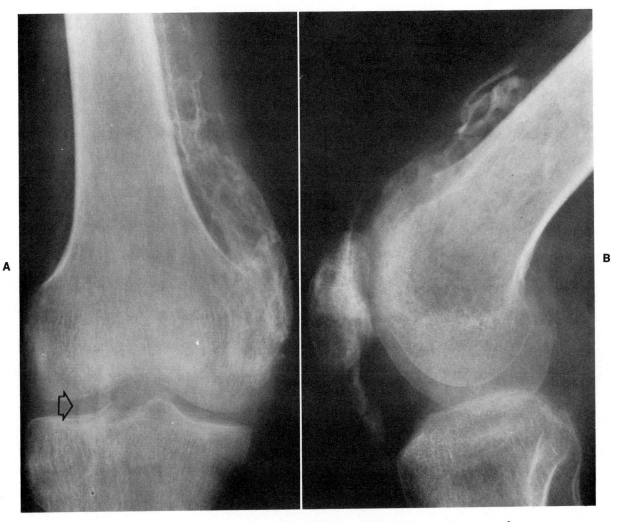

Fig. 16-11. Ectopic bone formation in knee of 22-year-old man with paraplegia secondary to L2 fracture. **A,** Ectopic bone can be seen crossing lateral joint compartment immediately lateral and inferior to patella *(arrow)*. Medial ectopic bone is seen in its usual position. **B,** Ectopic bone can be seen anterior to distal femur but is also present inferior to patella adjacent to patellar ligament, possibly involving periphery of ligament.

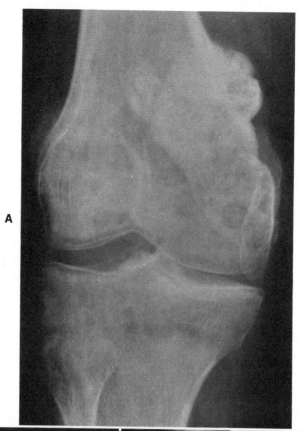

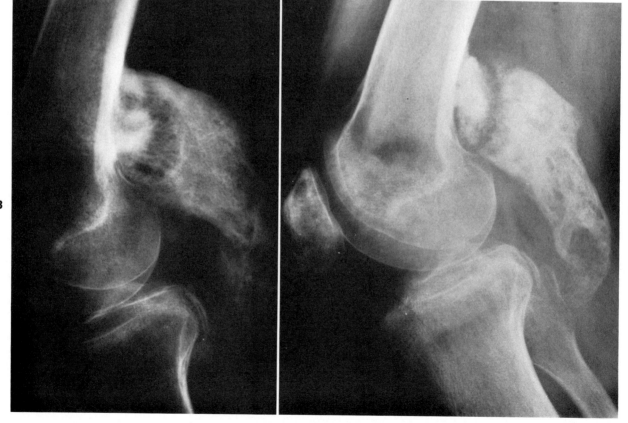

Fig. 16-12. For legend see opposite page.

Fig. 16-12. Ectopic bone formation in knee of 24-year-old complete T5 paraplegic man 17 months after thoracic fracture-dislocation. **A,** Ectopic bone can be seen in what appears to be its usual position anteromedial to distal femur. Metaphyseal band of demineralization is seen in proximal tibia, and subarticular demineralization is present in femoral condyles. **B,** Lateral view demonstrates that ectopic bone has formed posterior to joint, which is an infrequent finding. Lack of additional ectopic bone anywhere adjacent to knee makes this a quite unusual finding. Trabeculae within bone mass are indistinct, indicating that bone is immature. **C,** Four years after injury the ectopic bone has matured significantly. Bone is continuous with cortex of distal femur and has resulted in significant loss of flexion. This motion loss is less significant than the same degree of loss in a hip joint. This patient had identical ectopic bone formation in opposite knee (see Fig. 15-5).

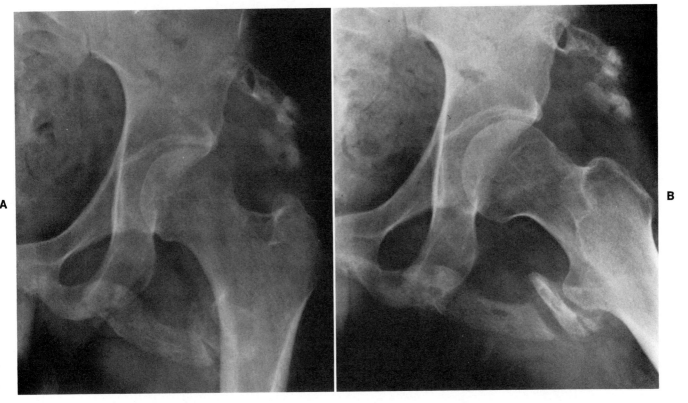

A   B

Fig. 16-13. Ectopic bone formation in 23-year-old complete T5 paraplegic man 15 months after injury. **A,** Medially, ectopic bone forms a bridge between lesser trochanter and ischiopubic junction, a common site of such ossification. A less common site superior and lateral to joint also contains ectopic ossification. **B,** Frog-leg lateral view demonstrates no impairment of abduction in spite of ectopic bone.

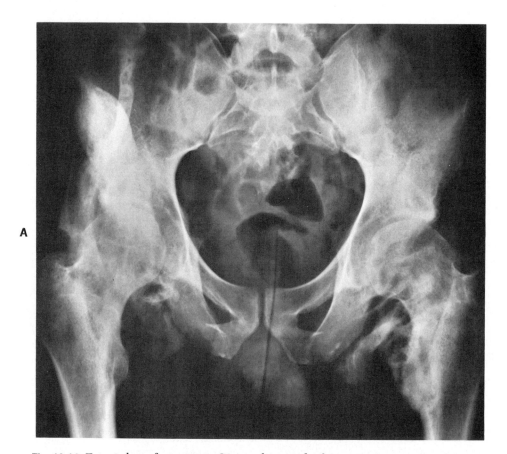

Fig. 16-14. Ectopic bone formation in C6 complete quadriplegic man 2 years, **A,** and 9 years, **B,** after an automobile accident. **A,** Ectopic bone formation can be seen adjacent to both hips. Lateral and posterior to right hip joint is a long band of ectopic bone in distribution of gluteus medius muscle, extending from greater trochanter to iliac crest. Ectopic bone is also present adjacent to right ischial tuberosity and immediately inferior to hip joints bilaterally. Erosion of a portion of right ischium from a pressure sore can be seen along its inferior margin.

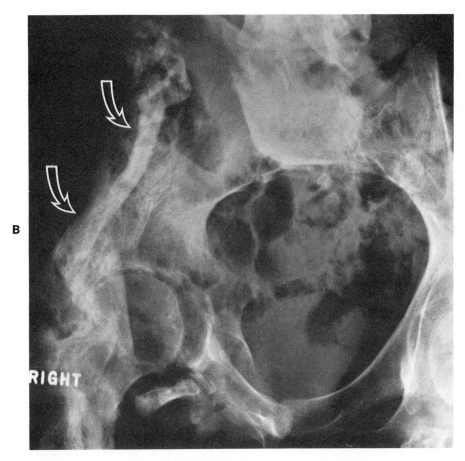

Fig. 16-14, cont'd. B, Right posterior oblique projection demonstrates well the long thin band of ectopic bone in gluteus medius muscle *(arrows)*. Patient is now 40 years old. There has been narrowing of hip joint superiorly, as well as osteophyte formation of articular margins of femoral head. There is now calcification in articular cartilage of femoral head. Partial right ischiectomy was performed because of pressure sore.

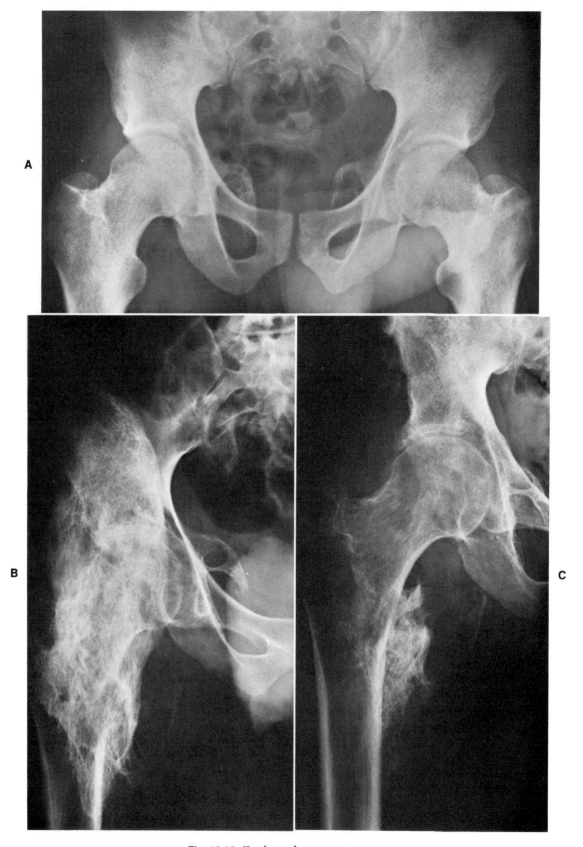

Fig. 16-15. For legend see opposite page.

D

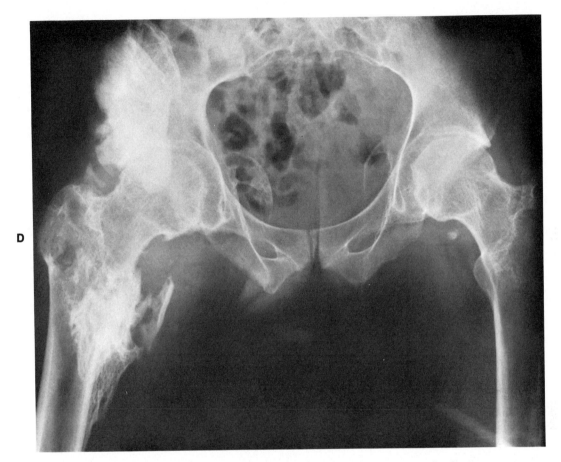

Fig. 16-15. Evolution and surgical resection of ectopic bone in C6 quadriplegic man. **A,** Ectopic ossification is present adjacent to left greater trochanter. Bilateral ossification adjacent to and continuous with posterior inferior iliac spines is unusual and has appeared within 1 year of patient's injury. **B,** Six years after injury. Extensive ectopic bone has formed anterior to right hip, resulting in extra-articular ankylosis of joint. There is superior narrowing of joint space. **C,** One month later, most of ectopic bone has been surgically removed with restoration of joint motion. Superior narrowing of hip joint can be better appreciated. **D,** Three years and six months later. As is always true even after resection of mature ectopic bone, there is at least a small amount of recurrence, which is seen here superior and anterior to joint.

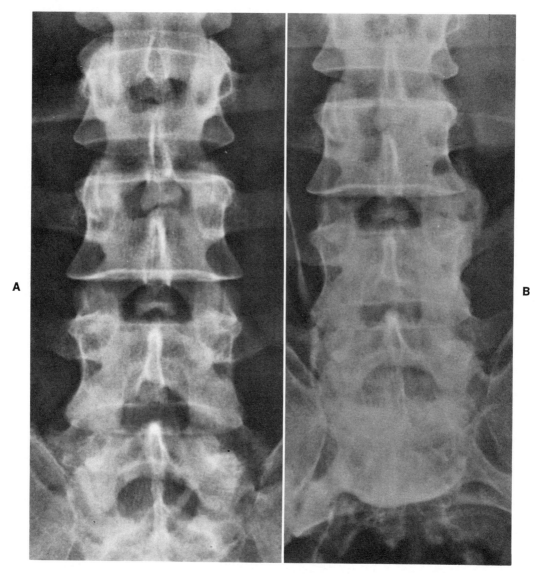

Fig. 16-16. Ectopic bone formation in spine of complete C5 spastic quadriplegic man. **A,** Normal lumbar spine 2 years after initial injury at 24 years of age. **B,** Four years after injury. Amorphous fluffy calcification can be seen superimposed on left side of the L3 and L4 vertebral bodies and L3-4 disc space.

ECTOPIC BONE FORMATION IN THE SPINE

Paraspinal ossification is included in this chapter with the soft tissue changes under the assumption that it most likely shares in the overall process of ectopic bone formation although it demonstrates some unique differences, which will be explained. Extensive ossification in the lumbar spine may cause ankylosis of multiple vertebrae in a small number of spinal cord injured patients. The mechanism of this ossification and the identity of predisposing factors are not known. There have been a few references in the literature to such findings,[3,6,80] but no detailed description has been pub-

lished. No definite clinical complaints related to the ossification were noted in the cases reported or in those patients whom we have examined.

Radiologic findings

Ossification forms between the vertebrae of the lumbar spine and eventually leads to ankylosis. The distal lumbar spine is more often affected than the proximal levels. Initially amorphous, fluffy or cloudlike calcification is seen, which eventually matures and forms a cortex and a spongiosa with the appearance of normal bone (Figs. 16-16 and 16-17). The ossification has an appear-

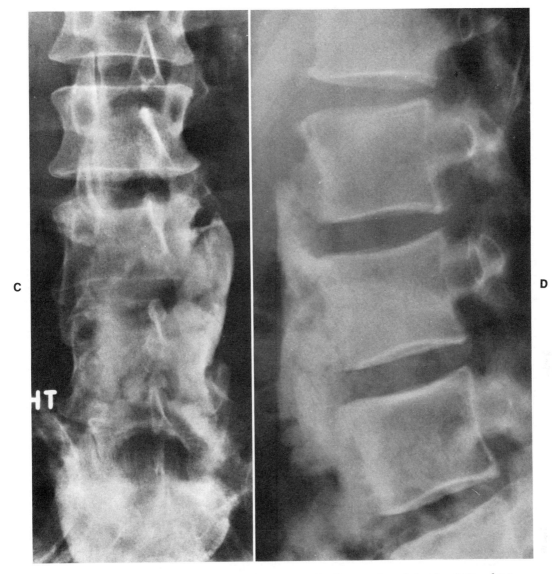

Fig. 16-16, cont'd. C and **D,** Nine years after injury. Ossification along left side of L3 and L4 vertebrae has matured with a well-defined cortex and distinct trabeculation within bony mass. On lateral projection, ectopic bone is seen to be anterior to L2, L3, and L4 vertebrae. Anterior margin of each of these vertebrae is indistinct, indicating that ectopic bone attaches to cortex. Disc spaces are unaffected. No ectopic bone can be seen involving posterior elements of these vertebrae.

ance very similar to that of flowing candle wax. It is attached to the margins of the vertebral bodies and usually has an asymmetric distribution in the spine. The location along the anterolateral margins of the bodies has much the same appearance as is seen with diffuse idiopathic skeletal hyperostosis (DISH). Bone may also form bridges between the transverse processes, the spinous processes, and the lamina of the vertebrae (Fig. 16-18). The vertebral disc spaces retain their normal vertical height with no evidence of degenerative disc

disease. The spinal ossification has not been identified above the level of the cord injury in our material. Facet joint narrowing has not been observed in the involved vertebrae. Ectopic bone formation has been identified elsewhere in the soft tissues in each of the patients with lumbar spine bone bridging. Concomitant ankylosis of the sacroiliac joints was seen in one of our patients, but the sacroiliac joints were normal in the remaining six patients. All of these patients were less than 30 years old at the onset of this ossification.

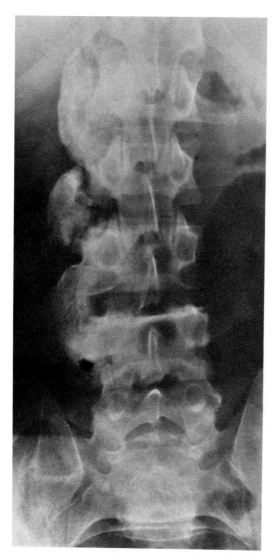

Fig. 16-17. Massive ectopic bone formation in 20-year-old man with paraplegia. Ectopic bone has formed anteriorly and has become continuous with L1, L2, L3, and L4 vertebrae with obliteration of portions of their cortices. Posterior elements can be seen clearly, indicating that they are not affected.

The ectopic ossification of the lumbar spine has a similar appearance and distribution to that seen in DISH.[27,60-62] The flowing nature of the ossification and its location along the anterior lateral margins of the vertebral bodies is similar in both of these entities. The disc spaces retain their normal vertical dimension with both entities. The posterior elements of the vertebrae can be affected in patients with DISH but are significantly less frequently involved than the anterior portions of the vertebrae.[60] The relative frequency of involvement in the spinal cord injured patients has not been established.

There are differences between DISH and the lumbar

ossification of spinal cord injured patients. DISH occurs in an older age group usually in the sixth decade or older.[60] Spinal cord injured patients with lumbar spine hyperostosis tend to be in the third and fourth decades. In older spinal cord injured patients (in the sixth and seventh decades) we have seen changes like those of DISH that extend above the level of the cord lesion. These cases have not been included in the above description. The lower third of the lumbar spine is most frequently involved in spinal cord injured patients. However, it is the least frequently involved area of the spine with DISH although the entire spine can be affected. We have not seen ectopic ossification of the spine extending above the level of a spinal cord lesion in any of the patients in the third and fourth decades.

Ossification involving the lumbar spine differs in several important respects from the ectopic bone formation seen in the soft tissues adjacent to the hips, knees, elbows, and shoulders. Its onset is much later after the spinal cord injury. In our patients it has usually appeared more than 2 years after injury. The ectopic bone elsewhere occurs almost always within the first year after a spinal cord injury.[80] Our patients had been rehabilitated and were active at the time the ossification was occurring in the lumbar spine. This ossification led to ankylosis of multiple vertebrae in all of our seven patients with spine involvement. Ankylosis of a large joint by ectopic bone occurs far less frequently than that seen in the lumbar spine even though most of the ectopic bone occurring in the soft tissues of the appendicular skeleton lies adjacent to large joints.

So far we have not seen any complications from the lumbar ossification. No history of stiffness or loss of range of motion could definitely be elicited. As a result no treatment was necessary. Perhaps when more patients are seen with these findings, clinical manifestations may be identified. To date we have only seen lumbar ossification in patients several years after spinal cord injury. We have not seen definite evidence of changes in the appendicular skeleton in these patients similar to those described in patients with DISH.[62] Also, we have not seen ossification in the thoracic spine but feel certain that this is possible with a high thoracic or cervical lesion.

It is possible that ectopic bone formation in the lumbar spine is caused by the same mechanism causing ossification in other soft tissues of spinal cord injured patients. We are unable to explain why this ossification appears at a later time than the ectopic bone adjacent to the hips and knees. The similar appearance and similar distribution to DISH in the lumbar spine suggest the possibility of a common mechanism being responsible for both entities. Patients with spinal cord injury have a negative calcium balance, which lasts several

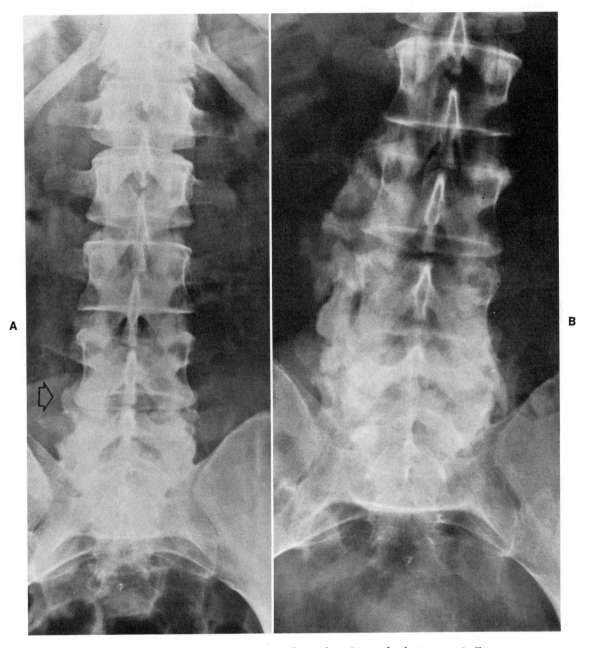

Fig. 16-18. Ectopic bone formation in spine of complete C6 quadriplegic man. **A,** Five years after injury. Lumbar spine and sacroiliac joints are essentially normal. Small amount of ectopic bone has formed at L4-5 level on right *(arrow)*. Patient is 23 years old. **B,** Eleven years after injury. Extensive ectopic bone formation is present along right side of lumbar spine (L3 to L5). Ectopic bone is located posteriorly, which can be appreciated on AP projection because lateral margin of bodies of involved vertebrae can be clearly seen. Comparison should be made with Fig. 16-17, in which bone formation involves vertebral bodies.

Continued.

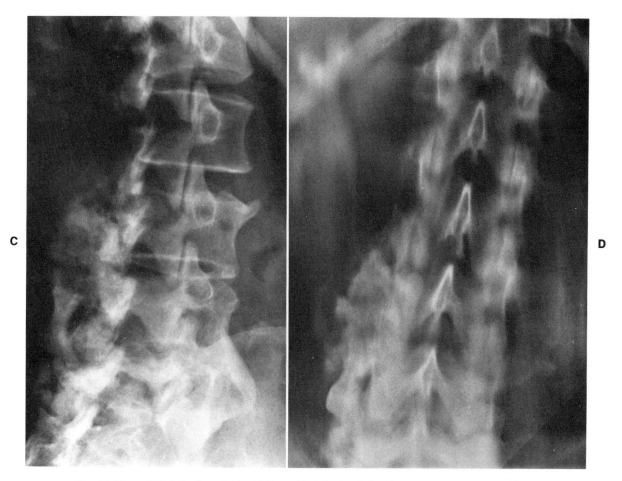

Fig. 16-18, cont'd. C, Left posterior oblique film obtained during intravenous urogram demonstrates posterior position of ectopic bone with ankylosis of transverse processes and bases of spinous processes. **D,** Tomogram obtained in AP projection demonstrates ectopic bone located posteriorly with involvement of transverse processes, lamina, and spinous processes.

months but returns to normal usually by approximately 18 months.[13] By the time the ectopic bone is forming in the lumbar spine of spinal cord injured patients, the calcium balance should have returned to a steady state.[13] The sympathetic nervous system is frequently damaged in the spinal cord injured patient. Vascular changes do occur below the level of the cord lesion with formation of arteriovenous fistulae.[31,66] However, there is no reason to suspect a similar abnormality in patients with DISH. More work will be necessary to determine the similarities and differences between the ectopic bone formation in these two abnormal states. It is possible that the radiologic similarities arise because the soft tissues adjacent to the spine have a limited number of ways to respond. The tissue response may be from totally different mechanisms.

In a group of ten of our patients with extensive ectopic bone formation, including some with lumbar spine ossification, tissue typing was done for the HLA-B27 antigen.[68] This antigen is present in a large percentage of patients with ankylosing spondylitis, psoriatic arthritis, and Reiter's arthritis.[69] It was absent in all ten of our patients, a finding that concurs with that of Bhate.[6]

PRESSURE SORES

The breakdown of soft tissue because of pressure plagues the spinal cord injured patient. Treatment of soft tissue breakdown is one of the most difficult problems faced by physicians dealing with these patients. This soft tissue breakdown is known by multiple names, such as bed sore, decubitus ulcer, pressure ulcer, or pressure sore. *Pressure sore* and *pressure ulcer* are the most accurately descriptive terms. Not all of the lesions occur from assuming the decubitus position or occur while the patient is in a bed, but all do occur secondary

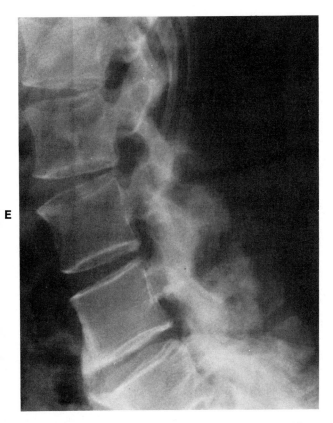

E

Fig. 16-18, cont'd. E, On lateral projection, margins of laminae and spinous processes from L3 to S1 are indistinct because ectopic bone has caused a posterior fusion throughout this area. Patient has had no previous lumbar surgery. Note anterior osteophytes at L4-5.

to pressure. Pressure sores occur at sometime in almost all spinal cord injured patients. They hinder rehabilitation of the patient, are difficult to treat, and take a long time to heal at a great expense in terms of hospitalization and lost time for the patient. Pressure sores can lead to sinus formation, abscesses, osteomyelitis, malnutrition, anemia, and amyloidosis. Their most discouraging characteristic is that they usually recur although not necessarily in the same spot.

Pathogenesis

To acquire an adequate understanding of pressure sores, it is necessary to know the mechanism by which they occur. Many intrinsic and extrinsic factors of varying importance participate in the formation of a pressure sore. The most important factors are extrinsic pressure and its duration. The body presses on a supporting surface such as a bed or a chair with a force proportional to its weight. There is nonuniform transmission of the pressure into the underlying soft tissues because of the inhomogeneity of the tissues. This pressure is eventually transmitted to the skeleton.[52,70] Bony

prominences cause compressive and shearing forces in the adjacent soft tissues when there is weight bearing. The soft tissues are compressed between the bone and the bed or chair on which the patient rests.[34] This compression exceeds the pressure in the skin capillaries and cuts off skin circulation.[49,52] The pressure is also transmitted into the underlying soft tissues, resulting in ischemia there as well.[47,70] Capillary pressure ranges from 12 to 33 mm Hg in normal skin and can increase to 60 to 70 mm Hg during hyperemia.[50] Pressures exceeding 300 mm Hg over the ischial tuberosities have been measured during sitting.[49] Maximal capillary pressures may also be exceeded over the sacrum, occiput, heels, rib margins, and knees when the patient is prone or supine.[52] Such pressure for as little as 2 to 4 hours can lead to pressure necrosis.[41,82] The magnitude and duration of the pressure are the important factors and are inversely related.[24,47] The greater the pressure, the shorter is the time necessary for pressure sore formation. The skin tolerates high pressures for a short time but not for a sustained time interval. Blood flow to a compressed area is greatly increased when pressure is relieved, allowing restoration of nutrition and removal of toxic metabolic wastes. If this pressure release occurs frequently, high pressures such as are borne by the soles of the feet can be tolerated.[52]

Additional extrinsic factors are important in the formation of pressure sores. Maceration of the skin from exposure to moisture from perspiration, urine, or feces greatly accelerates soft tissue necrosis.[24,36,82] Friction is another important factor. A pressure sore will form after a shorter time and at a lower pressure if friction has damaged the epidermis, such as with a sheet burn.[24] Shearing forces occur when one layer of soft tissue moves with respect to another, causing stretch on the small vessels, which can result in thrombosis.[24,59] Venules are the most likely site of thrombi produced in this manner.[23] Shearing force can produce dissection or cleavage in the soft tissues parallel to the skin surface and may be part of the reason for undermining of pressure sore margins in addition to being a factor in their development.

Several intrinsic factors promote and predispose to the formation of pressure sores. The most important of these factors is the loss of sensation. In a healthy person numbness, pain, or a pins-and-needles sensation from anoxia and local chemical irritation occurs after sitting in one position too long. This causes the person to change position slightly, long before anoxia of the skin and soft tissues results. In the spinal cord injured patient this protection is lost. The loss of vasomotor control also is thought to cause a decrease of resistance to pressure.[36] Poor nutrition occurs as a result of anorexia from a lack of physical activity, constipation, or psychologic factors[78] and promotes the development of pressure sores.[56] The not infrequent presence of chronic alcoholism, drug addiction, or a desire for self-destruction can further aggravate this problem.[16,41] Appetite can also be affected after a pressure sore develops because of resulting infection, abscess formation, fever, and malaise. Thus a vicious cycle can result. Anemia predisposes the patient to pressure sore formation in that it decreases the body's ability to deal with the resulting infection and to repair the soft tissue necrosis. It can originate from blood loss from the pressure sore or from malnutrition. Hematopoiesis is suppressed secondary to poor nutrition or infection.[41] Arteriovenous shunting has been demonstrated by arteriography[31,66] in the paralyzed regions of the body, which leads to decreased oxygen delivery to the local tissues. This should make the soft tissues more susceptible to pressure necrosis and more resistant to healing of any resulting ulceration.

Changes in the skin are determined by the degree of ischemia. Typically necrosis of the skin and underlying soft tissue occurs within a few hours after abnormal pressure. Skin ulceration is first noted two to three days after the application of pressure.[48] The necrotic tissue sloughs or is debrided after several days or even weeks, leaving an ulcer. Superimposed infection accelerates the process of tissue necrosis and ulcer formation. The skin, subcutaneous fat, deep fascia, muscle, and periosteum may participate in the ischemia secondary to the extrinsic pressure. Necrosis may occur in each of the soft tissues, and eventually an underlying bony prominence becomes exposed and may become infected.[34] Not all pressure sores, however, extend down to bone. A given lesion may terminate at any point between the dermis and the underlying bony prominence. A superficial ulcer may heal with conservative therapy, but a deep ulcer through the fascia will not heal satisfactorily without surgery.[70] No pressure sore should be taken lightly.[42] Vigorous conservative management must be undertaken or a superficial ulcer will develop into a deep lesion. Necrosis of the deeper soft tissues is frequently more extensive than that of the skin, particularly over the sacrum, trochanters, and ischium.[36,47] The skin margins are usually undermined in pressure sores of these three areas.

The body attempts to heal a pressure sore with granulation tissue that covers the entire raw surface of the ulcer.[15,41,42] This tissue will also cover a bony prominence if all the overlying soft tissues are sloughed. Granulation tissue is an immature vascular connective tissue that will erode bone when it comes in contact with it. Most of the bone erosions seen adjacent to pressure sores are not caused by osteomyelitis,[51] but probably result from granulation tissue that has come

into contact with the bone (see Chapter 15). The granulation tissue will mature and form a tough, relatively avascular fibrous scar over the adjacent bony prominence which becomes adherent to the bone.[26] If surgery is not performed, a thin, avascular epithelium may form over this scar. This epithelium only offers temporary healing because it will break down easily when subjected to pressure.[9,70]

Closed pressure sores, or bursae, are a less frequent occurrence than the open type described above. Compression and shear forces cause ischemic necrosis in the subcutaneous fat[70,82] with formation of a fluid-filled bursalike cavity containing necrotic debris. Usually a sinus tract develops from the bursa to the skin with a deceptively small opening on the skin surface (Fig. 16-25). Because the large underlying cavity may not be clinically suspected or is larger than expected, all sinus tracts should be examined by a sinogram to determine the size, extent, and proximity to the underlying bone and joints.[58] A different type of bursa will be referred to sometimes and can be confused with the above lesion. This is seen primarily when dealing with trochanteric ulcers. There are two bursae that are normal anatomic structures superficial to the greater trochanter. An adjacent pressure sore can penetrate into these bursae and cause hypertrophy of the bursa wall, which will form part of the base of a trochanteric pressure sore.[26] Frequent reference is made to this remnant of the bursa at the base of the pressure sore. It is definitely different from the pseudobursa, or closed pressure sore, discussed above.

Sinus tracts may form especially from trochanteric and ischial pressure sores. The sinus tracts may communicate with unilocular or multilocular abscess cavities or with an adjacent joint. Computed tomography is useful to determine the actual size and extent of a large pressure sore and its adjacent fibrotic scar. Its relation to local anatomic structures and the position of any local ectopic bone are also clearly delineated. This information is useful to the surgeon when he plans a surgical closure. Magnification radiography is useful in such cases to obtain maximal bone detail when there is questionable erosion of the underlying bone by the pressure sore.[40]

Pressure sores always become infected and contain a mixed flora such as *Staphylococcus, Streptococcus, Escherichia coli, Proteus,* and *Pseudomonas.*[41] The infected sore or ulcer can cause a periostitis in the underlying bony prominence.[36] The adjacent bone may be eroded by granulation tissue from the pressure sore or by osteomyelitis.[40] The osteomyelitis usually progresses slowly. The patient may have a temperature elevation, malaise, anorexia, and depressed hematopoiesis. Usually any elevated temperature is mistakenly attributed to a urinary tract infection. In the past amyloidosis was seen rather frequently in patients with chronic osteomyelitis. With improvement of surgical techniques and the use of antibiotics, chronic osteomyelitis is seen far less commonly and is treated much more aggressively. As a result amyloidosis is now very rarely seen. Epithelial tumors occurring in the wall of a sinus tract have been reported.[32,36] These occurrences are extremely rare to the point of being medical curiosities.

A pressure sore is similar to a third-degree burn in that extensive protein loss can occur from fluid weeping from its raw surface.[9] A large ulcer can lose up to 50 g of protein per day.[78] This protein loss becomes a major factor causing a negative nitrogen balance; poor intake of protein is a less significant factor.

Location

Pressure sores occur most commonly over the ischia, the sacrum, the greater trochanters, and the heels.[16,82] The most important factor determining the site of a pressure sore is merely the site where abnormal pressure occurs due to the patient's most frequent position or positions. In patients who remain in bed, pressure sores most commonly occur over the sacrum, the trochanters (Fig. 16-19), and the heels (Fig. 16-20). Patients who remain prone are most likely to develop ul-

cers over the costal margins, anterior iliac spines, the knees, and the dorsum of the feet. Patients in wheelchairs are most likely to develop ulcers over the ischia. Patients who do any walking may develop ulcers from braces. Ulcers over the coccyx or sacrum can occur from a patient's slouching down in a chair. The placement of the television or the patient's roommate in relation to his bed can determine the side on which a pressure sore will develop. Patients in whom spasticity develops are likely to develop ulcers over the malleoli, elbows, and knees from the knees or ankles rubbing together or against bed sheets during spasm.[41] Ischial pressure sores can penetrate along the ramus of the ischium anteriorly into the groin area or inferiorly down the posterior fascial compartment of the thigh. Pressure sores over the trochanter tend to form sinuses that extend into the adjacent hip joint.[9,36]

Prevention

There are several principles that are followed when dealing with pressure sores. Prevention is always the most important way of dealing with this problem. All patients must be turned at least every 2 hours, 24 hours per day.[34] Waterbeds, air mattresses, and air beds have been developed that markedly reduce the amount of pressure on the skin.[43,63] Such equipment is expensive

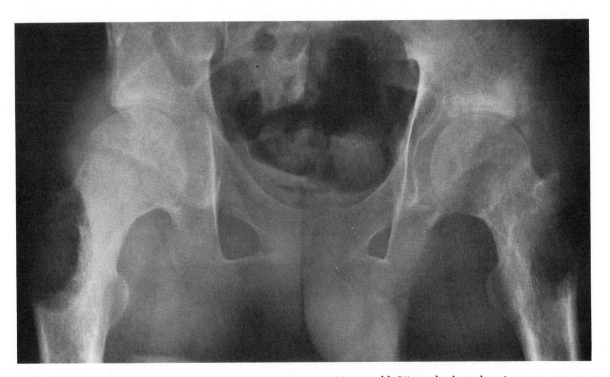

Fig. 16-19. Bilateral trochanteric pressure sores in 18-year-old C5 quadriplegic boy 1 year after gunshot wound. Air can be seen in pressure sores. Bone detail of greater trochanters is poorly visualized because of superimposed air in ulcers. Definite erosion of cortex of right greater trochanter has occurred. Both hip joints are significantly narrowed superiorly.

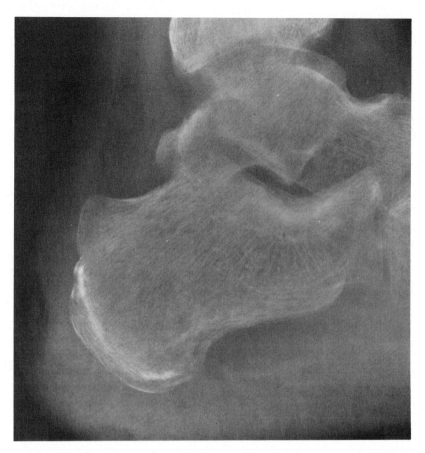

Fig. 16-20. Heel pressure sore in 30-year-old T9 paraplegic man. Underlying bone is intact. There is undermining of skin margins of pressure sore. This is a typical characteristic of pressure sores and is not unique for this location. This patient has a companion pressure sore in same spot on opposite heel.

and is not available everywhere. On a regular hospital bed, pressure of 50 to 70 mm Hg occurs over some of the dependent portions of the body.[25,52] With a water mattress, pressure can be reduced to 15 to 20 mm Hg and with an air bed this can be further reduced to approximately 10 mm Hg.[83] Soilage of skin by urine must be prevented by catheterization or reflex emptying of the bladder routinely. Routine bowel care must be maintained.[33] Once pressure sores do occur, they must be dealt with quickly. Usually they will not heal spontaneously unless they are quite superficial, and surgery will be necessary.[83]

Presurgical preparation

Prior to a surgical procedure, any nitrogen imbalance or nutritional deficiency should be treated by a high-protein, low-fat, low-carbohydrate diet with the addition of multiple vitamins. Anemia must be treated, if necessary by transfusion up to 12 g/100 ml. Urinary tract infection and calculi must be treated. If spasm is not eliminated, it usually leads postoperatively to

breakdown of the skin flap over the trochanters, ischia, or sacrum.[34] Treatment of spasm is a particularly difficult problem because it occurs in 50% of paraplegic patients and even more often in quadriplegic patients. Spasm can be treated by rhizotomy or intrathecal injection of alcohol or phenol. If there is any residual reflex bladder function or sexual function, such procedures will ablate them. This may further discourage the patient and remove his motivation for rehabilitation.[41,42] The problem is further complicated because the ethanol or phenol block and even the rhizotomy are only temporary helps in combating spasm in approximately 50% of the patients. Thus some investigators think that these procedures should be abandoned completely.[37] This view, however, is not universally held.[34]

Surgical treatment

The surgical treatment of pressure sores must be meticulous, and a group of principles has evolved for the treatment for these lesions. The pressure sore is debrided carefully, irrigated one to three times daily with

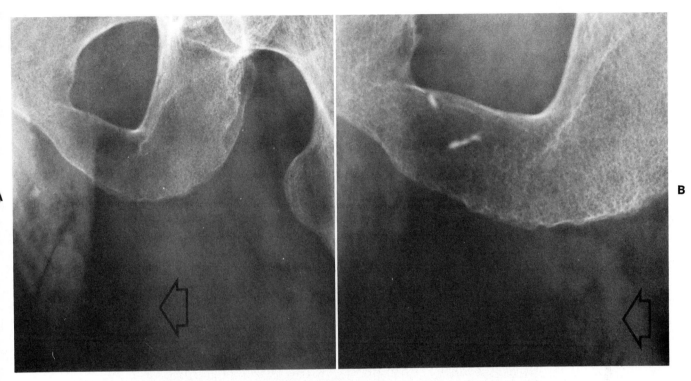

Fig. 16-21. Ischial pressure sore in 28-year-old paraplegic man. **A,** Air within pressure sore can be seen in soft tissues superficial to ischiopubic junction *(arrow)*. Radiologic examination was requested to determine whether adjacent bone cortex was affected. Cortex has a wavy appearance, which is normal for this area, but there was uncertainty with this routine radiograph whether cortex was definitely intact. **B,** View of same area, obtained by using direct radiographic magnification, clearly demonstrates that adjacent bone cortex is intact and not affected by pressure sore. Air can be seen in pressure sore *(arrow)*.

saline, peroxide, or a similar antiseptic solution, and packed with gauze.[9,41] The entire pressure sore is excised with removal of the underlying bony prominence. There is excision of any ectopic ossification if it is present in the adjacent area. Careful hemostasis is achieved and wound suction is maintained to prevent hematoma formation under the skin flap. A large flap of muscle or fascia is turned over the underlying bone partially as a cushion but also to fill in the large defect created by excision of the pressure sore. The wound is covered with a large, regional, full-thickness skin flap. The patient is not allowed to put pressure on this flap for 2 to 6 weeks.[34,41,42] Radical excision of any underlying bony prominence[7,10,16] has been advocated by a number of investigators. Ischiectomy on one side has resulted in pressure sore formation on the opposite side because of the resulting imbalance of weight bearing.[16,78,82] Pelvic tilt and scoliosis have occurred due to the resulting asymmetry from a radical ischiectomy.[78] Posterior urethral diverticulum or fistula formation is a common complication after radical ischiectomy.[14] Perineal and coccygeal pressure sores can occur after bilat-

eral radical ischiectomy.[16,42,78] Because of these complications with radical ischiectomy, less extensive excision of the underlying bone has been subsequently advocated with elimination of the complications.[9,42]

Amputation

Bilateral amputation of the lower extremities has been advocated as a method of eliminating many of the problems with pressure sores, fractures, edema, and osteomyelitis occurring in these limbs.[12] Also, weight reduction and maneuverability are improved. Spasticity also may be improved after such surgery. The loss of the lower extremities has a cosmetic disadvantage that usually is aesthetically undesirable for the patient. Although most paraplegics can achieve crutch walking, only a small percentage of them continue to use this form of mobility outside the hospital. The possibility of crutch walking is lost after bilateral amputation, and once the surgery occurs, it is irreversible. In some cases recurrent pressure sores cannot be covered by the existing skin, and amputation of a lower extremity is necessary to obtain a large enough skin flap to cover

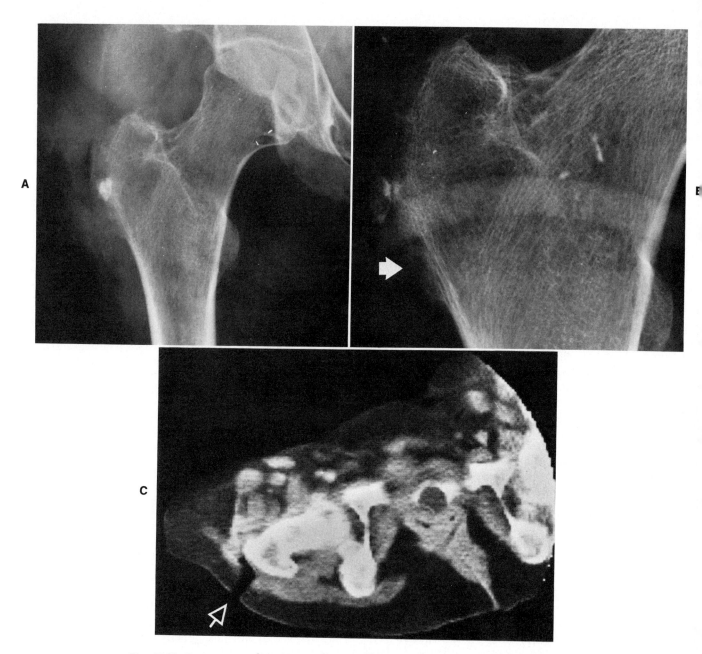

Fig. 16-22. Pressure sore formation in 24-year-old T4 paraplegic woman. **A,** Air is present in soft tissues adjacent to right greater trochanter. Ectopic bone formation is also present in same area. Cortex of greater trochanter is indistinct. **B,** Direct magnification view shows air in pressure sore and ectopic bone. Cortical margin of greater trochanter is completely gone, and bare bone trabeculae can be seen. Cortex has been eroded by adjacent pressure sore. Microscopic and histologic study of bone from this area did not demonstrate osteomyelitis. A large amount of granulation tissue was present at base of pressure sore, and this is thought to cause the erosions. At inferior aspect of greater trochanter, erosions extend beyond eroded cortex and include underlying bone trabeculae *(arrow)*. **C,** CT scan at level of greater trochanter demonstrates pressure sore *(arrow)* and its relationship to greater trochanter. CT scan offers less information about cortical integrity than does direct magnification technique. (From Hendrix, R. W., et al.: Radiology **138:**351, 1981.)

the ulceration.[8] Intractable infection of an underlying bone or joint may also necessitate amputation or disarticulation.[35,70]

In cauda equina lesions there is saddle anesthesia and ischial or perineal pressure sores may occur. Rotational skin flaps from the lateral buttocks have been used for treatment; this restores partial sensation to the affected area, effectively decreasing the anesthetic area. Thus the patient is aware of pressure, and the possibility of recurrence is greatly reduced.[36]

Radiologic findings

The presence of pressure sores is quite simple for the clinician to detect visually. Radiology has no place in the detection of these lesions. Routine radiographs will demonstrate no abnormalities in the soft tissues in a majority of patients.[40] In other patients a collection of air is seen in the soft tissues (Fig. 16-21), which alerts the radiologist that a pressure sore is present. Radiology contributes to the management of pressure sores in three ways. The first is determining whether there is ectopic bone formation present; this could be the bony prominence leading to initial formation of the pressure sore. The second is determining whether there are changes of osteomyelitis in the underlying bone. Most often the clinician obtains radiographs of the pressure sore area, desiring to learn whether osteomyelitis is present. The third contribution occurs only in the presence of a sinus tract. In such cases a sinogram should be performed to determine the extent of the sinus and of underlying soft tissue necrosis. Computed tomography may be used to determine the extent of an abscess cavity and of its proximity to local anatomic structures. We have made attempts to use ultrasonography to evaluate pressure sores, but the findings have not been useful and thus it was abandoned for this purpose.[40] Hindrances such as the pressure sore opening and air in the pressure sore led to nondiagnostic ultrasound studies.

Direct magnification radiography (see Chapter 15) is a technique that is used for optimal visualization of bone detail in a thick body part (Fig. 16-22). This technique provides the best detail of bone in body parts such as the pelvis, sacrum, and hips. Therefore bone erosions may be detected earlier with this technique than with any other radiologic modality.[40]

Sinography

Pressure sores of the sacral, ischial, and trochanteric areas are the three most difficult sites to treat.[36] They are also the three sites most likely to have associated sinus tracts (Figs. 16-23 to 16-25). The only external manifestation sometimes is a small innocent-appearing opening that connects with a large abscess cavity in the

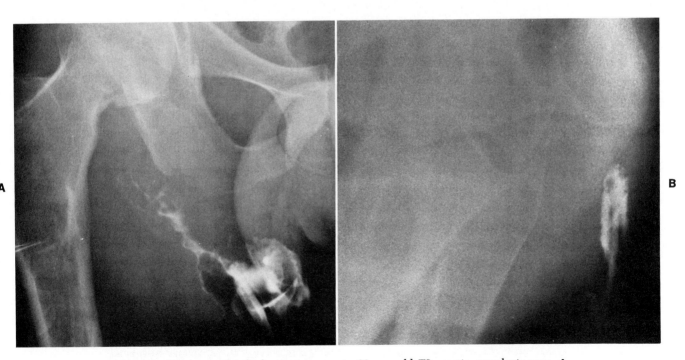

Fig. 16-23. Sinogram of ischial pressure sore in 26-year-old T8 spastic paraplegic man. **A,** Erosion of cortical margin of right ischium is seen. Contrast agent in sinus tract lies close to eroded bone. Prior to sinogram, length and size of sinus tract were unknown. **B,** Lateral view shows sinus tract extending all the way to surface of ischium.

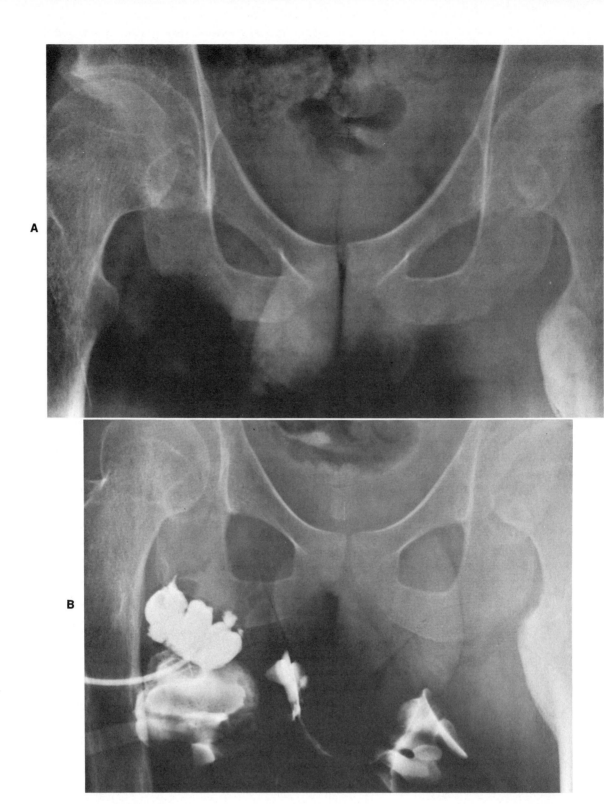

Fig. 16-24. Sinograms of bilateral ischial pressure sores in 19-year-old T11 paraplegic man 16 months after gunshot wound. **A,** A large erosion of right ischium and a smaller erosion of left ischium are present. A minimal amount of air is seen in right pressure sore and none on left, which is frequently the situation. **B,** Both ischial pressure sores were injected simultaneously. Foley balloon was blown up on the right side and a straight catheter was used on the left side with resulting spill onto adjacent soft tissues. On left side, pressure sore is superficial; on right side it is quite deep and extends all the way to surface of eroded bone. Biopsy of this bone demonstrated osteomyelitis.

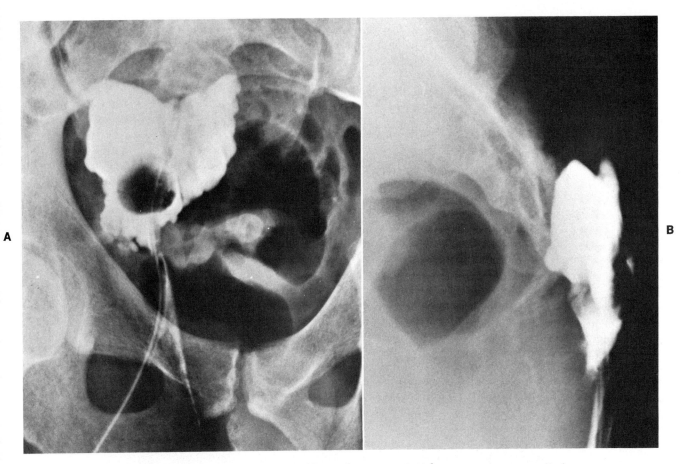

Fig. 16-25. Sacral sinogram in 27-year-old paraplegic man. **A,** A large pressure sore cavity is outlined by contrast agent. Note inflated Foley balloon used to perform sinogram. **B,** Lateral view demonstrates contrast agent in intimate contact with distal tip of underlying sacrum. Patient has had a partial sacrectomy as part of treatment for previous sacral pressure sores.

underlying soft tissues (Fig 16-25). It is always important to determine the size and the extent of the sinus tract. It is especially important to know whether a sinus tract communicates with an adjacent joint.

It can also be useful to know whether the sinus extends down to the surface of underlying bone. Sinography is the easiest way to determine the size and extent of the sinus tract.[9,30,36,58] The technique used is to insert a Foley catheter into the sinus tract with the balloon blown up outside the patient.[58] A balloon blown up inside the sinus tract may rupture the tract and extend the infection into additional soft tissues. The Foley balloon is held against the skin occluding the sinus opening during injection of a water-soluble iodinated contrast material (Fig. 16-25). The examination is done in the radiology department using intermittent fluoroscopy to determine the course of the contrast agent. In addition, it can be used to position the patient for the radiographs. In particular, fluoroscopy is useful to determine the best projection and the proximity of the

contrast medium to the underlying bone. At least two radiographs are obtained at 90° to one another while the opening of the sinus tract is farthest from the table or is the least dependent portion of the patient. In this position contrast agent does not leak out of the tract. Radiographs are obtained in the vertical and horizontal projections without moving the patient (Fig. 16-23). A lateral radiograph is always obtained shooting horizontally across the table. By obtaining radiographs taken at 90° from one another, a satisfactory three-dimensional idea of the size and extent of the sinus can be obtained in most cases. Turning the patient for additional views can also be done if there are questions about the proximity of contrast material to adjacent bones. This question is most likely to occur in association with the greater trochanters. The sinogram gives an idea of the extent of the lesion so that any surgical procedure can be planned appropriately (Fig. 16-26). Also, any bones adjacent to the sinus tract should be scrutinized for erosive changes, which can be caused by either granulation

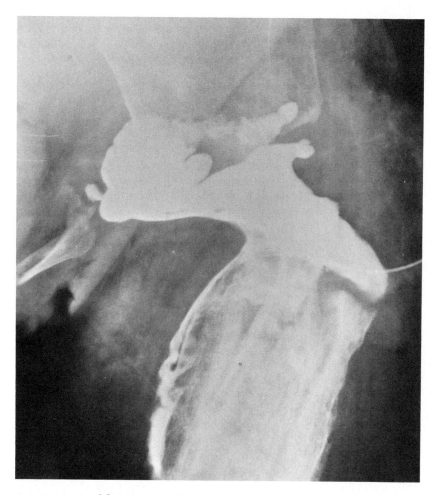

Fig. 16-26. Sinogram of draining sinus that has been present for 7 years. This is same patient as in Fig. 15-11. Chronic osteomyelitis in proximal femur developed after Girdlestone procedure was performed. Large portion of pelvis has been resected for osteomyelitis. Contrast agent is in intimate contact with proximal end of femur and also with a portion of remaining left iliac wing.

tissue or osteomyelitis. In cases with very large subcutaneous cavities or with multiple loculations, sinography may not demonstrate the full extent of the area involved. Computed tomography (CT) may be useful in such cases. Experience using this modality for such an application is still limited; however, it is most useful in determining the extent of lesions and their association with adjacent anatomic structures (Fig. 16-27).[40] It is anticipated that this modality will be invaluable in selected cases, especially those with extensive dissecting lesions, with formation of large abscesses, and in whom surgery is contemplated.

DEEP VEIN THROMBOSIS

Deep vein thrombosis is treated in detail in Chapter 10. It is a soft tissue abnormality in which clinical diagnosis is confirmed using one or more special diagnostic modalities. Its importance to the present discussion is that it may have clinical findings of localized swelling, erythema, and heat identical to those of early ectopic bone formation or of a long bone fracture. A point of differential diagnosis is that ectopic bone occurs with frequency in limited areas anterior to the hip or anteromedial to the distal femur. Venous flow studies and venography can quickly determine the presence or absence of deep vein thrombosis. If such studies are negative, the early onset of ectopic bone formation is the most likely diagnosis. Confusion is most likely to occur in the proximal thigh. If the clinical findings are in the calf of the leg, there is no diagnostic difficulty because ectopic bone does not occur in this area. In the event that the venography and flow studies are negative, a bone scan and radiographs, particularly in the lateral projection of the involved area, should be obtained. Long bone fractures most frequently occur adjacent to the knee. They may cause greater and more diffuse

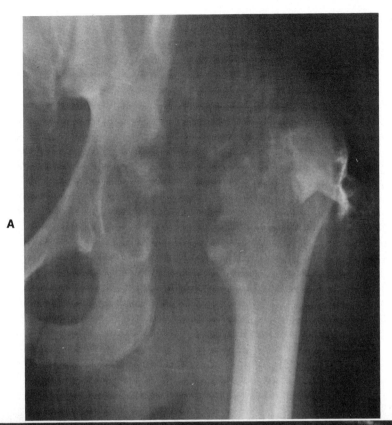

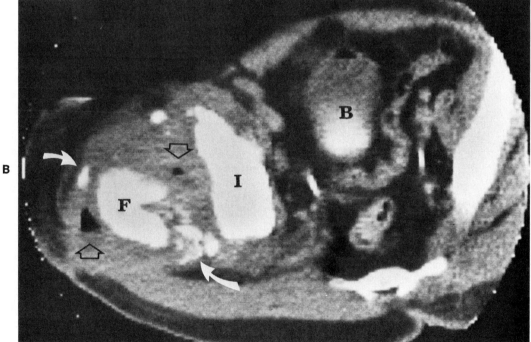

Fig. 16-27. Recurrent pressure sore in 26-year-old T6 paraplegic man 10 months after injury. **A,** Girdlestone procedure was done secondary to infected joint from adjacent pressure sore. Procedure was performed 2 months prior to present study. Pressure sore was excised at that time but has recurred. Air and iodinated contrast material outline pressure sore over greater trochanter. **B,** CT scan through level of proximal femoral shaft demonstrates considerable ectopic bone *(closed arrows)* adjacent to proximal end of femur. Exact relation of ectopic bone to adjacent bones and muscles can best be seen with this imaging modality. Air can be identified in soft tissues *(open arrows)* both medial and lateral to proximal femur. Patient was examined in prone position. *I,* Ilium; *F,* femur; *B,* urinary bladder containing contrast agent. (From Hendrix, R. W., et al.: Radiology **138:**351, 1981.)

swelling than ectopic bone. If deformity is present, the diagnosis is not difficult and a radiograph of the area will clearly demonstrate the pathology. A routine radiograph of an area of swelling and erythema is a rapid method of ruling out bone and soft tissue abnormalities before more sophisticated time-consuming special studies are performed.

CLUBBING

Radiographs of the hands and feet are not frequently obtained in most spinal cord injured patients. Clubbing of fingers and toes was reported to occur frequently in one study.[81] Clubbing is primarily a clinical diagnosis and is infrequently identified radiographically . Wright and co-workers[81] identified clubbing in 11 of 25 patients in whom paralysis had been present for more than 1 year. They did not see clubbing in patients less than 1 year after injury. The clubbing was also present in 8 of 13 patients with pressure sores, which was suggested as a possible cause or predisposing factor. The status of the cardiovascular and pulmonary systems of these patients was not indicated.

Radiologic findings

The radiologic findings caused by clubbing are nonspecific. The distal ends of the digits have a bulbous appearance. The soft tissues may appear slightly more dense than usual. Atrophy of the terminal tuft of the digit has not been reported in clubbing associated with spinal cord injury but has been seen in association with other causes.[64] Usually the underlying bone is normal.

REFERENCES

1. Abramson, A. S.: Bone disturbances in injuries to spinal cord, and cauda equina (paraplegia): their prevention by ambulation, J. Bone Joint Surg. [Am.] 30:982, 1948.
2. Abramson, A. S., and Delagi, E. F.: The contribution of physical activity to rehabilitation, Res. Q. 31:365, 1960.
3. Abramson, D. J., and Kamberg, S.: Spondylitis, pathological ossification, and calcification associated with spinal-cord injury, J. Bone Joint Surg. [Am.] 31:275, 1949.
4. Armstrong-Ressy, C. T., Weiss, A. A., and Ebel, A.: Results of surgical treatment of extraosseous ossification in spinal cord injuries, Proc. Clin. Paraplegia Conf. 6:12, 1957.
5. Benassy, J., Mazabraud, A., and Diverres, J.: L'osteogenese neurogene, Rev. Chir. Orthop. 49:95, 1963. 1963.
6. Bhate, D. V., Pizarro, A. J., Seitam, A., and Mak, E. B.: Axial skeletal changes in paraplegics, Radiology 133:55, 1979.
7. Blocksma, R., Kostrubala, J. G., and Greeley, P. W.: The surgical repair of decubitus ulcer in paraplegics: further observations, Plast. Reconstr. Surg. 4:123, 1949.
8. Burkhardt, B. R.: An alternative to the total-thigh flap for coverage of massive decubitus ulcers, Plast. Reconstr. Surg. 49:433, 1972.
9. Campbell, R. M.: The surgical management of pressure sores, Surg. Clin. North Am. 39:509, 1959.
10. Cannon, B., O'Leary, J. J., O'Neil, J. W., and Steinsleck, R.: An approach to the treatment of pressure sores, Ann. Surg. 132:760, 1950.
11. Chantraine, A. L.: Clinical investigation of bone metabolism in spinal cord lesions, Paraplegia 8:253, 1971.
12. Chase, R. A., and White, W. L.: Bilateral amputation in rehabilitation of paraplegics, Plast. Reconstr. Surg. 24:445, 1959.
13. Claus-Walker, J., Singh, J., Leach, C. S., et al.: The urinary excretion of collagen degradation products by quadriplegic patients and during weightlessness, J. Bone Joint Surg. [Am.] 59:209, 1977.
14. Comarr, A. E., and Bors, E.: Perineal urethral diverticulum—complication of removal of ischium, J.A.M.A. 168:2000, 1958.
15. Conway, H., et al.: The plastic surgical closure of decubitus ulcer in patients with paraplegia, Surg. Gynecol. Obstet. 85:321, 1947.
16. Conway, H., and Griffith, B. H.: Plastic surgery for closure of decubitus ulcers in patients with paraplegia, based on experience with 1000 cases, Am. J. Surg. 91:946, 1956.
17. Costello, F. V., and Brown, A.: Myositis ossificans complicating anterior poliomyelitis, J. Bone Joint Surg. [Br.] 33:594, 1951.
18. Couvee, L. M. J.: Heterotopic ossification and the surgical treatment of serious contractures, Paraplegia 9:89, 1971.
19. Damanski, M.: Heterotopic ossification in paraplegia. A clinical study, J. Bone Joint Surg. [Br.] 43:286, 1961.
20. Davis, R.: Spasticity following spinal cord injury, Clin. Orthop. 112:66, 1975.
21. Deitrich, J. E., Whedon, G. D., and Shorr, E.: Effects of immobilization upon various metabolic and physiologic functions of normal men, Am. J. Med. 4:3, 1948.
22. Dejerine, Mme., and Ceillier, A.: Para-osteo-arthropathies des paraplegiques par lesion medullaire (étude clinique et radiographique), Ann. Med. (Paris) 5:497, 1918.
23. Dinsdale, S. M.: Decubitus ulcers in swine: light and electron microscopy study of pathogenesis, Arch. Phys. Med. Rehabil. 54:51, 1973.
24. Dinsdale, S. M.: Decubitus ulcers: role of pressure and friction in causation, Arch. Phys. Med. Rehabil. 55:147, 1974.
25. Dowling, A. S.: Pressure sores—their cause, prevention and treatment, Md. State Med. J. 19:131, 1970.
26. Elson, R. A.: Anatomical aspects of pressure sores and their treatment, Lancet 1:884, 1965.
27. Forestier, J., and Rotes Querol, J.: Senile ankylosing hyperostosis of the spine, Ann. Rheum. Dis. 9:321, 1950.
28. Freehafer, A. A., Yurick, R., and Mast, W. A.: Para-articular ossification in spinal cord injury, Med. Serv. J. Can. 22:471, 1966.
29. Furman, R., Nicholas, J. J., and Jivoff, L.: Elevation of the serum alkaline phosphatase coincident with ectopic

bone formation in paraplegic patients, J. Bone Joint Surg. [Am.] **52**:1131, 1970.

30. Gage, H. C., and Williams, E. R.: Radiological exploration of sinus tracts, fistulae and infected cavities, Br. J. Radiol. **16**:8, 1943.

31. Galibert, P., Fossati, P., Lopez, C., et al.: Etude angiographique de la circulation des membres inferieurs aux differents stades evolutifs d'une paraplegie, Neurochirurgie **7**:181, 1961.

32. Gillis, L., and Lee, S.: Cancer as a sequel to war wounds, J. Bone Joint Surg. [Br.] **33**:167, 1951.

33. Griffith, B. H.: Advances in treatment of decubitus ulcers, Surg. Clin. North Am. **43**(1):245, 1963.

34. Griffith, B. H.: Pressure sores, Mod. Trends Plast. Surg. **2**:150, 1966.

35. Griffith, B. H., and Schultz, R. C.: Prevention and surgical treatment of recurrent decubitus ulcers in patients with paraplegia, Plast. Reconstr. Surg. **27**:248, 1961.

36. Guttmann, L.: The problem of treatment of pressure sores in spinal paraplegics, Br. J. Plast. Surg. **8**:196, 1955.

37. Harding, R. L.: Analysis of one hundred rehabilitated paraplegics, Plast. Reconstr. Surg. **27**:235, 1961.

38. Hardy, A. G., and Dickson, J. W.: Pathological ossification in traumatic paraplegia, J. Bone Joint Surg. [Br.] **45**:76, 1963.

39. Hassard, G. H.: Heterotopic bone formation about the hip and unilateral decubitus ulcers in spinal cord injury, Arch. Phys. Med. Rehabil. **56**:355, 1975.

40. Hendrix, R. W., Calenoff, L., Lederman, R., and Neiman, H. L.: Radiology of pressure sores, Radiology **138**:351, 1981.

41. Herceg, S. J., and Harding, R. L.: Surgical treatment of pressure sores, Pa. Med. **74**:45, 1971.

42. Herceg, S. J., and Harding, R. L.: Surgical treatment of pressure ulcers, Arch. Phys. Med. Rehabil. **59**:193, 1978.

43. Hofstra, P. C.: Air fluidized bed utilized for spinal cord injury patients, Proc. Ann. Clin. Spinal Cord Injury Conf. **18**:215, 1971.

44. Hossack, D. W., and King, A.: Neurogenic heterotopic ossification, Med. J. Aust. **1**:326, 1967.

45. Hsu, J. D., Sakimura, I., and Stauffer, E. S.: Heterotopic ossification around the hip joint in spinal cord injured patients, Clin. Orthop. **112**:165, 1975.

46. Irving, J., and LeBrun, H.: Myositis ossificans in hemiplegia, J. Bone Joint Surg. [Br.] **36**:440, 1954.

47. Kosiak, M.: Etiology and pathology of ischemic ulcers, Arch. Phys. Med. Rehabil. **40**:62, 1959.

48. Kosiak, M.: Etiology of decubitus ulcers, Arch. Phys. Med. Rehabil. **42**:19, 1961.

49. Kosiak, M., Kubicek, W. G., Olson, M., et al.: Evaluation of pressure as factor in production of ischial ulcers, Arch. Phys. Med. Rehabil. **39**:623, 1958.

50. Landis, E. M.: Micro-injection studies of capillary blood pressure in human skin, Heart **15**:209, 1930.

51. Lewis, V.: Unpublished data, 1979.

52. Lindan, O.: Etiology of decubitus ulcers: an experimental study, Arch. Phys. Med. Rehabil. **42**:774, 1961.

53. McLennan, C. E., McLennan, M. T., and Landis, E. M.: The effect of external pressure on the vascular volume of the forearm and its relation to capillary blood pressure and venous pressure, J. Clin. Invest. **21**:319, 1942.

54. Miller, L. F., and O'Neill, C. J.: Myositis ossificans in paraplegics, J. Bone Joint Surg. [Am.] **31**:283, 1949.

55. Muheim, G., Donath, A., and Rossier, A. B.: Serial scintigraphies in the course of ectopic-bone formation in paraplegic patients, Am. J. Roentgenol. **118**:865, 1973.

56. Mulholland, J. H., Co Tui, Wright, A. M., et al.: Protein metabolism and bed sores, Ann. Surg. **118**:1015, 1943.

57. Nicholas, J. J.: Ectopic bone formation in patients with spinal cord injury, Arch. Phys. Med. Rehabil. **54**:354, 1973.

58. Putnam, T., Calenoff, L., Betts, H. B., and Rosen, J. S.: Sinography in management of decubitus ulcers, Arch. Phys. Med. Rehabil. **59**:243, 1978.

59. Reichel, S. M.: Shearing force as a factor in decubitus ulcers in paraplegics, J.A.M.A. **166**:762, 1958.

60. Resnick, D., and Niwayama, G.: Radiographic and pathologic features of spinal involvement in diffuse idiopathic skeletal hyperostosis (DISH), Radiology **119**:559, 1976.

61. Resnick, D., Shapiro, R. F., Wiesner, K. B., et al.: Diffuse idiopathic skeletal hyperostosis (DISH), Semin. Arthritis Rheum. **7**:153, 1978.

62. Resnick, D., Shaul, S. R., and Robins, J. M.: Diffuse idiopathic skeletal hyperostosis (DISH): Forestier's disease with extraspinal manifestations, Radiology **115**:513, 1975.

63. Reswick, J. B., and Simoes, N.: Application of engineering principles in management of spinal cord injured patients, Clin. Orthop. **112**:124, 1975.

64. Rimoin, D. L.: Pachydermoperiostosis (idiopathic clubbing and periostosis): genetic and physiologic considerations, N. Engl. J. Med. **272**:923, 1965.

65. Roberts, P. H.: Heterotopic ossification complicating paralysis of intracranial origin, J. Bone Joint Surg. [Br.] **50**:70, 1968.

66. Rossier, A. B., Bussat, P., Infante, F., et al.: Current facts on para-osteo-arthropathy (POA), Paraplegia **11**:36, 1973.

67. Russell, R. G. G., and Smith, R.: Diphosphonates, J. Bone Joint Surg. [Br.] **55**:66, 1973.

68. Sahgal, V.: Personal communication, 1979.

69. Schumacher, T. M., Genant, H. K., Kellet, M. J., et al.: HLA-B27 associated arthropathies, Radiology **126**:289, 1978.

70. Shea, J. D.: Pressure sores: classification and management, Clin. Orthop. **112**:89, 1975.

71. Silver, J. R.: Heterotopic ossification. A clinical study of its possible relationship to trauma, Paraplegia **7**:220, 1969.

72. Soule, A. B.: Neurogenic ossifying fibromyopathies: a preliminary report, J. Neurosurg. **2**:485, 1945.

73. Stover, S. I., Hataway, C. J., and Zeiger, H. E.: Heterotopic ossification in spinal cord injured patients, Arch. Phys. Med. Rehabil. **56**:199, 1975.

74. Stover, S. L., Niemann, K. W., and Miller, J. M.: Disodium etidronate in the prevention of postoperative re-

currence of heterotopic ossification in spinal cord injured patients, J. Bone Joint Surg. [Am.] **58:**683, 1976.

75. Tanaka, T., Rossier, A. B., et al.: Quantitative assessment of para-osteo-arthropathy and its maturation on serial radionuclide bone images, Radiology **123:**217, 1977.

76. Tibone, J., Sakimura, I., Nickel, V. L., and Hsu, J. D.: Heterotopic ossification around the hip in spinal cord-injured patients, J. Bone Joint Surg. [Am.] **60:**769, 1978.

77. Wakim, K. G.: A review of denervation atrophy with some comment on the results of electric stimulation in humans and in animals, Clin. Orthop. **12:**63, 1958.

78. Weiss, A. A.: Management of decubitus ulcers, N.Y. State J. Med. **60:**79, 1960.

79. Wharton, G. W.: Heterotopic ossification, Clin. Orthop. **112:**142, 1975.

80. Wharton, G. W., and Morgan, T. H.: Ankylosis in the paralyzed patient, J. Bone Joint Surg. [Am.] **52:**105, 1970.

81. Wright, V., Catterall, R. D., and Cook, J. P.: Bone and joint changes in paraplegic men, Ann. Rheum. Dis. **24:**419, 1965.

82. Yeoman, M. P., and Hardy, A. G.: Pathology and treatment of pressure sores in paraplegics, Br. J. Plast. Surg. **11:**179, 1954.

83. Zackin, H. J.: Management of decubitus ulcers in paraplegic patients, South. Med. J. **71:**574, 1978.

CHAPTER 17

Joint changes after spinal cord injury

RONALD W. HENDRIX, M.D.

Changes in the joints of spinal cord injured patients range from unimportant curiosities to potentially life-threatening problems. Joint contractures cause abnormal posture and limitation of transfers and may lead to pressure sore formation. A septic joint may lead to osteomyelitis of adjacent bones and will surely necessitate surgery in some form for its treatment. Joint subluxation and dislocation occur most often in the hip and usually have minor consequences for the patient. Joint narrowing and intra-articular ankylosis occur in specific joints but do not lead to patient debility. Neuropathic joints are rarely seen in spinal cord injured patients in spite of their neurologic deficit.

JOINT NARROWING

Joint narrowing in spinal cord injured patients occurs in several joints without any evidence of other pathology. These joints are below the cord level and are usually noted coincidentally on radiographs from urograms or cystourethrograms. The hips, the sacroiliac joints, and less frequently the symphysis pubis are the joints that become involved.[1] Sacroiliac joint narrowing probably reflects a stage in time that will eventually terminate in an ankylosed joint. Sacroiliac joint narrowing is asymptomatic, and no clinical significance has been determined to result from it.

The earliest time that sacroiliac joint abnormalities have been described after spinal cord injury is at 3 months.[44] No correlation between the sacroiliac changes and the presence of pressure sores or abnormal uro-

graphic findings could be demonstrated.[27,44] Urethral discharge was cultured from a group of these patients, but the findings did not correlate with sacroiliac joint changes.

Narrowing of the hip joints has also been described in patients with flaccid paralysis.[31] It is thought that this joint narrowing is due to atrophy of the articular cartilage. A large portion of the articular cartilage receives nutrition from the synovial fluid, and a smaller portion of the cartilage is nourished from diffusion from the adjacent bone. Cartilage is composed of scattered cells embedded in a sea of protein polysaccharide. The protein polysaccharide contains considerable water, which is driven from the protein complex with the pressure applied to it from weight bearing. With weight bearing the cartilage becomes slightly thinner but resumes its original shape when the stress is removed. Along with resuming its original shape, the amount of water that was previously lost is reabsorbed. Weight bearing, as in walking, accomplishes the pumping action necessary for the diffusion of synovial fluid through the protein polysaccharide and the consequent nutrition of the cartilage and carrying away of metabolic wastes. Presumably the cartilage atrophies because of less effective nutrition from lack of weight bearing in spinal cord injured patients. When hip joint narrowing does occur, it will do so within the first 2 years after spinal cord injury in at least half of the patients.[31] We have seen this occur in less than 1 year in many patients and as rapidly as 6 months in a few cases.

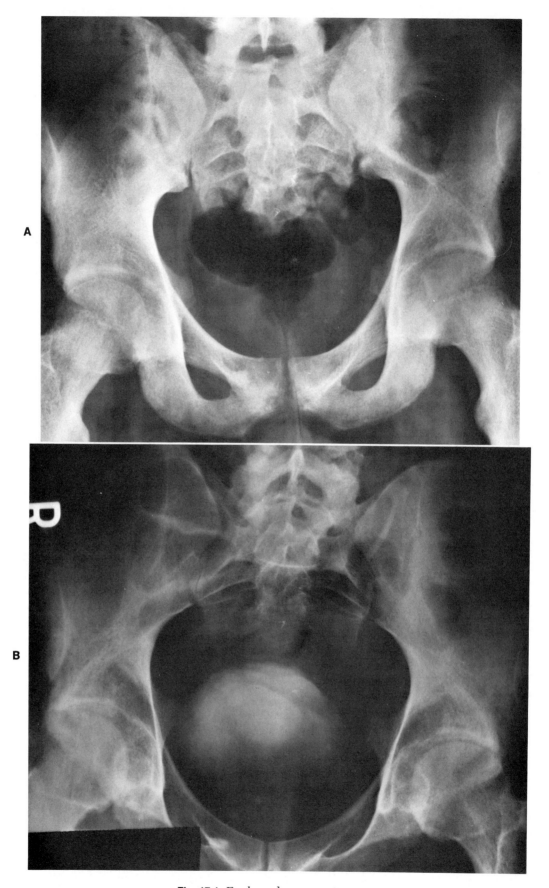

Fig. 17-1. For legend see opposite page.

Radiologic findings

The radiologic findings in the hip are those of a uniformly narrowed joint initially (Figs. 15-31 and 16-13). The joint is narrowed more superiorly and axially than horizontally. At this stage the narrowing usually stabilizes at approximately 2 mm width superiorly and axially. The normal joint space measures approximately 4.5 mm axially and superiorly.[15] The early joint narrowing characteristically occurs from 6 to 24 months after a cord injury. No osteophyte formation accompanies the narrowing at this stage. Usually the narrowing is stable for several years. In some patients irregular joint narrowing and marginal osteophyte formation are seen to

replace the uniform initial narrowing 5 to 10 or more years after a spinal cord injury. The joint space may become essentially obliterated in some areas (Fig. 17-1). We have not seen joint fusion result after such narrowing. Many patients surviving more than 10 years have had joint infection or a Girdlestone resection of the hip, which precludes seeing these changes. The joint narrowing is variable with more rapid evolution and more extensive changes in some patients than in others but without a satisfactory explanation.

The normal sacroiliac joint width measures 2 to 5 mm on radiographs.[32] Serial radiographs are needed to demonstrate narrowing with certainty (Fig. 17-2). The joint

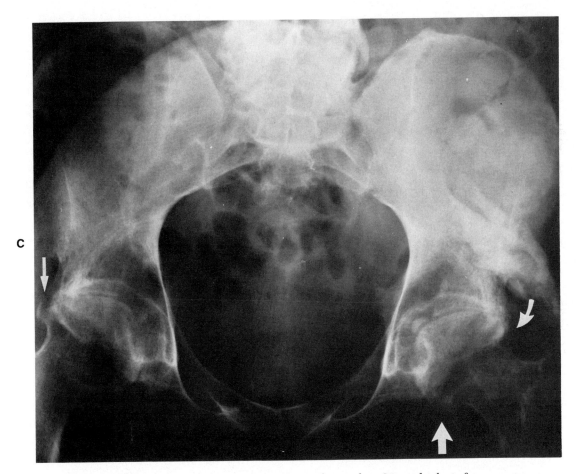

Fig. 17-1. Progression of joint changes in a man with complete C6 quadriplegia from a motor vehicle accident at 18 years of age. **A,** Two years after injury. Hip joints are normal. Bony erosions on both sides of symphysis pubis are present. Sacroiliac joint margins are somewhat indistinct. **B,** Four years after injury. There is definite narrowing of both hip joints superiorly. Erosions of symphysis pubis have resolved, with resultant narrowing. Both sacroiliac joints are narrower. **C,** Eleven years after injury. There has been further progression of hips joint narrowing. There is narrowing in horizontal axial and vertical directions with greatest narrowing superiorly. Osteophytes are forming at articular margins of femoral heads *(arrows)*, and there is change in shape of femoral heads. Symphysis pubis has fused completely. Sacroiliac joints are significantly narrow. Patient has had bilateral partial ischial resections for pressure sores.

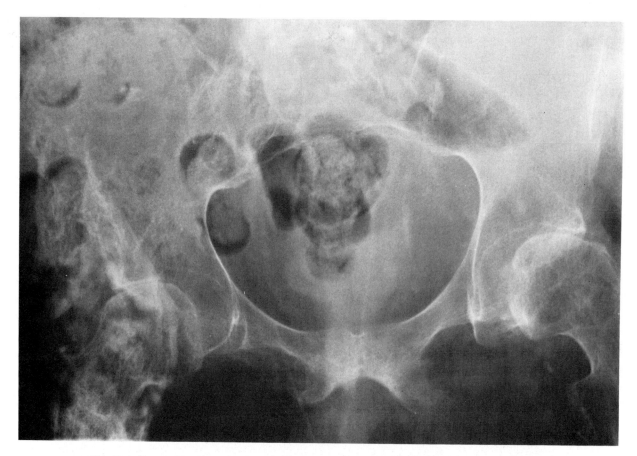

Fig. 17-2. Joint narrowing in 40-year-old male with C6 quadriplegia for 25 years. Definite narrowing of both sacroiliac joints is present. Joints measure approximately 1 mm in width. Symphysis pubis has completely fused. Left femoral head is deformed and subluxated. Both hip joints are markedly narrow.

can be measured from a routine anterior-posterior view of the pelvis. Oblique radiographs significantly magnify the size of the sacroiliac joints and will result in faulty measurements. Etiology of the joint narrowing is uncertain,[27] and no known clinical significance has been attached to narrowing of these joints.

JOINT CONTRACTURES

Daily range-of-motion exercises are necessary to prevent joint contractures. This prevents shortening of one muscle group and stretching of the opposing group. It also prevents capsular and pericapsular changes.[11] Usually joint contractures occur after the patient leaves the hospital and the daily exercises are not continued or are continued in an intermittent fashion. It is frequently difficult to convince the patient and his family of the importance of these exercises.

The contracture is most commonly caused by muscle imbalance. This also includes an imbalance of spasm in opposing muscle groups. In the upper extremity quadriplegic patients, flexion and supination contractures occur at the same time at the elbow.[17] In the shoulder there is shortening of the adductors and contraction with the shoulder in internal rotation.[11]

Spasticity greatly hastens the occurrence of contractures. The onset of a contracture must be dealt with quickly when it occurs or it will lead to a fixed deformity.[11] At times what is thought clinically to be the evolution of a joint contracture is an early stage in the development of ectopic ossification. If vigorous range-of-motion exercises are not performed, the joint will ankylose rapidly.[43] In the hips, adduction and flexion contractures are most commonly seen. However, extension contractures can occur less frequently. In the knee, flexion contractures are seen most commonly; however, occasionally an extension contracture occurs. Contractures of the hip joints lead to an asymmetric sitting position. This imbalance can lead to scoliosis or hyperlordosis of the lumbar and thoracic spine[19] and to ischial pressure sore formation.[26]

Radiologic findings

Radiography is not necessary to make the diagnosis of joint flexion contractures. The radiologic examination

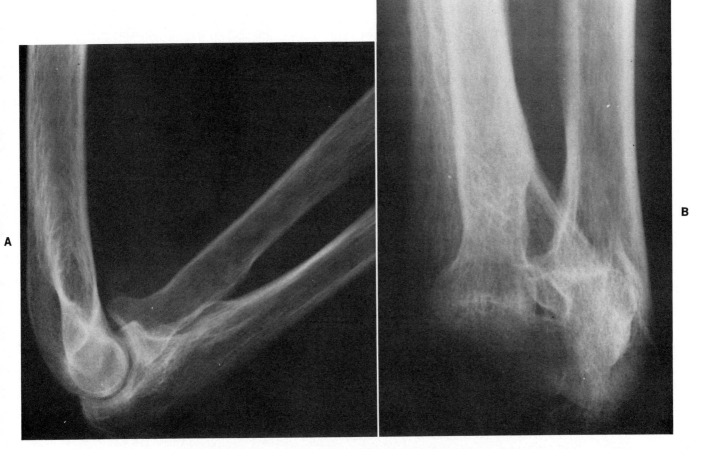

Fig. 17-3. Elbow flexion contracture in 39-year-old man with C5 quadriplegia for 15 years. **A,** Lateral projection demonstrates flexion of 125°. **B,** Anteroposterior view was obtained with film parallel to humerus along posterior surface of arm.

merely demonstrates the absence or presence of additional pathology in the region of the joint, such as ectopic bone formation or joint sepsis. Interpretation of the radiograph from such a joint is hindered because of the inability to obtain radiographs using standard radiographic positioning (Figs. 17-3 and 17-4). Normally one view, usually the lateral projection, of a major joint is relatively normal in appearance. If bilateral flexion contractures are present, obtaining even one view in nearly normal projection may be very difficult especially in the hips (Fig. 17-6, *E*).

Normally the lateral view of the elbow or knee and the AP view of the shoulder are relatively normal appearing. A contracture of the elbow or knee joints may demonstrate much greater flexion than is usually possible with a normal joint and much greater flexion than is seen with standard radiographic positioning (Fig. 17-3). The shoulder will be held in internal rotation, and it will be impossible to obtain the routine external rotation view. Gross distortion and magnification will oc-

cur on the AP views of the knees, hips, elbow, wrists, or digits. This appearance is quite foreign when compared to a normal joint. A radiologic examination with multiple normal views cannot be expected in a contracted joint. The examination will be limited because of the positioning difficulties. Except for the hip, these joints will appear narrowed on the AP projection (Figs. 17-4 and 17-5). In the AP or PA projection the x-ray beam does not traverse the joint tangential to the articular surfaces on both sides of the joint as it does with standard positioning. This results in overlapping of the joint surfaces and a suggestion of narrowing. A lateral film will demonstrate that the joint space is not narrow (Fig. 17-6, *A* and *B*). These findings apply only to flexion contractures but not to extension contractures. There should be little difficulty radiographing a joint with an extension contracture in the AP projection. Lateral views of the hips will be difficult to obtain if there are bilateral extension contractures because the opposite femur is in the way.

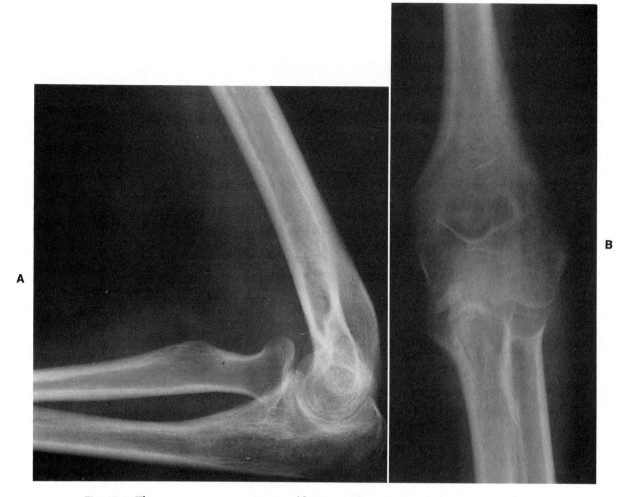

Fig. 17-4. Flexion contracture in 23-year-old C6 complete quadriplegic woman. **A,** Flexion contracture of 110° is present. **B,** AP view of elbow demonstrates overlap of capitellum and radial head because of contracture, preventing extension of elbow. This appearance of elbow because of contracture is less extreme but more common than appearance in Fig. 17-3, *B*.

JOINT ANKYLOSIS

Joint ankylosis in spinal cord injured patients occurs in two ways. The most common type is *extra-articular ankylosis*, which was disucssed in detail in Chapter 16. The less common form of ankylosis is an *intra-articular ankylosis*. This occurs in the sacroiliac joints and in the symphysis pubis but is not seen in other joints. In two large studies[1,28] intra-articular ankylosis has been reported in the sacroiliac joints in 11% and 28% of the patients. Ankylosis, narrowing, and erosions of the symphysis pubis were grouped together with a total incidence of 28% of patients in one study.[4]

No correlation could be made between the incidence of sacroiliac joint ankylosis and the patient's age, infection in the genitourinary tract, level of the cord lesion, pressure sores, bladder calculi, or joint contractures.[1,44]

Ankylosis in the sacroiliac joints occurred more frequently in patients who were confined to bed for longer-than-usual periods, in patients whose admission to a spinal cord facility was delayed, and in patients for whom mobilization was delayed.[44] We found such ankylosis occurred more frequently in patients with long-standing paralysis. However, there is disagreement in the literature on this point.[1,4]

The etiology of sacroiliac joint or symphysis pubis ankylosis is unknown. A suggestion that the changes are similar to those of ankylosing spondylitis[1] is not supported by changes in the lumbar spine.[44] Adjacent pressure sores as a possible cause[39] have not been supported by multiple investigators.[4,44] No significant correlation between genitourinary infection and sacroiliac joint changes has been demonstrated.[27,44] Severe mechanical

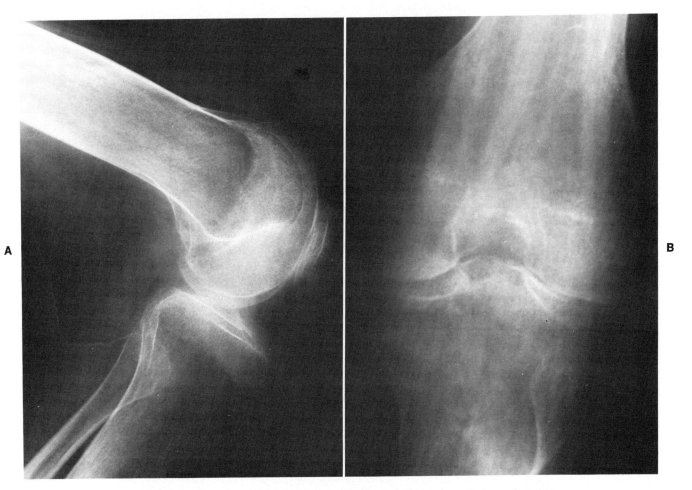

Fig. 17-5. Knee joint contracture in C6 16-year-old quadriplegic boy. **A,** Lateral projection demonstrates 90° flexion contracture. **B,** AP view shows marked positional magnification of bones, with overlapping of articular surfaces of femoral condyles and tibial plateau.

stress from transfers and crutch walking without adjacent muscle support has also been suggested as a possible etiology.[44]

Histologic material from ankylosed sacroiliac joints is almost nonexistent. One biopsy[1] revealed gross obliteration of the joint space and cartilage. The adjacent bone was atrophic and very vascular. Microscopically the joint was not completely obliterated, but the articular cartilage was destroyed and the bony surface was ragged.

Erosions of the bony margins of the sacroiliac joints and the symphysis pubis (Fig. 17-6, *C* and *D*) occur, but no definite disability has accompanied such erosions. This appears to be the earliest stage of a progression that ends in narrowing and ankylosis of the joint (Fig. 17-1).

No known clinical problems arise from ankylosis of the sacroiliac joints or symphysis pubis. This ankylosis is usually a coincidental findings on an urogram or lumbar spine radiograph.

Radiologic findings

The radiologic findings are straightforward. Usually portions of the sacroiliac joint space remain visible (Fig. 17-7). Bars of bony trabeculae crossing the joint space or complete obliteration of portions of the joint may be seen. The superior one third to one half of the sacroiliac joint is the interosseous sacroiliac ligament. The inferior one half to two thirds of the joint is a synovial joint.[32] Both parts of the joint may ankylose. Narrowing and ankylosis appear to occur earliest in the synovial portion of the joint (Fig. 17-2).

The symphysis pubis first narrows and later fuses (Fig. 17-2). The superior and inferior joint margins fuse first followed by eventual fusion of the entire joint (Figs. 17-1, 17-2, and 17-7).

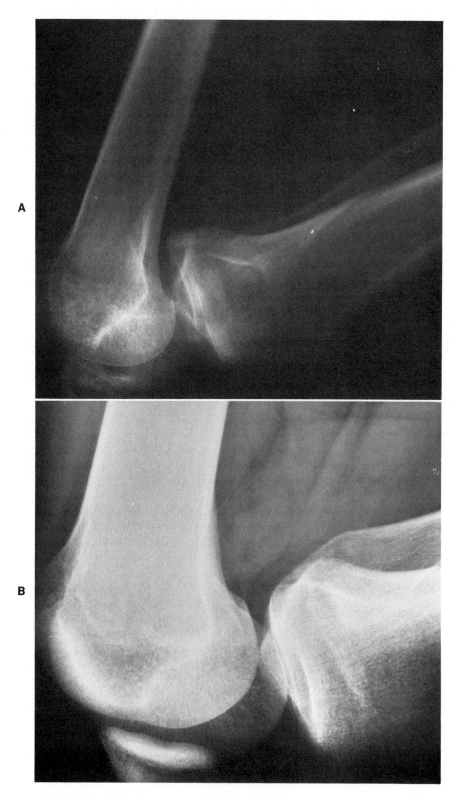

Fig. 17-6. A, Extreme flexion contracture of knee in 21-year-old quadriplegic man. Posterior margin of tibial plateau lies very close to shaft of femur. Significant loss of soft tissue mass from muscle atrophy allows joint to be flexed to this extreme. Shortening of flexor muscles and stretching of extensor muscles of knee are active factors in development of contracture. **B,** Maximal flexion in normal knee of 25-year-old man shown for comparison.

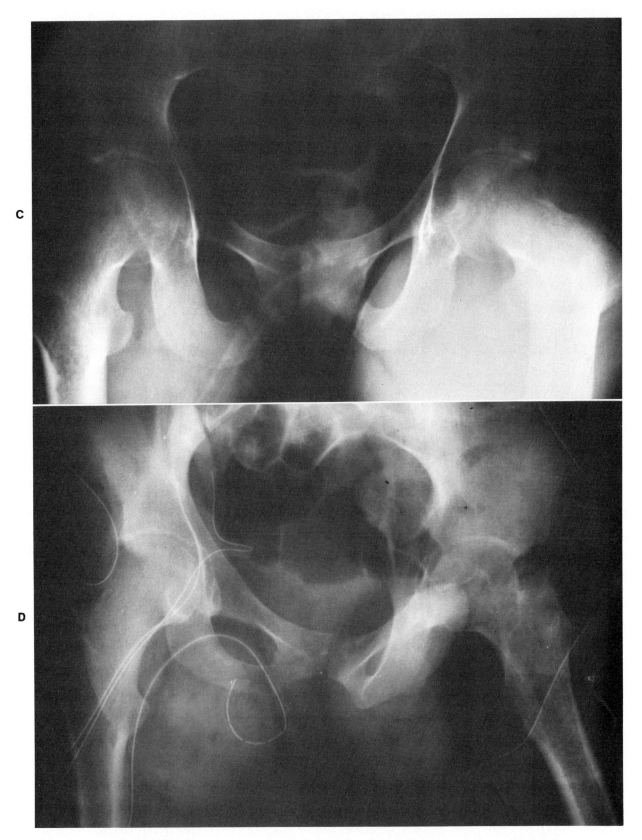

Fig. 17-6, cont'd. C, Flexion contracture of left hip in same patient as in **A.** Proximal left femur has an unusual appearance when compared to right hip. There is foreshortening of femoral neck and intertrochanteric area. **D,** Intertrochanteric area and femoral neck have returned to normal appearance after soft tissue surgical release was performed.

Continued.

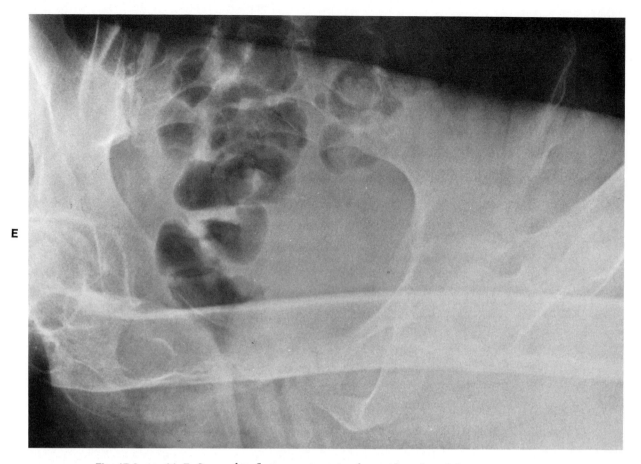

E

Fig. 17-6, cont'd. E, Severe hip flexion contractures but without hip dislocation in 25-year-old woman.

Fig. 17-7. Ankylosis of sacroiliac joints in 36-year-old man with T11 paraplegia for 19 years. **A,** Superior portion of each sacroiliac joint is seen but inferior two thirds are fused. There is narrowing of superior portion of symphysis pubis, which will probably progress to ankylosis in the future. **B,** Right posterior oblique view of left sacroiliac joint. Superior third of sacroiliac joint is preserved as can be seen on anterior view. There is severe narrowing of inferior two thirds, the synovial portion, of sacroiliac joint. The most inferior portion of joint demonstrates complete ankylosis.

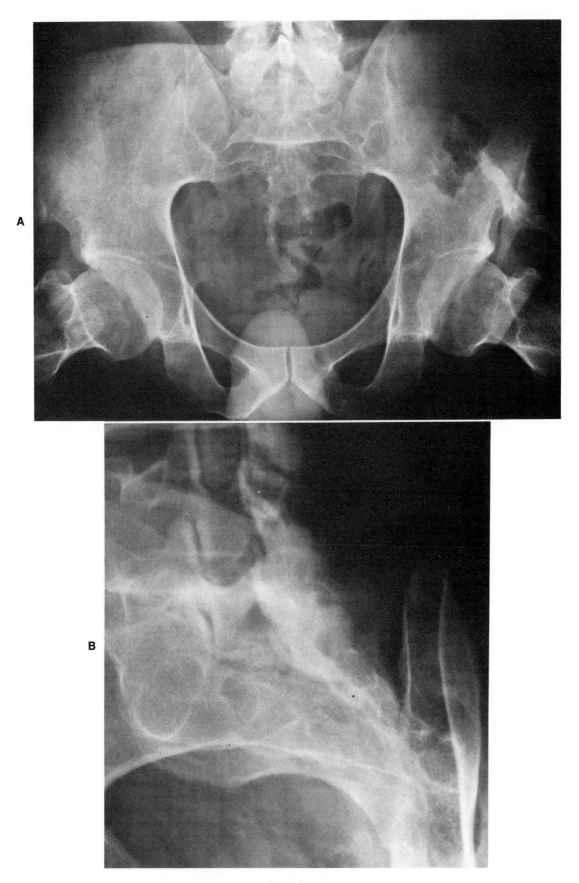

Fig. 17-7. For legend see opposite page.

JOINT INFECTION

Joint infection is not an infrequent complication in spinal cord injured patients. The hip is the most frequently infected joint with knee and ankle infection occurring considerably less often.[18,22] Joint infection is most often seen in patients with long-standing paralysis.[16,35] There is almost always an associated pressure sore, which may appear innocuous clinically. The joint usually becomes infected from a sinus tract penetrating into the joint. The sinus characteristically originates from a trochanteric or less frequently from an ischial pressure sore. Joint sepsis also occurs but less often after surgical treatment of an ischial or trochanteric pressure sore[18] or after excision of ectopic bone.[42] Sepsis of the knee or ankle joints occurs secondary to a pressure sore over the medial or less frequently over the lateral aspect of either joint in a patient with severe spasticity. Adductor and flexor spasms cause friction of the soft tissues of the medial aspect of the knees and ankles rubbing on one another or from the rubbing of soft tis-sues lateral to the joint on bed clothing. Friction increases the susceptibility of skin to ulceration at lower pressures than are otherwise necessary.[13] Pressure sores can also occur over the dorsal or plantar surfaces of the toes, particularly in patients with toe joint contractures. Joints of the feet, ankles, and knees are located superficially and can become infected relatively easily from extension of a pressure sore.[22]

Clinical findings

Pain sensation is diminished or absent in spinal cord injured patients. A pressure sore is clinically obvious, but there is a striking absence of local signs to suggest joint infection when the hip is involved. This is less of a problem with the knee, ankle, and toes because soft tissue swelling is obvious. Advanced infection of the hip can cause dislocation with lower extremity shortening, adduction, and internal rotation, which may suggest the diagnosis clinically. Elevated temperature, toxicity, and malaise are the most reliable clinical signs, but they are

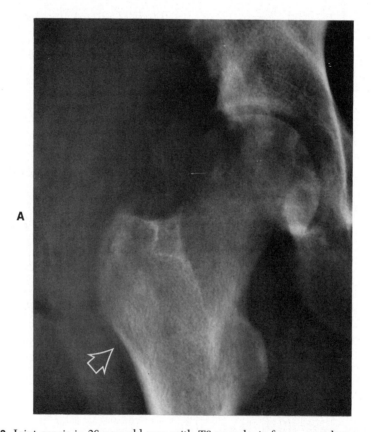

Fig. 17-8. Joint sepsis in 26-year-old man with T6 paraplegia from a gunshot wound. **A,** Six months after injury. Hip joint space is normal, and articular margins are smooth, regular, and well defined. Ectopic bone formation is present lateral to joint and greater trochanter. Air is present in trochanteric pressure sore. Greater tuberosity has a fuzzy appearance indicating bone erosion from adjacent pressure sore. Some periosteal new bone formation is present immediately inferior to greater trochanter (*arrow*).

usually misinterpreted as resulting from a urinary tract infection.[16] Joint aspiration is the earliest method to make a certain diagnosis.[34] Early detection of joint infection is of paramount importance for early treatment to prevent irreversible joint destruction in normal patients. Because virtually all spinal cord injured patients who develop a joint infection are unable to walk, a joint infection does not have the same catastrophic results that it does in normal patients. Severe complications, some of which may be related to subsequent treatment, may occur. Joint sepsis may lead to osteomyelitis, necessitating surgery (Fig. 17-8). Osteomyelitis may spread to adjacent bones after surgery (see Fig. 15-10). Surgical resection of the femoral head and neck[20] and acetabulum or disarticulation may be necessary for definitive treatment of a complicating osteomyelitis.[18,36]

Radiologic findings

The earliest radiologic finding of joint infection is diffuse soft tissue swelling from a joint effusion and local, nonspecific edema. Technetium pertechnetate joint scanning is the most sensitive imaging modality available for early diagnosis of abnormal synovial activity.[3,21] The joint scan is not specific for septic arthritis but will indicate any synovitis with resultant hyperemia. An adjacent pressure sore may cause increased activity, but usually this should not cause diagnostic difficulties. Local views in multiple projections over the area of interest should allow differentiation of joint activity from activity in the adjacent soft tissues in most cases. Radiologic findings specific enough to make a diagnosis of septic arthritis do not occur until after significant destructive change occurs in the joint.[6,10] Clinical suspi-

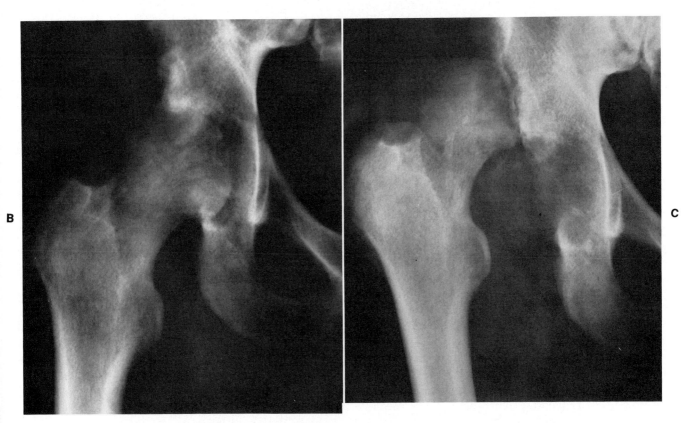

Fig. 17-8, cont'd. B, Eight months after injury. Articular cartilage of superior portion of joint has been completely destroyed as evidenced by narrowing of joint. Femoral head is subluxated laterally. Articular margin of femoral head and superior portion of acetabulum are less distinct, indicating direct erosion of these bones. Air is seen in soft tissues lateral to joint and greater trochanter. Joint infection followed extension of a fistula from pressure sore into joint. Periosteal new bone formation immediately inferior to greater trochanter has progressed. **C,** One week after **B.** Dislocation of femoral head has occurred. Superior margin of acetabulum is quite indistinct. Indistinctness of trabecular bone in right femoral head and neck is significantly different than that seen earlier, **A,** indicating that bone is being resorbed rapidly. Air is seen within pressure sore superimposed both on lateral femoral head and greater trochanter. Ectopic bone is again seen in soft tissues.

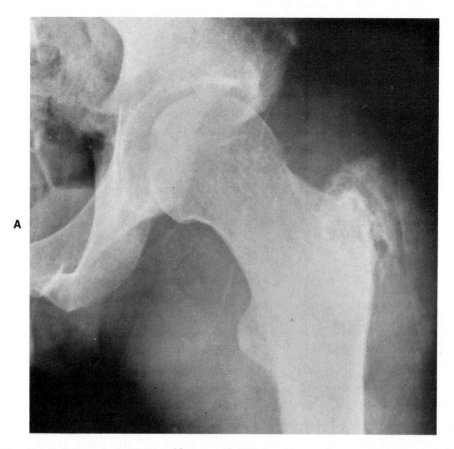

Fig. 17-9. Joint sepsis in 21-year-old man with T10 flaccid paraplegia secondary to gunshot wound. **A,** One year after injury. Ectopic bone is superimposed on greater trochanter, thus predisposing patient to pressure sore formation. Hip joint is normal.

cion of infection in the hip joint of spinal cord injured patients normally does not occur, if at all, until long after significant destructive changes have occurred. Usually the joint infection has progressed to the point of subluxation or complete dislocation before the radiologic diagnosis is made (Fig. 17-9). Frequently the dislocation is coincidentally detected on a routine urogram or cystogram. Nevertheless, it is important to know the sequence of radiologic changes that do occur in order to identify a septic joint as early as possible so treatment can be started and complications such as osteomyelitis held to a minimum.

Diffuse soft tissue swelling adjacent to the joint is the earliest radiologic finding and is easier to appreciate in the knee, ankle, or foot than in the hip especially in adults. A decrease of mineral in the bones adjacent to an infected joint occurs secondary to local hyperemia. This may not always be detectable because of existing bone atrophy. Patients in whom hip joint infection occurs usually have had paralysis long enough to develop some degree of disuse bone atrophy.[16] The articular cartilage is destroyed by an enzyme produced by the in-

fection.[6,8,9] The radiologic manifestation of this cartilage destruction is narrowing of the joint. Interpretation of hip joint narrowing as evidence for a septic joint in spinal cord injured pateints must be done with care. If joint narrowing occurs in a joint adjacent to a pressure sore, a sinus tract originating in the ulcer should be diligently sought. If a sinus is found, examination with a sinogram will determine its relation to the joint. Most hip and knee joint narrowing in spinal cord injured patients, however, is caused by cartilage degeneration that is probably secondary to disuse.[31] It is only rarely caused by a joint infection. The joint narrowing should be bilateral and symmetric if cartilage degeneration is the cause. Usually there is no adjacent pressure sore in such cases, making the diagnosis easy if clinical correlation is made with the radiologic findings.

Later, after cartilage destruction occurs, the underlying bone becomes involved and erosions of the cortical margin occur. Radiologically the normally smooth, sharply defined articular margin on both sides of the joint becomes fuzzy and indistinct. The bone erosions will be uneven and the bone margin will become irreg-

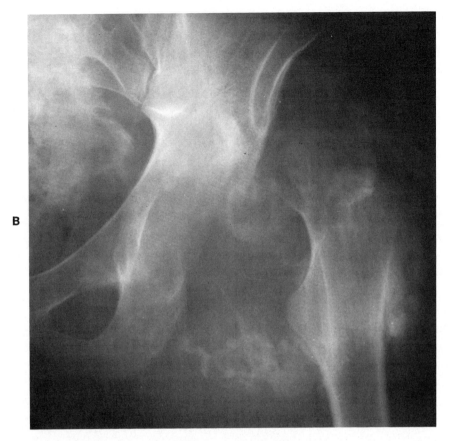

Fig. 17-9, cont'd. B, Two years after injury. Pressure sore formed over greater trochanter and eroded into joint. This caused a joint infection and led to hip dislocation. Superior margin of acetabulum has been eroded. Cortical margin of femoral head is indistinct and demineralized. These are radiologic findings of osteomyelitis that were present in femoral head and in acetabular margin. Surgical resection of infected bone was necessary for treatment.

ular (Fig. 17-8). The pressure in the joint increases with the duration of the infectious process, which in the hip eventually results in subluxation of the femoral head. This progresses usually until complete dislocation occurs with the femoral head occupying a position superior and posterior to the acetabulum.[16,18] Muscle spasms may also play an important role in such a dislocation. With dislocation the vascular supply to the femoral head can be significantly impaired and avascular necrosis may occur. If left untreated, disintegration and resorption of the femoral head may occur.[16]

Identification of the joint infection at any one of the above stages allows institution of appropriate treatment that will arrest the progress of the sepsis.

Treatment

Treatment of a septic joint is exemplified by the treatment that has been successful in the hip. Two different approaches have been used.[16,18] In the less extensively infected joint when osteomyelitis is not present

in the adjacent bones, incision and drainage are employed and are sufficient. In patients with infection involving adjacent bone, excision of the infected femoral head and neck, acetabulum, and adjacent necrotic soft tissues is necessary. In either case the wound is either packed open and allowed to granulate in or a rotational full thickness skin flap is used to cover the skin defect. Supportive measures as outlined for pressure sores in Chapter 16 are followed.[16,18]

JOINT DISLOCATION AND SUBLUXATION

Dislocation and subluxation differ by degree, and the terms should not be used interchangeably. Subluxation is an intermediate stage in a spectrum that includes a normal joint at one extreme and dislocation at the opposite extreme. Dislocation of a joint is complete disruption of the joint with displacement of opposing contiguous articular surfaces so that they are no longer in contact (Fig. 17-9, *B*). Subluxation, on the other hand, is an incomplete dislocation with a portion of the articular surfaces maintaining contact. The articular surface on one side of the joint is displaced from its usual position, causing the opposing articular surfaces not to mesh normally with one another (Fig. 17-8, *B*).

Joint subluxation and dislocation are seen primarily in the hip joints in spinal cord injured patients. The subluxation or dislocation may be unilateral or bilateral and usually occurs in bed-bound patients.[29] An exception occurs when the patient has paralytic scoliosis with a pelvic tilt.[30]

Pathogenesis

There are three mechanisms that can lead to dislocation of the hip joint. The most common cause is severe spasticity with resulting adductor spasm. Joint sepsis also causes subluxation. A combination of joint sepsis and adductor spasm may be present simultaneously with resulting dislocation (Figs. 17-8 and 17-9). Scoliosis with a pelvic tilt is the third mechanism. The tilted pelvis is the important feature. When scoliosis occurs, secondary curves in the opposite direction may

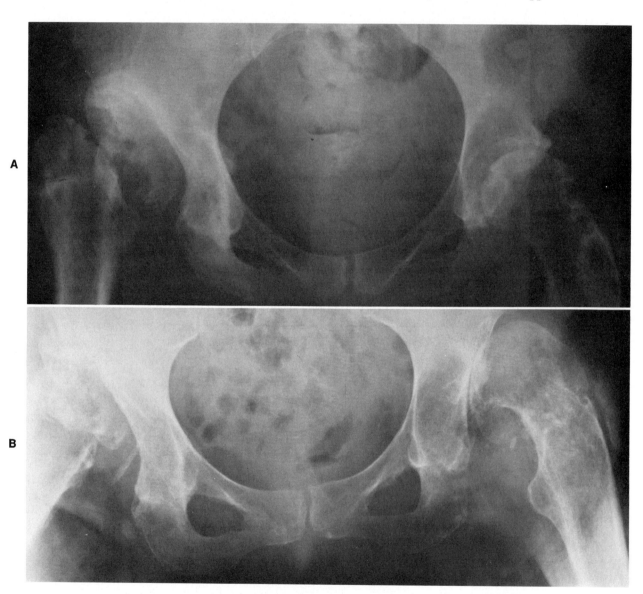

Fig. 17-10. Hip dislocation in woman with T8 paraplegia since 28 years of age. **A,** Eight years after motor vehicle accident. Girdlestone procedure has been performed on right because of pressure sores. Pseudoacetabulum has formed superior to normal joint. In left hip, marginal osteophyte formation affects superior margin of femoral head. Ectopic bone is present over partially resected greater trochanter. **B,** Twenty-two years after injury. Left hip has dislocated and articulates now with iliac wing. Huge osteophytes have formed at medial and lateral articular margins of femoral head. Pseudoacetabulum on the right has enlarged.

develop to compensate for the primary curve in order to maintain a level pelvis and level shoulders. As discussed in Chapter 15, the most common type of curve caused by paralysis is a long C-shaped curve without a compensatory curve. The pelvis may participate in this scoliosis and become tilted. A scoliosis with level shoulders and a level pelvis is called a compensated scoliosis and will not result in pelvic tilt and hip dislocation. With pelvic tilt the hip on the concave side of the scoliotic curve is adducted and the other hip is abducted. The pelvis comes to lie over the femoral head on the abducted side, and the hip on the opposite side goes into extreme adduction. This puts stretch on the superior aspect of the hip joint capsule, which eventually stretches and allows the femoral head to slide laterally first to subluxate and later to dislocate (see Fig. 15-27). The acetabular angle, which is usually approximately 45° with respect to the horizontal plane, may be rotated to 90° with the pelvis tilted due to scoliosis (see Fig. 15-25).

Joint sepsis, when it occurs, is almost always secondary to a fistula from a pressure sore eroding into the joint. The pressure sore is usually over the greater trochanter area and rarely from the ischial area. If the pressure sore erodes down to the joint and erodes a large hole in the joint capsule, purulent material can drain easily from the joint and dislocation is not expected to occur from pressure buildup. If, however, the joint becomes infected from a small-diameter fistula, the fistula can wall itself off and sufficient pus can form in the joint to result in a marked increase of joint pressure and lateral dislocation of the femoral head (Figs. 17-8 and 17-9).

Radiologic findings

Dislocation of a hip is easily identified radiographically (Figs. 17-10 and 17-11). The femoral head dislocates superiorly and posteriorly.[18] The femoral head then will articulate with the lateral aspect of the iliac wing, and if the patient is ambulatory, a pseudoacetab-

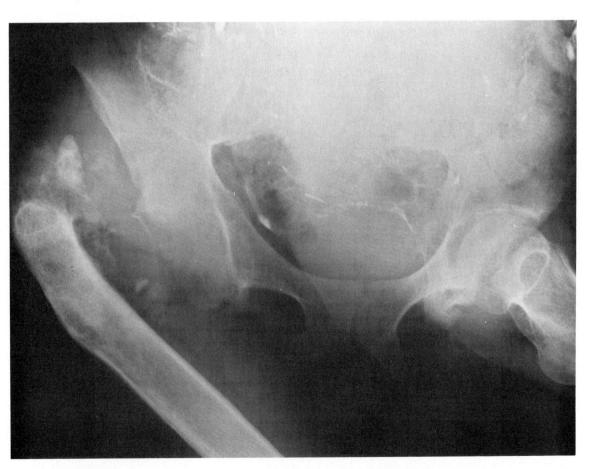

Fig. 17-11. Hip dislocation in 31-year-old man with T2 complete paraplegia for 11 years. Severe flexion deformity is present in both hips. Extreme adduction and flexor spasm led to dislocation of right hip. Because of severe flexion contracture, right femoral head does not articulate with iliac wing. Ectopic bone is superimposed on femoral head.

ulum will develop (Fig. 17-10). Eventually changes will occur in the femoral head and innominate bone. The femoral head will change shape because of its articulation with the iliac wing and osteophytes will form at the articular margins of the femoral head (Fig. 17-10). Avascular necrosis may occur in the femoral head from tearing of the nutrient vessels to the head because of dislocation.[41] The necrotic bone will appear dense compared to surrounding bone. If the dislocation occurs secondary to joint sepsis, destruction of the articular surface of the femoral head and acetabulum will probably occur. Radiographically the articular surfaces will appear indistinct and fuzzy (Fig. 17-8). Narrowing of the joint space may be detected prior to the dislocation if the latter is secondary to joint sepsis (Fig. 17-8). Usually this will be treated surgically by draining the joint or resection of the femoral head and neck or both.[18,20]

NEUROPATHIC JOINTS

Joint changes secondary to spinal cord injury were included in the original description of the neuropathic joint by Charcot in 1868.[7] Neuropathic joints have commonly been known as Charcot's joints since the publication of this description. In the past, tabes dorsalis and syringomyelia were the most common causes but diabetic neuropathy is now the most frequent etiology.[24] Charcot joints have been produced experimentally in cats by rendering a joint analgesic and anesthetic and then subjecting it to trauma.[14] Loss of sensation without trauma did not produce a neuropathic joint in the animals. Therefore a joint must lose sensation and then be subjected to repeated trauma in order to develop neuropathic changes.

Charcot joints may be seen initially as a spontaneous fracture or as an arthritis.[24,25] The arthritis is characterized as either hypertrophic or atrophic. Weight-bearing joints tend to demonstrate the hypertrophic characteristics, and non-weight-bearing joints tend to develop the atrophic characteristics.[37,38,40]

A controversy exists in the literature about the existence of neuropathic joints in patients with spinal cord injury. Multiple investigators indicate that they do not

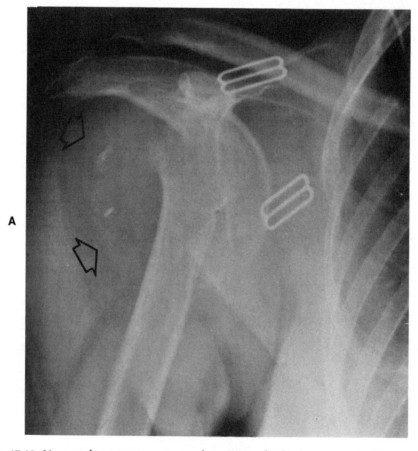

Fig. 17-12. Neuropathic joint in an incomplete C2 quadriplegic woman. **A,** Nineteen years after injury. Humeral head has been almost completely resorbed. Glenoid fossa is eroded and is several times larger than normal. A few small calcifications are seen lateral to joint in soft tissues. Soft tissue swelling is present from joint effusion *(arrows)*.

occur in these patients because the patients are not active enough to cause sufficient trauma to produce a neuropathic joint.[2,23,24] Other investigators[5,7,37] have reported a few neuropathic joints in spinal cord injured patients. The rare occurrence of Charcot joint following spinal cord injury may account for many investigators not reporting its occurrence and indicating that the lesion never occurs. Some confusion exists because ectopic bone formation as definitively described in 1918 by Dejerine and Ceillier[12] was originally ascribed to an incomplete neuropathic arthropathy. Some investigators[37] since that time have followed Dejerine's example and have called ectopic bone formation adjacent to a joint a Charcot joint. This is incorrect. The joint interior is not directly involved by ectopic bone formation in spinal cord injured patients,[33] and its etiology is unknown.

In a quadriplegic patient the most likely joints to develop Charcot features are the shoulder and elbow. Trauma of weight bearing occurs in the upper extremity during wheelchair push-ups and during transfers from bed to wheelchair, wheelchair to automobile, and so on. Quadriplegic patients with a complete cord level are never able to walk with any type of assistance so the lower extremity is not at risk to trauma from weight bearing or to development of a Charcot joint. An incomplete quadriplegic or a paraplegic patient who can ambulate with at least partial weight bearing on the lower extremities may develop a neuropathic joint in the knee, ankle, or foot. This is more likely to develop in a patient with significantly greater sensory than motor impairment. Nevertheless, the extreme infrequency of Charcot joints in spinal cord injured patients makes generalization somewhat uncertain.

Radiologic findings

A hypertrophic-type joint may demonstrate findings consisting of diffuse sclerosis of adjacent bone ends, fragmentation and erosion of the articular cortex, marginal osteophytes, loose bone fragments within the joint, and bone formation in the adjacent soft tissues.[24,38] An atrophic joint, usually the shoulder, hip,

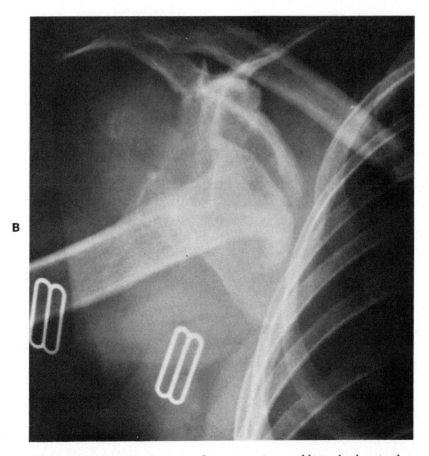

Fig. 17-12, cont'd. B, Twenty-one years after injury. Some additional sclerotic changes and erosion are present in humeral head. Position of humeral head gives an idea of how much erosion of scapula has occurred to result in enormous enlargement of glenoid fossa. Margin of eroded glenoid appears more sclerotic. A small calcification lateral to joint has increased in size.

or elbow, demonstrates erosive enlargement of the glenoid fossa, the acetabulum, or the trochlear notch and erosive absorption of the humeral or femoral side of the joint (Fig. 17-12).[37,38] Periarticular ossification is minimal in the atrophic form. Joint effusion and subluxation or dislocation are associated with both types of Charcot joints. Spontaneous fractures occur frequently in Charcot joints and may be the earliest sign of a developing neuropathic joint.[24,38] Spontaneous fractures are also common in spinal cord injured patients because of osteoporosis. A given fracture should not be assumed to imply the presence of a neuropathic arthropathy in these patients because neuropathic joints are rare.

REFERENCES

1. Abel, M. S.: Sacroiliac joint changes in traumatic paraplegics, Radiology 55:235, 1950.
2. Abramson, D. J., and Kamberg, S.: Spondylitis, pathological ossification and calcification associated with spinal-cord injury, J. Bone Joint Surg. 31:275, 1949.
3. Bekerman, C., Genant, H. K., Hoffer, P. B., et al.: Radionuclide imaging of the bones and joints of the hand, Radiology 118:653, 1975.
4. Bhate, D. V., Pizarro, A. J., Seitam, A., and Mak, E. B.: Axial skeletal changes in paraplegics, Radiology 133:55, 1979.
5. Brailsford, J. F.: Changes in bones, joints and soft tissues associated with disease or injury of the central nervous system, Br. J. Radiol. 14:320, 1941.
6. Butt, W. P.: Radiology of the infected joint, Clin. Orthop. 96:136, 1973.
7. Charcot, J. M.: Sur quelques arthropathies qui paraissent dépendre d'une lésion du cerveau ou de la moelle épinière, Arch. Physiol. Norm. Path. 1:161, 1868.
8. Clawson, D. K., and Dunn, A. W.: Management of common bacterial infections of bones and joints, J. Bone Joint Surg. [Am.] 49:164, 1967.
9. Curtiss, P. H.: Cartilage damage in septic arthritis, Clin. Orthop. 64:87, 1969.
10. Dalinka, M. K., Lally, J. F., Koniver, G., et al.: The radiology of osseous and articular infection, C. R. C. Crit. Rev. Diagn. Imaging 7:1, 1975.
11. Damanski, M.: Heterotopic ossification in paraplegia. A clinical study, J. Bone Joint Surg. [Br.] 43:286, 1961.
12. Dejerine, Mme., and Ceillier, A.: Para-ostéo-arthropathies des paraplégiques par lésion médullaire (etude clinique et radiographique), Ann. Med. (Paris) 5:497, 1918.
13. Dinsdale, S. M.: Decubitus ulcers: role of pressure and friction in causation, Arch. Phys. Med. Rehabil. 55:147, 1974.
14. Eloesser, L.: On the nature of neuropathic affections of joints, Ann. Surg. 66:201, 1917.
15. Fredensborg, N., and Nilsson, B. E.: The joint space in normal hip radiographs, Radiology 126:325, 1978.
16. Freehafer, A. A.: Sepsis of the hip in patients with advanced neurologic disease, Clin. Orthop. 29:180, 1963.
17. Freehafer, A. A.: Flexion and supination deformities of the elbow in tetraplegics, Paraplegia 15:221, 1977.
18. Freehafer, A. A., and Herndon, C. H.: Infection of the hip as a complication of advanced neurologic disease, Clin. Orthop. 64:135, 1969.
19. Gassler, R.: Differential diagnosis of hip contractures in paraplegics and their treatment, Paraplegia 11:86, 1973.
20. Girdlestone, G. R.: Acute pyogenic arthritis of the hip: operation giving free access and effective drainage, Lancet 1:419, 1943.
21. Green, F. A., and Hays, M. T.: The pertechnetate joint scan. II. Clinical considerations, Ann. Rheum. Dis. 31:278, 1972.
22. Guttmann, L.: The problem of treatment of pressure sores in spinal paraplegics, Br. J. Plast. Surg. 8:196, 1955.
23. Heilbrun, N., and Kuhn, W. G., Jr.: Erosive bone lesions and soft-tissue ossifications associated with spinal cord injuries (paraplegia), Radiology 48:579, 1947.
24. Johnson, J. T. H.: Neuropathic injuries of the hip, Clin. Orthop. 90:29, 1973.
25. Katz, I., Rabinowitz, J. G., and Dziadiw, R.: Early changes in Charcot's joints, Am. J. Roentgenol. 86:965, 1961.
26. Kilfoyle, R. M., Foley, J. J., and Norton, P. L.: Spine and pelvic deformity in childhood and adolescent paraplegia, J. Bone Joint Surg. [Am.] 47:659, 1965.
27. Liberson, M., and Mihaldzic, N.: Sacro-iliac changes and urinary infection in patients with spinal cord injuries, Br. J. Vener. Dis. 42:96, 1966.
28. Lodge, T.: Bone, joint and soft tissue changes following paraplegia, Acta Radiol. 46:435, 1956.
29. Miller, L. F.: Orthopedic problems in patients with spinal cord injuries, Proc. Clin. Paraplegia Conf. 5:19, 1956.
30. O'Brien, J. P., Dwyer, A. P., and Hodgson, A. R.: Paralytic pelvic obliquity, its prognosis and management and the development of technique for full correction of the deformity, J. Bone Joint Surg. [Am.] 57:626, 1975.
31. Pool, W. H.: Cartilage atrophy, Radiology 112:47, 1974.
32. Resnick, D., Niwayama, G., and Goergen, T. G.: Comparison of radiographic abnormalities of the sacroiliac joint in degenerative disease and ankylosing spondylitis, Am. J. Roentgenol. 128:189, 1977.
33. Rossier, A. B., Bussat, P. H., Infante, F., et al.: Current facts on para-osteo-arthropathy (POA), Paraplegia 11:36, 1973.
34. Russell, A. S., and Ansell, B. M.: Septic arthritis, Ann. Rheum. Dis. 31:40, 1972.
35. Schneider, M., and Kreeg, A. J.: Dislocation of the hip secondary to trochanteric decubitus: a complication of multiple sclerosis, J. Bone Joint Surg. [Am.] 42:1165, 1960.
36. Shea, J. D.: Pressure sores: classification and management, Clin. Orthop. 112:89, 1975.
37. Solovay, J., and Solovay, H. U.: Paraplegic neuroarthropathy, Am. J. Roentgenol. 61:475, 1949.
38. Steindler, A.: The tabetic arthropathies, J.A.M.A. 96:250, 1931.

39. Stepanek, V., and Stepanek, P.: Changes in bones and joints of paraplegics, Radiol. Clin. (Basel) **29:**28, 1960.

40. Tatkow, R. W.: Charcot disease of the wrist and the carpus, Clin. Orthop. **46:**115, 1966.

41. Theron, J.: Superselective angiography of the hip, Radiology **124:**649, 1977.

42. Wharton, G. W.: Heterotopic ossification, Clin. Orthop. **112:**142, 1975.

43. Wharton, G. W., and Morgan, T. H.: Ankylosis in the paralyzed patient, J. Bone Joint Surg. [Am.] **52:**105, 1970.

44. Wright, V., Catterall, R. D., and Cook, J. P.: Bone and joint changes in paraplegic men, Ann. Rheum. Dis. **24:**419, 1965.

PART IV

Miscellaneous aspects of spinal cord injury

CHAPTER 18

Spinal cord injury in children

LAXMAN S. KEWALRAMANI, M.D., M.S., Orth.

Spinal cord injury resulting in paraplegia or tetraplegia is a devastating affliction since present methods of treatment offer very little hope for restoration of neurologic function. The impact of permanent paralysis in an otherwise normal child often results in severe psychologic trauma to the child as well as to the parents and elicits a feeling of guilt in our society. In the United States at present the annual incidence of paralysis from spinal cord injuries is greater than the total incidence of paralytic polio during the last decade, yet the national determination to eliminate this form of catastrophic disability appears to be lacking. In the literature there is a paucity of references to spinal cord injuries in children, and most of the reported clinical series are small. Some authors have used 12 years as the upper age limit whereas others have included an age limit of 18 years without any explanation. This has added considerable confusion and controversy regarding the incidence of radiologic abnormalities, pathomechanism of injury, and prognosis. The comparison of the mechanism of injury, severity of trauma, methods of management, complications, and outcome of various series has been difficult. Since ossification of the ring apophysis of vertebral bodies starts at the age of 14 or 15 years and since most of the hospitals in the United States admit children under 15 years of age on the pediatric service, we have used 15 years as the upper age limit.

EPIDEMIOLOGIC FEATURES

The occurrence of acute spinal cord lesions in children has been reported to be rare, accounting for less than 1% to 3.3% of all cases of spinal cord injuries.[2,11,40] In Switzerland, Gehrig and Michaelis[22] carried out a survey and reported an estimated annual incidence of 15 spinal cord injuries per million population; 5% of these were children under 14 years of age, that is, there were 0.75 new cases per million children per year. According to Burke[13] 4% of all spinal cord injuries admitted to the Spinal Injuries Unit of the Austin Hospital in Heidelberg, Australia, were children. In most of these reports the term *incidence* refers only to those cases admitted to a hospital with a diagnosis of spinal cord injury. Children with a spinal cord lesion who died prior to admission or during hospital emergency treatment were probably not included with the survivors. In an epidemiologic study of spinal cord injuries in 18 counties of northern California with a population of 5.8 million for the years 1970 and 1971, we were able to identify 617 cases, 58 of which were children. Only 30 of these children were admitted; the other 28 died prior to their admission to a hospital or were dead on arrival.[33]

The average annual incidence of acute spinal cord injuries in children in this epidemiologic study was 18.2 per million population, or 9.4% of all spinal cord injuries. The incidence of hospital-admitted cases of spinal cord injuries was 8.9 per million children, or 4.8% of all spinal cord injury cases. Projected nationally this rate indicates that about 1065 children sustain an acute lesion of the spinal cord each year, and about 550 of these are admitted to a hospital. At the Regional Spinal Cord Center located in the Institute for Rehabilitation and Research, Houston, from 1970 through 1977, 733

503

Table 18-1. Spinal cord injuries by age and etiology

Etiology	Age (yr) <5	6-10	11-15	All ages (total)
Motor vehicle	22	13	45	80
Auto crash	13	6	27	46
Pedestrian-automobile	9	6	6	21
Bike-automobile	—	1	6	7
Motorcycle	—	—	6	6
Sports and recreation	—	1	41	42
Diving	—	1	28	29
Football/wrestling	—	—	10	10
Horseback riding	—	—	3	3
Firearms	5	5	11	21
Falls	—	1	8	9
Others*	1	—	2	3
TOTAL	28	20	107	155

*Airplane crash, go-carting, battered child.

patients with spinal cord injury were admitted, 97 (14%) of whom were children.[35] This apparent increase may be caused by (1) an increasing number of motor vehicle collisions and more competitive outdoor sports and recreation-related activities, (2) better quality of medical care provided during the acute phase with low case fatality rate, or (3) selective referral of children with spinal cord injuries to this center.

To draw any meaningful conclusions about the cause of spinal cord injury, neurologic patterns of deficit, radiologic features, management, and outcome in children, we have combined the California epidemiologic study (58 children) and The Institute for Rehabilitation and Research (TIRR), Houston, patient population (97 children)—a total of 155 cases (Table 18-1).

Fifty-two percent (80 children) of the spinal cord injuries were from motor vehicle collisions. In this group 57% were passengers in an automobile or pickup truck, 26% were pedestrians, 9% were bicyclists, and 7% were riding motorcycles. Spinal cord injuries from sports and recreation-related activities—diving, football, wrestling, boxing, and horseback riding, and so on—occurred in 27%. Firearms accounted for 13% of spinal cord injuries, all from accidental firing. Falls from various heights caused spinal cord injury in only 6% of cases. One child sustained a spinal cord injury in a plane crash, one was injured while riding a go-cart, and the other one was a battered child. This 2-year-old battered boy was admitted in a comatose state and died 48 hours after admission. On autopsy he was found to have a fracture of the C7 vertebral body and dislocation of C7 on T1 along with prevertebral hemorrhages. In addition, he had subdural hematoma, sagittal sinus thrombosis, old fractures of ribs, and a fracture of the distal tibia. The most common cause of spinal cord in-

jury during the first decade was motor vehicle accidents (73%) followed by firearm injuries (21%). During the second decade (11 to 15 years of age), motor vehicles accounted for only 42%, and sports and recreation-related activities accounted for 38% of injuries. Firearm injuries were about equally distributed in the two groups. Burke[13] reported no spinal cord injuries from surfing, football, trampoline, and horseback riding, and there was only one injury from diving, as compared to 27% from these activities in the present series.

Hubbard[27] reported a higher incidence of trauma in girls than in boys and a greater susceptibility to thoracic and thoracolumbar spine injuries in children and adolescents (1 to 17 years of age). Similarly other authors[11,26,40,50] have reported a higher incidence of thoracic and lumbar lesions and a slightly larger number of girls with spinal cord injury. However, in the present series there was a higher incidence of spinal cord injuries in boys than in girls (male:female ratio of 2:1), and cervical spinal cord trauma was more frequent than trauma to the thoracic and lumbar regions (ratio cervical injuries to thoracic and lumbar injuries: approximately 3:1). This difference might be due to the fact that most of the previous series[11,12,26,40,50] are from countries with fewer motor vehicles, fewer firearms, and relatively less competitive sports and recreational activities, or it may be due to the selective referral of patients to TIRR.

Fatal spinal cord lesions

In the epidemiologic study of spinal cord injuries in children, the fatality rate was 59%. Thirteen of 34 deaths occurred within 20 minutes of the injury, none occurred within 20 to 60 minutes, and seven occurred within 1 to 24 hours after trauma. An additional four deaths occurred in 1 to 30 days; and one child died 953 days after injury. All children with spinal cord injury from falls, firearms, or sports and recreation-related activities survived at least 4 years following the date of injury. Seventy-six percent of children involved in automobile-pedestrian accidents and 83% of children involved in motor vehicle crashes died. All children involved in motorcycle crashes and automobile-bicycle collisions also died.

Victims of automobile-pedestrian accidents on autopsy were found to have maceration and transection of the spinal cord at the atlanto-occipital or atlantoaxial level with fractures and/or subluxation at C1-2. In most of these patients skull fracture along with lacerations of the cerebral cortex and brain-stem region were also noted. Six children involved in bicycle-automobile collisions and motorcycle accidents were also found to have dislocation of atlanto-occipital joints, fracture of the rim of the foramen magnum along with transection of the spinal cord at the cervicomedullary junction, and laceration of the cerebral cortex. About one third of the children who died were observed to have severe intrathoracic or intra-abdominal injuries or both in addition to fatal craniovertebral trauma.

PATHOMECHANICS OF SPINAL CORD INJURY

An extensive search of the literature revealed little information about the pathologic changes in the spine and spinal cord of children after trauma. This paucity of references has been attributed to the relative rarity of spinal injuries in children as well as the fact that the majority of them survive. In some countries difficulty in obtaining the permission for autopsy coupled with poor cooperation from the coroner's office has probably slowed down research. However, in an attempt to analyze the mechanism of spinal cord injury a careful review of the history, neurologic findings, evolution of deficit, radiologic abnormalities, operative findings, and in some instances, pathologic evidence obtained at autopsy is necessary.

It has been shown in autopsy specimens that the spinal canal increases in length in ventroflexion (flexion) and decreases in retroflexion (extension). The range of elongation in ventroflexion and shortening in retroflexion is relatively greater for the posterior contour of the spinal canal than for the anterior and posterior walls.[61] In addition, Breig[9] has shown that there is actual elongation of the spinal cord in ventroflexion; and individual cord segments may change in length by as much as 25%. The spinal cord, because of its elastic recoil and plasticity, adapts to these changes in the length of the spinal canal. Leventhal[37] demonstrated that the infantile spinal canal could be stretched about 5 cm but the cervical spinal cord could be pulled down only 5 mm before rupturing. The elastic recoil and plasticity of the spinal cord are limited by the pia mater, and once the maximal length of the cord is reached, further axial tensile forces possibly disrupt the neuronal tissue, leaving the arachnoid and the dura mater in continuity. The disruption of the spinal cord would be facilitated by the extruded disc material, dislocated vertebral bodies, and fractured fragments of vertebrae compromising the canal. Because of the relative hypermobility of the cervical region and dorsolumbar junction, the injuries to the spinal cord are more frequent in these regions. The horizontal direction of nerve roots in the cervical region, the attachment of the dura mater at the foramen magnum and intervertebral foramina, and the formation of the brachial plexus tend to anchor the cervical spinal cord and reduce its mobility and ability to elongate in the canal. All these factors make the cervical cord more prone to axial disruptive as well as compressive forces. Distally the spinal cord is anchored by the lumbar

roots, but in the thoracic region there is little anchoring support. Some authors believe that this lack of support makes the upper thoracic cord prone to trauma. However, in the present series and in others[3,11,12] there were more cervical cord injuries than injuries to the thoracic and lumbar cord.

Burke[12] recorded a constricted area of 4 cm above the cervical enlargement in a C5 tetraplegic 11-month-old child who died 3½ months after the trauma. Glasauer and Cares[23] recorded thinning and atrophy of the spinal cord (during surgery in one instance and at autopsy in the other instance) along with marked discrepancy between the neurologic deficit and the vertebral level of injury. LeBlanc and Nadell[36] noted the complete absence of spinal cord and dura mater from T2 to T5 on surgery and have also recorded segmental atrophy of the spinal cord at autopsy. In our series total transection of the spinal cord and dural sac occurred in one cervical and three thoracic lesions. In the other 26 patients, during laminectomy the spinal cord was found to be macerated or lacerated or both in 11 patients; contused and swollen in seven patients; and "normal appearing" in eight patients. These findings support the hypothesis of "longitudinal axial traction" in a number of children with upper thoracic spinal cord lesions and total absence of osteoarticular injury on plain radiographs.

In children involved in high-velocity motor vehicle injuries, at impact there could be retroflexion preceded or followed by forcible ventroflexion of a relatively large head and mobile neck over the fixed trunk. This might cause longitudinal axial traction on the cervical spinal cord, whereas compression of the cord might result from dislocation and fracture fragments of the vertebrae. With compromise of the spinal canal in the anteroposterior axis, there could also be occlusion of the anterior spinal artery or vertebral arteries producing ischemia of the spinal cord.

Of the 21 patients with spinal cord (four cervical and 17 thoracic lumbar) from firearm injuries (Table 18-1), eight were found to have fractures of the vertebral body or neural arch or both; and in three of these patients the spinal cord was found to be lacerated on laminectomy. Two other patients with normal radiographs were found to have, on laminectomy, total transection of the spinal cord. Thus in ten patients with firearm injuries there was evidence of direct traumatic disruption of the cord. In the remaining 11 patients in the absence of any radiologic abnormalities, paralysis was probably caused by indirect high-velocity tissue deformation and ischemia of the spinal cord.

Of the nine patients without any radiologic evidence of osteoarticular injury (excluding firearm injuries), one was found to have laceration of the dura mater on laminectomy, although the spinal cord and nerve roots were reported to be normal. The tear in the dura mater might have resulted from transient dislocation or from traction on the dural sac during acute flexion. In another patient at laminectomy, dislocation of T2 and T3 was detected and the spinal cord was reported to be macerated. In the other seven patients in the absence of any evidence of osteoarticular injury, the neurologic deficit (two cervical and five thoracic) was probably produced by axial traction or ischemia or both.

Based on the clinical and radiologic findings an attempt was made to classify the mechanism of injury. An additional 58 cervical lesions were considered to be due to ventroflexion/rotation (hyperflexion/rotation), seven were due to retroflexion rotation (hyperextension), and three were due to the vertical loading mechanism of injury. In ten cervical lesions, the mechanism of injury could not be satisfactorily classified. Of the 17 thoracolumbar lesions, 13 were due to ventroflexion/rotation mechanism. In the remaining four patients the mechanism of injury was probably lateral flexion, rotation, and shearing.

From these data it is evident that the compressive and disruptive forces are the most common mechanisms of spinal cord lesions in children with osteoarticular trauma. Longitudinal axial traction appears to be the most common cause of neurologic deficit in patients without osteoarticular lesions.

NEUROLOGIC FEATURES

Precise neurologic examination to ascertain the level of lesion and degree of sensory and motor preservation in children with spinal cord injury requires considerable patience and perseverence on the part of the examiner. Very frequently the examination may have to be repeated several times when the child is awake and asleep.

Audic and Maury[2] did not attempt to distinguish complete from incomplete lesions in children with spinal cord injuries and merely classified them as paraplegics and tetraplegics. Melzak[40] reported two incomplete cervical lesions, six complete and no incomplete upper thoracic lesions (T1-5), 15 complete and three incomplete lower thoracic lesions (T6-12), and three with cauda equina injuries. Burke[13] adopted a similar pattern of classification and reported nine complete and five incomplete cervical lesions, 11 complete and no incomplete upper thoracic lesions, and six complete and three incomplete lower thoracic lesions.

Neurologically the patients we reviewed could be classified as listed in Table 18-2. Of the 80 cervical lesions, 49 were complete transverse myelopathy and there were 31 children with incomplete lesions of the cervical cord. Fifteen were observed to have acute central cervical cord syndrome. Three patients had neurologic findings compatible with Brown-Séquard syndrome, and six had anterior cervical cord syndrome. The remaining five children with patchy sensory and motor preservation below the level of lesion were classified as having incomplete transverse myelopathy. These incomplete lesions were difficult to classify and required repeated examination on several occasions. Two girls (6 and 14 years old) had transient paralysis, sharp shooting pain starting in the lower part of their neck, tingling, and a feeling of pins and needles in all four extremities. At the time of admission except for the complaint of paresthesias, there were no other neurologic abnormalities.

There were 14 complete upper thoracic (T1-6) and 18 lower thoracic (T7-12) spinal cord lesions. One T5 and the other T9 paraplegic patient had preservation of sensation and trace voluntary motion in the distal muscles of lower limbs. There were eight children with a cauda equina pattern of injury. Melzak[40] and Burke[13] reported an absence of incomplete spinal cord lesions in upper and lower thoracic spinal cord injuries and a lower incidence of incomplete spinal cord lesions in children. However, in our experience on repeated examination approximately 35% of spinal cord lesions in children have been incomplete.

In addition to spinal cord trauma, 23 surviving patients were reported to be unconscious for 30 minutes or longer and eight of them had parietal and basal skull fractures. Thirty-four children in the epidemiologic study died from severe intracranial and cervicomedullary injuries associated with other visceral trauma.

There are a number of distinct neurologic features in children with spinal cord injury that are not seen in adults with a similar injury. In children the duration of spinal shock characterized by hypotonia, areflexia, and sensory/motor loss below the level of lesion is shorter than in adults. Often, in complete lesions within 10 to 14 days after trauma, hyperactive or physiologic deep

Table 18-2. Neurologic status in children with spinal cord injury

Injury	Complete	Incomplete
Cervical lesions (80)	49	31
Paresthesias	—	2
Central cord syndrome	—	15
Anterior cord syndrome	—	6
Brown-Séquard syndrome	—	3
Transverse myelopathy	49	5
Thoracic and lumbar lesions (42)	32	10
T1-6	14	1 (T5)
T7-12	18	1 (T9)
Cauda equina	—	8

tendon reflexes in lower limbs are noted along with normal muscle tone, as compared to a spinal shock period of 4 to 6 weeks in adults. The plantar response, although extensor more frequently, is also present, as compared to its absence during the early period in adult spinal cord injuries. Bulbocavernous reflex, anocutaneous response, and reflex bladder function in children also return much earlier than in the adults. This may be due to the lack of development and maturation of advanced cortical inhibitory mechanisms resulting in the more autonomous nature of the spinal cord in children.

RADIOLOGIC FEATURES

There is considerable confusion in the literature regarding the terminology of various osseous and articular spinal lesions.[6,7] We use the following terminology:

1. *Wedge fracture:* radiologic evidence of compression of the anterior part of the vertebral body leading to reduction of height as compared to its posterior portion, without any evidence of comminution (Fig. 18-1)
2. *Bursting fracture:* fracture of vertebral body with dispersion and comminution (Fig. 18-2)
3. *Teardrop fracture:* the anterior part of the caudal vertebral body chiseled away as a result of compressive forces delivered by the cephalad vertebra; larger part of the vertebra often projects into the spinal canal (Fig. 18-3)
4. *Sagittal fracture:* vertical fracture line in the sagittal plane seen in AP view of the spine, with or without reduction in the height of its vertebral body (Figs. 18-4 and 18-5)
5. *Chip fracture:* a small triangular piece of bone avulsed from the anterior inferior angle of ce-

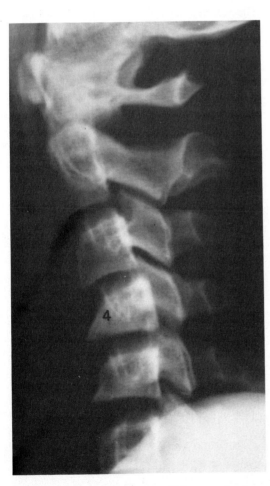

Fig. 18-1. Cervical spine of 13-year-old boy involved in a motorcycle crash. Wedge fractures of C4 and C5 vertebral bodies and increase in interfacetal and interspinous spaces between C3 and C4.

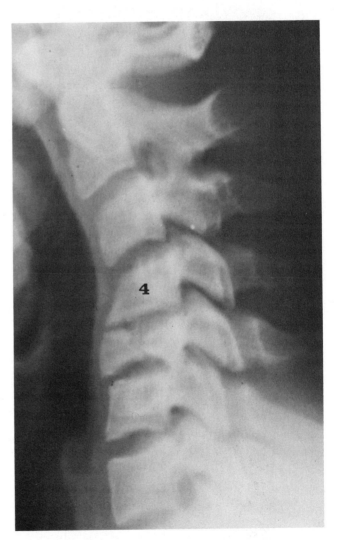

Fig. 18-2. Cervical spine of 14-year-old boy following automobile accident. Note wedge fracture of C4 and bursting fracture of C5. C5 vertebral body is split in the middle, and there is reduction in its vertical height at the center. There is also increase in anteroposterior diameter of C5.

phalad vertebra or the anterior superior angle of caudal vertebra

6. *Subluxation:* a partial loss of contact of the two articular surfaces; first-degree subluxation: 25% of articular surfaces have lost contact (i.e., greater than 75% of articulating surfaces remain in contact); second-degree subluxation: 26% to 50% of articulating surfaces have lost contact; third-degree subluxation: 51% to 75% of articulating surfaces have lost contact (The term *dislocation* is preferred if more than 75% of one vertebral body has moved away from the others.) (Figs. 18-6 to 18-8)

7. *Neural arch fracture:* fracture of pedicle, lamina, or spinous processes

Frequently diagnostic errors are made if there is no familiarity with certain constitutional peculiarities of the spine in children, such as horizontal position of facets, pseudodislocation, congenital anomalies, and epipyseal lines. While the examiner is reviewing the radiographs of a child, the following special features must be kept in mind:

1. The distance between the anterior arch of the atlas and the intact odontoid process is 4 to 5 mm in children as compared to 2 to 3 mm in adults. Normally the AP diameter of the atlas is 1 to 3 mm greater than that of the axis.

2. Os odontoideum, a congenital anomaly, shows evidence of reduction of deformity only with flexion while a fracture of the base of the odontoid process usually shows reduction with extension.

3. Minor angulation and step deformity of vertebrae at C2-3 and C3-4 are not unusual in children as a result of immature musculature and hypermobility.

4. The absence of normal lordotic curvature of the cervical spine and the absence of uniform angulation between the adjacent vertebrae should be

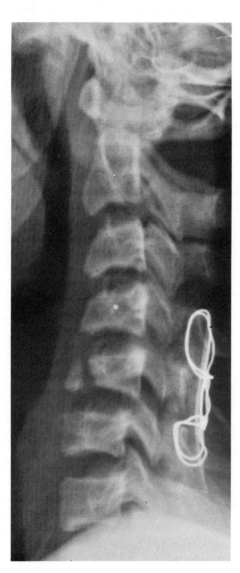

Fig. 18-3. Cervical spine of 13-year-old C6 tetraplegic boy after wrestling injury. Note teardrop fracture of C5 and wedge fracture of C4. Patient underwent posterior fusion and wiring.

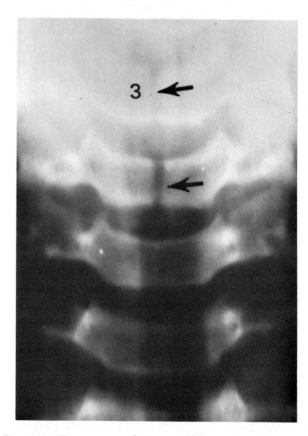

Fig. 18-4. AP tomogram of 14-year-old boy with acute central cervical cord syndrome from diving injury. Sagittal fractures of C3 and C4 vertebral bodies *(arrows)* are evident.

carefully analyzed and correlated with the clinical findings.

5. The vertebral apophyseal ossification centers should not be confused with chip fractures.

It is difficult to say how many of the dead patients in our series would have shown radiologic evidence of injury to the spine on adequate examination. Since most of these patients died within 24 hours and had multiple–organ system involvement, an adequate search for radiologic evidence of osteoarticular injuries to the spine could not have been done. However, of the 122 surviving spinal cord injured children, there was evidence of fracture or subluxation or both in 91 patients on plain radiography or tomography. An additional 21 patients with spinal cord injury from firearms showed metal stippling, the bullet tract, pellets, or fracture of the neural arches.

Vertebral body fractures

There were 102 fractures of the vertebral bodies with or without dislocation in 77 patients (Table 18-3). Fifty-six patients had fractures of a single vertebral body, 18 had fractures of two vertebral bodies, and three had fractures of three contiguous vertebral bodies. Seventy-two fractures occurred in the cervical region and approximately 48% of the fractures involved C5 and C6 vertebrae. Teardrop and bursting fractures accounted for approximately 12% each, and sagittal fractures were observed in 9% children. Wedge fractures were observed in 63% of cases and "chip" fractures in only 2%. In the remaining 2% of cases the fractures on lateral view appeared as wedge or teardrop whereas on AP views they appeared as sagittal fractures.

There were 21 fractures of thoracic vertebrae. The fractures of the lumbar spine in children at or below

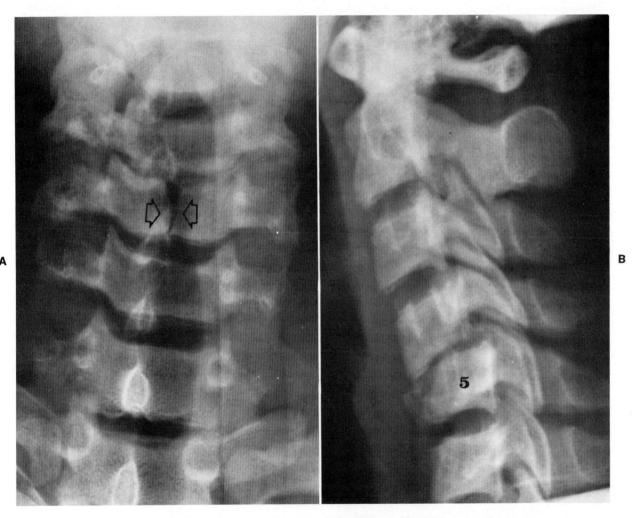

Fig. 18-5. Cervical spine of 15-year-old C4 tetraplegic boy. **A,** Sagittal fracture of C5 vertebral body *(arrows)*. C4-5 intervertebral space is obliterated, and C5-6 intervertebral space is asymmetric. **B,** Fracture of C5 vertebral body appears similar to a wedge fracture with first-degree subluxation of C4-5.

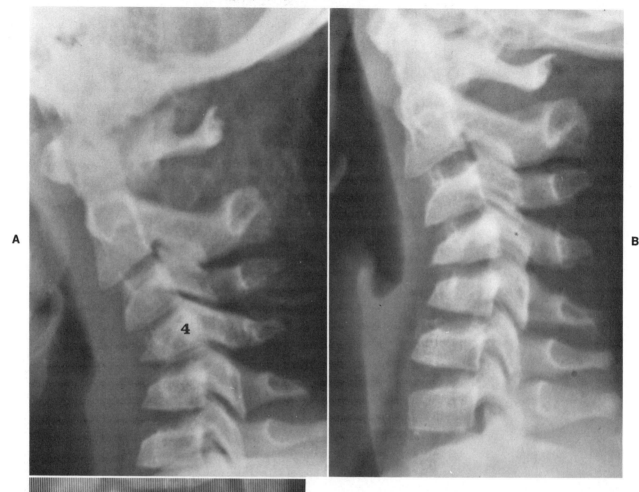

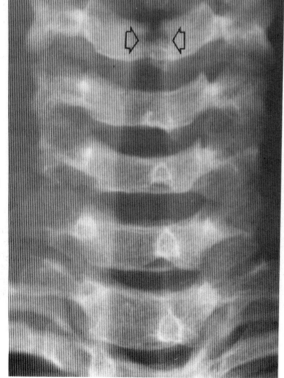

Fig. 18-6. Cervical spine radiographs of 10-year-old C4 tetraplegic boy. **A,** Lateral view shows disruption of arch of atlas, wedge fractures of C4, C5, and C6 and first-degree subluxation of C3-4. Retropharyngeal space is increased because of prevertebral hematoma. **B,** Lateral view of cervical spine 3½ months later shows fractures and cervical kyphosis. Prevertebral space appears normal. **C,** AP view shows reduction in height of vertebral bodies of C5 and C6. Vertebral body of C4 shows sagittal fracture *(arrows).*

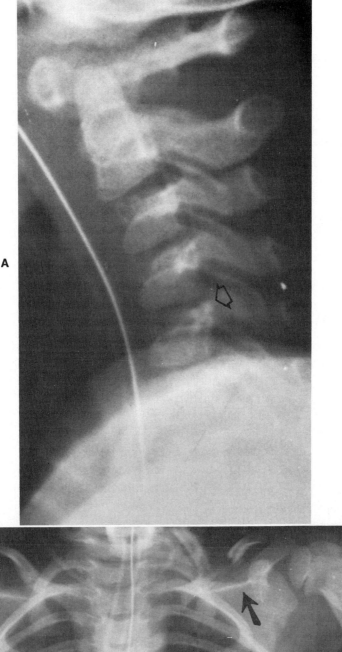

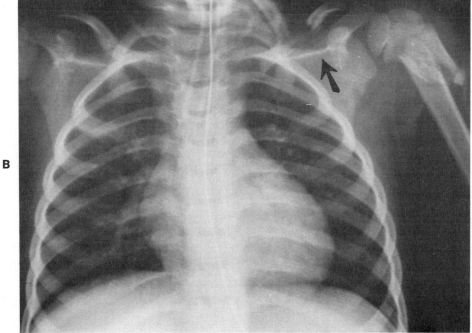

Fig. 18-7. Girl, 2½ years old, who was involved in automobile accident and sustained C4 tetraplegia. **A,** Lateral cervical spine radiograph shows first-degree subluxation of C4-5 *(arrow).* **B,** AP view of chest shows displaced fracture of left clavicle *(arrow)* and fracture of upper left humerus.

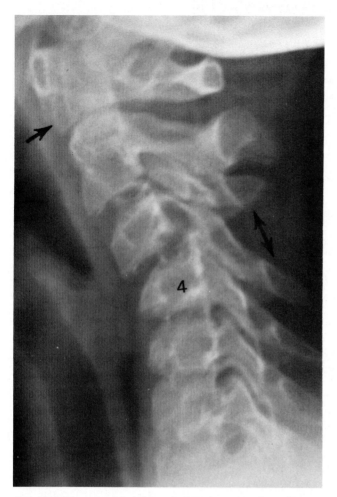

Fig. 18-8. Six-year-old child with C4 anterior cord syndrome, wedge fracture of C4, first-degree subluxation of C3-4, and increase in interspinous space between C3 and C4 (*double arrow*). There is a fragment (*arrow*) in front of odontoid process suggestive of injury to atlantoaxial periarticular structures.

the first lumbar segment are very rare, and in the present series there were only nine fractures of the lumbar vertebrae. Of these 30 fractures, 20 were wedge, eight were bursting, and two were chip fractures of the vertebral bodies.

Neural arch fractures

Fifteen children were observed to have 21 fractures of neural arches at various levels. In 11 patients fractures of the neural arch were associated with fractures of vertebral bodies, and in two patients the fractures of the neural arch were associated with dislocations. There were only two patients with fractures of the neural arch without a fracture of a vertebral body or dislocation.

Dislocations

There were 67 children with dislocation. Sixty-two children were noted to have subluxations, 54 had a single-level subluxation, and eight had subluxations at two levels. Another five patients were found to have total dislocations. Approximately 84% of the dislocations involved the cervical region and two thirds of these occurred at the C4-5 and C5-6 levels. Only ten subluxations and four dislocations were observed in the thoracic and lumbar regions.

Several authors have emphasized "minimal" or "very often" total absence of radiologic abnormalities in most of the cases of traumatic lesions of the spine in children. Cheshire[15] has attempted to define separately a "pediatric syndrome of traumatic myelopathy without demonstrable vertebral injury." In an analysis of 29 children with traumatic spinal lesions admitted at the National Spinal Injuries Center, Stokes Mandeville Hospital, Melzak[40] found no evidence of vertebral fracture or dislocation in 16; in another 18 cases fracture was present from the beginning, and one other case the

Table 18-3. Osteoarticular injuries in 92 children with spinal cord injury

	Fractures			Dislocations	
Level	Vertebral body	Neural arch	Level	Subluxation	Complete dislocation
C1 and C2	1	2	C1-2	2	—
C3	3	2	C2-3	2	—
C4	14	3	C3-4	8	—
C5	31	3	C4-5	22	—
C6	17	2	C5-6	18	—
C7	6	2	C6-7	8	—
T1-6	7	2	C7-T1	—	1
T2-12	14	3	T1-6	2	1
L1-5	9	2	T7-12	3	2
			L1-5	5	1
TOTAL	102 (77)*	21 (15)*	TOTAL	70 (62)*	5 (5)*

*Number of patients.

fracture was detected after laminectomy. Four children sustained gunshot injuries. Audic and Maury[2] reported that "very often no fracture of the vertebral column was detected" in 21 traumatic paraplegic children. Thirteen of 31 spinal cord injured children reported by Burke[11,12] had no evidence of radiologic abnormality. Minimal or major bone injury, however, was detected in 15 patients, and in another three patients myelographic abnormalities in the absence of a fracture were also demonstrated. Similarly of the 16 spinal cord injured children reported by Scher[50] seven were found to have fractures and/or dislocation of the vertebrae on radiographs. A detailed analysis of the literature* clearly indicates that there were only a slightly over 47 cases out of 196 children (1 to 18 years old) with spinal cord injury without any radiologic abnormalities, if seven cases of firearm and stab injuries to the spine were excluded. In at least 119 cases (61%) there was definite evidence of osteoarticular injury on plain radiographs. In addition, there were more than six patients with normal radiographs but abnormal myelograms, and the abnormalities were confirmed at the time or surgery.

Absence of radiologic abnormalities

In our series there were only nine patients out of 101 without any radiologic evidence of osteoarticular injury (if 21 firearm injuries are excluded). Seven were paraplegic, one was tetraplegic below C2, and one had acute central cervical cord syndrome. Six patients were 10 years old or under and three were 11 to 15 years old.

The radiographs are only static recordings of a dynamic situation and do not necessarily indicate the exact alignment at the time of trauma. However, these findings do indicate that the resultant damage from the initial injury could be seen in approximately 70% of children with spinal cord injury on a careful analysis of good-quality radiographs. The absence of radiologic abnormalities in about 30% of children with spinal cord injuries is about the same as reported for adults, and the appearance of these fractures is in no way different from that observed in acute traumatic spinal cord lesions in adults.

Myelography

The role of myelography in patients without any evidence of osteoarticular injury on plain radiographs after spinal cord trauma has been questioned. Some authors feel that if satisfactory plain radiographs of the spine show no abnormality, tomography and myelography are of no value. Burke[11,12] reported normal findings on myelogram in seven, partial block in two, and complete

*References 2, 11, 15, 23, 25-27, 36, 40.

block in one of the ten patients with clinical evidence of major spinal cord trauma but normal plain radiographs. At the time of surgery the partial myelographic block in these patients was believed to be due to edema and contusion of the spinal cord; and the complete extradural block was due to a hematoma six segments below the level of lesion. Similarly a number of other children with normal plain radiographs and abnormal myelograms at the time of surgery were found to have significant damage to the spinal cord.[23,36,50]

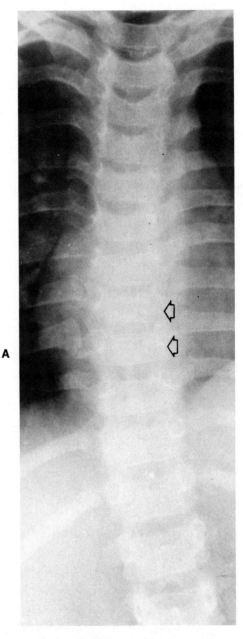

Fig. 18-9. Radiographs of 6-year-old T11 paraplegic. **A,** Fractures of T8 and T9 (*arrows*) along with reduction in height of these vertebrae and right thoracic scoliosis.

Continued.

In the present series myelography was not performed with any regularity and only ten patients had myelograms performed. Of the seven patients with evidence of osteoarticular spinal trauma on plain radiographs, six were found to have complete block at the corresponding levels. Three of these patients on laminectomy were found to have maceration of the spinal cord, and one was reported to have edematous and hyperemic cord. Of the three patients with normal plain radiographs, only one showed a block at T2 level and on laminectomy this patient was reported to have dislocation at T2-3 with transection of the spinal cord.

Myelography is an invasive procedure of limited value in complete lesions of the spinal cord. We believe that in selected cases after carefully examining the patient's radiographs if questions or inconsistencies exist, myelography should be performed at a later date. In the meantime children without any evidence of fracture or dislocation on radiographs but clinically suspected of spinal cord trauma must be treated very carefully until such time when definite decision can be made by appropriate studies.

MANAGEMENT OF SPINAL CORD INJURIES

The management of spinal cord injuries in children is as controversial as in adults. The main objective of treatment of acute spinal cord injuries is restoration of the patient's condition to the highest level of function in the shortest possible time with the least morbidity and mortality. A wide difference of opinion exists over the best way to achieve this objective. For acute cervical dislocations in children some authors have advised manipulation without anesthesia in an attempt to achieve relaxation of muscle spasm and possibly spontaneous correction without the need for excessive force and neck motion. However, spinal manipulation with or without anesthesia carries a risk of neurologic deterioration. Application of continuous cervical traction with a head halter to alleviate the paraspinal muscle spasm and reduce the subluxation has also been recommended. After 1 or 2 weeks the traction is replaced by a cervical collar for 2 to 3 weeks in patients with subluxations, and after about 6 weeks for patients with dislocations. We believe that application of a well-padded halo-fixation apparatus in older children with spinal cord injury is very effective in minimizing the time spent in bed and the adverse effects of immobilization, hypercalcemia, and boredom. Crutchfield, Gardner-Wells, or Vinke tongs can also be used in children.

According to Sharrard[51] fractures in the thoracic region are rarely very unstable, compression is not usually great, and it does not require reduction. The youn-

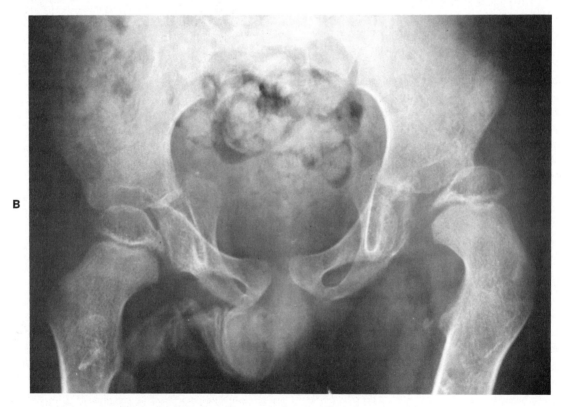

B

Fig. 18-9, cont'd. B, Approximately 1 year after spinal cord injury, patient developed subluxation of left hip from spasticity and hip flexion contracture.

ger children may need to be immobilized in a plaster cast or brace, while older children can be treated by simple bed rest until pain subsides. Burke[13] also strongly advocated similar conservative approach to the spine of young children based on his observations that a large number of these patients have no bone injury associated with spinal cord trauma. Although we strongly favor the nonoperative approach, in certain selective cases with progressive neurologic deterioration or in cases with persistent significant malalignment with

incomplete lesion, operative intervention is needed. Initially all patients were immobilized by halter or skull tong traction. Nonsurgical techniques (Fig. 18-9) were also used to treat 25 of 42 thoracic and lumbar lesions. In most of these patients a molded plastic body jacket was used to immobilize the spine and permit active participation in daily activities out of bed.

Several authors have recommended early anterior spondylodesis of the cervical spine in order to decompress the spinal cord anteriorly, stabilize the spine, and

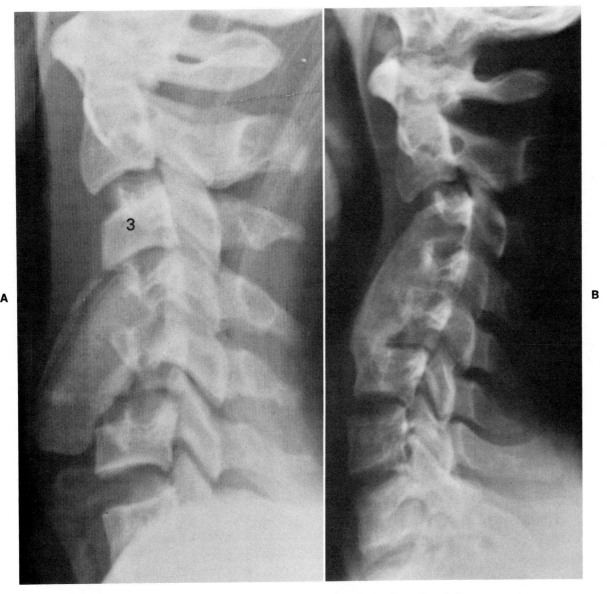

Fig. 18-10. Cervical spine radiographs of 14-year-old C5 tetraplegic boy following anterior cervical fusion using Smith-Robinson technique. **A,** Extrusion of bone graft at caudal end of C6. Upper end of graft is also partially extruded. **B,** Approximately 1 year after reoperation there was solid fusion of C3 to C6. Marked "swan neck" deformity of cervical spine is evident.

permit early mobilization,* whereas other authors have reported a number of complications of this procedure in traumatic lesions of spine[29,34,42] and have suggested that this procedure has very little to offer in acute traumatic lesions. Eleven patients in the present series underwent anterior interbody fusion; graft extruded in two, and severe deformity occurred in other two. Nine other patients initially had cervical laminectomy but later underwent anterior interbody fusion for stabilization (Figs. 18-10 and 18-11).

In an attempt to minimize the neurologic deficit and facilitate neuronal recovery after traumatic lesions of the spinal cord, "decompression laminectomy" has been recommended and practiced frequently in the United States. In several instances the presence of a myelographic block even in the absence of a fracture has been used as an indication for this procedure. In the present series 19 children underwent cervical laminectomy alone or combined with posterior or anterior fusion for stability. In two of these patients the neurologic status deteriorated from C5 to C2 tetraplegia. Significant angular cervical deformity was also observed in another four patients (Figs. 18-12 to 18-14).

Open reduction of locked facets and posterior fusion and wiring have also been performed frequently in an attempt to reduce the deformity, stabilize the spine, and mobilize the patient faster. However, in a number of instances this has failed to provide adequate stability (Figs. 18-15 to 18-17). In our series posterior fusion and wiring were performed in five patients. In another four patients with posterior fusion and wiring, anterior interbody fusion was necessary for stability.

Of the 17 children with thoracic and lumbar lesions who had surgery, 11 had laminectomy, three had posterior fusion and Harrington instrumentation, and two had posterior fusion and wiring. One patient underwent L3 laminectomy immediately after the injury, but later on underwent anterior interbody fusion of L2 and L3 for stabilization. One T2 paraplegic patient became C4 tetraplegic after laminectomy.

*References 5, 17-19, 43, 44, 47.

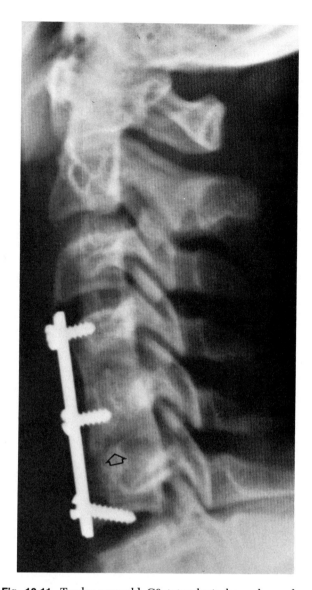

Fig. 18-11. Twelve-year-old C6 tetraplegic boy who underwent excision of C6 vertebra and anterior interbody fusion of C4-6 with iliac strut graft and Egger's plate fixation. Two months after surgery there is fracture *(arrow)* of strut graft between C5 and C6. Lower screw appears loose, without adequate fixation at inferior anterior angle of C6 vertebra.

Fig. 18-12. Cervical spine of 13½-year-old boy with C6 incomplete transverse myelopathy. **A,** Lateral view showing burst of C5 vertebral body and obliteration of cervical lordosis. Prevertebral space is markedly increased because of hematoma. **B,** Myelogram. Lateral view shows posterior indentation *(arrow)* in contrast material at C4-5. **C,** AP view shows widening of spinal cord at C4 and C5 levels consistent with hematomyelia. **D,** Lateral view of cervical spine 6 months after laminectomy shows severe deformity of cervical spine.

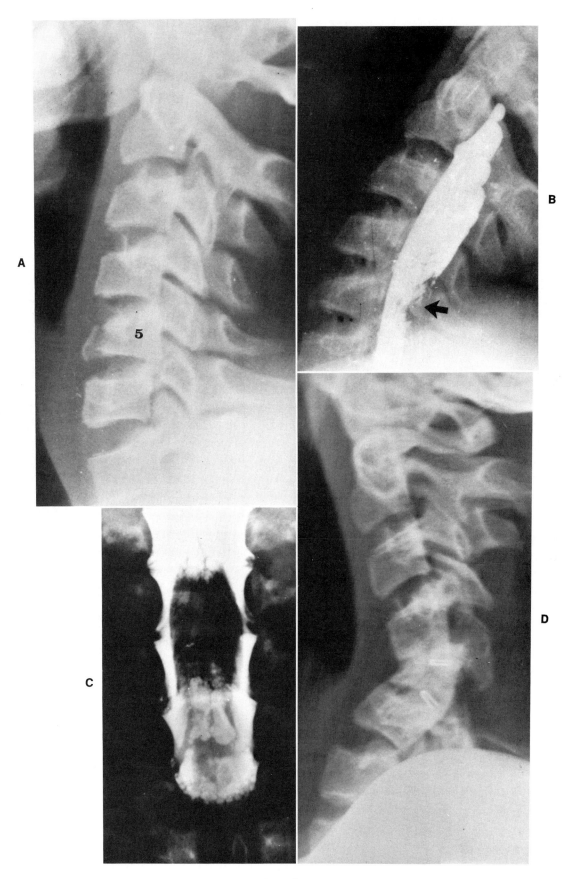

Fig. 18-12. For legend see opposite page.

These data indicate that 58 (47% of total series) children underwent some operative procedure; 13 (10% of total series) of these made a good recovery, and three deteriorated. However, all those patients who improved had incomplete lesions initially and would have possibly improved without surgery. Of the 64 children who were not operated on, 15 (12% of total series) showed good return, but these were again incomplete lesions. Thus neurologic improvement was about the same in the two groups, but the incidence of complications and extent of spinal deformity were significantly greater in the group that had surgery.

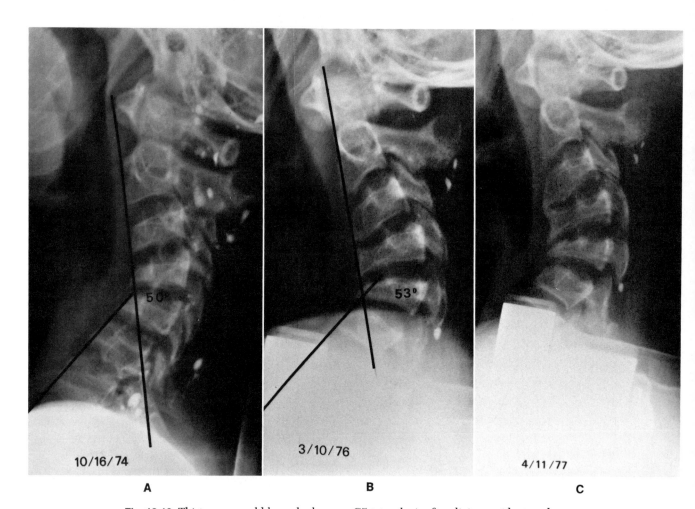

A **B** **C**

Fig. 18-13. Thirteen-year-old boy who became C5 tetraplegic after diving accident underwent laminectomy of C3-5. **A,** Lateral view 4 months after surgery shows wedge fractures of C3, C4, and C5 and anterior kyphosis of 50°. **B,** Seventeen months after surgery there is a significant increase in AP diameter of C4, reduction in vertical height of C4 and C5, and anterior bridging along C3-5. There is cervical kyphosis of 53°. **C,** At 34 months after surgery there is bony bridging of C3-5 and altered trabecular pattern in vertebral bodies. Articular facets show sclerosis and obliteration of joint spaces.

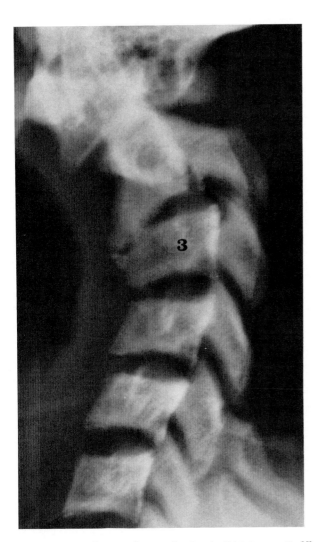

Fig. 18-14. Lateral view of cervical spine in C4 tetraparetic 15-year-old boy taken approximately 3 years after laminectomy of C1-4 shows significant cervical deformity, persistent anterior atlantoaxial subluxation, and C2-3 first-degree subluxation.

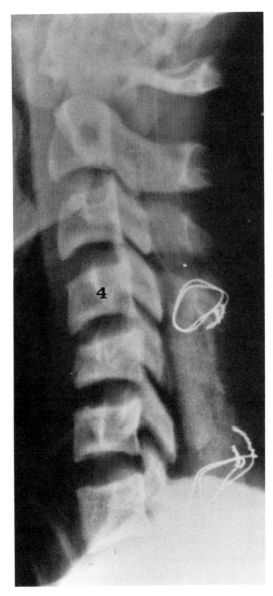

Fig. 18-15. Laminectomy and posterior strut grafting done at same time in 15-year-old C5 tetraplegic boy after a fall while wrestling. Following surgery, patient was noted to be C2 tetraplegic and remained on respirator. Lateral view of cervical spine shows wedge fracture of C5. Bone graft has been retained with wires at C4 and C7.

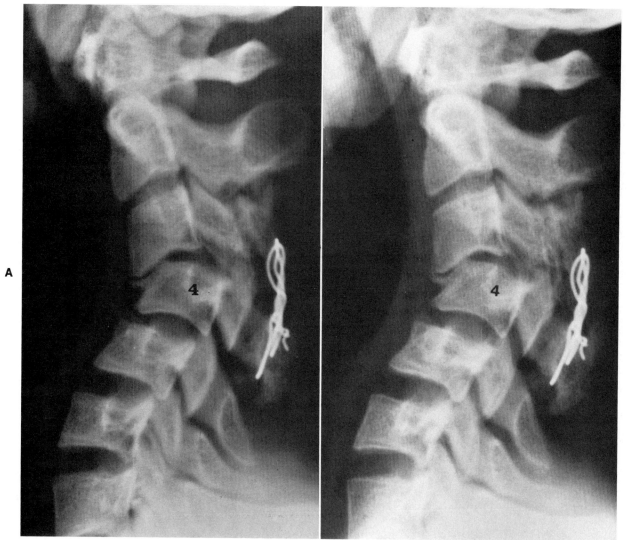

Fig. 18-16. A, Posterior fusion and wiring of C3 and C4 performed without adequate reduction of second-degree subluxation at C3-4. Step deformity and cervical kyphosis persisted. There is compensatory opening of intervertebral spaces at C5-6 and C6-7. **B,** Lateral view of cervical spine 11 months later. Although posterior fusion is solid, cervical deformity appears to be more prominent. Anterior longitudinal ligament is also ossified.

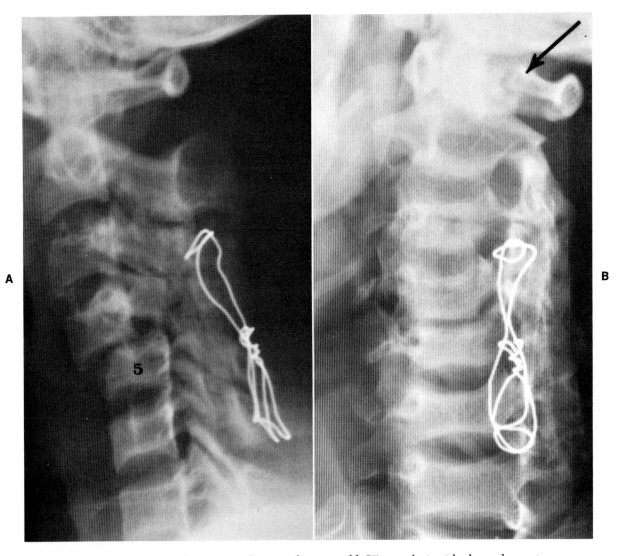

Fig. 18-17. Radiographs of cervical spine of 14-year-old C5 tetraplegic girl who underwent open reduction and posterior fusion and wiring (C3-6) 2 months after injury. **A,** Lateral view approximately 4 months after surgery shows wedge fracture of C5 and second-degree subluxation of C4-5. There is fracture of pedicle of C4. Subluxation was not helped by posterior fusion and wiring. **B,** Oblique view shows fractures of arch of atlas (*arrow*) and pedicle of C4.

REHABILITATION AND PHYSICAL RESTORATION

Rehabilitation of children with spinal cord injury is directed toward achieving maximal independence in activities of daily living commensurate with their lesion level, developmental stage, and ability to learn. In younger children efforts must be concentrated on achieving the basic motions of sitting, feeding, and drinking. With growth, these activities may be advanced to transfers, dressing, and possibly standing and walking with braces. These goals must be evaluated at 3- to 6-month intervals and advanced with growth and development of the child. Once the patient's medical condition is stabilized, therapeutic exercises directed toward strengthening the functioning groups of muscles, maintaining the range of motion at various joints of paralytic limbs, and minimizing the development of edema, contractures, and deformities must be started. During the early phase of spinal instability these exercises could be carried out in bed and subsequently in the physical therapy department. Adduction internal rotation contracture at the shoulders, flexion contractures at elbows, pronation contractures of forearms, ra-

dial deviation at wrists, flattening of palmar arches, tightness of web spaces, and flexion contractures at the metacarpophalangeal joints must be avoided by a regular program of range of motion initially performed by the physical therapist and nurse and later taught to the patient and family members. In the lower limbs flexion contractures at hips and knees and tightness of Achilles tendon must also be vigorously treated. If the patient's spine is stable, lying prone should be encouraged since this will stretch the hip flexion contractures and provide postural drainage of pulmonary secretions as well as better aeration of lower posterior lobe alveoli. Hydrotherapy in the form of swimming has proved invaluable for the development of movement patterns that promote good postural control. Children with spinal paralysis can start swimming lessons at the age of $2\frac{1}{2}$ to 3 years. However, for these children to overcome their fear and anxiety of water requires great patience, firmness, and perseverance on the part of the instructor.

Standing and walking in children can begin once the postural control and vasomotor control in sitting position have improved sufficiently. As a preliminary to ambulation, the paraplegic child should first be taught to

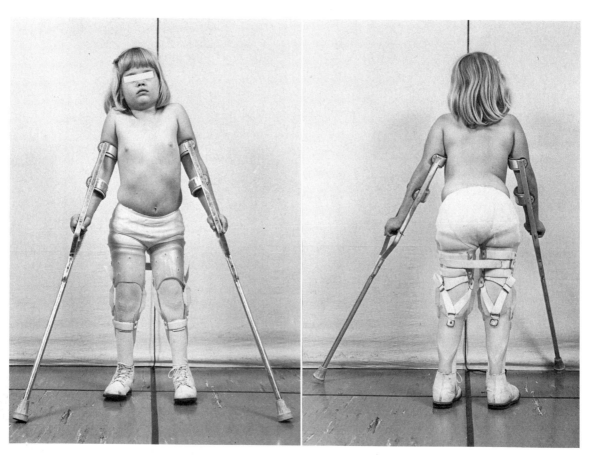

Fig. 18-18. Polypropylene above-knee, ankle-foot orthosis (Engen type).

stand up from the wheelchair with braces. Initially they should be tried in posterior splints extending from mid-thigh to ankles and subsequently in customized long leg braces with double upright bars, drop-lock-knee joints, and limited ankle motion. To avoid foot drop a simple toe-raising spring can be attached with a D-ring, or a Klenzak or Becker spring-loaded ankle joint can be incorporated into the brace. Children with varus deformity of heels would require an outside T strap, whereas those with valgus deformity will need an inside T strap. The proper fit and light weight of these braces are essential. Since most of the metal braces weight 2.25 to 3.2 kg (5 to 7 lb), I have successfully used a long leg brace with a plastic thigh cuff connected to a short leg polypropylene Engen-type brace (Fig. 18-18) with metal knee joints weighing about 0.45 kg (1 lb). Similarly in cauda equina lesions, a below-knee polypropylene ankle-foot orthosis weighing only 140 to 200 g (5 to 7 oz) has proved invaluable (Fig. 18-19). Severity of spasticity, total contact, and adequacy of the fit of these polypropylene above-knee or blow-knee braces must be checked periodically. Children with spinal paralysis learn walking even with high levels of paralysis more

frequently than adults; however, a majority of them discontinue walking in their teens because of slowness of speed compared to the wheelchair and the relatively high energy requirement for walking with braces. In the beginning gait training should be started in parallel bars and gradually with forearm or underarm crutches outside the parallel bars. In our experience children with lesions above T6 have been able to stand with braces or in a standing box but were not able to achieve functional walking. Children with lesions at T6 to T12 have been able to walk a short distance (150 to 450 m) (500 to 1500 ft) with long leg braces and forearm crutches. Those with lesions at T12 to T13 required long leg braces but they could walk a longer distance with swing-through, swing-to, or four-point gait. Children with lesions at or below L4 have been able to walk very well with a polypropylene short leg brace.

Most of the children with permanent paralysis need a wheelchair as a major mode of transportation. In tetraplegic children under 5 years of age usually a manual wheelchair is prescribed, while in older tetraplegic children attending school an electrically propelled wheelchair should be recommended. In paraplegic chil-

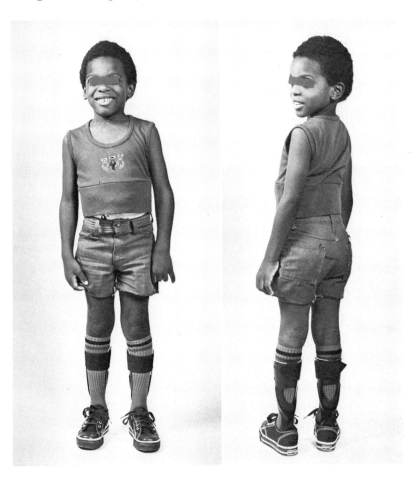

Fig. 18-19. Polypropylene ankle-foot orthosis (Engen type) used by patient with cauda equina lesion.

dren a manual wheelchair with detachable desk arms, swinging detachable footrests with foot straps, pneumatic tires, extended toggle brakes, and a lapboard is often prescribed. A good-quality seat cushion (7.5 cm [3 in] thick Sorbo rubber or Temper foam) covered with an absorbent cloth material is also essential.

Burke[13] reported that children adapt far better psychologically to disability than the adults. However, this has not been our experience. Children with chronic physical disease have been invariably depressed with subtle or obvious signs of sadness. Chronic handicap seems to have undermined their self-image and self-esteem. Their responses can be categorized as depression, aggression and acting out, regression, increasing dependence, a feeling of inferiority, and withdrawal from social contacts. Some type of reward mechanism, patience, and perseverance when dealing with younger children have been helpful in pulling them out of depression. Goal setting, verbal or written contractual agreement, and reward mechanisms have also been successful in teenaged children with postinjury maladaption. Distortion of body image, return to peer group, socialization, and sexuality also require intense psychologic rehabilitation in adolescent spinal cord injured patients.

Education of spinal cord injured children during hospitalization should be continued by bedside teaching and by the homebound teacher during their period of convalescence. These children should be enrolled in regular classes and schools in order that they will be integrated with able-bodied children and have the same opportunity to compete for the highest scholastic achievements. All schools have been given a federal mandate that they should be accessible to the handicapped, and physical rehabilitation sessions should be available for them in the school. The desks for children in wheelchairs should be high enough and bathrooms should be wide enough to accommodate the wheelchairs. In school dormitories at least a few rooms should be architecturally designed for handicapped students.

COMPLICATIONS AND MANAGEMENT
Urologic complications

The prevention of urologic complications (Table 18-4) is one of the most important objectives of successful rehabilitation of children with spinal cord injury (Fig. 18-20). During the first 48 hours, since a number of neurosurgical team use steroids or diuretics in an attempt to minimize the spinal cord edema, an indwelling urethral catheter should be placed to avoid overdistention of the bladder. However, this catheter must be removed as soon as possible and the patient should be started on an intermittent catheterization program. Depending on the level of spinal cord lesion in children,

Table 18-4. Medical complications in 97 children with spinal cord injury

Area	Complication	No.
Gastrointestinal tract	Gastroduodenal bleeding/ulcerations	12
	Paralytic ileus	9
	Mesenteric artery syndrome	1
Genitourinary tract	Bacteriuria (100,000/ml)	97
	Urolithiasis	28
	Hydronephrosis	8
Metabolic	Hypercalcemia	21
	Osteoporosis	33
Respiratory	Insufficiency	20
	Pneumonia/atelectasis	23
	Pulmonary embolism	1
Soft tissues	Pressure sores	26
	Ectopic ossification	13
Vascular	Deep venous thrombosis (lower limbs)	26
	Septicemia	1

as in adults, the neurogenic bladder could be upper motor neuron, mixed motor neuron, or lower motor neuron type. The duration of spinal shock in the upper motor neuron lesions is shorter than in adults. The period of bladder hypotonicity after acute spinal cord injury is also shorter in complete lesions. Reflex voiding in children with upper motor neuron and mixed motor neuron bladder involvement following intermittent catheterization program also develops much sooner (3 to 10 weeks in 70% of children) than in adults. Sterile urine could be obtained in 86% of the boys in the present series. Occasionally the young age of the child, lack of high standards of personal hygiene, and an inability because of the age to empty the bladder regularly may pose considerable difficulty in bladder training; under these circumstances parents may have to assume the total responsibility in the beginning. In younger boys vesicostomy bags or other external 24-hour urine collection devices can be used instead of paper diapers. Spinal cord injured girls pose more difficult problems because a satisfactory external collecting system is not available. Although Comarr[20] reported that female paraplegic patients of any age could satisfactorily manage in diapers without any difficulty with excoriation or ulceration of the skin from urine, we feel that the malodor of urine and the need to change the wet diapers periodically are psychologically unacceptable. In most of the spinal cord injured girls under 5 years of age we have used diapers and intermittent catheterization by clean technique done four times a day by parents; in older girls self-clean catheterization has worked well. In

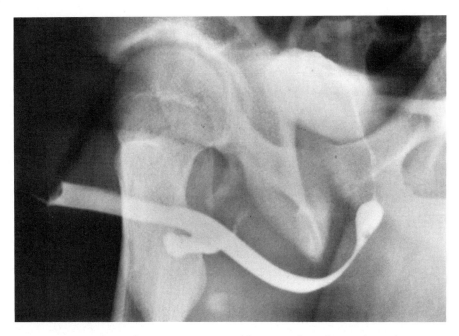

Fig. 18-20. Retrograde urethrogram in 14-year-old T6 paraplegic boy with urethrocutaneous fistula. Sacular diverticulum-like structure at penoscrotal junction has irregular walls, and there is extravasation of contrast material.

undependable children and suboptimal family-support situations, we have used a Silastic or silicone-coated Foley catheter that is changed at least once a month. Meatus care and cleaning of the catheter are done at least once a day.

In the present series of 83 boys with spinal cord injury, 17 developed good volitional control and did not require any external collecting system. Forty-two of the boys developed reflex voiding and emptied their bladder satisfactorily with external collecting systems; 16 had indwelling Foley catheters; three emptied the bladder by Credé's method; and five had suprapubic catheters or tubes. Of the 39 spinal cord injured girls, 11 developed good volitional control, 20 had indwelling catheters, and only six developed reflex voiding and stayed dry.

Urolithiasis. The incidence of urolithiasis in children has been reported to be 28%[58] as compared to less than 2% in adults with spinal cord injury.[24,46,54] This higher frequency is probably due to the higher incidence of hypercalciuria and hypercalcemia. Fifty-two percent of hypercalcemia spinal cord injured children developed predominantly renal calculi as compared to 22% of normocalcemic children who developed predominantly vesical calculi. The pathogenesis of nephrolithiasis in children with spinal cord injury seems to be directly related to hypercalcemia, and the pathogenesis of vesicolithiasis seems to be related to hypercalciuria, urinary stasis, and urinary tract infection. Only 15% of children

treated with intermittent catheterization developed lithiasis, whereas 45% of those with indwelling catheters developed this complication. Since it is easier to achieve a catheter-free state early, especially in boys, it must be started as soon as possible to minimize the risk of urinary tract infection and lithiasis.

Hydronephrosis. Only eight children (six boys and two girls) were found to have evidence of hydronephrosis and hydroureter on routine intravenous urography 3 to 6 months after the injury (Fig. 18-21). In two patients it was associated with lithiasis. Five of these eight patients were treated nonsurgically and three were operated on—one underwent dilatation of the urethra, one required nephrostomy and suprapubic cystostomy, and one required left ureteral reimplantation.

Autonomic dysreflexia. There is a paucity of references about autonomic dysreflexia associated with myelopathy in children. The characteristic symptoms and signs of autonomic dysreflexia in children—excessive sweating, flushing of the face, pilomotor erection, headache, congestion of nasal passages, and paroxysmal hypertension—are similar to those of adults with minor exceptions. The elevation of blood pressure is less severe and hyperhydrosis less frequent.[2]

In younger children restlessness, nausea, vomiting, thrashing of the head and neck, facial flushing, sweating, tightening of abdominal muscles, and penile erection should raise the suspicion of autonomic dysreflexia. Paroxysmal elevation of bood pressure alone in a child

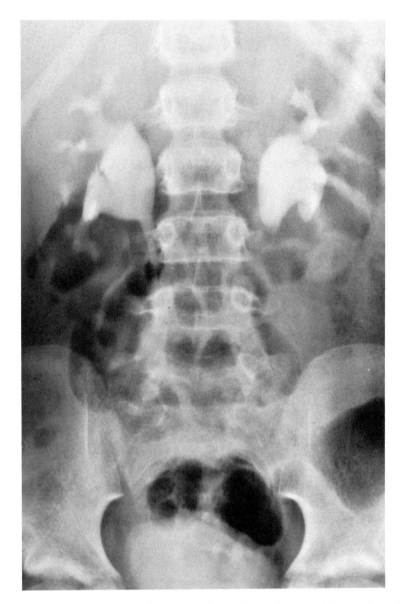

Fig. 18-21. Intravenous urogram of 10-year-old tetraplegic showing dilation of renal pelvis and large kidneys.

with a lesion of spinal cord at or above T5 warrants prompt alleviation of bladder and colorectal distention. The prevalence of autonomic dysreflexia in children is slightly lower than that in adults; in our series 24% of the children developed this problem. In older children regular use of guanethidine sulfate (Ismelin), 5 mg, and/or mecamylamine hydrochloride (Inversine), 2.5 mg, twice daily has been helpful in preventing the recurrence of these episodes.

Respiratory problems

Children with lesions of the cervical and high thoracic cord may have vital capacity less than one third of the predicted normal value because of paralysis of the intercostal and abdominal muscles. In individuals with lesions of the cervical cord at or above C4, the diaphragmatic paralysis along with intercostal and abdominal muscles might necessitate permanent mechanical ventilatory assistance. The ability to forcibly exhale, sigh, and cough is significantly impaired. This results in accumulation of bronchopulmonary secretions, atelectasis, and pneumonitis, causing more respiratory insufficiency. An active respiratory therapy program must be instituted in all children with cervical and high thoracic lesions on the day of injury. Intermittent positive pressure breathing for 10 to 15 minutes at least four times a day must be continued until vital capacity reaches 2500 cc or above. The use of an incentive respirometer instead of intermittent positive pressure breathing has been equally effective. Vital capacity during the first 2 to 3 weeks must be recorded daily and later on at least twice a week. With the slightest evidence of further respiratory compromise, chest percussion and postural drainage should be started. If secretions cannot be cleared by active percussion therapy and positive pressure breathing, tracheostomy might be necessary. The inspissated mucous plugs responsible for atelectasis may need to be removed with fiberoptic bronchoscopy. Use of an elastic abdominal binder during the early stage has been helpful in assisting diaphragmatic breathing. During the early stage 23 of 97 patients in our series (Table 18-4) developed atelectasis or pneumonitis or both, and only one patient developed pulmonary embolism. There is also a high risk of inhalation of vomitus, aspiration pneumonitis, and death during the early phase in young children. Upper respiratory tract infection in spinal cord injured children who go to school must be carefully watched and vigorously treated.

The young spinal cord injured child has a higher risk of developing spinal deformity, namely, kyphoscoliosis, which would reduce pulmonary capacity and reserve, especially on the concave side. This condition may require operative correction of the deformity to minimize further compromise of respiratory functions.

Venous thrombosis and embolism

Venous thrombosis in spinal cord injured patients still remains a common and poorly understood complication. Several authors have reported 12% to 100% incidence of deep venous thrombosis and a 5% to 15% incidence of pulmonary embolism, with less than 2% to 5% fatalities. Whether this difference in incidence is due to the differences in patient samples or patient care or is related to the different sensitivity of various diagnostic techniques is not clear. Although clinical findings, impedance plethysmography, Doppler ultrasound technique and ^{125}I fibrinogen scan have been used to diagnose deep venous thrombosis, contrast venography still remains the definitive diagnostic test for clinically suspected cases of venous thrombosis. In the present series 48 of 97 children (Table 18-4) admitted at The Institute for Rehabilitation and Research underwent venography—33 had cervical lesions and 15 had thoracic lesions. Sixteen of 33 (48%) cervical cord lesions and ten of 15 (66%) thoracic cord lesions were found to have unilateral or bilateral occlusion of deep venous channels in the lower extremities (Figs. 18-22 to 18-24). Children with complete spinal cord lesions had a higher incidence of venous thrombosis. Since routine venography in children under 5 years of age was not performed in the present series, the incidence of venous

thrombosis in this group is not known. Pulmonary embolism occurred in only one patient with positive venogram. It is quite possible that children with minor clinically insignificant pulmonary emboli were not recognized. This 26% incidence of deep venous thrombosis on venography and 2% incidence of pulmonary embolism in children is significantly lower than that reported for adult spinal cord injured patients.

Since the objectives of treatment of deep venous thrombosis are to prevent pulmonary embolism, to relieve the symptoms of acute thrombosis, and to prevent chronic venous insufficiency, prophylactic anticoagulant therapy has been recommended by some authors.[14,23,52,65] Hachen[25] used 10,000 IU of heparin for 3 weeks followed by Cintron orally until wheelchair activity was achieved; he recorded a reduction in the incidence of deep venous thrombosis from 21% to 6%. By using Phenindione during a period of 12 weeks, Silver[52] recorded a comparable reduction from 25% to 5%. However, Watson[64] reported an incidence of deep venous thrombosis of only 12% with physical therapy and continuous observation without using any prophylactic anticoagulants. Van Hove[62] also concluded that passive mobilization, massage, and elastic stocking compression started on the day of injury and done twice daily provided adequate prophylaxis for thrombophlebitis and pulmonary embolism in his 27 paraplegic patients, none of whom were clinically found to have evidence of thrombophlebitis or pulmonary embolism. From these series, however, we cannot draw any meaningful conclusions about deep venous thrombosis in children. None of the children in the present series had prophylactic anticoagulation therapy. All children with positive venograms were initially treated with intravenous heparin for 7 to 10 days and later switched to warfarin (Coumadin) for at least 3 months. The foot of the bed was elevated by 20° to facilitate venous drainage. The use of elastic stockings or ace wraps while in bed has not been effective in reducing venous thrombosis. Since the total incidence of deep venous thrombosis on venography in children is only 26% and the incidence of pulmonary embolism is only 2%, significantly lower rates than in adults, the prophylactic use of anticoagulants is not warranted in light of the complications of anticoagulant therapy and the need for constant monitoring.

Gastrointestinal problems

Gastrointestinal problems after complete spinal cord lesions in children are not uncommon (Table 18-4). After cervical and high thoracic lesions there is a loss of sympathetic inhibitory influence to viscera and interruption of vasoconstrictor pathways, which result in paralytic vasodilation and vagotonia. Paralytic vasodila-

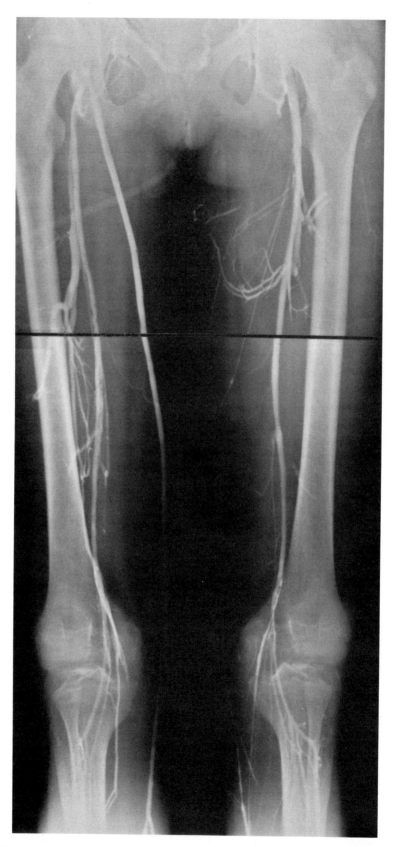

Fig. 18-22. Lower limb venogram of 11-year-old C5 tetraplegic girl shows occlusion of superficial femoral venous channels on left side. There is also an increase in collateral vessels in left calf and thigh.

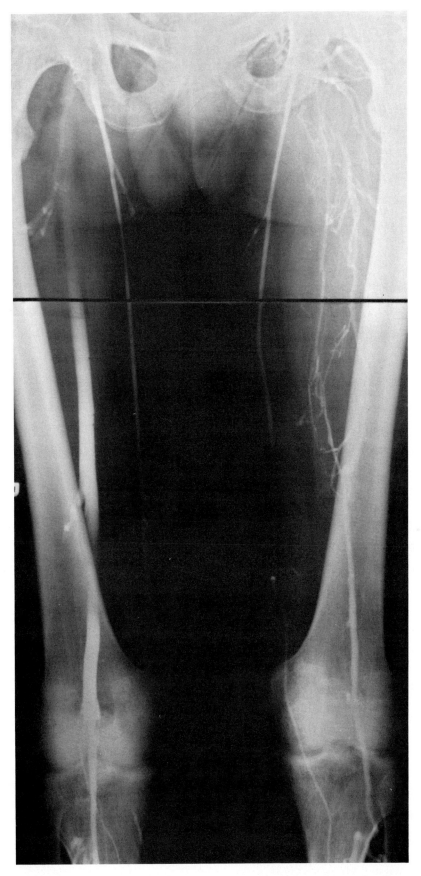

Fig. 18-23. Fifteen-year-old C6 tetraplegic. Venogram of lower limbs 3 months after onset of paralysis shows complete obstruction of deep femoral veins on left side and marked increase in collateral vessels in left thigh consistent with venous obstruction of more than 6 to 8 weeks' duration.

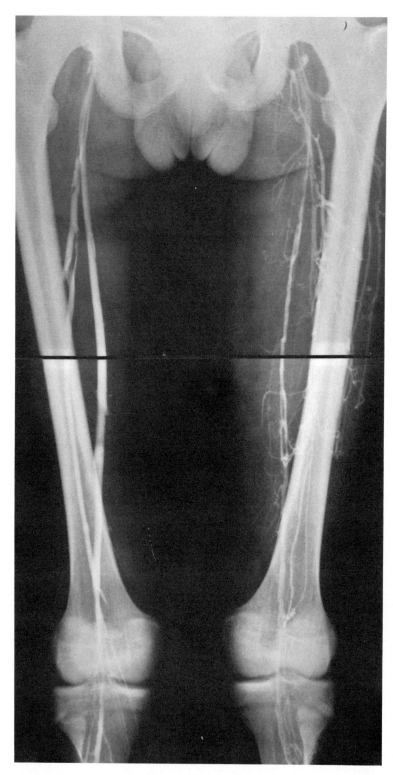

Fig. 18-24. Venogram of lower limbs of 14-year-old C6 tetraplegic boy 10 weeks after injury. There is occlusion of superficial and deep venous channels on left side and marked increase in collaterals in thigh.

tion has been known to produce hemorrhages, necrotic areas, and eventually ulcerations of gastroduodenal mucosa. Vagotonia leads to liberation of large volumes of gastric juice rich in acid and enzymes. Also, elevated levels of catecholamines following the "stress" of trauma (and often of surgery as well) cause a reduction of blood flow to gastric mucosa. In addition, the use of steroids during the acute phase of injury may thin the protective gastric mucin coating. When acted on by excessive amounts of acid and enzyme-rich gastric juices in the absence of mucin these ischemic as well as hemorrhagic foci may further produce erosions and necrosis of the mucosa. The incidence of gastrointestinal bleeding and ulceration in patients of all ages with traumatic lesions of the spinal cord has been reported to be 0.5% to 22%.[10,31,41,45,48] However, the incidence of neurogenic gastroduodenal ulceration and bleeding in children in the present series was 12%. The onset of bleeding in most of these patients occurred during the first 2 weeks following trauma. An acute episode of hypotension, a drop in hematocrit level, and tachycardia were the most common manifestations. Sharp pain in the epigastric region radiating to the back of shoulder, and "shoulder tip" pain occurred in two children. Abdominal distention and paralytic ileus associated with gastroduodenal bleeding were observed in three other children. Six patients underwent laparotomy to control the bleeding or repair the perforated viscus. During surgery multiple ulcers (1 to 5 mm in diameter) in the anterior wall of the stomach were observed in three patients, and in two other patients giant perforated posterior duodenal ulcers were found. Awareness of gastrointestinal hemorrhage and ulceration as a complication of spinal cord injury and very close observation from the time of initial blood loss in children are necessary to minimize the fatalities.

During an intermittent catheterization program, most of the children with spinal cord injury and upper motor neuron bladder require bethanechol chloride (Urecholine Chloride) or other cholinergic drugs, which may mean the possibility of gastroduodenal ulceration; and they must be carefully observed for epigastric discomfort, hyperacidity, and a drop in hematocrit level.

The incidence of paralytic ileus in the present series was 7%. It was successfully treated by placement of nasogastric tube and gravity drainage in two children and by continuous mild suction and drainage of gastric contents in the others. One patient developed symptoms and signs of acute intestinal obstruction on the thirteenth day after injury and underwent a laparotomy but no pathology was found. The cause was probably hypercalcemia. In our experience, during the second and third weeks paralytic ileus has been associated with gastrointestinal hemorrhage and perforated ulcer, whereas during the first week it has been associated with spinal shock. One patient also developed superior mesenteric artery syndrome.

Children with complete spinal cord injury invariably develop fecal incontinence. From the beginning, attention should be focused on developing a regular habit of emptying bowels daily or every other day with the assistance of stool softeners and a rectal suppository. Hardening of stools, impaction, strong purgatives, and enemas must be avoided. After observing the bowel program of a child for 3 days, we start them on low dose dioctyl sodium sulfosuccinate (Colace) and use glycerin or Vacuetts suppositories. It takes about 15 minutes for the suppository to melt and act on the lower intestinal tract. Whether or not there is emptying of the bowels following administration of the suppository, digital stimulation is done in an attempt to obtain more complete evacuation. The regular evacuation of bowel contents is the only key for avoiding erratic bowel accidents and embarassment for the child. In about half the children with spinal cord injury, eventually with improved eating habits and a high-residue diet the bowels can be emptied with only digital stimulation.

Metabolic problems

Sensory deprivation, motor paralysis, and protracted confinement in bed, as well as stress following traumatic injuries of the spinal cord, produce significant metabolic alterations (Table 18-4). An imbalance between osteoblastic and osteoclastic activity is produced. With immobilization osteoblastic activity is considerably decreased and osteoclastic activity with bone resorption is accelerated, which results in mobilization of the calcium pool from the bones, causing hypercalcemia and hypercalciuria. Under these circumstances the levels of serum calcium depend on the efficiency of the renal calcium clearance mechanism. Hypercalcemia in adult spinal cord injured patients is rare, and in children in the present series it occurred in 23% patients. The severity of hypercalcemia had little relationship to the severity of paralysis. Hypercalcemia was observed in most of the cases during the first 3 months and was no longer present 18 months after spinal cord trauma. Children with serum calcium levels of 12 mg/100 ml or above had malaise, anorexia, nausea, vomiting, abdominal distention, constipation, polyuria, polydipsia, and weight loss. Five patients were noted to have fever, vomiting, abdominal distention, hypoactive or absent bowel sounds, and constipation, mimicking acute intra-abdominal pathology; serum calcium levels in four of these patients were above 13.5 mg/100 ml. Fifty-five percent of the hypercalcemia children with spinal cord injury developed urolithiasis, mostly in the kidneys.

Awareness that hypercalcemia is a complication of spinal cord injury in children and regular determination of serum calcium levels at least at 1-month intervals during the first 6 months are essential to make the diagnosis and minimize its complications. Adequate hydration and combination of furosemide and infusion of saline, oral phosphate therapy, and a low-calcium diet have been recommended in the management of hypercalcemia.[55] We have successfully used oral prednisone, 1 to 2 mg/kg/day, in four divided doses in six patients with close monitoring for any evidence of gastrointestinal bleeding. The beneficial effect of prednisone therapy in hypercalcemic patients has also been reported by others,[38,58] but the mechanism of action is not clear. Active mobilization of spinal cord injured children must be pursued; active and passive range of motion, sitting, and weight bearing of extremities must be carried out regularly. Continuous electric stimulation of paralytic muscles to produce stress on long bones in an attempt to minimze bone resorption, osteoporosis, and hypercalcemia is being investigated by the author.

The second common metabolic problem in children is osteoporosis. With increased bone resorption within a few days after the onset of tetraplegia, increased urinary excretion of calcium, phosphorus, and hydroxyproline has been reported.[16] Resumption of total bed rest in tetraplegic patients has also been known to result in increased excretion of collagen metabolites. Infection and toxemia have been shown to increase the severity of osteoporosis. Nevertheless, the role of neurohumeral and trophic factors, nutritional components, and altered circulatory dynamics in inducing osteoporosis in spinal cord injured children needs to be defined. A severe degree of osteoporosis in spinal cord injured children has always been distal to the level of the neurologic lesion—predominantly in the pelvic region and the distal third of the femora. Osteoporosis has been observed less frequently in the ankle region—involving the distal fourth of the tibia, the fibula, and the os calcis. Osteoporosis in some cases might also result in pathologic fractures during severe spasms, physical therapy, and transfer activities. Adequate nutrition and positive nitrogen balance along with active resistive exercises of functioning groups of muscles and passive movements of paralytic limbs are beneficial in improving bone mineralization along the stress trajectories and reducing osteoporosis.

The posttraumatic catabolic state coupled with relatively poor eating habits and lack of proper knowledge in children and adolescents requires careful observance since individuals with low serum albumin levels tend to heal slowly, to form poor osteoid matrix, and to be potential candidates for severe osteoporosis. In the early acute phase a low-calcium diet with high protein and high roughage should be recommended. Children should be taught proper dietary selection and given the choice of picking out their food; they should be encouraged to eat in the dining room instead of in bed.

Spinal deformity

Progressive spinal deformity, although rare in adults, is relatively more common in children with traumatic lesions of spinal cord. The true incidence of this problem is not known. According to Bedbrook[8] all children under 11 years of age sustaining complete or partial paralysis above T10 inevitably develop scoliosis. Babcock[4] also felt that a high proportion of children with cervical and upper thoracic lesions develop scoliosis. Burke[13] in a review of 40 children under 13 years of age with spinal cord trauma reported an incidence of 50% of some degree of spinal deformity between 1 to 18 years after the injury. Paeslack and von Bazan[63] observed scoliosis greater than 15° in 29 of 63 (46%) traumatic lesions of spine in children. The severity of curvatures and degree of deformity increased with the survival time, and there was no relationship between the deformity and the radiologic evidence of osteoarticular trauma to the spines (Figs. 18-25 and 18-26).

There were at least 37 children with thoracic and/or lumbar scoliosis in our series: 21 had mild scoliosis (less than 40°) and 16 had moderate to severe scoliosis (greater than 40°). There were 21 cervical, 7 upper thoracic (T1-6), and 9 lower thoracic and thoracolumbar lesions. Approximately 60% of patients with thoracolumbar scoliosis were 10 years old or younger at the time of injury with progressively increasing kyphoscoliosis. Although all levels of neurologic lesions were at risk in the development of scoliosis, the cervical lesions were more frequently associated with scoliosis than were the thoracic and lumbar segments. There was definitely a higher incidence of laminectomy in the group with more severe scoliosis, but at the same time they were younger (less than 10 years of age). Approximately 80% of children with scoliosis more than 40° had moderate to marked spasticity, whereas 60% of children with scoliosis less than 40° had mild to moderate spasticity.

It is difficult to pinpoint a single etiologic factor responsible for spinal deformity after traumatic injury to the spine. The damage to the vertebral epiphyseal growth plate, or loss of bone height and asymmetric growth of vertebral segments; and the paralysis or muscle imbalance in paraspinal, abdominal, and pelvic muscles, coupled with flexion abduction contractures in the hip region, and in some instances laminectomy following trauma, alone or in combination might initiate the deformity.

Asymmetric pull and loading of the growing spinal column (from asymmetric collapse of the vertebral body from trauma, asymmetric incomplete neurologic lesions, and different degrees of spasticity on the two sides) are the most important factors in the production of progressive spinal deformity. McSweeny[39] stressed the importance of the effect of imbalance of muscles that are not equally innervated from both sides. Roaf[49] has also stressed that the asymmetric action of deep muscle fibers of erector trunci may be the only important factor in initiating the rotational deformity of the vertebral bodies. Similarly, von Bazan and Paeslack[63] have observed that with thoracic paralysis a small asymmetry in the neurologic level of paralysis may produce a difference in muscle tone or spasticity, which often plays a significant role in the production of scoliosis. Varying degrees of spasticity in paraspinal, abdominal, and intercostal muscles produce asymmetric loading of

the spinal column, and the magnitude of deforming forces depend on the degree of spasticity, the level of neurologic lesion, and its completeness. Asymmetric paralysis in children occurs more frequently than in adults, which may produce different degree of spasticity on the two sides. Also, in patients with a higher level of neurologic lesion, a longer segment of spinal column is exposed to the intrinsic spastic musculature and its deforming influence. Unilateral flexion contracture or abduction–external rotation and/or adduction–internal rotation contractures at the hip would produce pelvic obliquity and compensatory thoracolumbar scoliosis and lordoscoliosis. A tight iliotibial band would also produce pelvic tilt, obliquity, and scoliosis. Contracture of the iliopsoas muscle may exert significant deforming forces from its upper attachment to the spine, predominantly

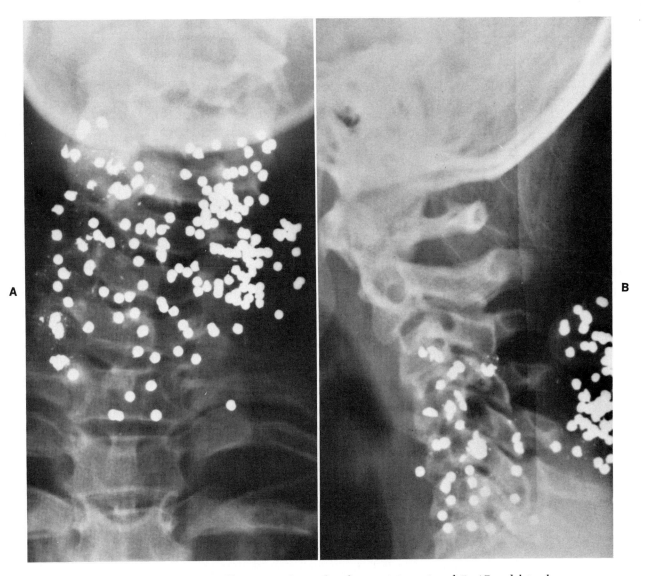

Fig. 18-25. Thirteen-year-old C5 tetraplegic after firearm injury. **A** and **B,** AP and lateral views of cervical spine show multiple pellets in cervical region.

Continued.

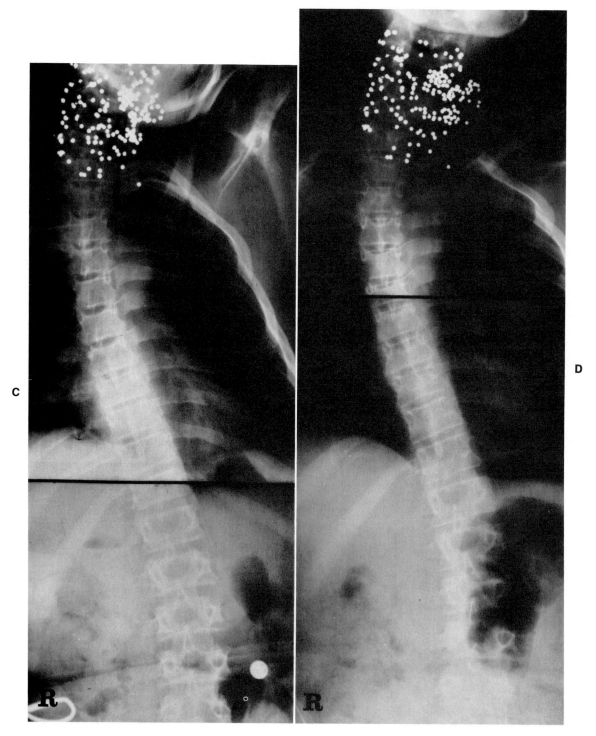

Fig. 18-25, cont'd. C, Scoliosis series 15 months after injury shows right thoracic scoliosis of 22°. **D,** Scoliosis series 2 years after injury shows right thoracic scoliosis of 29°.

resulting in lordosis or lordoscoliosis. Over a period of 18 to 24 months these deforming forces coupled with greater plasticity and flexibility of the spine in approximately 40% of children after spinal paralysis produce varying degrees of kyphoscoliosis, lordosis, and lordoscoliosis. There is often an increase in the deformity with continued growth of the spine and poor sitting posture. The incidence is even higher in children sustaining injury before 10 years of age. We have observed that the progression of spinal deformity has been directly proportional to the period left between the age at the time of injury and the ossification and fusion of the ring apophysis, which starts at 14 to 15 years of age. The younger the child is at the time of injury, the greater the chances are for spinal deformity.

Unreduced or inadequately reduced vertebral fractures and dislocations associated with ligamentous tears very frequently produce a segmental deformity of the spine in children. Often, compressive and disruptive

forces at the time of initial injury produce asymmetric damage to the vertebral body and its growth plate, which results in asymmetric growth and progression of deformity. Operative procedures, such as laminectomy in the presence of unilateral fracture of pedicle and facet or anterior cervical fusion with asymmetric placement of the bone graft, also add to spinal instability and deformity. In the present series slightly over 50% of the children had varying degrees of local spinal deformity.

Complete prevention of spinal deformities after paralysis is not possible. By active awareness that children frequently develop significant spinal curvatures following paralysis and by careful monitoring at regular intervals, the progression and severity of these deformities may be slowed. During the acute stage good anatomic alignment, preferably by nonoperative methods or by judicious surgery, must be obtained and maintained for an adequate length of time to allow good healing of soft

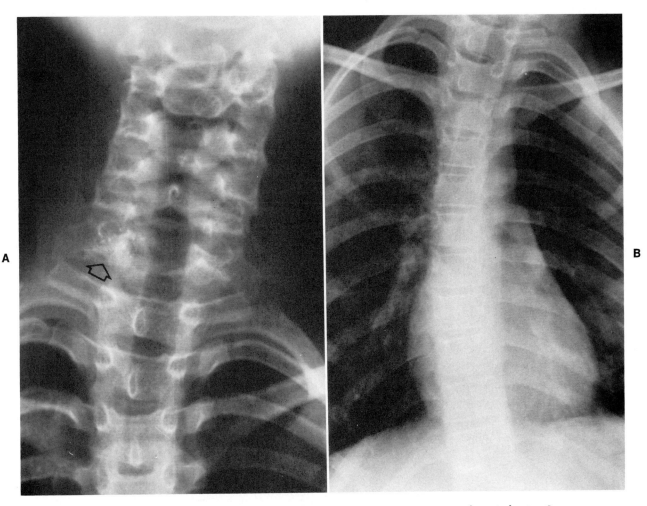

Fig. 18-26. Nine-year-old C7 tetraplegic after gunshot injury. **A,** AP view of cervical spine 8 months after paralysis shows metal stippling along right pedicle of C7 *(arrow)* and torticollis. **B,** AP view of chest shows right thoracic scoliosis.

tissue and osteoarticular lesions. Since traumatized collagen tissue takes about 14 to 21 days to develop adequate tensile strength, static (isometric) exercises of the paraspinal muscles should be started at that time in an attempt to develop good muscle strength and endurance. The patient should be started on a graded sitting program as soon as the spine is stabilized in an adequate brace or by operative means. Good sitting posture at all times must be emphasized and demanded by the treating personnel. Hip and knee flexion contractures should be prevented by an active program of range-of-motion and stretching exercises and prone lying. Standing in a "stand alone" frame with bilateral braces would also provide better vertical tolerance and better control of neck-body reflex mechanisms, in addition to the correction of hip and knee flexion contractures and tight heel cords. Postural methods such as active participation in sports and recreational activities to maintain adequate spinal alignment should be introduced early. If significant spasticity is present, it should be treated promptly by drug therapy and by a regular stretching and corrective splinting program. Regular examination and full-length spine radiographs, sitting and standing, must be done at least once each year. If there is progression of deformity then an examination and radiographs may have to be done more frequently.

Mild scoliosis (less than 40°) can be treated conservatively by a Milwaukee brace, Boston bucket, or corrective plastic or plaster jackets.[4,7] However, the Milwaukee brace, or body jacket along with corrective therapeutic exercises, has been relatively less effective in spinal paralytics than in the management of idiopathic scoliosis. In moderate to severe thoracolumbar scoliosis with or without lumbar lordosis, the Dwyer procedure by anterior approach alone or in combination with Harrington instrumentation can also be used. In fact, Bedbrook[7] suggested that fusion either posteriorly with instrumentation or anteriorly with instrumentation may not be sufficient to maintain the correction in the face of extraordinary forces and extra mobility affecting the paraplegic spine. In spite of better surgical corrections obtained, surgical failure from pseudoarthrosis and recurrence of deformity has been observed frequently in these children.

PROGNOSIS

There seems to be lack of general agreement among those involved in the management of children with traumatic lesions of the spinal cord regarding the prognosis and long-term sequelae. Some authors have reported a benign course and total absence of long-term sequelae in children and adolescents after injuries to spine,[27] and they have indicated that the younger patients have a better prognosis than the adults.[6,27]

According to Tachdjian[56] the prognosis is excellent for full recovery. However, this has not been the experience of other investigators.[11,12,23,36] In our experience the clinical features, radiographic abnormalities, operative findings, and outcome in children with spinal cord injuries are quite similar to those seen in adults with minor exceptions.

In our series, of the 80 patients with cervical spinal cord injury, 59 remained tetraplegic without any improvement in motor function below the level of lesion. Twelve of the 15 patients with central cervical cord syndrome pattern showed good return and were ambulatory on subsequent examination, and three patients remained tetraparetic and confined to wheelchair. All three patients with Brown-Séquard syndrome also made good motor recovery and were ambulatory. The motor status of six patients with anterior cord syndrome pattern remained unchanged. Only one of five patients with incomplete transverse myelopathy showed functional recovery below the level of lesion in the lower limbs and was able to ambulate with braces. The neurologic status of 49 patients with complete transverse myelopathy remained unchanged. Although the patients with complete motor lesions did not show any significant improvement in neurologic return, that is, there was no return of function in new groups of muscles, there was definitely improvement in their functional ability commensurate with the level of injury and age following admission to rehabilitation program. Only two of 36 patients with thoracic cord lesions showed functional return in the lower limbs and became ambulatory with braces, whereas 33 remained paraplegic. After laminectomy one T2 paraplegic patient became a C3-4 tetraplegic. None of the patients with complete lesions of the thoracic spinal cord showed any motor return. Of the eight patients with cauda equina and conus lesions, six showed motor and sensory improvement and became ambulatory with short leg braces; however, none of these patients gained enough strength to ambulate without braces and none developed complete bladder and bowel control.

The autonomic dysfunction triad (hypotension [systolic pressure below 90 mm Hg] hypothermia, and bradycardia [pulse rate of 60/min or below]) was noted in 26 patients at the time of admission and all remained tetraplegic.

Thus in the present series 66% of the children had complete lesions and their status remained unchanged. Of the 41 patients with incomplete lesions, only 19 (15% of total series) showed good functional return and seven (6%) showed some motor return such that they were able to ambulate with braces. The neurologic outcome in children after spinal cord injuries in our experience has been no different than that of adults. Often the prognosis has been worse because of the higher mortality during the acute phase from the associated injuries to other organ systems and the higher frequency of urolithiasis, gastrointestinal bleeding, and ulceration.

NEONATAL SPINAL CORD INJURY

Although neonatal spinal cord injury was first described by Kennedy in 1836[30] under the term *spinal apoplexy* (i.e., spinal cord trauma resulted in death of the neonate), the significance of intrapartum spinal cord trauma is still not realized. When examiners are pursuing the problem of birth injuries during autopsies of newborns, the contents of the spinal canal are not examined regularly and the spinal cord lesions are thus overlooked. According to Towbin[59] in the United States approximately 50,000 pregnancies per year terminate in neonatal death and greater than 10% of these at autopsy show evidence of brain-stem or spinal cord trauma. Ep-

idural and subdural hemorrhages, laceration of dura and nerve roots, distortion of the spinal cord, myelomalacia, and trauma to the vertebral arteries have been reported frequently at autopsy. An awareness that intrapartum spinal cord injury can occur and a high suspicion index are necessary, since such injuries in the newborn asphyxiated infants might be overlooked mainly because attention is directed toward cerebral lesions.

Breech, brow, face, occipitoposterior, and other intrauterine malpositions may render the fetus vulnerable to nonphysiologic forces. Similarly, congenital craniocervical malformations may also predispose the neonate to trauma during mechanical manipulation of the head and trunk, especially during breech delivery and during the application of forceps. Asphyxiated babies are usually hypotonic and therefore particularly vulnerable to spinal injury during difficult delivery. In utero

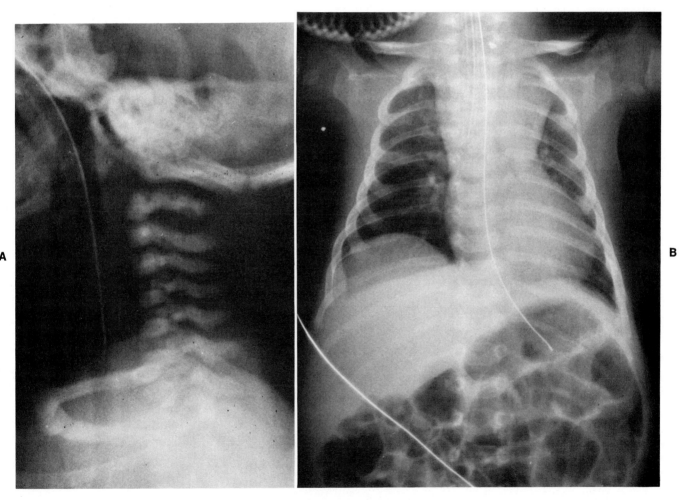

Fig. 18-27. Radiographs of 4-week-old neonate delivered full-term by cesarean birth with C4 central cervical cord syndrome. **A,** Lateral view of cervical spine shows no osteoarticular injury. There is some increase in prevertebral space. **B,** AP view of chest shows bell-shaped chest from paralysis of intercostal muscles.

spinal cord injury without the application of excessive obstetric force is very rare, and well-documented cases are few. Amine[1] reported the birth of a girl who was paraplegic from a stab wound with a barbecue fork sustained by her mother 1 week before the spontaneous delivery. Laminectomy at the age of 7 months in this infant revealed dense scarring of the spinal cord and arachnoid membranes.

The pathomechanism of injury depends on the method of delivery, the type of malposition, and the direction of forces applied. Excessive axial traction during breech and forceps delivery appears to be the single most important and frequent mechanism of intrapartum injury. Thus far the amount of force necessary to produce spinal column and cord damage has not been studied adequately. Experimental studies in fresh, mature stillborn fetuses about the tensile strength of the spinal column were carried out by Duncan in 1874,[21] who reported that the application of 41 kg (90 lb) of longitudinal traction force on the vertebral column resulted in vertebral trauma and 55 kg (120 lb) of force resulted in decapitation. From these data it appears that the longitudinal traction applied during difficult breech extraction is probably more than 41 kg (90 lb). This needs to be critically evaluated in the future. Recently it has been demonstrated that the neonatal spinal column at autopsy can be stretched by 5 cm (2 in) whereas the cervical spinal cord can be pulled down by only 0.64 cm (0.25 in).[59] This "differential elasticity" of the spinal cord and the vertebral column on application of traction might result in significant neurologic deficit without any evidence of osteoarticular trauma. Acute ventroflexion, retroflexion, and trunk rotation during delivery can produce disruption of posterior ligamentous structures, dislocation of vertebrae, and epidural or subdural hematoma, which might cause direct compression of the spinal cord and/or occlusion of radicular, vertebral, and anterior spinal arteries.

In our small series of four intrapartum spinal cord injuries, two were breech deliveries, one was a cephalic presentation, and one was a cesarean delivery. All neonates had involvement of the cervical cord: one was C6 tetraplegic and two had C8-T1 lesions. One neonate with respiratory insufficiency showed a clinical picture of central cervical cord syndrome. Radiographs of the spine showed no evidence of osteoarticular injury or congenital vertebral abnormalities. The chest roentgenograms showed a bell-shaped thorax indicative of intercostal paralysis (Fig. 18-27). We feel that spine radiographs in neonates with spinal cord injury should be used more to rule out any congenital vertebral anomalies than to diagnose osteoarticular trauma.

LIFE EXPECTANCY

Patients with spinal cord injuries have been known to have a higher mortality and lower average life expectancy than individuals of similar age and sex in the general population. Greater susceptibility to pressure sores, urinary tract infection, hypertension, and other metabolic and respiratory complications have been considered to be the common causes of death in these patients. There are few publications about the life expectancy in adult spinal cord injured patients, and there is a paucity of references on this subject in pediatric population. Analysis of the mortality trends for spinal cord injured patients indicates that the age of the patient at the time of trauma and the severity of injury are the two important determinants of the likelihood of survival. In general, the younger the patient, the better are the prospects for a longer life span. Similarly the less severe the injury, the better the chances are for patients enjoying a near-normal life expectancy. This is only true after the initial 4 weeks following spinal injury in children, since the initial mortality from associated injuries and their complications is higher in the pediatric population. By using the relative mortality ratios

Table 18-5. Life expectancies of spinal cord injured children

| Age at discharge | General population* | | Paraplegic | | | | Tetraplegic | | | |
| | | | Incomplete | | Complete | | Incomplete | | Complete | |
	Boys	Girls	Boys	Girls	Boys	Girls	Boys	Girls	Boys	Girls
9	60.3	67.8	58.2	65.1	43.1	51.2	50.8	59.0	29.4	38.7
10	59.3	66.8	57.2	64.1	42.2	50.9	49.9	58.1	28.6	37.8
11	58.3	65.8	56.3	63.1	41.3	50.0	48.9	57.1	27.8	36.9
12	57.3	64.8	55.3	62.1	40.4	49.1	48.0	56.1	26.9	36.1
13	56.4	63.8	54.3	61.2	39.4	48.1	47.0	55.2	26.1	35.2
14	55.4	62.8	53.3	60.2	38.5	47.2	46.1	54.2	25.2	34.3
15	54.5	61.9	52.4	59.2	37.6	46.2	45.1	53.2	24.4	33.4
16	53.5	60.9	51.5	58.2	36.8	45.3	44.3	52.3	23.8	32.7

*Figures used for comparison.

developed by Jousse and co-workers[28] and the annual mortality for the general population derived from the 1973 United States life tables,[60] it is possible to estimate the survival probabilities and life expectancy for spinal cord injured children of either sex, at various ages between 9 and 15 years, with paraplegia or tetraplegia, and with a complete or an incomplete lesion. Standard life table techniques may be also used to accomplish the calculations.[53] Table 18-5 shows life expectancies for male and female spinal cord injured patients based on the available data. However, with continued research and improvements in the quality of medical care a significant improvement and a close to normal life expectancy should be expected in the future.

FOLLOW-UP AND READMISSION PLAN

After discharge from the spinal unit, children must be observed at regular intervals in an attempt to minimize the medical complications. The family physician or pediatrician can also participate in continued care. Readmission to the spinal cord unit at least once a year is strongly recommended. During this admission a thorough medical check-up, including liver and renal function tests, urodynamic studies, intravenous urography, and spinal scoliosis series, should be done. The upper and lower limb orthotic equipment must be checked for proper fit and functional efficacy. The wheelchair must also be checked for its fit and signs of wear and tear. The patient's ability to perform day-to-day activities should be evaluated, and efforts must be made to upgrade those activities commensurate with the level of lesion and age and development of the child. For this purpose hospitalization of 10 to 14 days is necessary, which can be arranged during the summer vacation or winter holidays for children attending school.

REFERENCES

1. Amine, A. R. C.: Spinal cord injury in a fetus, Surg. Neurol. 6:369-370, 1976.
2. Audic, B., and Maury, M.: Secondary vertebral deformities in childhood and adolescence, Paraplegia 7:10-16, 1969.
3. Aufdermauer, M.: Spinal injuries in juveniles, J. Bone Joint Surg. [Br.] 56:513-519, 1974.
4. Babcock, J. B.: Spinal injuries in children, Pediatr. Clin. North Am. 22:487-500, 1975.
5. Bailey, R. W., and Badgley, C. E.: Stabilization of the cervical spine by anterior fusion, J. Bone Joint Surg. [Am.] 42:565-594, 1960.
6. Beatson, T. R.: Fractures and dislocations of the cervical spine, J. Bone Joint Surg. [Br.] 45:21-35, 1963.
7. Bedbrook, G. M.: Stability of spinal fractures and fracture dislocations, Int. J. Paraplegia 9:23-32, 1971.
8. Bedbrook, G. M.: Correction of scoliosis due to paraplegia sustained in pediatric age group, Paraplegia 15:90-97, 1977.
9. Breig, A.: Biomechanics of the central nervous system, Stockholm, 1960, Almqvist & Wiksell.
10. Brock, J. S.: X-ray survey—upper gastrointestinal disease—284 spinal cord injury patients. Proceedings of the Veterans Administration Spinal Cord Injury Conference, Oct. 1964.
11. Burke, D. C.: Spinal cord trauma in children, Paraplegia 9:1-14, 1971.
12. Burke, D. C.: Traumatic spinal paralysis in children, Paraplegia 11:268-276, 1974.
13. Burke, D. C.: Injuries of the spinal cord in children. In Vinken, P. J., and Bruyn: Handbook of clinical neurology, vol. 25, New York, 1976, American Elsevier Publishing Co., pp. 175-195.
14. Casas, E. R., Sanchez, M. P., Arias, C. R., and Masip, J. P.: Prophylaxis of venous thrombosis and pulmonary embolism in patients with traumatic spinal cord lesions, Paraplegia 15:209-214, 1977.
15. Cheshire, D. J. E.: The pediatric syndrome of traumatic myelopathy without demonstrable vertebral injury, Paraplegia 15:74-85, 1977.
16. Claus-Walker, J., Spencer, W. A., Carter, R. E., et al.: Bone metabolism in quadriplegia: dissociation between calciuria and hydroxyprolinuria, Arch. Phys. Med. Rehabil. 56:327-332, 1975.
17. Cloward, R. B.: Surgical treatment of dislocations and compression fractures of the cervical spine by the anterior approach. Proceedings of the Seventh Annual Clinical Spinal Cord Injury Conference, Sept. 29-30 and Oct. 1, 1969, pp. 26-34.
18. Cloward, R. B.: Skull traction of cervical spine injury: should it be abandoned, J.A.M.A. 226:1008, 1973.
19. Cloward, R. B.: Treatment of spinal cord injury, J.A.M.A. 228:1096-1097, 1974.
20. Comarr, A. E.: Conservative management of the urinary bladder among children with spinal cord injury, Paraplegia 10:232-241, 1972.
21. Duncan, J. M.: Laboratory note: on the tensile strength of the fresh adult foetus, Br. Med. J. 2:763, 1874.
22. Gehrig, R., and Michaelis, L. S.: Statistics of acute paraplegia and tetraplegia on a national scale, Paraplegia 6:93-95, 1968.
23. Glasauer, F. E., and Cares, H. L.: Traumatic paraplegia in infancy, J.A.M.A. 219:38-41, 1972.
24. Guttmann, L., and Frankel, H. L.: Value of intermittent catheterization in the early management of traumatic paraplegia and tetraplegia, Paraplegia 4:63-84, 1969.
25. Hachen, H. J.: Anticoagulant therapy in patients with spinal cord injury, Paraplegia 12:176-187, 1974.
26. Hegenbarth, R., and Ebel, K. D.: Roentgen findings in fractures of vertebral column in childhood. Examination of thirty-five patients and its results, Pediatr. Radiol. 5:34-39, 1976.
27. Hubbard, D.: Injuries of the spine in children and adolescents, Clin. Orthop. 100:56-65, 1974.
28. Jousse, A. T., Wynne-Jones, M., and Breithaupt, D. J.: A follow-up study of life expectancy and mortality in trau-

matic transverse myelitis, Can. Med. Assoc. J. **98**:770-772, 1968.

29. Kempe, L.: Anterior decompression in spinal cord injury: a follow up report. Proceedings of the Thirteenth Annual Clinical Spinal Cord Injury Conference, Oct. 1964, pp. 64-65.

30. Kennedy, E.: Observations on cerebral and spinal apoplexy, paralysis and convulsions of new-born infants, Dublin J. Med. Sci. **10**:419, 1836.

31. Kewalramani, L. S.: Neurogenic gastroduodenal ulceration and bleeding associated with spinal cord injuries. Trauma **19**:259-265, 1979.

32. Kewalramani, L. S.: Autonomic dysreflexia in traumatic myelopathy, Am. J. Phys. Med. **59**:1-21,1980.

33. Kewalramani, L. S., Kraus, J. F., and Sterling, H. M.: Acute spinal cord lesions in a pediatric population—epidemiological and clinical features, Paraplegia **18**:206-219, 1980.

34. Kewalramani, L. S., and Riggins, R. S.: Complications of anterior spondylodesis for traumatic lesions of the cervical spine, Spine **2**:25-38, 1977.

35. Kewalramani, L. S., and Tori, J. A.: Spinal cord trauma in children—neurological patterns, radiological features and pathomechanics of injury, Spine **5**:11-18, 1980.

36. LeBlanc, H. J., and Nadell, J.: Spinal cord injuries in children, Surg. Neurol. **2**:411-414, 1974.

37. Leventhal, H.: Birth injuries of the spinal cord, J. Pediatr. **56**:447-453, 1960.

38. Maynard, F., and Imaii, K.: Immobilization hypercalcemia in spinal cord injury, Arch. Phys. Med. Rehabil. **58**:16-24, 1977.

39. McSweeny, T.: Spinal deformity after spinal cord injury, Paraplegia **6**:212-221, 1969.

40. Melzak, J.: Paraplegia among children, Lancet **2**:45-48, 1969.

41. Mihaldzic, N., and Frederick, W.: Peptic ulcer in paraplegia. Proceedings of the Thirteenth Spinal Cord Injury Conference, Oct. 1964, pp. 68-71.

42. Myers, P. W., and Buckley, R. E.: Management of the complications of anterior cervical fusion. Proceedings of the Sixteenth Annual Clinical Spinal Cord Injury Conference, Sept. 1967, pp. 33-38.

43. Norrell, H. A.: The role of early vertebral body replacement in treatment of certain cervical fractures. Proceedings of the Eighteenth Annual Clinical Spinal Cord Injury Conference, Oct. 1971, pp. 35-39.

44. Norrell, H. A., and Wilson, C. B.: Early anterior fusion for injuries of the cervical portion of the spine, J.A.M.A. **214**:525-530, 1970.

45. Nusiebeh, I. M.: Stress ulceration in spinal injuries. In Vinken, P. J., and Bruyn: Handbook of clinical neurology, vol. 26, New York, 1976, American Elsevier Publishing Co., pp. 351-353.

46. Pearman, J. W.: Urological follow up of 99 spinal cord injured patients initially managed by intermittent catheterization, Br. J. Urol. **48**:297, 1976.

47. Perret, G., and Greene, J.: Anterior interbody fusion in the treatment of cervical fracture dislocation, Arch. Surg. **96**:530-539, 1968.

48. Perret, G., and Soloman A.: Gastrointestinal hemorrhage and cervical cord injuries. Proceedings of the Seventeenth Veterans Administration Spinal Cord Conference, 1969.

49. Roaf, R.: Vertebral scoliosis secondary to paraplegia, Paraplegia **8**:42-47, 1970.

50. Scher, A. T.: Trauma of the spinal cord in children, South Afr. Med. J. **50**:2023-2025, 1976.

51. Sharrard, W. J. W.: Pediatric orthopaedics and fractures, Oxford, England, 1973, Blackwell Scientific Publications.

52. Silver, J. R: The prophylactic use of anticoagulant therapy in the prevention of pulmonary embolism in one hundred consecutive spinal injury patients, Paraplegia **12**:188-196, 1974.

53. Smart, C. N., and Sanders, C. R.: The costs of motor vehicle related spinal cord injuries, Washington, D.C., 1976, Insurance Institute for Highway Safety.

54. Smith, P. H., Cook, J. B., and Robertson, W. G.: Stone formation in paraplegia, Paraplegia **7**:77, 1969.

55. Suki, W. N., Yium, J., Von Minden, M., et al.: Acute treatment of hypercalcemia with furosemide, N. Engl. J. Med. **283**:836-840, 1970.

56. Tachdjian, M. O.: Pediatric orthopedics, vol. 2, Philadelphia, 1972, W. B. Saunders Co.

57. Tori, J. A., and Hill, L. L.: Hypercalcemia in children with spinal cord injury, Arch. Phys. Med. Rehabil. **59**:443-447, 1978.

58. Tori, J. A., and Kewalramani, L. S.: Urolithiasis in children with spinal cord injury, Paraplegia **16**:357-365, 1979.

59. Towbin, A.: Latent spinal cord and brain stem injury in newborn infants, Dev. Med. Child Neurol. **11**:54-68, 1969.

60. U.S. Department of Health and Human Services, National Center for Health Statistics: Life tables. Vital statistics of the United States, vol. 2, sec. 5, 1973.

61. Vakili, H.: The spinal cord, New York, 1967, International Medical Book Corporation, Publishers.

62. Van Hove, E.: Prevention of thrombophlebitis in spinal injury patients, Paraplegia **16**:322-335, 1978.

63. von Bazan, U. K. B., and Paeslack, V.: Scoliotic growth in children with acquired paraplegia, Paraplegia **15**:65-73, 1977.

64. Watson, N.: Anticoagulant therapy in the treatment of venous thrombosis with pulmonary embolism in acute spinal injury, Paraplegia **12**:197-201, 1974.

65. Watson, N.: Anticoagulant therapy in the prevention of venous thrombosis and pulmonary embolism in spinal cord injury, Paraplegia **16**:265-270, 1978.

CHAPTER 19

Nuclear medicine in spinal cord injury

STEWART SPIES, M.D.

The patient who has suffered a spinal cord injury is susceptible to a variety of coexistent abnormalities incurred at the time of the initial injury or which develop secondary to prolonged hospitalization. The use of radioisotope techniques in the assessment of the traumatized patient is well established. These methods offer the advantage of ease of performance and relative independence from patient cooperation. In addition, the rapid advance in mobile scintillation camera technology over the past few years has made it possible to obtain the highest quality clinical images at the patient's bedside. The availability of portable studies has been particularly welcome in view of the difficulty in transporting patients with spinal cord injury to the nuclear medicine department.

The radiation burden to a patient undergoing diagnostic imaging procedures is the same magnitude as that received during conventional radiologic examinations and generally less than the exposure from special procedures, such as angiography and fluoroscopy. Idiosyncratic or true allergic reactions to radiopharmaceuticals are rare; thus these procedures may be employed in all age groups and in patients with a variety of allergic histories with relative safety. As with any examination using ionizing radiation, the use of isotope techniques in pregnant women should be done only after careful consideration of the potential risks and the reasonably expected benefits.

ASSESSMENT OF SKELETAL ABNORMALITIES

In the early days of radioisotope bone imaging, these procedures were applied almost exclusively to the evaluation of patients with known or suspected malignant disease. With the rapid improvement in radiopharmaceuticals and imaging equipment, the use of bone imaging in patients with a variety of benign bone disorders began to increase. Today it is feasible to identify fractures and assess the skeletal healing process, identify and follow areas of active bone infection, and detect and quantitate areas of ectopic ossification in the trauma patient through the use of radioisotope techniques.

Bone imaging is performed using one of the phosphate ^{99m}Tc compounds, including pyrophosphate (PYP) ^{99m}Tc, hydroxyethylidene diphosphate (HEDP) ^{99m}Tc, and methylene diphosphonate (MDP) ^{99m}Tc. Following intravenous injection of these bone-seeking radiopharmaceuticals, approximately 50% of the injected dose is deposited in the skeletal system by chemisorption to calcium-hydroxyapatite crystals within the bone. The remainder of the dose is excreted by glomerular filtration, and the combined plasma clearance through excretion and bone extraction has a half-life of less than 30 minutes for most modern bone imaging agents. Although the precise mechanism of localization in pathologic conditions is still the subject of investigation, it seems certain that alteration in local blood flow plays an important role in the increased accumulation of these compounds in areas of abnormal bone.[22,25]

541

A typical clinical protocol for performing a whole-body bone scintigram begins with the intravenous injection of 15 mCi of one of the previously described radiopharmaceuticals. The site of injection is recorded on the patient record so that an extravasation of the dose will not be interpreted as a pathologic process. A 2- to 3-hour delay prior to imaging allows for adequate bone localization and renal excretion of background activity in patients with near-normal renal function. During this delay the patient is encouraged to take fluids if clinically feasible. If an indwelling bladder catheter is not present, the bladder should be emptied before imaging commences. The images themselves may be performed in one of two ways. Individual scintiphotographs of various parts of the skeleton may be obtained using a standard or large-field-of-view scintillation camera. Alternatively, the patient may be placed on a whole-body imaging couch interfaced to a scintillation camera. In the latter instance a single view of the entire skeleton can be recorded on one film. In the case of whole-body imaging, anterior and posterior projections are generally obtained. Suspicious or confusing areas on the original set of images can often be clarified by obtaining additional views using either a pinhole or converging collimator to increase the effective spatial resolution of the imaging system.

Fractures

Although the diagnosis of skeletal fractures is generally within the domain of conventional radiologic procedures, there are certain instances in which radioisotope bone imaging may be useful.[2,16,27] The metabolic and accompanying perfusion changes that occur within 1 to 2 days after traumatic fracture of a bone result in enhanced concentration of bone-seeking radiopharmaceuticals. In parts of the skeleton where detection of fracture is difficult, such as the sternum, scapula, facial bones, and ribs, bone imaging can be useful. In addition, whole-body imaging to survey for unsuspected bone injury is feasible. In the typical case, increased uptake at the fracture site will first be seen 48 hours after injury. This uptake may increase in intensity over several weeks to months. At this time the uptake at the fracture site will gradually decrease, although the rapidity and extent of this decrease depend on fracture location, patient age, and the presence of underlying bone disease. In addition, the immobilization of the spinal cord injured patient will result in persistence of abnormal uptake at the fracture site beyond what is usual. Trauma severe enough to result in periosteal reaction in the affected bone will be detected by bone imaging (Figs. 19-1 and 19-2). In addition, minor bone trauma not seen on conventional radiographs will frequently be detected on bone images.[7]

Osteomyelitis

Active bone infection results in changes in regional bone perfusion not unlike those described for traumatic fractures, and as a result, increase bone uptake in and around a region of infected bone is the rule. There are two major indications for using radionuclide imaging techniques for detection of osteomyelitis. Because the abnormal bone uptake precedes radiographic changes by several days, isotope imaging may give the first indication of a developing infection.[6,20] In addition, the whole-body survey can be useful in identifying clinically unsuspected lesions. A second indication for bone imaging is as an aid in distinguishing cellulitis from cellulitis with underlying osteomyelitis. The immobilized victim of a spinal cord injury is more susceptible to developing local areas of skin inflammation. The distinction of these areas from areas overlying osteomyelitis[4,10] has important therapeutic implications. In patients with active bone inflammation in addition to overlying cellulitis, multiple scintillation camera views of the affected region will demonstrate increased activity along the course of the bone (Fig. 19-3). In addition, the uptake in osteomyelitis tends to become more prominent

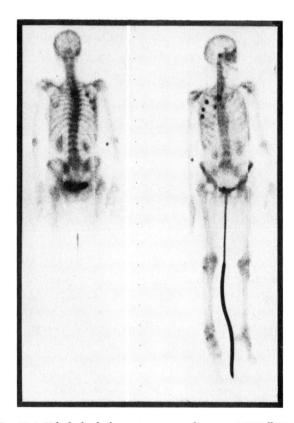

Fig. 19-1. Whole body bone images made using MDP ^{99m}Tc in the posterior *(left)* and anterior projections. Multiple areas of increased uptake in right anterior ribs are typical of recent rib fracture.

on delayed (2 to several hours) views whereas the blood pool activity typical of cellulitis decreases with the passage of time. Thus comparison of early and delayed images following a single intravenous injection can be of considerable help in the differential diagnosis of osteomyelitis. The interpretation of bone images in patients with bone infection can be complicated by concurrent antibiotic therapy or corticosteroid administration, and thus a careful medication history should be obtained in all cases.[11]

Ectopic ossification

It is generally accepted that the timing of surgery for the removal of ectopic bone deposits in the paralyzed patient is critical. Surgical intervention prior to complete maturation of such bony deposits is associated with a high recurrence rate. Conventional radiographs, arteriographs, and blood gas determinations have not been found to be reliable in determining when the process of ectopic ossification has stabilized and therefore are not sufficient to determine when surgery should be

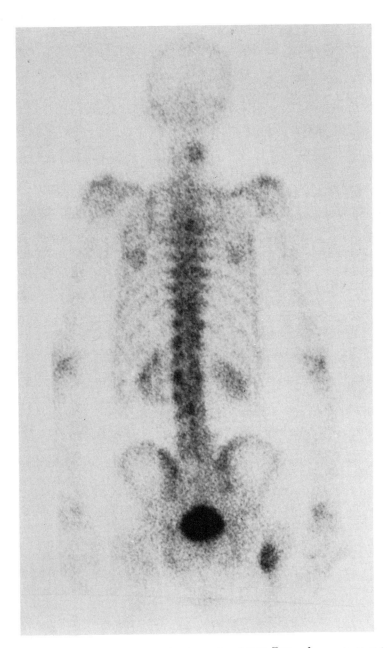

Fig. 19-2. Bone image in posterior projection using MDP ⁹⁹ᵐTc, demonstrating increased uptake in right medial cervical region and proximal right femur both secondary to traumatic fracture.

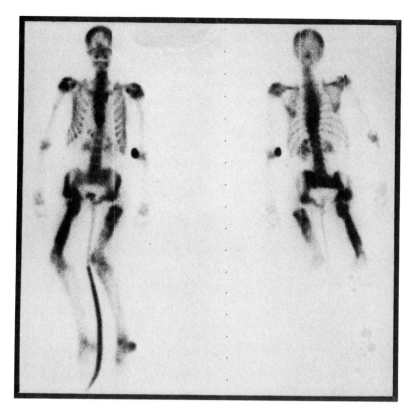

Fig. 19-3. Whole body bone images in anterior *(left)* and posterior projections, demonstrating striking increased accumulation of MDP ^{99m}Tc in both femurs secondary to acute osteomyelitis.

undertaken. Measurements of serum alkaline phosphatase, when performed serially, can be useful in this regard.[14,18] Recently, radioisotopic bone scans have been employed to detect and quantitate the presence of ectopic bone.[1,13] These bony deposits generally result in intense uptake of ^{99m}Tc bone imaging agents (Fig. 19-4). If images are stored on a dedicated digital computer, regions of interest around areas of abnormal accumulation can be assigned. The uptake in these regions can be compared with uptake in nearby normal bone, and the resulting ratio can be compared with ratios obtained on previous and subsequent studies to assess the activity of the abnormal ossification. Some investigators feel that this is the most reliable way of determining when stabilization has occurred.

ABDOMINAL INJURY
Spleen

The significant incidence of splenic abnormality after abdominal trauma and the potentially serious consequences of allowing such injury to go undetected are well known.[9] Since splenic injury almost invariably results in disruption of the normal splenic architecture, techniques that reveal the morphology of the spleen

can be useful in evaluating patients for the presence of splenic trauma. Conventional radiologic examination of the abdomen may not reveal small subcapsular or intrasplenic hematomas, and yet a low clinical index of suspicion may preclude the use of the more sensitive but more invasive arteriographic techniques. Splenic imaging using ^{99m}Tc sulfur colloid (SC) can be performed quickly, inexpensively, and with minimal discomfort to the patient. Following intravenous injection of 2 to 4 mCi of the radiopharmaceutical, greater than 90% of the activity is cleared from the plasma by reticuloendothelial cells within 30 minutes. Using a gamma camera equipped with a high resolution collimator, images of the spleen are obtained in the anterior, left lateral, posterior, left anterior oblique, and left posterior oblique projections. The importance of obtaining multiple views when looking for splenic injury must be stressed. Each image will typically contain 500,000 events and take only a few minutes to acquire. Interpretation of the resulting images is based on finding displacement of the organ or focal defects in sulfur colloid distribution (Figs. 19-5 and 19-6). As with any imaging technique, a knowledge of the variability of normal anatomy is required to accurately interpret the re-

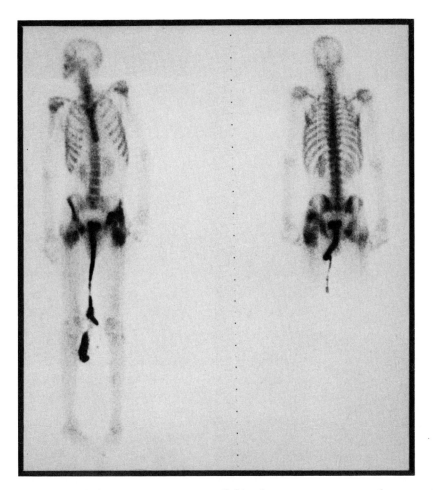

Fig. 19-4. Whole body bone images in anterior *(left)* and posterior projections, demonstrating increased MDP 99mTc uptake in ectopic bone in region of left hip.

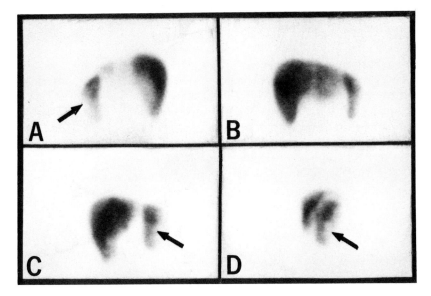

Fig. 19-5. 99mTc SC liver-spleen scintiphotographic study in posterior, **A**, anterior, **B**, left anterior oblique, **C**, and left lateral, **D**, projections, demonstrating defect in splenic uptake secondary to acute subcapsular hematoma *(arrows)*.

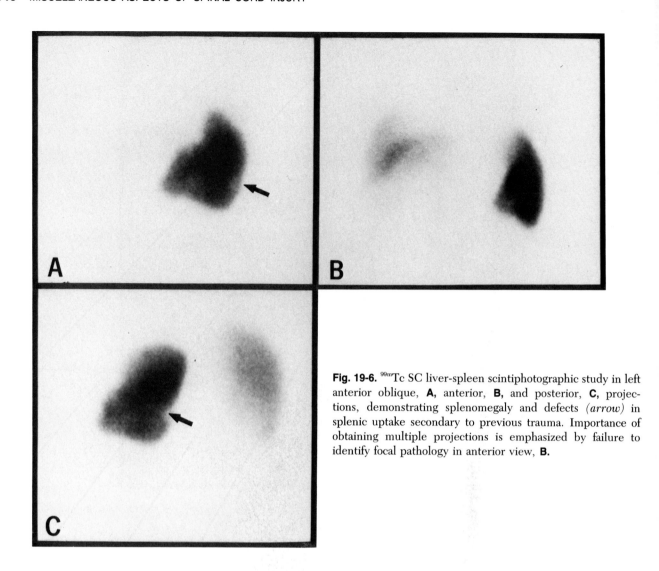

Fig. 19-6. ^{99m}Tc SC liver-spleen scintiphotographic study in left anterior oblique, **A,** anterior, **B,** and posterior, **C,** projections, demonstrating splenomegaly and defects *(arrow)* in splenic uptake secondary to previous trauma. Importance of obtaining multiple projections is emphasized by failure to identify focal pathology in anterior view, **B.**

sults. The presence of costal grooving or unusual "defects" in areas where the left lobe of the liver and the spleen overlap must not be confused with pathologic areas of decreased uptake. With careful attention to technique and interpretation, the sensitivity of imaging for detection of significant splenic trauma is approximately 90%.[15,17,23,28] False positive scans resulting from splenic abscess or neoplasm or from congenital variation in splenic shape are not commonly seen and do not seriously affect the clinical utility of the procedure.[3]

Liver

Although splenic injury is twice as common as hepatic injury in blunt abdominal trauma, significant damage to the liver is frequent enough to warrant diagnostic procedures to identify or exclude this possibility. The same technique of using ^{99m}Tc sulfur colloid (SC) for

splenic imaging can be used to obtain high-resolution images of the liver. Once again, multiple projections are employed to optimize the likelihood of finding defects in uptake. Typically, anterior, posterior, right lateral, and right and left anterior oblique images are obtained. Subcapsular hematoma, hepatic lacerations, and intrahepatic hemorrhage can all be identified by imaging techniques.[5,21] It is generally accepted that scintigraphy of the liver and spleen should be among the first imaging procedures obtained in patients with abdominal trauma. Normal results in the examination will effectively rule out significant liver and spleen trauma in the majority of cases (false negative rate less than 1%). Questionable abnormalities will allow subsequent arteriography to concentrate on suspicious areas. The finding of defects typical of significant hepatic or splenic injury may preclude the need for more invasive procedures.

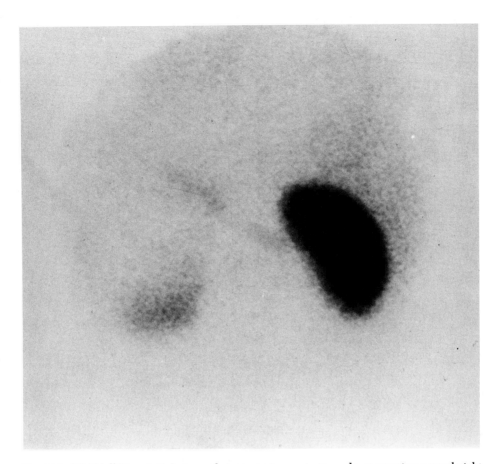

Fig. 19-7. DMSA ^{99m}Tc scintiphotograph in posterior projection, demonstrating normal right kidney and large cyst in left kidney with little functioning parenchyma.

RENAL MORPHOLOGY AND FUNCTION

Radioisotopes have long been employed for the assessment of structural and functional anomalies of the urinary tract. Trauma affecting the vascular supply to the kidneys at the level of the abdominal aorta can be evaluated using isotope aortography. A bolus injection of erythrocytes labeled with ^{99m}Tc or human serum albumin ^{99m}Tc can be used to obtain a dynamic sequence of images over the abdominal aorta. Significant abnormalities including aneurysmal dilatation and thrombosis can be readily appreciated. Static "blood pool" images obtained after the dynamic sequence have also been shown to be useful in evaluating the abdominal aorta.

The use of renal localizing agents labeled with ^{99m}Tc, such as DTPA, glucoheptonate, and dimercapto succinic acid (DMSA), facilitates the rapid assessment of parenchymal trauma, including renal laceration and hematoma. The use of DMSA with its high percentage of irreversible renal cortical binding allows one to obtain high-resolution images of the renal parenchyma. Typically, 5 to 7 mCi of this agent is injected intravenously and images in multiple projections are obtained after a delay of 1 to several hours (Fig. 19-7). An additional dividend of DMSA imaging occurs if the camera data can be recorded and stored using a small digital computer. In such cases it is possible to calculate the fraction of renal blood flow perfusing each kidney. This technique can be used to clarify findings on the isotope aortogram described above as they relate to renal perfusion. Perhaps the most useful applications of radioisotopes in the evaluation of spinal cord injured patients both immediately after trauma and during convalescence are those that relate to the assessment of renal function. The principal radiopharmaceutical used for renal function analysis is orthoiodohippurate (OIH) ^{131}I. After intravenous injection of 200 μCi of OIH ^{131}I, a timed sequence of images is obtained using a gamma camera. If the camera is interfaced to a digital computer, quantitative assessment of renal function including calculation of effective renal plasma flow is possible. Analysis of scintillation images in conjunction with the quantitative data can be helpful in evaluating the extent and location of significant renal trauma and also in detection of urinary extravasation (Fig. 19-8).[12]

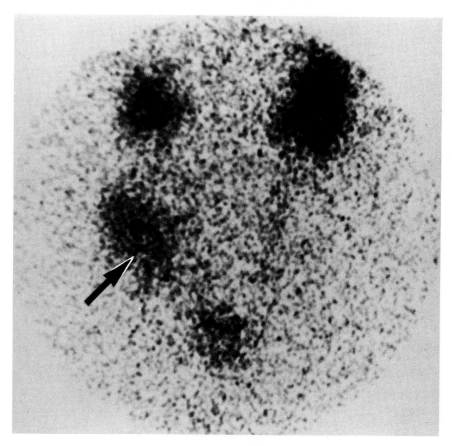

Fig. 19-8. Sodohippurate sodium ^{131}I in posterior projection, demonstrating area of urinary extravasation adjacent to middle third of left ureter *(arrow)*.

DETECTION OF DEEP VENOUS THROMBOSIS

Because of relative immobility, the spinal cord injured patient is at risk for the development of deep venous thrombosis, and recent data suggest that the incidence of deep venous thrombosis in this patient population is extremely high. There are two nuclear medicine procedures that can be employed in evaluating patients for the presence of deep venous thrombosis: the radionuclide venogram and the fibrinogen uptake test.

Radionuclide venography is a simple procedure for evaluating the patency of the deep venous system. The test is performed by injecting 2 mCi of albumin ^{99m}Tc microspheres or macroaggregated albumin simultaneously into each foot and obtaining sequential images of the ascent of each bolus through the venous system of the legs, thighs, and into the pelvis. Delayed images over these same areas are obtained to look for areas of radionuclide retention ("hot spots"). In the presence of deep venous thrombosis, one or more abnormal observations will be made: retained activity in the region of a thrombus, collateral circulation, or decreased flow through the involved area (Figs. 19-9 and 19-10). Re-

sults of isotope venography have been compared with conventional contrast venography with good agreement between the two techniques.[26] However, radionuclide venography is of limited value in the calf, where stasis and collateral flow may be observed in the absence of thrombosis. Nonetheless, the simplicity and accuracy of this technique make it a useful diagnostic tool, and the ability to perform the examination at the bedside using a mobile scintillation camera adds to its value in patients with spinal cord injury (Fig. 19-9). More recently, the availability of human fibrinogen labeled with ^{125}I has resulted in a highly sensitive and easily performed method of detecting active thrombosis in the lower extremities. The commercially available fibrinogen is obtained from a highly screened donor population, and the risk of hepatitis is considered remote. The test is performed by injecting 100 μCi of fibrinogen ^{125}I intravenously after appropriate blockade of the thyroid gland with oral potassium iodide. Counting over the legs is performed on the day after injection and every 24 hours thereafter until a diagnosis of thrombosis has been made or the count rate is too low to continue. This counting is generally performed with a portable

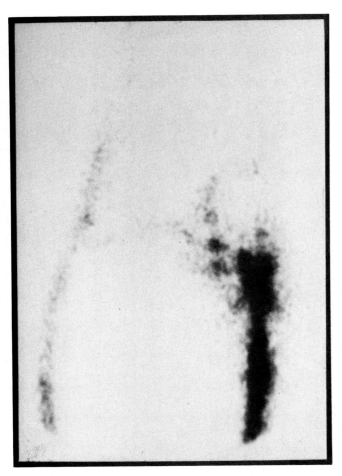

Fig. 19-9. Human albumin microsphere (HAM) ^{99m}Tc image from dynamic flow study over region of pelvis and proximal thighs. Anterior projection demonstrates decreased flow through left illiac vein with collateral circulation.

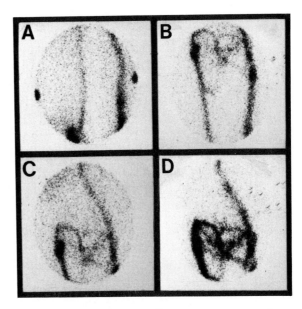

Fig. 19-10. Images from HAM ^{99m}Tc venogram over calves, **A,** thighs, **B,** and pelvis, **C** and **D,** demonstrating right iliac vein occlusion with extensive collateral formation secondary to deep vein thrombosis.

NaI detector system specifically designed for the task. Marks are made on each lower extremity at each counting position to ensure that the same areas are counted at each daily measurement. These marks are placed at 5 cm intervals along the course of the major venous channels of each extremity. The interpretation of the test rests with the comparison of count rates of adjacent sites on the same limb and corresponding sites on opposite limbs. A 20% or greater difference in count rate in either of these two situations, which persists for at least 24 hours, is considered positive at the site with the elevated uptake. Using these criteria, the sensitivity for detection of thrombosis in the lower extremities is greater than 90%. False positive results of the examination can occur in the presence of hematoma, cellulitis, ulceration, and surgical procedures; however, these conditions are usually evident clinically and therefore are not a major source of inaccuracy. In the majority of patients with active thrombosis, a positive

result will be obtained after the first two sets of measurements (i.e., within 48 hours).[8] Because of the small size of the counting equipment, the fibrinogen uptake test is easily performed at the bedside, even in patients with a variety of orthopedic hardware. Should human fibrinogen labeled with ^{123}I become readily available, the detection of deep venous thrombosis with radioisotopes will have the added dimension of imaging active thrombi. This will likely result in improved specificity for the examination.

DIAGNOSIS OF PULMONARY EMBOLISM

Because of the high incidence of deep venous thrombosis in patients with spinal cord injuries, as noted in the previous section, it follows that this patient population is at risk for the development of pulmonary embolism (see Chapter 8). The conventional radionuclide pulmonary perfusion image remains the initial test of choice for screening for this disorder. Images of the lungs in various projections are obtained following the injection of 3 mCi of albumin ^{99m}Tc particles, either macroaggregated albumin or albumin microspheres. These particles are approximately 35 μm in diameter and thus lodge in pulmonary precapillaries proportional to the regional lung perfusion. The classic findings in acute pulmonary embolism are multiple segmental or lobar perfusion defects. Although the perfusion lung scan is quite sensitive, an abnormal finding is not specific for pulmonary embolism. There are two additional examinations that can improve the specificity greatly.

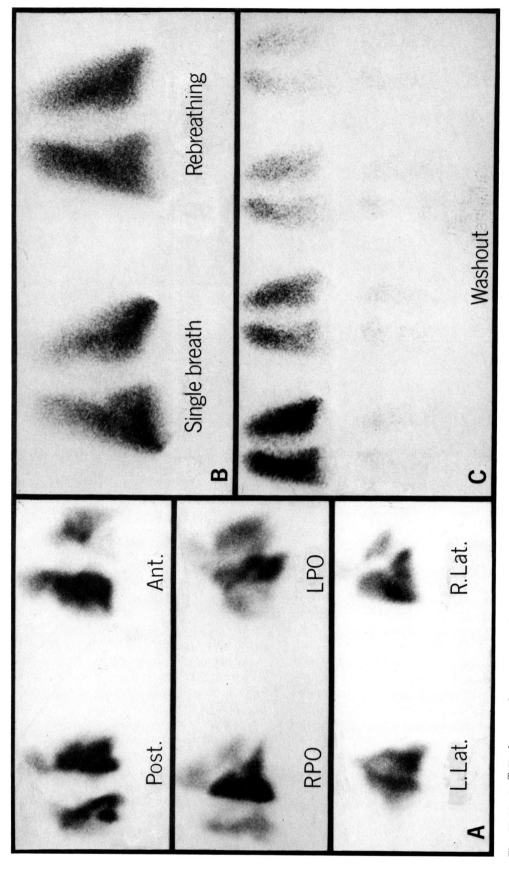

Fig. 19-11. A, ^{99m}Tc lung perfusion images demonstrating multiple segmental defects. **B,** Single breath ^{133}Xe ventilation image and subsequent rebreathing image, demonstrating minimal ventilatory impairment in upper lung field with normal lung volume. **C,** ^{133}Xe washout study at 15 seconds per image, corroborating minimal impairment in ventilation. This mismatch of perfusion and ventilation is typical of pulmonary thromboembolism. *RPO,* Right posterior oblique; *LPO,* left posterior oblique.

The first is a conventional chest radiograph, which should be obtained prior to and within 24 hours of lung images and must be available during scintiphotographic interpretation. The second study is pulmonary ventilation imaging, performed with ^{133}Xe, ^{127}Xe, or ^{81m}Kr. The

findings of segmental or lobar perfusion abnormalities in a radiographically normal area, which show normal ventilation on the inert gas study, are highly suggestive of pulmonary embolism (Fig. 19-11).[19] Although the finding of normal ventilation and perfusion images effectively excludes the diagnosis of significant pulmonary embolism, patients with equivocal images in the face of a moderate to high clinical index of suspicion should be evaluated by conventional contrast pulmonary arteriography.

BILIARY TRACT IMAGING

Until recently, evaluation of the biliary system using radionuclide imaging techniques was limited to the use of rose bengal sodium ^{131}I. The unfavorable dosimetry and imaging characteristics of ^{131}I yielded poor quality images in which visualization of the intrahepatic ducts and even the common bile duct was marginal in many patients. With the introduction of biliary radiopharmaceuticals labeled with ^{99m}Tc, the clinical utility of biliary imaging has increased greatly. The short physical half-life and absence of particulate radiation allow the use of millicurie quantities of ^{99m}Tc, and the 140 keV photon energy is well suited to imaging with modern day scintillation cameras.

After the intravenous injection of 5 mCi of iminodiacetic acid (IDA) ^{99m}Tc, images of the abdomen are obtained throughout the first hour. In cases that exhibit pathology of the hepatobiliary system, delayed images may be required, and imaging as long as 24 hours after injection can prove valuable. In the typical normal study, the liver uptake is prompt, excretion into the common duct is noted within 15 to 30 minutes, and both gallbladder visualization and intestinal visualization are noted within the first hour (Fig. 19-12). In the presence of complete biliary obstruction, there is failure to visualize bowel activity even in 24-hour delayed images. Intermediate degrees of obstruction result in

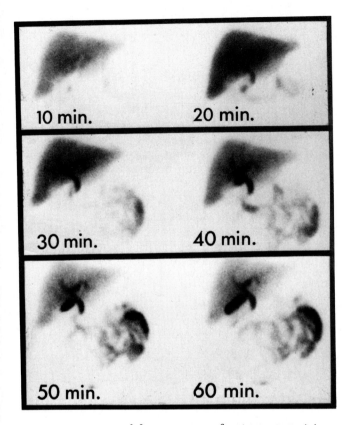

Fig. 19-12. Anterior abdomen images after intravenous injection of IDA^{99m}Tc, demonstrating normal appearance of common duct activity in 20-minute image along with evidence of proximal jejunal activity. Gallbladder is well visualized at 40 minutes. Much of injected dose is in gut at 1 hour. These findings are characteristic of a normal hepatobiliary tract.

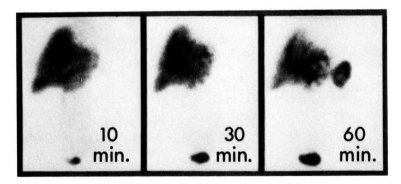

Fig. 19-13. Anterior IDA ^{99m}Tc study, demonstrating dilatation of intrahepatic ducts secondary to partial common duct obstruction. Note gut activity in 60-minute image, which effectively rules out complete obstruction.

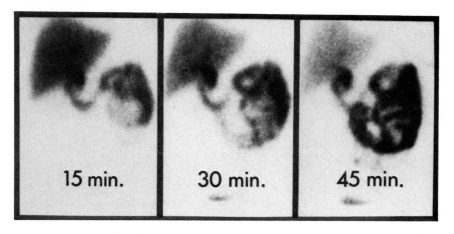

Fig. 19-14. Anterior IDA ^{99m}Tc study, demonstrating prompt common duct and gut visualization with failure to visualize gallbladder. This constellation of findings is very sensitive in detection of acute cholecystitis.

delayed appearance of gut activity. The caliber of intrahepatic biliary ducts can also be qualitatively assessed on scintillation images (Fig. 19-13). A characteristic pattern of common duct and gut visualization with failure to visualize the gallbladder is seen in patients with acute cholecystitis (Fig. 19-14). Gallbladder function can be further evaluated by noting the response to cholecystokinin (CCK) injection. The normal gallbladder will empty promptly following CCK administration, whereas the diseased gallbladder may have an attenuated or absent response.[24]

Visualization of biliary structures in the absence of anatomic obstruction is possible despite high serum bilirubin concentrations. At bilirubin levels below 5 mg/100 ml, technically satisfactory studies are the rule. With some of the newer IDA derivatives, adequate visualization is possible even at bilirubin levels exceeding 20 mg/100 ml.

SUMMARY

In summary, radioisotope techniques have much to offer in the evaluation of victims of spinal cord injury. The tests are minimally invasive, easily performed, and can frequently be done at the patient's bedside. Adverse reactions are rare. In addition to evaluating the immediate results of trauma, such as fracture, splenic and hepatic injury, and renal injury, these techniques can be useful in evaluating some of the late sequence of trauma, including infection, ectopic bone formation, deep venous thrombosis, pulmonary embolism, and biliary tract disorders.

REFERENCES

1. Beauchamp, J. M., Belanger, M. A., and Neitzschman, H. R.: The diagnosis of subcapsular hematoma of the liver by scintigraphy, South. Med. J. **69:**1579-1581, 1976.
2. Berg, B. C.: Radionuclide studies after urinary-tract injury, Semin. Nucl. Med. **4:**371-393, 1974.
3. Carretta, R. F., DeNardo, S. J., DeNardo, G. L., et al.: Early diagnosis of venous thrombosis using I-125 fibrinogen, J. Nucl. Med. **18:**5-10, 1977.
4. Danzl, D. F., and Berg, B. C.: Peritoneal lavage and scintigraphic evaluation of blunt abdominal trauma, J.A.C.E.P. **6:**397-404, 1977.
5. Davis, M. A., and Jones, A. G.: Comparison of Tc-99m labeled phosphate and phosphonate agents for skeletal imaging, Semin. Nucl. Med. **6:**19-31, 1976.
6. Duszynski, D. O., Kuhn, J. P., Afshani, E., et al.: Early radionuclide diagnosis of acute osteomyelitis, Radiology **117:**337-340, 1975.
7. Evans, G. W., Curtin, F. G., McCarthy, H. F., et al.: Scintigraphy in traumatic lesions of liver and spleen, J.A.M.A. **222:**665-667, 1972.
8. Fordham, E. W., and Ramachandran, P. C.: Radionuclide imaging of osseous trauma, Semin. Nucl. Med. **4:**411-429, 1974.
9. Geslien, G. E., Thrall, J. H., Espinosa, J. C., et al.: Early detection of stress fractures using Tc-99m polyphosphate, Radiology **121:**683-687, 1976.
10. Gilday, D. L., Paul, D. J., and Peterson, J.: Diagnosis of osteomyelitis in children by combined blood pool and bone imaging, Radiology **117:**331-335, 1975.
11. Handmaker, H., and Leonards, R.: The bone scan in inflammatory osseous disease, Semin. Nucl. Med. **6:**95-105, 1976.
12. Harris, B. H., Morse, T. S., Weidenmier, C. H., et al.: Radioisotope diagnosis of splenic trauma, J. Pediatr. Surg. **12:**385-389, 1977.
13. Hsu, J. D., Sakimura, I., and Stauffer, E. S.: Heterotopic ossification around the hip joint in spinal cord injured patients, Clin. Orthop. **112:**165-169, 1975.
14. Jones, A. G., Francis, M. D., and Davis, M. A.: Bone scanning: radionuclide reaction mechanisms, Semin. Nucl. Med. **6:**3-18, 1976.
15. Kewalramani, L. S.: Ectopic ossification, Am. J. Phys. Med. **56:**99-121, 1977.

16. Lisbona, R., and Rosenthall, L.: Observation on the sequential use of Tc-99m phosphate complex and Ga-67 imaging in osteomyelitis, cellulitis and septic arthritis, Radiology 123:123-129, 1977.

17. Lutzker, L., Loenigsberg, M., Meng, C., et al.: The role of radionuclide imaging in spleen trauma, Radiology 110:419-425, 1974.

18. McNeil, B. J.: A diagnostic strategy using ventilation-perfusion studies in patients suspect for pulmonary embolism, J. Nucl. Med. 17:613-616, 1976.

19. Muheim, G., Donata, A., and Rossier, A. B.: Serial scintigrams in the course of ectopic bone formation in paraplegic patients, Am. J. Roentgenol. Radium Ther. Nucl. Med. 118:865-869, 1973.

20. Nebasar, R. A., Rabinovla, R., and Potsaid, M. S.: Radionuclide imaging of the spleen in suspected splenic injury, Radiology 110:609-614, 1974.

21. Patten, D. D., and Wodfenden, J. M.: Radionuclide bone scanning in diseases of the spine, Radiol. Clin. North Am. 15:177-201, 1977.

22. Popovsky, J., Wiener, S. N., Felder, P. A., et al.: Liver trauma, Arch. Surg. 108:184-186, 1974.

23. Rosenthall, L., Hill, R. O., and Chuong, S.: Observation on the use of Tc-99m phosphate imaging in peripheral bone trauma, Radiology 119:637-641, 1976.

24. Rosenthall, L., Shaffer, E. A., Lisbona, R., et al.: Diagnosis of hepatobiliary disease by Tc-99m HIDA cholescintigraphy, Radiology 126:467-474, 1978.

25. Rossier, A. B., Byssat, P. H., Infante, F., et al.: Current facts on para-osteo-arthropathy (POA), Paraplegia 2:36-78, 1973.

26. Ryo, U. Y., Oazi, M., Srikantaswamy, S., et al.: Radionuclide venography: correlation with contrast venography, J. Nucl. Med. 18:13-17, 1977.

27. Treves, S., Khettry, S., Broker, F. H., et al.: Osteomyelitis: early scintigraphic detection in children, Pediatrics 57:173-186, 1976.

28. Witek, J. T., Spencer, R. P., Pearson, H. A., et al.: Diagnostic spleen scans in occult splenic injury, J. Trauma 14:197-199, 1974.

CHAPTER 20

Autonomic dysreflexia

JOEL S. ROSEN, M.D.

Autonomic dysreflexia is a syndrome of uncontrolled massive autonomic reflex response occurring in spinal cord injured patients during stimulation below the level of injury. Various radiologic procedures, namely, intravenous urogram, cystography,[1] ileal loopography,[2] barium enema, angiography,[3] fistulography, and others, can precipitate the autonomic crisis. The dramatic clinical manifestations, the serious complications, and treatment should be known to anyone involved in radiologic procedures in spinal cord injured patients.

The syndrome of autonomic dysreflexia, also known as hyperreflexia or paroxysmal hypertension,[11] was well documented as early as 1917.[5] It is a term applied to a clinical syndrome of an uninhibited mass outpouring of autonomic reflexes because of a spinal cord lesion above T5. Below this level there is enough intact innervation to the splanchnic vascular bed to compensate for the symptoms. About 85% of quadriplegics develop this problem at some time during the course of their rehabilitation. There are no good statistics available as to how high-level paraplegics develop the syndrome, but it is certainly not uncommon. The tendency toward dysreflexia decreases with time and is relatively infrequent although not rare after about 3 years following the injury.

There is no scientific method available to predict the sensitivity to this syndrome in a given patient, nor can it be predicted how severe a reaction will be or how long the patient will remain sensitive. Autonomic dysreflexia occurs in complete and *incomplete* lesions. The more incomplete the lesion, the less the likelihood of sympathetic response, because of remaining compensatory mechanisms. Patients with vascular compromise or massive damage to multiple sections of the spinal cord below the level of the lesion do not develop autonomic dysreflexia. In order to develop autonomic crisis, it is necessary that the distal stump of spinal cord (below the lesion) be viable and functioning.

ETIOLOGY

The whole syndrome can be elicited by any noxious stimulus at the skin or viscera below the level of the lesion. The most common stimulus is a relative overdistention of a hollow viscus, such as the urinary bladder, the bowel, or the uterus. The least likely stimulus comes from the skin. There are many other potential causes: ingrown toenails, pressure sores, menstrual cramps, flatus, fecal impaction, tracheal suctioning in high quadriplegics, bronchoscopy, gastrointestinal ulcerations, gastritis secondary to medications, traction on a catheter, urethral scrotal abscess, fractures, abscesses, and certainly all of the already mentioned radiologic procedures.

In regard to a hollow viscus, there are other possible noxious stimuli in addition to overdistention, such as hemorrhage into the bladder, severe spasms secondary to genitourinary manipulations,[8] inflation of the Foley catheter balloon in the urethra.

Overdistention of a viscus is related to the capacity of the organ. About 90% of the autonomic dysreflexia

554

cases develop from overdistention of the urinary bladder.[4] If the capacity of a bladder is approximately 100 ml, a sudden influx of 150 ml of contrast medium would cause a relative overdistention and initiate this reflex in spite of the total volume being only 150 ml. If the normal capacity of the bladder is 400 ml, a sudden influx of 600 ml might be needed before the reflex would be initiated.

During pregnancy the enlargement of the uterus occurs slowly enough over a prolonged period of time; there is a gradual accommodation and seldom do we see the dysreflexia syndrome. When the pregnant woman with a spinal cord injury goes into labor, the uterine contractions trigger the reflex arc and produce autonomic dysreflexia. The afferent stimuli from the uterus are similar to those arising from sudden overdis-

tention of a hollow viscus. With delivery of the fetus, the cause of the dysreflexia is removed and the symptoms subside unless there is an ongoing source of noxious stimuli, such as uterine hemorrhage, spasms, or retained placenta.

MECHANISM

The major splanchnic outflow of the sympathetic system is from approximately T5-L2, and a lesion of the spinal cord above this level will prevent the normal reflex inhibition of the system from the higher centers, permitting a massive outpouring of autonomic sympathetic stimuli. After the start of the stimulus and its afferent arc leading to the cord, the thoracolumbar sympathetic trunks, the outflow portion of this reflex arc, are activated. This leads to an intense sympathetic

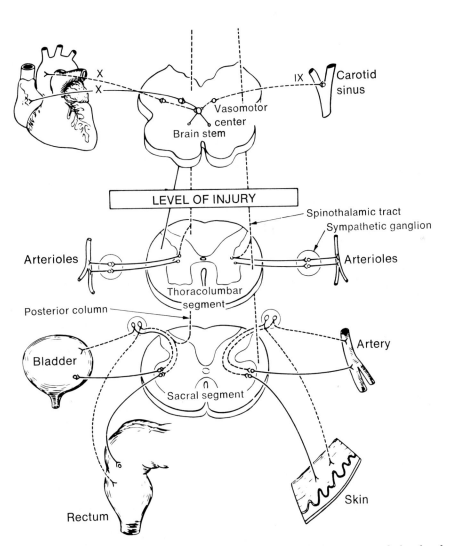

Fig. 20-1. Pathways affecting blood pressure after stimulation to various organs below level of cord lesion. Afferent pathways shown by interrupted lines. Efferent pathways shown by solid lines. (From Fleischman, S., and Shah, P.: Radiology **124**:695, 1977.)

outpouring from below the level of the lesion, causing an intense splanchnic vasoconstriction and spasticity of the abdominal viscera with an increased outpouring of blood into the system.

The peripheral circulation of the lower limbs diminishes because of vasoconstriction and a dramatic rise in blood pressure occurs because of increased peripheral resistance. This increase in blood pressure is reflex mediated by the sympathetic nervous system and is mediated by a release of norepinephrine from the sympathetic nerve endings. Studies have been done during this stage, and there is indeed an increase in the concentration of norepinephrine breakdown products.[9]

If the bladder or rectum is the initiating organ, the actual anatomic pathways for this relfex include afferent stimuli entering the cord at the sacral or lower thoracic regions via the hypogastric (sympathetic) and pelvic (parasympathetic) nerves (Fig. 20-1). Mucosal (pain and touch) impulses pass up the cord via the spinothalamic tract. Detrusor stretch impulses pass up the cord via the posterior columns.[7] There are multiple segmental synapses within the intermediolateral cell column that do lead to efferent effects on the vasculature and the resulting vasoconstriction. The activation is uninhibited from the higher nerve centers because of the presence of the spinal cord lesion and the blockage in the transmission of nerve impulses down the spinal cord. The thoracic sympathetic ganglia form the main efferent pathway for the reflex sympathetic outpouring. The increase in peripheral resistance then leads to a dramatic hypertension, which may be as high as 300 mm Hg systolic. This usually produces a throbbing occipital headache resulting from overdistention of the intracranial pial arteries. If not treated immediately, it can lead to convulsions, subarachnoid hemorrhage, and even death. Late changes include seizures and encephalomalacia.

SYMPTOMS

The reflex hypertension is monitored by the carotid and aortic pressure receptors, which relay inhibitory impulses via the brain stem, causing intense vagal stimulation of the heart and resulting bradycardia. This is monitored from the vasomotor center in the brain stem along the ninth cranial nerve from the carotid sinus and the tenth cranial nerve from the aortic receptors. In addition to the bradycardia, other cardiac changes occur, such as bigeminal pulse, extrasystoles of artrial and ventricular origin, and increased magnitude of the T and U waves on the cardiogram.

In addition to severe hypertension and bradycardia, the patient frequently has profuse sweating, piloerec-

tion (gooseflesh), and marked flushing of all skin with normal sensory innervation, namely, the skin above the level of the lesion. Some of the other symptoms that can occur include congestion of the nasal mucosa, dilated pupils, nausea, apprehension, and dyspnea, primarily due to a marked bronchospasm but can also be due to abdominal distention with resultant splinting of the diaphragm. There is diffuse, severe vasoconstriction below the level of the lesion with reduction of the fluid available to the sweat glands.

TREATMENT

When the patient is known to be prone to autonomic dysreflexia, radiologic procedures must be carried out with caution. The bladder and rectum should be distended slowly and progressively. If the urinary catheter is removed during the voiding part of a voiding cystourethrogram, a sterile catheter should be handy for immediate insertion in the bladder if symptoms develop. During barium enema, the barium-containing bag should be lowered to the floor to drain the rectum. Premedication with 15 mg mecamylamine (Inversine) by mouth 30 minutes prior to the procedure has been advocated.[3] The bladder and rectal mucosa can be anesthetized with a local anesthetic prior to the procedure, thus blocking the afferent arc of the reflex.

If symptoms of autonomic dysreflexia occur, the following treatment is recommended:

1. Stop the radiologic procedure immediately.
2. If lesion is stable, sit patient up at 90°, thus causing postural hypotension and alleviation of symptoms.[6]
3. Check to see that urine is draining freely from bladder. If any question exists or present catheter is plugged, insert Foley catheter to empty bladder.
4. Check rectum for fecal impaction; if impaction is present, insert local anesthetic ointment prior to removing impaction.
5. If above measures do not immediately alleviate the symptoms, give chlorpromazine, 50 mg intramuscularly, for temporary relief.
6. Start intravenous fluids and be prepared to give diazoxide (Hyperstat), 300 mg intravenously as a bolus injection.

Further measures include emergency suprapubic cystotomy with an angiocatheter or emergency spinal anesthetic.[10] The severe headache that accompanies autonomic dysreflexia can frequently be relieved by manual pressure on the carotid sinuses or by artificially increasing intracranial pressure. Neither of these methods is used very often.

REFERENCES

1. Arieff, A. J., Tigay, E. L., and Pyzik, S. W.: Acute hypertension induced by urinary bladder distension, Arch. Neurol. **6**:248-256, 1962.
2. Barbaric, F. L.: Autonomic dysreflexia in patients with spinal cord lesions: complication of voiding cystourethrography and ileal loopography, Am. J. Roentgenol. **127**:293-295, 1976.
3. Fleischman, S., and Shah, P.: Autonomic dysreflexia: an unusual radiologic complication, Radiology **124**:695-697, 1977.
4. Guttmann, L., and Whitteridge, D.: Effects of bladder distension and autonomic mediastinum after spinal cord injuries, Brain **70**:361-404, 1947.
5. Head, H., and Riddoch, J.: The automatic bladder, excessive sweating and some other reflex conditions in gross injuries of spinal cord, Brain **40**:188-263, 1917.
6. Kurnick, N. B.: Autonomic hyperreflexia and its control in patients with spinal cord lesions, Am. Intern. Med. **44**:678-686, 1956.
7. Nathan, P. W., and Smith, M. C.: Centripetal pathway from the bladder and urethra within the spinal cord, J. Neurol. Neurosurg. Psychiatry **14**:267-280, 1951.
8. Nieder, R. M., O'Higgins, J. W., and Aldrete, J. A.: Autonomic hyperreflexia in urologic surgery, J.A.M.A. **213**:867-869, 1970.
9. Sell, G. H., Naftchi, N. E., Lowman, E. W., and Rusk, H. A.: Autonomic hyperreflexia and catecholamine metabolites in spinal cord injury, Arch. Phys. Med. Rehabil. **53**:415-417, 1972.
10. Sizemore, G. W., and Winternitz, W. W.: Autonomic hyperreflexia—suppression with alpha-adrenergic blocking agents, N. Engl. J. Med. **282**:795, 1970.
11. Thompson, C. E., and Witham, A. C.: Paroxysmal hyperflexia in spinal cord injuries, N. Engl. J. Med. **239**:291-294, 1948.

Index

558